Integrative Women's Health

Integrative Medicine Library

Published and Forthcoming Volumes

SERIES EDITOR

Andrew Weil, MD

Donald I. Abrams and Andrew Weil: *Integrative Oncology*

Robert Bonakdar and Andrew W. Sukiennik: *Integrative Pain Management*

Richard Carmona and Mark Liponis: *Integrative Preventive Medicine*

Timothy P. Culbert and Karen Olness: *Integrative Pediatrics*

Stephen DeVries and James Dalen: *Integrative Cardiology*

Randy Horwitz and Daniel Muller: *Integrative Rheumatology*

Mary Jo Kreitzer and Mary Koithan: *Integrative Nursing*

Victoria Maizes and Tieraona Low Dog: *Integrative Women's Health*

Daniel A. Monti and Bernard D. Beitman: *Integrative Psychiatry*

Gerard Mullin: *Integrative Gastroenterology*

Robert Norman, Philip D. Shenefelt, and Reena N. Rupani: *Integrative Dermatology*

Myles D. Spar and George E. Munoz: *Integrative Men's Health*

Integrative Women's Health

SECOND EDITION

EDITED BY

Victoria Maizes, MD
Executive Director
Arizona Center for Integrative Medicine
Professor of Clinical Medicine, Family Medicine and Public Health
The University of Arizona
Tucson, Arizona

Tieraona Low Dog, MD
Fellowship Director
Academy of Integrative Health & Medicine
Chair, US Pharmacopeia Dietary Supplements & Botanicals Admissions Panel
Pecos, New Mexico

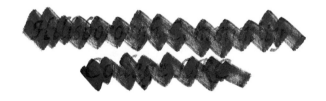
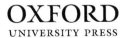

OXFORD
UNIVERSITY PRESS

OXFORD

UNIVERSITY PRESS

Oxford University Press is a department of the University of
Oxford. It furthers the University's objective of excellence in research,
scholarship, and education by publishing worldwide.

Oxford   New York

Auckland   Cape Town   Dar es Salaam   Hong Kong   Karachi
Kuala Lumpur   Madrid   Melbourne   Mexico City   Nairobi
New Delhi   Shanghai   Taipei   Toronto

With offices in

Argentina   Austria   Brazil   Chile   Czech Republic   France   Greece
Guatemala   Hungary   Italy   Japan   Poland   Portugal   Singapore
South Korea   Switzerland   Thailand   Turkey   Ukraine   Vietnam

Oxford is a registered trademark of Oxford University Press
in the UK and certain other countries.

Published in the United States of America by
Oxford University Press
198 Madison Avenue, New York, NY 10016

Library of Congress Cataloging-in-Publication Data
Integrative women's health / edited by Victoria Maizes, Tieraona Low Dog.—
Second edition.
p. ; cm.
Includes bibliographical references and index.
ISBN 978-0-19-021479-1 (alk. paper)
I. Maizes, Victoria, editor.   II. Low Dog, Tieraona, editor.
[DNLM: 1. Women's Health.   2. Integrative Medicine. WA 309.1]
RA778
613'.04244—dc23
2015002839

CONTENTS

FOREWORD

ANDREW WEIL, MD

Series Editor

As the only male contributor to this excellent volume on *Integrative Women's Health,* I feel both honored and intimidated.

Throughout history, medicine was a fraternal guild that excluded women. As recently as 1964, when I entered my first year at Harvard Medical School, my class of 125 included only 12 women. Even into the 20th century, women were considered unfit for the profession, and very few were allowed to become doctors. Of course, times have greatly changed, with female students now often outnumbering males in colleges of medicine. But the influence of centuries of tradition lingers in medical thinking and practice.

Ancient Greek physicians, the godfathers of Western medicine, thought female patients were peculiarly prone to disorders that simulated genuine dysfunction of internal organs. They called this class of ailments "hysteria," from their word for uterus (*hystera*), believing that the womb could detach from its moorings and travel elsewhere in the body, pressing on the diaphragm, throat, or other structures to cause symptoms. In their view, the probable cause of uterine wandering was that the organ became light and dry as a result of lack of sexual intercourse.

It is now 2,000 years later, and here is the definition of *hysteria* in a contemporary edition of Webster's Revised Unabridged Dictionary:

Hys*te"ri*a\, n. [NL.: cf. F. hyst['e]rie. See Hysteric.] (Med.) A nervous affection, occurring almost exclusively in women, in which the emotional and reflex excitability is exaggerated, and the will power correspondingly diminished, so that the patient loses control over the emotions, becomes the victim of imaginary sensations, and often falls into paroxism or fits.

Note: The chief symptoms are convulsive, tossing movements of the limbs and head, uncontrollable crying and laughing, and a choking sensation as if a ball were lodged in the throat. The affection presents the most varied symptoms, often simulating those of the gravest diseases, but generally curable by mental treatment alone.

In fact, even into our times, male physicians have tended to dismiss the somatic complaints of female patients as hysterical, especially when symptoms are generalized, vague, and difficult to diagnose.

When the first anti-anxiety drugs came on the market in the middle of the past century, they seemed just right for managing the disordered emotionality of women that was believed to be the cause of their headaches, listlessness, and various aches and pains. I have one pharmaceutical advertisement from the period in my files that shows a clearly hysterical woman—just the sort of patient you would not want to have to deal with—under the banner, "Emotional Crisis? Calm her immediately with injectable Valium (diazepam)!" In the 1960s, the manufacturer of Ritalin (methylphenidate) targeted women in a noteworthy series of ads in leading journals. On the left-hand page of each two-page spread was a black-and-white photograph of a depressed housewife contemplating a sink full of dirty dishes, a messy living room, or some other household disaster. "What can you do for this patient?" the physician–reader was asked. "Write 'Ritalin' on your prescription pad!" was the answer on the adjoining page—this over a full-color photograph of the same woman, now cheerful and energetic, standing proudly by spotlessly clean dishes or an ordered living room. The unwritten subtext was clear: Here is an easy way to get rid of complaining female patients, who take up your time, probably have nothing really wrong with them, and are so emotionally unbalanced that they are likely not even doing their housework.

The first oral contraceptive pills were becoming popular when I did my clinical rotations as a medical student. I remember a preceptor I had—a cocky, young internist—who urged us to prescribe them not just for contraception. "You know these women who just never feel right?" he told us. "You just put them on the pill, and they feel like a million bucks." In my OB/GYN rotation, I assisted in a lot of hysterectomies, many of them not necessary by today's standards. Hysterectomy was the "final solution" to female complaints.

How much have things changed? Today we experience a booming anti-depressant industry; when we look back will we see it as any different from the Valium or Ritalin chapters? At the same time, there is growing acknowledgment that men and women are different and that the differences extend beyond reproduction to physiology and virtually every organ system. While female reproductive physiology is undeniably complex, it does not sufficiently explain why women are at greater risk for autoimmune disorders, process information differently in the brain, or react differently to pharmaceutical drugs than men. As the caregivers in our society, women experience particular forms of stress. Yet women throughout the world live longer than men; why they do is unknown. Gender-based medicine is a nascent field and it is growing.

Women have been vocal about their desire to be seen as more than just physical bodies. They have pushed for a broader view of health and wellness. Women are the major consumers of health care and are also much more health conscious than men in our society. They take better care of themselves and are more likely to seek professional help for symptoms that demand attention. Women are the chief buyers of books about health and self-care, and women's magazines have been major outlets for information on these subjects. Over the past few decades, women have led the consumer movement for holistic and alternative medicine, because they are more open than men to natural therapies, mind/body interventions, and the healing traditions of other cultures. That consumer movement, which is still gaining strength, laid the foundation for acceptance of integrative medicine.

Integrative medicine, as this series of volumes from Oxford University Press demonstrates, has much broader goals than simply bringing alternative and complementary therapies into the mainstream. It aims to restore the focus of medicine on health and healing, especially on the human organism's innate capacity for maintaining and repairing itself; to foster whole-person medicine that includes the mental/emotional and spiritual dimensions of human life; to train physicians to attend to all aspects of lifestyle in working with patients; and to protect the practitioner/patient relationship as a key contributor to the healing process. Because integrative medicine stresses the individuality of patients and encourages real partnerships between doctors and patients, it is able to recognize and discard the limiting, paternalistic attitudes, and concepts that have dominated medicine for centuries and give women's health issues the attention and care they demand.

As women have moved toward equality with men in the medical profession, both in terms of numbers and status, the field of women's health has come into its own. I believe that integrative medicine and women's health are a perfect fit. Therefore, it gives me great pleasure to introduce this updated edition of *Integrative Women's Health,* an outstanding compilation of practical information. Included here is a powerful new chapter on "Environmental Exposures and Women's Health," a topic that clinicians need to know and don't; it dovetails nicely with an expanded "Preconception Counseling and Fertility" chapter that presents an integrative strategy for advising women and their partners not only on conceiving but on healthy conception. With growing research showing that many adult disorders originate in the womb, this is an important subject. Also new is a chapter on "Lesbian, Bisexual, and Transgender Health," a topic the editors feel they were remiss in not including last time. All chapters have been updated with the latest information.

The editors are long-time friends and colleagues. Drs. Victoria Maizes and Tieraona Low Dog are leading voices in the emerging field of women's integrative health. Victoria Maizes, a pioneer graduate of the integrative medicine fellowship that I founded at the University of Arizona, has been the executive director of the Arizona Center for Integrative Medicine for the past decade. Dr. Tieraona Low Dog, is one of the world's leading authorities on botanical medicine and dietary supplements. I congratulate them for the excellence of their editorial work and thank them for asking me to add my words to theirs.

PREFACE

We are delighted to present the 2nd edition of *Integrative Women's Health*. It is our hope that you will continue to find it of value as you care for your patients. As the largest group of healthcare consumers, women have made it abundantly clear that they desire a broader, more integrative approach to their care. In response to this need, Integrative Women's Health addresses women's reproductive health as well as conditions that manifest differently in women. Thus you will find perspectives on spirituality and sexuality, perspectives for lesbian and bisexual women, integrative approaches to premenstrual syndrome, pregnancy, menopause, and endometriosis and treatment of cardiovascular disease, hypothyroidism, rheumatoid arthritis, depression and cancer in women.

We honor the clinical experience and heartfelt connection that clinicians share with their patients. We have intentionally designed this book to present the latest scientific evidence within a clinically relevant framework. Woven together are conventional treatments, mind-body interventions, nutritional strategies, acupuncture, manual medicine, herbal therapies and dietary supplements. Careful attention is given to the art of medicine; clinical pearls include language that helps motivate patients, questions that enhance a health history, and the spiritual dimensions of care. Unlike many primers on women's health that emphasize either an alternative or conventional approach - this text is truly integrative.

While gender specific medicine is growing as a field, it tends to focus on the biological differences between men and women and, at times, turns normal life events such as pregnancy and menopause into medical problems that need to be managed. We have worked with our authors to convey care that addresses the medical issue addressing the fullness of a woman's body, mind and spirit; acknowledging the therapeutic relationship that exists between patient and provider, and making use of the best of conventional and complementary medicine. To this end, we have intentionally chosen only female authors as a tribute to the growing influence of women providers and their unique perspective.

It has been a great joy working together to conceptualize, write, edit and birth this second edition. We pass it on to you hoping you will find a life-affirming perspective that honors the many paths to healing.

Victoria Maizes and Tieraona Low Dog

CONTRIBUTORS

Priscilla Abercrombie, RN, NP, PhD, AHN-BC
Clinical Professor
UCSF Department of Obstetrics, Gynecology and Reproductive Sciences
Osher Center for Integrative Medicine
Women's Health & Healing
San Francisco, California

Lise Alschuler, ND, FABNO
Executive Director, TAP Integrative
Co-founder, Five to Thrive, LLC
Practitioner, Naturopathic Specialists, LLC
Tucson, Arizona & Chicago, Illinois

Iris R. Bell, MD, PhD
Professor of Family and Community Medicine, Psychiatry, Psychology, and Public Health
Department of Family and Community Medicine
Tucson, Arizona

Maria Benito, MD
Princeton Integral Endocrinology, LLC
Princeton, New Jersey

Rita Benn, PhD
Director, Faculty Scholars Program in Integrative Healthcare
Department of Family Medicine
University of Michigan
Ann Arbor, Michigan

Manijeh Berenji, MD, MPH
Assistant Professor
Division of Occupational and Environmental Medicine
Department of Community and Family Medicine
Duke University Medical Center
Durham, North Carolina

Bridget S. Bongaard, MD, FACP
Retired Medical Director of Integrative Medicine
Carolinas Healthcare System North East
Charlotte, North Carolina
Medical Director of Islands Hospice
Maui, Hawaii

Ann Marie Chiasson, MD, MPH
Assistant Clinical Professor of
   Medicine
Arizona Center for Integrative
   Medicine
University of Arizona
Tucson, Arizona

MargEva Morris Cole, MD
Clinical Assistant Professor
Division, Durham Obstetrics and
   Gynecology
Department of Obstetrics and
   Gynecology
Duke University Medical Center
Durham, North Carolina

Barbara Eckstein, MD
Assistant Professor
University of North Carolina
Chapel Hill, North Carolina

Louise Gagné, MD
Clinical Assistant Professor
Department of Community Health
   and Epidemiology
University of
   Saskatchewan
Saskatoon, Canada

Mary L. Hardy, MD
Wellness Works
Los Angeles, California

Cheryl Hawk, DC, PhD, CHES
Executive Director
Northwest Center for Lifestyle and
   Functional Medicine
University of Western States
Portland, Oregon

**Bettina Herbert, MD, FAAPMR, IFMCP,
DABOIM**
Director, Biodetoxification Program
Center for Occupational and
   Environmental Medicine
North Charleston, South Carolina
Clinical Instructor
Department of Rehabilitation Medicine
Jefferson Medical College
Thomas Jefferson University Hospital
Philadelphia, Pennsylvania

Tori Hudson, ND
Clinical Professor
National College of Natural Medicine
Bastyr University
Medical Director, A Woman's Time
Program Director, Institute of Women's
   Health and Integrative Medicine
Portland, Oregon

Raheleh Khorsan, MA
Department of Planning, Policy
   and Design
University of California
Irvine, California

Karen Koffler, MD
Medical Director, Carillon Hotel
   and Spa
Adjunct Faculty, University of Miami
   School of Medicine
Miami, Florida

Wendy Kohatsu, MD
Associate Clinical Professor
Department of Family and
   Community Medicine
University of California San Francisco
Director, Integrative Medicine Fellowship
Santa Rosa Family Medicine Residency
Santa Rosa, California

Vivian Kominos, MD, FACC
Mount Sinai Beth Israel Center for
    Health and Healing
New York, New York

Naomi Lam, MD
San Francisco Department of
    Public Health
Tom Waddell Urban Health Clinic
San Francisco, California

Marnie Lamm, MD
Family Medicine
Alamance Regional Medical Center
Moses Cone Health
Mebane, North Carolina

Beverly Lanzetta, PhD
Religious Studies Professor (retired)
Independent Scholar
San Diego, California

Patricia Lebensohn, MD
Professor of Family and Community
    Medicine
Department of Family and
    Community Medicine
University of Arizona
Tucson, Arizona

Roberta Lee, MD
Clinical Assistant Professor of Medicine
Arizona Center for Integrative
    Medicine
University of Arizona
Tucson, Arizona

Dawn Lemanne, MD, MPH
Oregon Integrative Oncology
Ashland, Oregon

Irina Lisker, MD
Family Medicine Resident, PGY2
Hunterdon Family Medicine
    Residency
Hunterdon Medical Center
    Flemington, New Jersey

Elizabeth R. Mackenzie, PhD
Adjunct Assistant Professor, Applied
    Psychology - Human Development,
    Graduate School of Education
Associated Faculty, Health and
    Societies Program, School of Art
    and Sciences
University of Pennsylvania
Philadelphia, Pennsylvania

Nisha Manek, MD, FACP, FRCP (UK)
Kingman Rheumatology
Kingman Regional Medical Center
Member, Mayo Clinic Care Network,
    Arizona
Kingman, Arizona

Kelly McCann, MD, MPH&TM
Program Development Director
Integrative Medicine and Wellness
    Program
Hoag Memorial Hospital
    Presbyterian
Newport Beach, California

Hilary McClafferty, MD, FAAP
Interim Director of the Fellowship
Associate Professor of Medicine and
    Pediatrics
Arizona Center for Integrative Medicine
University of Arizona
Tucson, Arizona

Leslie McGee, RN, LAc
Diplomate in Acupuncture
Diplomate in Chinese Herbology
(NCCAOM)
East-West Acupuncture &
  Chinese Herbs
Tucson, Arizona

Daphne Miller, MD
Adjunct Associate Clinical Professor
Department of Family and
  Community Medicine
University of California, San
  Francisco
San Francisco, California

Pamela A. Pappas, MD, MD(H)
Private Practice
Optimal You
Scottsdale, Arizona

Premal Patel, MD
Wellness Director, Banyan Botanicals
Integrative Health Consultant
Houston, Texas

Jacquelyn M. Paykel, MD, FACOG
Director of the Sexual Health,
  Incontinence & Pelvic Pain Clinic
Women's Health Division
James A. Haley Veterans' Hospital &
  Clinics
Tampa, Florida

Joanne L. Perron, MD, MPH, FACOG
Lecturer, College of Health Sciences
  and Human Services, Nursing
California State University,
  Monterey Bay
Seaside, California

Sudha Prathikanti, MD, ABIHM
Integrative Psychiatrist
Clinical Professor
Department of Psychiatry
University of California
San Francisco, California

Birgit Rakel, MD
Assistant Professor
Department of Family and
  Community Medicine
Department of Emergency Medicine
Sidney Kimmel Medical College at
  Thomas Jefferson University
Director of Women's Health
Myrna Brind Center for Integrative
  Medicine
Philadelphia, Pennsylvania

Melinda Ring, MD, FACP
Medical Director
Osher Center for Integrative Medicine
Drs. Pat and Carl Greer Distinguished
  Physician in Integrative Medicine
Northwestern University Feinberg
  School of Medicine
Chicago, Illinois

Carolyn Coker Ross, MD, MPH
Eating Disorder, Addiction Medicine,
  and Integrative Medicine Specialist
Denver, Colorado

Kathie Madonna Swift, MS, RDN, LDN, FAND
Co-Founder, Integrative and
  Functional Nutrition Academy
Education Director, Food as Medicine,
  Center for Mind Body Medicine
Adjunct Faculty, Saybrook University
  School of Mind Body Medicine
San Francisco, California

PART I

Lifestyle

1

Integrative Approach to Women's Health

VICTORIA MAIZES AND TIERAONA LOW DOG

Traditionally, women have served as healers. They often hold family and community rituals and determine many aspects of family life. Women are defined as much by their roles as mothers, sisters, daughters, wives, and friends as by their occupations. Having experienced triumphs and losses, joys and sorrows, they bear the hidden scars and treasured trophies as their stories.

We believe that healthcare professionals who seek to fully understand their patients' lives provide the finest possible healthcare. Exploring not only a woman's symptoms and medical history, but also her beliefs, intuitions, and preferences sets the foundation for a healing partnership. By acknowledging the value of this partnership, we bring our presence fully to each interaction. As health professionals, we set an intention to serve and together with our patients craft a unique treatment plan that fits this woman and her particular story and situation.

Our professional lives are enriched when we listen to our patients' stirring narratives. In so doing, we provide each patient the opportunity to hear her own story, sometimes for the very first time, while serving as witness to her triumphs and challenges. As a woman's story unfolds, connections can be made, insights gained, and the groundwork for healing laid. An intimacy develops, which is one of the supreme privileges of being a healer.

The root of "health" is "hale" or "whole." The purpose of medicine, then, is to restore wholeness. To do so requires an investigation into all factors that may be interfering with healing whether they arise from physical, emotional, mental, or spiritual distress.

Taking a broader history helps elucidate the roots of an illness. Integrative medicine professionals pose thought-provoking questions that deepen understanding and augment the conventional medical history. "Tell me about your typical day" reveals patterns in a woman's life. "What brings you joy?" evokes tales of a child, a pet, or even a hobby that lights the teller's eyes and spirit. "Imagine that a decade has gone by. What would you like to have accomplished?" exposes a longer trajectory. "What is most important to you at this point in your life?" can illuminate a patient's values. When asked "What are your strengths?" a woman has the opportunity to disclose who she is quite differently than she would at a typical doctor's appointment. The answer may reveal significant aspects of her character. Should she find it challenging to answer, a follow-up question—"What would your friends say they adore about you?"—may elicit more information.

With life-threatening illness, it may be appropriate to ask, "What is your understanding of your health condition?" followed by "What do you fear most?" Another question that opens the doorway into rich conversation and may reveal spiritual beliefs is "What do you believe happens after we die?" When a woman replies, "There is nothing more," or "I'd like to believe in an afterlife but I don't," a second question might be gently posed, such as "Have you ever had an experience of awe, or mystery, or something you just can't explain?" Sometimes remarkable experiences are shared.

This broader set of questions creates a framework for a broader set of treatment options. When barely a moment of quiet can be found in her typical day, rest or meditation can be recommended. A crisis of spirit can be identified and may require a referral to priest, minister, rabbi, or spiritual director. Journaling is an option when a woman is unclear as to what she wishes to unfold.

An integrative provider honors her patients' beliefs and weighs them as she suggests treatment recommendations. Therefore, it is essential to ask women "What is your belief about…." For example, one woman choosing to use hormone therapy for menopausal symptoms tells us, "I want to continue to take hormones because they keep me young." Another patient says nearly the opposite: "Every time I swallow one of those pills I feel as if I am feeding a breast tumor." Women have a unique set of experiences and beliefs that informs their decisions; integrative medicine seeks to understand and validate them.

Women have the capacity to see the sacred in everyday life. In the laughter of a child, the changing colors of the mountains at sunset, or the quiet at the end of day women may be reminded of the ineffable. Faith, religion, and spirituality are often core sources of strength. In seeking to understand our patients, it is vital to capture women's connection to spirit.

A 72-year-old woman calmly shares her life story filled with tremendous challenges. She has overcome the loss of her mother at 14, the death of her 37-year-old son, years of alcoholism in her husband, and a personal history of breast cancer. Her story provides a natural segue to inquire into her spiritual history. When asked what has given her the strength to carry on, she describes her deep connection to the Catholic Church. "It is my faith," she says, "that has allowed me to survive." Rather than being broken by these many losses, it has drawn her closer to God, her husband, and her friends.

Eliciting a history is a reductive exercise. Over the course of a complete history, we ask about the parts of a story, the details of a particular medical condition, and the review of systems. In an integrative medicine encounter, we are listening as well for the inner wholeness, seeking to understand the very essence of a person.

To let our patients know that we have listened closely, it is often useful to briefly summarize back what we have heard. For example, we might say, "You are a 42-year-old woman with a close relationship to your husband, two children whom you adore, a strong commitment to your spiritual practice, and a 10-year history of rheumatoid arthritis. While the arthritis is controlled with ibuprofen and Enbrel, you are eager to see whether nutritional changes would allow you to reduce your dose of Enbrel, as you are concerned about its long-term use." When hearing her own story reflected back, our patient's motivation might get stronger; she can correct any error or add to the list of concerns. It also provides an opportunity to emphasize her strengths, thereby reinforcing her ability to make necessary changes. Assembling this summary is a synthetic process. Not only do we reveal interconnections between symptoms but also we remind our patients of their fundamental wholeness.

Our philosophical orientation is to look for roots of the illness. When recognizable patterns emerge, they provide guidance for treatment recommendations in novel conditions. For example, many diseases have inflammation as an underlying root cause. A treatment plan that combines an anti-inflammatory diet and herbs as well as mind-body approaches that reduce inflammation, can serve as a cornerstone of treatment in a disease for which there is not yet a solid body of evidence.

We are struck by how frequently the synergism of multiple, simple, low-tech interventions can be powerful medicine. A 53-year-old woman with gastroesophageal reflux who had been treated for some time with a proton pump inhibitor (PPI) came to the clinic for advice. The PPI worked well, but she was concerned about the long-term risks of the medication including hip fractures and pneumonia. She had tried to stop taking the PPI on multiple occasions but experienced rebound symptoms that led her back to the medication. We advised eliminating triggers of acid reflux in her diet, a trial off dairy, and the use of dietary supplements including deglycyrrhizinated licorice (DGL), melatonin, and D-limonene. We questioned her about sources of stress and her coping skills and taught her a simple breathing exercise that elicits the relaxation response. Gradually, she was able to taper off PPI, then her supplements, and manage her symptoms with only occasional DGL.

The vastness of an integrative medicine toolbox helps us in many ways, not least of which is the mindset that we always have something to offer. Should one intervention be unsuccessful, there is another that can be attempted, creating a hopeful perspective. Where Western medicine has been unsuccessful, a traditional Chinese medicine or Ayurvedic approach might offer a unique therapeutic strategy.

As healthcare providers, there is always something we can do to be of service. Our very calling to medicine sets us apart from most others who turn away from human suffering. Instead we lean in, seeking to be of help. It is our passionate belief that there are multiple routes to healing. An integrative practitioner possesses a larger toolbox and can offer many treatment options beyond pharmaceutical approaches. While numerous healing strategies are discussed in the chapters that follow, integrative medicine is not simply about learning to use these new tools. It is about a different way *of being* with a patient.

Suggested Reading

Maizes, V., Koffler, K., & Fleishman, S. (2002). Revisiting the health history: An integrative approach. *Adv Mind Body Med, 18*(2), 32–34.

Miller, W. R., & Rollnick, S. (2002). *Motivational interviewing: Preparing people for change* (2nd ed.). New York, NY: Guilford Press.

Muller W. (1996). *How then shall we live: Four simple questions that reveal the beauty and meaning of our lives.* New York, NY: Bantam Books.

Remen, R. N. (1996). *Kitchen table wisdom.* New York, NY: Riverhead Books.

Walsh, R. (1999). *Essential spirituality: The 7 central practices to awaken heart and mind.* New York, NY: Wiley.

2

Nutrition

WENDY KOHATSU

CASE STUDY

Helen is a 29-year-old busy professional woman who approached me about her weight. She had gained weight steadily over the past 2 years and felt it was affecting her energy levels and causing more fatigue. Helen was a frequent soda drinker, and due to her hectic work schedule tended to eat big meals, when she could, at her desk. Typically, she complained of being "ravenous" by the time she got home for dinner and then indulged in overeating. Helen felt trapped in a vicious cycle.

Together, we worked on a plan to restructure her diet and exercise plan. I advised her to phase out soft drinks, and space out her calories with regular healthy snacks between meals to avoid binge eating. Helen added a healthy snack between 3 and 4 pm—usually a ¼ cup of nuts, a couple of whole-grain crackers with hummus or hard-boiled egg, or low-fat plain yogurt with fresh fruit. We also discussed the Okinawan philosophy of *hara hachi bu* ["eat until you are eight parts [out of ten] full"]—stopping when nearly full and paying attention to hunger and satiety signals. Helen also committed to one yoga class per week, and walking her dogs for 20 minutes a couple of days after work.

Eight months after adopting this gradual lifestyle change, her weight dropped from 173 to 161 pounds, and in another eight months down to 153 pounds, dropping her BMI from 27.1 to a healthy 23.6. Helen is happy with her weight and lifestyle and notes that she has more energy with moderating her carb intake and increasing protein. She is also willing to explore incorporating new healthy foods and exercise into her daily life.

Introduction

N utrition is a cornerstone of health, and food is necessary for energy, growth, repair, and renewal. Hippocrates's dictum "Let food be thy medicine and medicine be thy food" still holds value today. The subject of nutrition is vast; emphasis in this chapter will include the basics of nutrition—carbohydrates, proteins, fats, and water; key micronutrients; and the healthiest whole-food eating styles.

Carbohydrates

Carbohydrates ("carbs") can provide the bulk of the body's energy needs and are available in the form of starches, sugars, and fibers. When evaluating the health benefits of carbohydrates, the following questions are important to address:

1. How is the carbohydrate processed? To what extent is the carbohydrate processed?
2. What is the fiber content?
3. What is the glycemic index/load?

PROCESSED OR UNPROCESSED CARBOHYDRATES

Wheat can be served as a cracked whole-grain entree or as bleached white flour in a cookie. Unfortunately, refining strips away the nutrient-dense bran and germ, and 70%–80% of the iron, fiber, B vitamins, magnesium, and zinc, which do not always get added back via "enrichment" (Sizer & Whitney, 2014a). In women, intake of whole grains, but not refined carbohydrates, decreases the risk of type 2 diabetes (de Munter et al., 2007).

FIBER

Fibers are commonly described as being soluble (able to dissolve in water) or insoluble (roughage). Soluble fibers, such as pectins and gums—found naturally in oat bran, fruits, legumes, seaweed, and psyllium—lower serum cholesterol by reducing the absorption of dietary cholesterol. Insoluble fibers, such as cellulose and lignin—found in wheat bran and fruit skins—increase the sense of fullness, slow the rate of absorption of food across the small intestine, slow the rise in blood glucose levels, and act as bulking agents. Both soluble and insoluble fibers are valuable and are often found together in the same food. Whole oats, prunes, and black beans contain roughly equal amounts of soluble and insoluble fiber. Women should aim for 20 to 35 g of total fiber per day from whole grains, fruits, and vegetables.

Note: a word of caution about added fibers. Many manufactured food products tout themselves as "high fiber" by adding isolated fibers such as polydextrose and maltodextrin—mostly pulverized powders, but evidence is unconvincing that they have the same benefits as naturally occurring intact fibers (Liebman, 2008).

The glycemic index (GI) is a measure of how quickly a carbohydrate food raises blood sugar levels. The scale ranges from 1 to 100, with 100 representing pure glucose. Fiber, protein, and fats in food slow the rate of absorption of carbohydrates and the subsequent rise in blood glucose.

Foods with an index value ≥ 70 are considered high glycemic, 56–69 medium glycemic, and ≤ 55 low glycemic. Foods naturally high in fiber have a lower GI, as do foods that are less processed. Studies have shown a decreased risk of diabetes (Bhupathiraju et al., 2014) and cardiovascular disease with low-GI diets (Jenkins et al., 2002; Esfahani et al., 2009). Higher GI and glycemic load (GL) diet scores have been significantly associated with breast cancer risk in postmenopausal women (Woo, Park, Shin, & Kim, 2013). A meta-analysis of many chronic diseases supports the hypothesis that higher postprandial glycemia is a unifying mechanism for disease progression (Barclay et al., 2008).

Numerous scientists have criticized the GI, as it does not account for the fiber and water content of a food. A related, but more practical measure is the GL, which takes into account the *amount* of carbohydrates in a typical serving size plus its GI. Glycemic load values ≥ 20 are considered high glycemic load, 11–19 medium load, and ≤ 10 low load. For example, pasta has a medium-level GI, but is so dense in carbohydrate calories that the GL is high at 27. The carbs in watermelon have a high GI of 72; however, watermelon contains mostly water and only a small amount of carbohydrate, making its GL low at 4. It is recommended that women incorporate more low GL foods into their diets (Table 2.1).

Table 2.1. International Table of Glycemic Index and Glycemic Load Values: 2002

Food Items	Glycemic Index [Glucose = 100] High GI ≥ 70 Med GI 56–69 Low GI ≤ 55	Glycemic Load High GL ≥ 20 Med GL 11–19 Low GL ≤ 10
White baguette	95	15
Cornflakes	92	24
Watermelon	72	4
Rye crackers, wholegrain	63	11
Spaghetti, white	61	27
Cracked whole wheat bread	58	12
Apple, raw	40	6
Garbanzo beans	28	8
Black beans	20	5

Source: From Foster-Powell, Holt, & Brand-Miller (2002).

Clinical Pearl

Think of GI/GL as a tool for comparing carbohydrates. When counseling patients, I use the analogy of "food as fuel." Eating low GL foods (with more fiber, naturally occurring fat, etc.) provides more consistent and sustained energy (Figure 2.1 dotted line in the graph) than ingesting the same amount of high-GL carbs, having the fuel supply spike and then crash 90 minutes later (Figure 2.1, solid black line where sugar drops).

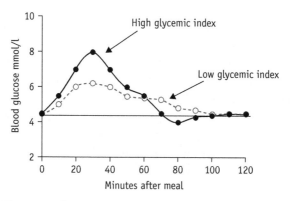

FIGURE 2.1. Glycemic index curve.

SUGAR—NOT SO SWEET FOR YOUR HEALTH

While sugars are naturally occurring components of carbohydrates, Americans consume excessive amounts of sugar, especially in the form of added sweeteners. From 2001 to 2004, the average intake of added sugars was 22 teaspoons per day (355 calories). High soft drink intake is associated with higher calorie intake, weight gain, obesity (Malik, Schulze, & Hu, 2006), and lower intake of essential nutrients. It is also linked to higher body fat, diabetes, hypertension, kidney disease, and metabolic syndrome. In 2009, the American Heart Association issued its recommendations that women consume no more than 100 calories (25 grams) per day from added sugars (American Heart Association, 2009). This is equal to 6 teaspoons, so enjoy sweets in moderation. Artificial sweeteners, despite their lack of calories, have a mixed record with regard to weight loss (Gardner et al., 2012), and studies in women suggest they may increase the risk of kidney dysfunction (Lin & Curhan, 2011).

Fructose, the most abundant sugar found in fruits, is metabolized in the liver, which lengthens the time it takes to raise blood sugar. Naturally occurring fructose in fruits is accompanied by fiber that slows digestion, further slowing the rise in blood sugar. However, when ingested as isolated fructose or high-fructose corn syrup, it can pose a real health hazard. Fructose metabolism within liver cells is complex. It can generate increased amounts of triglycerides (TGs), uric acid, and free radicals, ultimately increasing the risk of nonalcoholic fatty liver disease and, in severe cases, cirrhosis (R. J. Johnson, Sanchez-Lozada, & Nakagawa, 2010).

Fructose content is high in many common natural sweeteners: 50% of the sugar in honey and sucrose (table sugar) is fructose, whereas high-fructose corn syrup is modestly higher at 55% fructose. Surprising to most is the fact that the sugar in apple juice is 60% fructose, and in agave syrup 82% fructose (US Department of Agriculture [USDA], 2012). Even though the sugar is from a natural source, women still need to be mindful of the total sugar load they are consuming. This should not deter women from enjoying fresh, antioxidant-rich berries and fruit in season; women should simply be mindful of avoiding excess added sweeteners in food.

FRUITS AND VEGETABLES

While fruit contains variable amounts of fructose, nature also packs fruit with water, fiber, vitamins, minerals, and other micronutrients. Vegetables contain the highest concentrations of vitamins, minerals, and other protective phyto-chemicals, with a lower caloric density compared with other foods. Rich in biochemical complexity, whole vegetables and fruits are superior to any single isolated nutrient. Citrus fruit for example, contains not only vitamin C but also some 60 flavonoids and 20 carotenoids. A recent meta-analysis found that higher consumption of fruits and vegetables was significantly associated with a lower risk of all cause mortality (Wang et al., 2014). In these studies, it was shown that the threshold amount was five servings of vegetables and fruit per day.

Proteins

MINIMAL PROTEIN NEEDS

A common dietary concern for many women is getting enough protein. However, the average American diet provides ample, or even excessive, protein. The recommended daily allowance (RDA) of protein in women aged 13 and older (excluding pregnancy) is 46 g/day. For reference, a 3-ounce serving (size of a deck of cards) of chicken breast provides about 23 g of protein, ½ cup of firm tofu provides 20 g, and one slice of whole-grain bread about 4 g. Eating a well-balanced diet should provide plenty of protein. Indeed, the 2012 National Health and Nutrition Examination Survey (NHANES) revealed that women in the United States are eating an average of 68 grams of protein (US Department of Agriculture, Agricultural Research Service, 2012).

OPTIMAL PROTEIN AMOUNT

The optimal amount of protein varies with health status (i.e., less for women with kidney disease), activity (more protein may be advantageous during resistance training), and age. In the United States, guidelines recommend 0.8 g protein/kg of *ideal* body weight per day, thus for a fit 70-kg/154-lb woman, this would equal 56 g of protein. According to the Institute of Medicine, women should get at least 10% but not more than 35% of daily calories from protein.

Another important consideration is the source of protein: plant or animal. Plant sources of protein tend to be high in fiber, potassium, folate, and magnesium. Plant-based diets are associated with lower risk of chronic disease, including cardiovascular disease (F. B. Hu, 2003), whereas a diet high in red meat (one serving per day) increases the risk of diabetes (Fung, Schulze, Manson, Willett, & Hu, 2004), cardiovascular disease (Pan et al., 2012), colorectal cancer, and possibly other cancers (Farvid, Cho, Chen, Eliassen, & Willett, 2014; Xu et al., 2013). The American Institute for Cancer Research (AICR) recommends eating no more than 18 oz. (cooked weight) per week of red meats, like beef, pork, and lamb, and avoiding processed meat such as ham, bacon, salami, hot dogs, and sausages (AICR, 2011). Results from large prospective cohort trials recommend no more than half a serving of red meat per day. Substitution of other healthy protein sources for red meat is associated with a lower mortality risk (Pan et al., 2012).

BOTTOM LINE ON PROTEINS

Two to three servings of high-quality, protein-rich foods per day are adequate to meet most women's needs. If consuming animal protein, emphasize fish, chicken, turkey, and eggs—organic whenever possible. Limit red meat to once or twice a week. Plant sources of protein (legumes and nuts) are excellent choices and should be considered.

A QUICK WORD ABOUT SOY

Soy contains a full complement of essential amino acids, making it a complete protein. It also contains isoflavones (genistein, daidzein, glycitein), compounds that can act as weak estrogens or antiestrogens. Many concerns about soy's effect on breast cancer, osteoporosis, and thyroid function have been raised. A review by D'Adamo and Sahin (2014) showed that soy may provide relief from menopausal symptoms and protect against breast cancer and heart disease but does not appear to offer protection from osteoporosis. In their study, soy variably affected thyroid function—it can either increase or decrease thyroid function. Large epidemiologic studies in Asian countries have shown that lifelong, traditional consumption of soy may offer some protection against menopausal symptoms and breast cancer (Zhang et al., 2005). Other trials supported that eating soy foods at levels comparable to women in Asia has no detrimental effect on breast cancer, and may even reduce recurrence (Guha et al., 2009; Magee & Rowland, 2012). The review's authors conclude that consuming moderate amounts of traditionally prepared and minimally processed soy foods may offer modest health benefits while minimizing potential for adverse health effects.

The Skinny on Fats

There are three major categories of dietary fats—saturated, monounsaturated, and polyunsaturated—based on the number of double bonds within the lipid molecule. All fats found in nature are composite fats. For example, olive oil is 77% monounsaturated, but also contains 14% saturated fat and 9% polyunsaturated fats (Figure 2.2). High-quality fats are essential in the diet. While saturated fats have long been thought to increase the risk of heart disease, a recent meta-analysis revealed no increased risk of cardiovascular disease (Siri-Tarino, Sun, Hu, & Krauss, 2010). Furthermore, more data is emerging about the different types (carbon chain lengths) of saturated fats. Long-chain saturated fats with carbon length of 16 or greater will raise TG levels and lower HDL, and short-chain saturated fats do not appear to have these effects (*Vannice & Rasmussen*, 2014). Meat and animal fats contain higher amounts of long-chain saturated fats, while plant sources such as coconut oil contain about 60% MCTs (Schardt, 2012). Medium-chain TGs are more rapidly absorbed and can be burned by muscles and organs for immediate fuel.

Trans-fats are the big dietary "no-no." They increase serum levels of LDL, lipoprotein(a), TGs, and inflammatory mediators in women, and reduce HDL cholesterol (Micha & Mozaffarian, 2008). Foods containing *trans*-fats, usually in the form of partially hydrogenated fats, should be completely eliminated from the diet. While the data are mixed regarding saturated, monounsaturated, and omega-6 fats; *trans*-fats are clearly associated with heart disease (Chowdhury et al., 2014).

Extra-virgin olive oil contains antioxidants and LDL-lowering sterols and favorably affects anti-inflammatory mediators (Perona, Cabello-Moruno, & Ruiz-Gutierrez, 2006). Due to its high monounsaturated content, olive oil is less susceptible to conversion to *trans*-fatty acids, thus reducing risk of cardiovascular disease. In the PREDIMED study, higher baseline total olive oil consumption was associated with 48% reduced risk of cardiovascular mortality (Guasch-Ferré et al., 2014). Olive oil is a good choice for low-temperature cooking, but for temperatures > 350° F, oils with a higher smoke point, such as grapeseed or organic canola oils, are a better choice.

Omega-3 fats come from plant sources such as flaxseed, hempseed, walnuts, and canola and animal sources such as fatty fish and fortified. Fish oils, in particular, have high concentrations of eicosapentaenoic acid (EPA) and docosahexaenoic acid (DHA), which are the most biologically active omega-3 fats. Plant sources have high amounts of alpha-linolenic acid, of which only about 15% is converted into EPA and DHA.

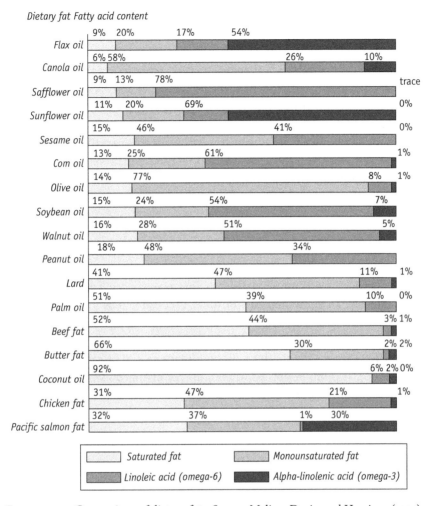

Dietary fat Fatty acid content

FIGURE 2.2. Comparison of dietary fats. *Source*: Melina, Davis, and Harrison (1995).

Women should eat two to three servings of fatty fish per week in order to obtain adequate omega-3 fats. Higher circulating levels of EPA and DHA are associated with lower coronary risk (RR 0.75), however supplementation with fish oil capsules containing EPA and DHA have shown mixed results. Higher doses of at least 1–6 grams of omega-3 oils as a supplement were shown to reduce risk of cardiac death, sudden death, and myocardial infarction in patients with a history of cardiovascular disease (Casula, Soranna, Catapano, & Corrao, 2013; Chowdhury et al., 2014; Kotwal, Jun, Sullivan, Perkovic, & Neal, 2012).

AVOIDING MERCURY IN FISH

Although a source of high-quality protein, fish often swim in waters contaminated with heavy metals such as cadmium, lead, mercury, and other pollutants such as polychlorinated biphenyls (PCBs), dioxins, and DDT. Large predatory fish that eat other fish accumulate higher levels of contaminants in their flesh. Fish highest in mercury include king mackerel, swordfish, shark, tilefish, orange roughy, grouper, and tuna. Some of the safest fish are tilapia, anchovies, and wild salmon. The Natural Resources Defense Council website offers more detailed information to help women make the best choices. (http://www.nrdc. org/health/effects/mercury/guide.asp).

Water

The Institute of Medicine recommends that women drink about 2 liters of water per day; an additional 20% of water is consumed as moisture in food. Herbal tisanes, tea, and coffee can be added to daily fluid intake, although there is an initial small diuretic effect with caffeine. Sugar-sweetened beverages are associated with obesity, and their intake should be minimized (Malik et al., 2006). It is important for women to stay hydrated as thirst signals can be mistaken for hunger. Fun ways to flavor water include adding mint leaves, sliced oranges, cucumbers, or raspberries.

Key Micronutrients

According to the latest NHANES data (National Center for Environmental Health, Division of Laboratory Sciences, 2012), five of the most common micronutrient deficiencies are iron and vitamins B6, B12, C, and D. Women are also often deficient in magnesium and selenium. Selecting vitamin- and mineral-rich foods can help women prevent these deficiencies, but a burning question exists: Can we get adequate micronutrients from our food?

- Well, yes if everyday we consume:
  - 9 oz sockeye salmon
  - 5 cups of blanched fresh spinach
  - 4 oz pumpkin seeds
  - 1 Brazil nut
  - 5 cups milk, 10 eggs, OR 2 teaspoons nutritional yeast

Because obtaining all our micronutrient needs from food alone is difficult (Table 2.2), supplementation may be warranted. However, studies are mixed with regard to the benefits and risks of taking a daily multivitamin (MVI) tablet (Muntwyler, Hennekens, Manson, Buring, & Gaziano, 2002; Neuhouser et al. 2009).The form of MVI supplementation may matter, and ingesting these same micronutrients from food is generally a safer bet. Bottom line: women should strive to eat a healthy, balanced diet rich in micronutrients and supplement when necessary. Women of child-bearing age are advised to take an MVI with folic acid. The Institute of Medicine states that women over the age of 50 should eat foods fortified with B12 or take a supplement. Vitamin D is difficult to get in diet alone (see Table 2.2); many women will need to supplement. See details in the chapters "Dietary Supplements," "Preconception Counseling and Fertility," "Pregnancy and Lactation," and "Osteoporosis." More information on vitamins and minerals, with references to studies, can be found at the National Institutes of Health Office of Dietary Supplements website (http://ods.od.nih.gov).

Therapeutic Diets

- Mediterranean-based diet
- Anti-inflammatory diet
- Low-carbohydrate diet
- Vegetarian diet
- Elimination diet
- Intermittent fasting

ABOUT THE MEDITERRANEAN DIET

The Mediterranean diet is based on traditional eating patterns of the Mediterranean region (Trichopoulou, 2001). It emphasizes a high intake of fruit, vegetables, and whole grains, moderate fish intake, moderate wine consumption, olive oil as the primary fat, and limited consumption of red meat and saturated fat. It has a favorable balance of polyunsaturated omega-6:omega-3 fatty acids of 2–4:1, whereas in the typical US diet this ratio is closer to 10–20:1. Fish, locally consumed wild greens, herbs, and walnuts (all sources of omega-3 fats) help contribute to a more favorable, anti-inflammatory balance (Manios, Detopoulou, Visioli, & Galli, 2006).

When combined with a healthy lifestyle, the Mediterranean diet has been shown to decrease all-cause mortality in women. The American Association of Retired Persons prospective study (Mitrou et al., 2007). showed that

Table 2.2. Micronutrients Available in Food

Vitamin /Mineral	RDA	Food Source /Amount Needed to Reach RDA
Iron	18 mg (women 20–50 years)	5 oz chicken liver 9.5 oz oysters 1 ¼ lb dark turkey meat 4–7 oz* pumpkin seeds 2–3.5 cups* edamame 2.5–5 cups* cooked spinach 5–9 Tbsp* blackstrap molasses
Vitamin D	600 IU	½ Tbsp cod liver oil 4 oz sockeye salmon 26 sardines, in oil 15 eggs, large 5.2 cups fortified milk OR 5–20 minutes of hands, face, and legs exposure to midday sunlight
Vitamin B12 (cobalamin)	6 mcg	1/10 oz clams 1/3 oz beef liver 6 oz rainbow trout, wild 5 cups milk, low-fat 10 eggs 2 teaspoons nutritional yeast
Vitamin B6	2 mg	2 cups chickpeas 7 oz tuna, fresh 9 oz sockeye salmon 5 bananas 5 cups potatoes 20 oz nuts 10 cups kale
Magnesium	400 mg	5 ounces of almonds or cashews 2 ½ cups cooked spinach 6 ½ cups black beans 16 Tbsp peanut butter 3 ½ lbs chicken breast 9 cups avocado 7.5 oz dark chocolate

*Vegan sources—may require 80% more intake due to impaired absorption

Vegetarians require 1.8 times more iron than nonvegetarians because of the lower bioavailability of plant-based iron. In addition, phytates in some plants, nuts, and grains inhibit iron absorption. Beans can be soaked and rinsed prior to cooking to reduce phytates and improve digestion. Vitamin B12 is only found in animal products and specially prepared yeast products; vegans will need to supplement.

all-cause mortality for women dropped by 20%. Similarly, the Healthy Ageing: A Longitudinal Study in Europe (HALE) study, confirmed that adherence to a Mediterranean diet and healthy lifestyle is associated with a >50% lower rate of all-cause and cause-specific mortality in healthy men and women more than 70 years of age (Knoops et al., 2004). While wine "in moderation" is a part of the Mediterranean food pyramid guidelines, it is recommended that women follow the CDC's recommendation of no more than one alcoholic beverage per day (5 ounces wine, or 12 ounces beer, or a 1.5 ounce shot of liquor).

Cardiovascular Disease

The Lyon Heart Study (De Lorgeril et al., 1999) reported that the Mediterranean diet reduced the risk of a second heart attack in people who had a previous heart attack by 70%. The Lyon diet was high in fruits, vegetables, whole grains, legumes, and fish. Forty percent of calories were from fat (olive oil and a special high monounsaturated spread), as compared with controls that consumed a 30% fat "heart-healthy" diet. The reduction in cardiac morbidity in the experimental group was so significant that the trial was stopped early. Similarly, in the GIZZI-Prevenzione study (Barzi et al., 2003), there was a 50% reduction of death in participants with high Mediterranean dietary scores compared with those in the lowest quartile. Of note, it appears that women with coronary artery disease (CAD) may be more responsive to the Mediterranean diet than men (Chrysohoou et al., 2003). A Mediterranean diet lowers lipids and blood pressure (Domenech et al., 2014), and significantly lowers risk of sudden cardiac death in women (Bertoia et al., 2014). Another primary prevention trial using the Mediterranean diet—rich in extra-virgin olive oil and nuts—was also stopped early due to significant reductions in cardiovascular events (Estruch et al., 2013).

Cancer

The overall cancer incidence in Mediterranean countries is lower than in northern European countries, the United Kingdom, and the United States. Several studies show that much of this may be attributable to dietary factors. The Lyon Diet Heart study was also analyzed for its impact on cancer; a 61% decrease in cancer incidence was noted (De Lorgeril et al., 1998). Another study (Trichopoulou et al., 2000) calculated that up to 25% of colorectal cancer, 15% of breast cancer, and 10% of pancreas and endometrial cancers could be prevented if Western populations shifted to the traditional Mediterranean diet. Indeed, a Western diet confers higher risk (OR 1.46) of breast cancer, while a Mediterranean diet lowers the risk of all breast cancer subtypes (OR 0.56) (Castelló et al., 2014; Mourouti et al., 2014).

Obesity

The Mediterranean diet has been associated with reduced obesity and risk of metabolic syndrome (Esposito et al., 2013). In a randomized, controlled trial on weight loss, despite a higher fat content (35% compared with 20%), participants eating a Mediterranean diet lost 4.1 kg, compared with the control group who gained nearly 3 kg over 18 months (McManus, Antinoro, & Sacks, 2001). The palatability of a higher fat diet may be the reason for greater long-term adherence—it tastes good, hunger signals are quieted, and people are satisfied. Women with diabetes following a Mediterranean diet had 23% higher levels of adiponectin, a hormone secreted by fat cells that is inversely correlated with body fat percentage (Mantzoros et al., 2006).

In a summary of the research on the Mediterranean diet, Dr. Walter Willett from the Harvard School of Public Health concluded that in nonsmoking individuals with regular physical activity, "over 80% of coronary heart disease, 70% of stroke, and 90% of type 2 diabetes can be avoided by healthy food choices that are consistent with the traditional Mediterranean diet" (Willett, 2006).

ABOUT THE ANTI-INFLAMMATORY DIET

It is now believed that chronic inflammation is the common pathophysiologic pathway underlying CAD, asthma, arthritis, Alzheimer's disease, autoimmune disorders, and some cancers. Obesity, saturated fat, *trans*-fat, and an inadequate amount of omega-3 fats have been shown to increase inflammatory biomarkers such as C-reactive protein (CRP), interleukin 6 (IL-6), and tumor necrosis factor (TNF) (Basu, Devaraj, & Jialal, 2006; Simopoulos, 2002). An *anti-inflammatory* diet increases dietary intake of foods that decrease inflammation while reducing foods that increase inflammation; two examples of these are the Mediterranean diet and the Okinawan diet. The Mediterranean diet, described above, has been shown to reduce inflammatory markers such as high sensitivity-CRP and IL-6 (Esposito et al., 2004). The Okinawan diet is similarly rich in anti-inflammatory foods, such as fish, deeply colored vegetables, sea plants, and turmeric (Muñoz & Costa, 2013; Murakami et al., 2005; Willcox, Willcox, Todoriki, & Suzuki, 2009), and Okinawans are among the longest-lived, healthiest people in the world.

Dr. Andrew Weil has published a patient-friendly and illustrative anti-inflammatory food pyramid (see http://www.drweil.com/drw/u/ART02995/Dr-Weil-Anti-Inflammatory-Food-Pyramid.html). This plan also features berries, Asian mushrooms, soy, tea, dark chocolate, and spices.

ABOUT LOW-CARBOHYDRATE DIETS

Popular diets vary in their carbohydrate recommendations: Less than 10% of total calories (Atkins), 40% (Zone), 55%–60% (LEARN), and 65%–75% (Ornish). Atkins-type, low-carb diets have been very popular since the late 1990s and are particularly promoted for weight loss. Over the past decade, many studies have been published on low-carbohydrate diets. A 2012 meta-analysis (T. Hu et al., 2012) examined more than 20 of these studies that were of at least six months duration. With isocaloric intakes of about 2,000 kcals, both low-carb and low-fat groups lost weight (-5 to 6 kg, and -6 cm waist circumference), but the low-carb groups overall fared better with slightly decreased LDL, TG, and improved HDL cholesterol levels. Low-carb diets ranged from 4% to 45% of the diet as carbohydrates (as compared with 60% in USDA guidelines). Based on these studies, women can safely choose a low-carb diet for weight loss and mild improvement in cardiac risk factors. In one of the best-conducted studies, women in the low-carb group lost more weight than the low-fat group and ate 250–500 calories less. One benefit of a low-carb diet is high palatability; fats and proteins tend to turn off hunger signals. Because low-carb diets are inherently higher in fat and protein, women should be counseled to choose high quality, minimally processed fats and organic proteins in order to maximize benefits of such a diet.

For a more comprehensive review of carbs, protein, fat, water, vitamins, and minerals, refer to *Nutrition—Concepts and Controversies* (Sizer & Whitney, 2014b) and *Krause's Food, Nutrition and Diet Therapy* textbooks (Mahan & Escott-Stump, 2004).

VEGETARIAN DIET

Women may choose to eat a vegetarian diet for health, spiritual, ethical, and/or environmental reasons. There are substantial data to recommend plant-based diets to promote health and reduce disease in women. Plant-based diets range from "flexitarian" diets (vegetarian diets with occasional meat), to complete veganism—avoiding all animal-based food. Vegetarian diets and low-meat diets are associated with decreased risk of heart disease, type 2 diabetes, and obesity and increased longevity (Marsh, Zeuschner, & Saunders, 2012; McEvoy, Temple, & Woodside, 2012).

Plant-based foods provide magnesium, vitamin C, and beta-carotene, with lower homocysteine and long-chain saturated fats. Dietary fiber comes exclusively from plant-based foods. With thoughtful planning, women on vegan diets will be able to obtain adequate iron, calcium, and folate from foods such as legumes, nuts, leafy greens, and nutritional yeast; vitamin B12 should be supplemented. Women interested in adopting a plant-based diet may start by eating vegetarian just 1 day a week, and reap the health and environmental benefits (Wannaveg, 2014). http://wannaveg.com

THE ELIMINATION DIET

The elimination diet is a clinical tool rather than a diet. It is defined as "an investigational short-term or possible lifelong eating plan that omits one or more foods suspected or known to cause an adverse food reaction or allergic response" (Mahan & Escott-Stump, 2004). Food allergy or intolerance may play a significant role in many chronic conditions including migraines, asthma, otitis media, skin conditions, attention deficit hyperactivity disorder (ADHD), arthritis, autoimmune diseases, and more. Clinical trials using food elimination diets have reported improvement rates as high as 58% for atopic dermatitis, 71% for irritable bowel syndrome (IBS), and 90% for migraines (Rindfleisch, 2012). Commonplace symptoms such as dyspepsia, flatulence, chronic fatigue, skin rashes, joint aches, and pains have all been linked to food sensitivities. Many integrative practitioners consider addressing dietary sensitivities as a critical first step to symptom amelioration.

Major Food Triggers

- Dairy products
- Wheat and other grains containing gluten (oats, barley, rye)
- Eggs
- Corn
- Soy and soy products
- Peanuts
- Citrus fruits
- Shellfish and fish
- Refined sugars
- Artificial additives, preservatives, and colorings

Skin-prick testing and serum immunoglobulin G (IgG) antibody measurements remain controversial. An empiric elimination diet will require advance planning and adherence, but is straightforward and specific to the individual being tested.

Phases of the Elimination Diet

1. *Elimination phase.* All suspected foods are omitted from the diet (i.e., refined sugar, dairy products, wheat, etc.) for 14 to 28 days. Clinical symptoms are monitored for resolution. For example, a woman may notice that she is less fatigued or bloated while eliminating dairy products from her diet.
2. *Reintroduction or challenge phase.* Suspected food triggers are reintroduced one at a time into the diet to see whether symptoms recur. For example, fatigue or bloating returns when the aforementioned woman resumes eating dairy.
3. *Maintenance phase.* Routinely eliminating foods from the diet that trigger symptoms.

The theory behind the elimination diet is simple, but as most of our diet consists of composite foods (e.g., pizza = bread + tomato sauce + cheese/dairy + various meat and vegetable toppings), it is often hard to practice. Women must learn to read labels carefully to identify hidden sources of allergens. For example, casein, lactose, and whey are all dairy products. Women testing for wheat sensitivity must avoid more obvious suspect foods such as breads, cookies, pasta, and cereals as well as the myriad of foods made with wheat, including "modified food starch," beer, caramel coloring, soy sauce, and more. [For a detailed list, visit www.celiac.com and search using the keywords "unsafe ingredients"]. Though the elimination diet requires diligence and patience, when it is properly done the results can be extremely beneficial.

A modified elimination diet is when *one* suspect food at a time is avoided for 14 to 28 days and then rotated back into the diet. It takes longer to test all the individual foods, however it is more practical for children and those who are reluctant to undergo the drastic dietary changes called for in the full elimination diet.

INTERMITTENT FASTING

Hippocrates, Galen, and Aristotle all advocated short fasts to clear the body and mind of disease. Religions from all over the world promote various practices of fasting for spiritual benefits. Science is now starting to confirm some of fasting's physical benefits. Intermittent fasting (IF) involves complete or partial calorie intake restriction (from 50% to 100%) one to three days per week. Studies have shown that IF can increase the resistance of neurons to injury and disease by stimulating adaptive cellular stress responses. Intermittent fasting may work via hypothalamic regulation: In one study, enhanced lipid oxidation was observed during fasting days, while eating days were accompanied by higher metabolic rates (Chausse et al., 2014).

Intermittent fasting produces substantial weight loss (5%–10% of baseline body weight) over 8 to 12 weeks; it has also been shown to decrease LDLs, TGs, blood pressure, and visceral fat and to increase insulin sensitivity and improve glucose tolerance (Rothschild, Hoddy, Jambazian, & Varady, 2014; Trepanowski et al., 2011). Other studies support improvement in seasonal allergies, autoimmune diseases, and menopausal hot flashes (J. B. Johnson, Laub, & John, 2006). Intermittent fasting may also protect the brain from neurodegenerative insults leading to Alzheimer's and Parkinson's diseases (Martin, Mattson, & Maudsley, 2006). Another form of IF is time-restricted feeding; food intake is limited to 3 to 12 hours per day with the remaining 12–21 hours spent fasting. Time-restricted feeding also shows promise of similar benefits (Rothschild, Hoddy, Jambazian, & Varady, 2014).

An IF regimen for an overweight woman trying to lose weight/gain health may look like this: normal calories and activity five days of week, limiting calories to 500 kcal on Mondays and Thursdays (Brown, Mosley, & Aldred, 2013). This approach is cost-effective, associated with low risk, and has been shown to be similarly or more effective than continuous modest calorie restriction, with less sense of deprivation.

ORGANIC FOOD

Many questions are posed about the value of organic food. Consumers pay 10%–40% more for certified organic food (Winter & Davis, 2006) because they perceive it as safer, more nutritious, and environmentally friendly. The evidence for nutritional advantages of consuming organic food is less clear than that for reducing pesticide exposure. While some studies have shown that organically grown crops have significantly higher levels of polyphenols and vitamin C, and lower nitrates and cadmium than conventionally grown crops (Barański et al., 2014; Benbrook, Zhao, Yanes, Davies, & Andrews, 2008; Worthington, 2001), a 2012 systematic review from Stanford pointed to minimal nutritional differences between organic and conventionally grown crops (Smith-Spangler et al., 2012), but did show reductions in pesticides (Holzman, 2012). Critics of that study assert there is considerable health risk reduction (94%) when one chooses an organic form of fruit that is not intensively pesticide-laden (Holzman, 2012). Children are especially vulnerable to pesticide exposure. Studies done with California farmworker communities show a 7-point deficit in IQ in children in the highest compared with the lowest quintile of in utero pesticide exposure (Bouchard et al., 2011). In October 2012, the American Academy of Pediatrics recognized that an organic diet definitely reduces exposure to pesticides while acknowledging lack of proof for relevant nutrition advantage over a conventional diet.

Raising animals for food takes a large toll on environmental resources— water, waste, fuel, increased greenhouse gases, and use of available land. For example, 1,850 gallons of water are needed to produce a single pound of beef, compared with 39 gallons for a pound of vegetables. The grain used to feed livestock would feed 840 million vegetarians (Pimentel & Pimental, 2008). For many reasons it is healthier to support and purchase grass-fed, humanely raised, organic meats. Organically raised beef has a more favorable ratio of omega 6 to omega 3 fats (Bjorklund, Heins, Dicostanzo, & Chester-Jones, 2014). By the USDA's definition, organic meat, poultry, eggs, and dairy products must come from animals that are not given growth hormones or routine antibiotics. It is estimated that 70% of the total amount of antibiotics used in the United States are given to poultry, swine, and beef cattle (Mellon, 2000). These antibiotic "food additives" are given to promote growth and to compensate for crowded animal conditions that place livestock at risk of infections. A major public health concern arising from these practices is the increase in antibiotic resistance.

Studies done on meat samples from supermarkets show that 6%–20% of samples were contaminated with Salmonella, the majority of which were resistant to at least one, and often three or more, antibiotics (White et al., 2001; Zhao et al., 2006). The World Health Organization, the American Public Health Association, and the Union of Concerned Scientists have confirmed that overuse of antibiotics in livestock contribute to the antibiotic resistance affecting humans and have called for their cessation. In 2012, the FDA issued a final, long-awaited guidance statement for the regulation of antibiotic use in food animal production (Alliance for the Prudent Use of Antibiotics, 2012).

Top 12 Fruits and Vegetables to Consume Organically Grown (USDA 2012)

1. Apples
2. Strawberries
3. Grapes
4. Celery
5. Peaches
6. Spinach
7. Sweet bell peppers
8. Imported nectarines
9. Cucumbers
10. Cherry tomatoes
11. Snap peas
12. Potatoes

Organophosphate (OP) residues, DDT by-products, and other products listed as endocrine disruptors or carcinogens were found in significant amounts in these foods. Because OP residues tend to concentrate in fat, it may be prudent to consume most if not all of your food oils (olive oil, butter, etc.) as organic.

Top Tips From Clinical Experience

- Remember to simply ask your patients what they eat. A 24-hour food recall may be a helpful snapshot of their intake and preferences, and can be done while patients are waiting.
- Encourage patients to double their vegetable intake and halve their refined carb intake—for example, eat an open-faced sandwich with one piece of bread with a small green salad, or a side of fresh vegetables. Stir in a cup of chopped leafy greens to a bowl of soup.
- Mindful eating + *hara hachi bu*—another tip that I teach patients is to simply check in with their level of hunger. Okinawan longevity is well-known, and one of their sayings, *hara hachi bu*, translates as "eat until you are eight parts full" (Willcox, Willcox, & Suzuki, 2001). This simple wisdom advises us to avoid stuffing our stomachs until they are bursting at the seams. It also teaches us be mindful of how much we eat and how are bodies are feeling. Often, we can be satisfied with less.
- Weight-loss guidelines recommend that obese women with BMI >35 cut out 500+ calories/day. Women with a BMI of 26–35 should reduce caloric intake by 300–500 calories/day.

- Successful "losers" engage in frequent exercise, eat an estimated 1,800 kcal/day, eat breakfast, and self-monitor their weight (Wing & Phelan, 2005).
- Getting adequate sleep and cutting back on alcohol and TV watching may help curb overeating (Chapman, Benedict, & Brooks, 2012).
- Healthy snacks under 200 calories: chopped vegetables (carrots, snow peas, cauliflower, radishes, cucumbers), one-quarter measuring cup of nuts, two whole-grain rye crackers with hummus, mini portions of leftover dinner, medium apple with 2 teaspoons of almond butter, half banana with 2 teaspoons of peanut butter, one 8-ounce cup of low-fat plain yogurt with a half-cup of fresh or frozen blackberries, 2-ounce string cheese, 2-inch square of smoked tofu with veggies.
- Chocolate—dark chocolate is rich in antioxidants as well as mood-enhancing phenylethylamine and anandamides. Despite its high saturated fat content, dark chocolate does not raise LDL, and indeed may lower it. One study showed that dark chocolate lowers blood pressure (Taubert et al., 2007). A small portion (about 1-inch flat square) of dark (70% cocoa or more) can be a healthy and happy treat.

Summary

- Eat whole, unprocessed foods with low glycemic load.
- Quality and quantity of fats, carbs, and proteins matter.
- Following a traditional Mediterranean diet is powerful medicine and has been proven to prevent or mitigate the onset or occurrence of multiple chronic diseases.
- Eat mindfully (*hara hachi bu*) and savor your food.
- Therapeutic use of specific plans—elimination diet, low-carb diets, plant-based diets, intermittent fasting—can yield health benefits for women.

Resources for Integrative Providers

- Oldways Preservation Trust—has the original Mediterranean Diet Pyramid, other culturally appropriate guidelines, recipes and research links.
  http://oldwayspt.org/resources
- The Healthy Eating Plate http://www.hsph.harvard.edu/nutritionsource/healthy-eating-plate/

- Portion size website—The National Heart Lung and Blood Institute of the NIH has a great downloadable website to teach people about portion size of foods. https://www.nhlbi.nih.gov/health/educational/wecan/eat-right/portion-distortion.htm
- *Eat, Drink, and Weigh Less* (Katzen & Willett, 2006): An excellent, no-nonsense, reader-friendly book with helpful tips and recipes to help people lose weight.
- *Nutrition—Concepts and Controversies* (Sizer & Whitney, 2014b): Basic textbook aimed at college level, but good review of nutrition basics for health practitioners.
- For excellent evidence-based information about vegetarian and vegan diets, read *Becoming Vegetarian* (Davis & Melina, 2013) and *Becoming Vegan* (Melina, Davis, & Harrison, 1995).
- Healthy at Every Size. http://www.haescommunity.org. Regardless of a woman's body size, she can maintain optimal health through lifestyle enhancement.
- Santa Rosa Family Medicine Residency website: Healthy Diet Essential handout. http://www.srfmr.org/integrative-medicine/im-handouts

REFERENCES

Alliance for the Prudent Use of Antibiotics. (2012). *Major developments in US policy on antibiotic use in food animals.* Retrieved Oct 10, 2014, from http://www.tufts.edu/med/apua/policy/policy_antibiotic_food_animals.shtml

American Heart Association. (2009). Dietary sugars intake and cardiovascular health. *Circulation, 120,* 1011–1020.

American Institute for Cancer Research. (2011). *Recommendations for cancer prevention.* Retrieved September 16, 2014, from http://www.aicr.org/reduce-your-cancer-risk/recommendations-for-cancer-prevention/recommendations_05_red_meat.html

Barański, M., Srednicka-Tober, D., Volakakis, N. et al. (2014). Higher antioxidant and lower cadmium concentrations and lower incidence of pesticide residues in organically grown crops: A systematic literature review and meta-analyses. *Br J Nutr, 112,* 794–811.

Barclay, A. W., Petocz, P., McMillan-Price, J., Flood, V. M., Prvan, T., Mitchell, P., & Brand-Miller, J. C. (2008). Glycemic index, glycemic load, and chronic disease risk: A meta-analysis of observational studies. *Am J Clin Nutr, 87,* 627–637.

Barzi, F., Woodward, M., Marfisi, R. M., et al. GISSI-Prevenzione Investigators. (2003). Mediterranean diet and all-causes mortality after myocardial infarction: Results from the GISSI-Prevenzione trial. *Eur J Clin Nutr, 57,* 604–611.

Basu, A., Devaraj, S., & Jialal, I. (2006). Dietary factors that promote or retard inflammation. *Arterioscler Thromb Vasc Biol, 26,* 995–1001.

Benbrook, C., Zhao, X., Yanes, J., Davies, N., & Andrews, P. (2008, March). New evidence confirms the nutritional superiority of plant-based organic foods. Available at www.organic-center.org

Bertoia, M. L., Triche, E. W., Michaud, D. S., et al. (2014). Mediterranean and dietary approaches to stop hypertension dietary patterns and risk of sudden cardiac death in postmenopausal women. *Am J Clin Nutr, 99,* 344–351.

Bhupathiraju, S. N., Tobias, D. K., Malik, V. S., et al. (2014). Glycemic index, glycemic load, and risk of type 2 diabetes: Results from three large US cohorts and an updated meta-analysis. *Am J Clin Nutr, 100,* 218–232.

Bjorklund, E. A., Heins, B. J., Dicostanzo, A., & Chester-Jones, H. (2014). Fatty acid profiles, meat quality, and sensory attributes of organic versus conventional dairy beef steers. *J Dairy Sci, 97,* 1828–1834.

Bouchard, M. F., Chevrier, J., Harley, K. G., et al. (2011). Prenatal exposure to organophosphate pesticides and IQ in 7-year old children. *Environ Health Perspect, 119,* 1189.

Brown, J. E., Mosley, M., & Aldred, S. (2013). Intermittent fasting: a dietary intervention for prevention of diabetes and cardiovascular disease? *Br J Diabetes Vasc Dis, 13,* 68–72.

Castelló, A., Pollán, M., Buijsse, B., et al. (2014). Spanish Mediterranean diet and other dietary patterns and breast cancer risk: Case-control EpiGEICAM study. *Br J Cancer, 111,* 1454–1462.

Casula, M., Soranna, D., Catapano, A. L., & Corrao, G. (2013). Long-term effect of high dose omega-3 fatty acid supplementation for secondary prevention of cardiovascular outcomes: A meta-analysis of randomized, placebo controlled trials. *Atheroscler Suppl, 14,* 243–251.

Chapman, C. D., Benedict, C., Brooks, S. J., & Schiöth, H. B. (2012). Lifestyle determinants of the drive to eat: a meta-analysis. *Am J Clin Nutr, 96*(3), 492–497.

Chausse, B., Solon, C, Caldeira da Silva, C. C., et al. (2014). Intermittent fasting induces hypothalamic modifications resulting in low feeding efficiency, low body mass and overeating. *Endocrinology, 155,* 2456–2466.

Chowdhury, R., Warnakula, S., Kunutsor, S., et al. (2014). Association of dietary circulating, and supplement fatty acids with coronary risk. *Ann Intern Med, 160,* 398–406.

Chrysohoou, C., Panagiotakos, D. B., Pitsavos, C, et al. (2003). Gender differences on the risk evaluation of acute coronary syndromes: The CARDIO2000 study. *Prev Cardiol, 6,* 71–77.

D'Adamo, C. R., & Sahin, A. (2014). Soy foods and supplementation: A review of commonly perceived health benefits and risks. *Altern Ther Health Med, 20*(Suppl 1), 39–51.

Davis, B., & Melina, V. (2013). *Becoming vegan.* Summertown, TN: Book Publishing Company.

De Lorgeril, M., Salen, P., Martin, J. L., et al. (1999). Mediterranean diet, traditional risk factors, and the rate of cardiovascular complications after myocardial infarction: Final report of the Lyon Diet Heart Study. *Circulation, 99,* 779–785.

De Lorgeril, M., Salen, P., Martin, J. L., Monjaud, I., Boucher, P., & Mamelle, N. (1998). Mediterranean dietary pattern in a randomized trial: Prolonged survival and possible reduced cancer rate. *Arch Intern Med*, *158*, 1181–1187.

de Munter, J. S., Hu, F. B., Spiegelman, D., et al. (2007). Whole grain, bran, and germ intake and risk of type 2 diabetes: A prospective cohort study and systematic review. *PLoS Med*, *4*, e261.

Domenech, M., Roman, P., Lapetra, J., et al. (2014). Mediterranean diet reduces 24-hour ambulatory blood pressure, blood glucose, and lipids: One-year randomized, clinical trial. *Hypertension*, *64*, 69–76.

Esfahani, A., Wong, J. M., Mirrahimi, A., Srichaikul, K., Jenkins, D. J., & Kendall, C.W. (2009). The glycemic index: physiological significance. *J Am Coll Nutr*, *28*, 439S–445S.

Esposito, K., Kastorini, C. M., Panagiotakos, D. B., et al. (2013). Mediterranean diet and metabolic syndrome: An updated systematic review. *Rev Endocr Metab Disord*, *14*, 255–263.

Esposito, K., Marfella, R., Ciotola, M., et al. (2004). Effect of a Mediterranean-style diet on endothelial dysfunction and markers of vascular inflammation in the metabolic syndrome: A randomized trial. *JAMA*, *292*, 1440–1446.

Estruch, R., Ros, E., Salas-Salvadó, J., et al. (2013). Primary prevention of cardiovascular disease with a Mediterranean diet. *N Engl J Med*, *368*, 1279–1290.

Farvid, M. S., Cho, E.,Chen, W. Y.,Eliassen, A. H.,& Willett, W. C. (2014). Dietary protein sources in early adulthood and breast cancer incidence: Prospective cohort study. *BMJ*, *348*.

Foster-Powell, K., Holt, S. H., & Brand-Miller, J. C. (2002). International table of glycemic index and glycemic load values: 2002. *Am J Clin Nutr*, *76*, 5–56.

Fung, T. T., Schulze, M., Manson, J. E., Willett, W. C., & Hu, F. B. (2004). Dietary patterns, meat intake, and the risk of type 2 diabetes in women. *Arch Intern Med*, *164*, 2235–2240.

Gardner, C., Wylie-Rosett, J., Gidding, S. S., et al. (2012). Nonnutritive sweeteners: Current use and health perspectives: A scientific statement from the American Heart Association and the American Diabetes Association. *Diabetes Care*, *35*, 1798–1808.

Guasch-Ferré, M., Hu, F. B., Martínez-González, M. A., et al. (2014). Olive oil intake and risk of cardiovascular disease and mortality in the PREDIMED Study. *BMC Med*, *12*, 78.

Guha, N., Kwan, M. L., Quesenberry, C. P., Jr., et al. (2009). LACE trial. *Breast Cancer Res Treat*, *118*, 395–405.

Holzman, D. C. (2012). Holzman, D. C. (2012). Organic food conclusions don't tell the whole story. *Environmental Health Perspectives*, *120*, A458. Retrieved August 1, 2014, from http://ehp.niehs.nih.gov/120-a458/

Hu, F. B. (2003). Plant-based foods and prevention of cardiovascular disease: An overview. *Am J Clin Nutr*, *78*, 544S–551S.

Hu, T., Mills, K. T., Yao, L, et al. (2012). Effects of low-carbohydrate diets versus low-fat diets on metabolic risk factors: A meta-analysis of randomized controlled clinical trials. *Am J Epidemiol*, *176*(Suppl 7), S44–S54.

Jenkins, D. J., Kendall, C. W., Augustin, L. S., et al. (2002). Glycemic index: Overview of implications in health and disease. *Am J Clin Nutr, 76*, 266S–273S.

Johnson, J. B., Laub, D. R., & John, S. (2006). The effect on health of alternate day calorie restriction: Eating less and more than needed on alternate days. *Med Hypotheses, 67*, 209–211.

Johnson, R. J., Sanchez-Lozada, L. G., & Nakagawa T. (2010). The effect of fructose on renal biology and disease. *J Am Soc Nephrol, 21*, 2036–2039.

Katzen, M., & Willett, W. (2006). *Eat, drink, and weigh less.* New York, NY: Hyperion.

Knoops, K. T., deGroot, L. C., Kromhout, D., et al. (2004). Mediterranean diet, lifestyle factors, and 10-year mortality in elderly European men and women. *JAMA, 292*, 1433–1439.

Kotwal, S., Jun, M., Sullivan, D., Perkovic, V., & Neal, B. (2012). Omega 3 fatty acids and cardiovascular outcomes: Systematic review and meta-analysis. *Circ Cardiovasc Qual Outcomes, 5*, 808–818.

Liebman, B. (2008, July/August). Fiber free for all. *Nutrition Action Newsletter,* 1–5.

Lin, J., & Curhan, G. C. (2011). Associations of sugar and artificially sweetened soda with albuminuria and kidney function decline in women. *J Am Soc Nephrol, 6*, 160–166.

Magee, P. J., & Rowland I. (2012). Soy products in the management of breast cancer. *Curr Opin Clin Nutr Metab Care, 15*, 586–591.

Mahan, L. K., & Escott-Stump, S. (Eds.). (2004). *Krause's food, nutrition and diet therapy* (11th ed.). Philadelphia: Saunders.

Malik, V. S., Schulze, M. B., & Hu F. (2006). Intake of sugar-sweetened beverages and weight gain: A systematic review. *Am J Clin Nutr, 84*, 274–288.

Manios, Y., Detopoulou, V., Visioli, F., & Galli, C. (2006). Mediterranean diet as a nutrition education and dietary guide: Misconceptions and the neglected role of locally consumed foods and wild green plants. *Forum Nutr, 59*, 154–170.

Mantzoros, C. S., Williams, C. J., Manson, J. E., et al. (2006). Adherence to the Mediterranean dietary pattern is positively associated with plasma adiponectin concentrations in diabetic women. *Am J Clin Nutr, 84*, 328–335.

Marsh, K., Zeuschner, C., & Saunders, A. (2012). Health implications of a vegetarian diet: A review. *Am J Lifestyle Med, 6*, 250–267.

Martin, B., Mattson, M., & Maudsley, S. (2006). Caloric restriction and intermittent fasting: Two potential diets for successful brain aging. *Ageing Res Rev, 5*, 332–353.

McEvoy, C. T., Temple, N., & Woodside, J. V. (2012). Vegetarian diets, low-meat diets and health: A review. *Public Health Nutr, 15*, 2287–2294.

McManus, K., Antinoro, L., & Sacks, F. (2001). A randomized controlled trial of a moderate-fat, low-energy diet compared with a low fat, low-energy diet for weight loss in overweight adults. *Intl J Obesity, 25*, 1503–1511.

Melina, V., Davis, B., & Harrison, V. (1995). *Becoming vegetarian.* Summertown, TN: Book Publishing Company.

Mellon M. (2000). *Hogging it: Estimates of antimicrobial abuse in livestock.* Cambridge, MA: Union of Concerned Scientists.

Micha, R., & Mozaffarian, D. (2008). Trans fatty acids: Effects on cardiometabolic health and implications for policy. *Prostaglandins Leukot Essent Fatty Acids, 79*, 147–152.

Mitrou, P. N., Kipnis, V., Thiebaut, A. C., et al. (2007). Mediterranean dietary pattern and prediction of all-cause mortality in a US population: Results from the NIH-AARP Diet and Health Study. *Arch Intern Med, 167*, 2461–2468.

Mourouti, N., Kontogianni, M. D., Papavagelis, C., et al. (2014). Adherence to the Mediterranean diet is associated with lower likelihood of breast cancer: A case-control study. *Nutr Cancer, 66*, 810–817.

Muñoz, A., & Costa, M. (2013). Nutritionally mediated oxidative stress and inflammation. *Oxidative Medicine and Cellular Longevity, 2013*. Article ID 610950.

Muntwyler, J., Hennekens, C. H., Manson, J. E., Buring, J. E., Gaziano, J. M. (2002). Vitamin supplement use in a low-risk population of US male physicians and subsequent cardiovascular mortality. *Arch Inter Med, 162*(13), 1472–1476.

Murakami, A., Ishida, H., Kobo, K., et al. (2005). Suppressive effects of Okinawan food items on free radical generation from stimulated leukocytes and identification of some active constituents. *Asian Pac J Cancer Prev, 6*, 437–448.

National Center for Environmental Health, Division of Laboratory Sciences. (2012). *Second national report on biochemical indicators of diet and nutrition in the U.S. population: Executive summary.* Available at http://www.cdc.gov/nutritionreport/pdf/ExeSummary_Web_032612.pdf#

Neuhouser, M. L., Wassertheil-Smoller, S., Thomson, C., et al. (2009). Multivitamin use and risk of cancer and cardiovascular disease in the Women's Health Initiative cohorts. *Arch Intern Med, 169*(3), 294–304.

Pan, A., Sun, Q., Bernstein, A. M., Schulze, M. B., Manson, J. E., Stampfer, M. J., … Hu, F. B. (2012). Red meat consumption and mortality: Results from two prospective cohort studies. *Arch Intern Med, 172*, 555–563.

Perona, J. S., Cabello-Moruno, R., & Ruiz-Gutierrez, V. (2006). The role of virgin olive oil components in the modulation of endothelial function. *J Nutr Biochem, 17*, 429–445.

Pimentel, D., & Pimental, M. (2008). *Food, energy and society* (3rd ed). Boca Raton, FL: CRC Press.

Rindfleisch, J. A. (2012). Food intolerance and elimination diet. In D. Rakel (Ed.), *Integrative medicine* (3rd ed.). Philadelphia, PA: Saunders Elsevier.

Rothschild, J., Hoddy, K. K., Jambazian, P., & Varady, K. A. (2014). Time-restricted feeding and risk of metabolic disease: A review of human and animal studies. *Nutr Rev, 72*, 308–318.

Rothschild, J., Hoddy, K. K., Jambazian, P., & Varady, K. A. (2014). Time-restricted feeding and risk of metabolic disease: A review of human and animal studies. *Nutr Reviews, 72*, 308–318.

Schardt, D. (2012). Coconut oil. *Nutrition Action Health Letter.* Retrieved September 24, 2014 from http://www.cspinet.org/nah/articles/coconut-oil.html

Simopoulos, A. P. (2002). Omega-3 fatty acids in inflammation and autoimmune diseases. *J Am Col Nutr, 21*, 495–505.

Siri-Tarino, P. W., Sun, Q., Hu, F. B., & Krauss, R. M. (2010). Meta-analysis of prospective cohort studies evaluating the association of saturated fat with cardiovascular disease. *Am J Clin Nutr.* doi: 10.3945/ajcn.2009.27725

Sizer, F., & Whitney, E. (2014a). The carbohydrates. In F. Sizer & E. Whitney (Eds.), *Nutrition: Concepts and controversies* (13th ed., p. 126). Belmont, CA: Thomson Wadsworth.

Sizer, F., & Whitney, E. (Eds.). (2014b). *Nutrition: Concepts and controversies* (13th ed.). Belmont, CA: Thomson Wadsworth.

Smith-Spangler, C., Brandeau, M. L., Hunter, G. E., et al. (2012). Are organic foods safer or healthier than conventional alternatives? A systematic review. *Ann Intern Med, 157,* 348–366.

Taubert, D., Roesen, R., Lehmann, C., et al. (2007). Effects of low habitual cocoa intake on blood pressure and bioactive nitric oxide: A randomized controlled trial. *JAMA, 298,* 49–60.

Trepanowski, J. F., Canale, R. E., Marshall, K. E., et al. (2011). Impact of caloric and dietary restriction regimens on markers of health and longevity in humans and animals: A summary of available findings. *Nutr J, 10,* 107.

Trichopoulou, A. (2001). Mediterranean diet: The past and the present. *Nutr Metab Cardiovasc Dis, 11*(Suppl 4), 1–4.

Trichopoulou, A., Lagiou, P., Kuper, H, et al. (2000). Cancer and Mediterranean dietary traditions. *Cancer Epidemiol Biomarkers Prev, 9,* 869–873.

US Department of Agriculture (USDA). (n.d.). *Nutrient database.* Retrieved September 13, 2014, from http://ndb.nal.usda.gov

US Department of Agriculture, Agricultural Research Service. (2012). Nutrient intakes from food: Mean amounts consumed per individual, by race/ethnicity and age. In *What We Eat in America, NHANES 2009–2010.* Available: www.ars.usda.gov/ba/bhnrc/fsrg.

Vannice, G., & Rasmussen, H. (2014). Position of the academy of nutrition and dietetics: dietary fatty acids for healthy adults. *J Acad Nutr Diet, 114*(1), 136–153.

Wang, X., Ouyang, Y., Liu, J., et al. (2014). Fruit and vegetable consumption and mortality from all causes, cardiovascular disease, and cancer: Systematic review and dose-response meta-analysis of prospective cohort studies. *BMJ, 349,* g4490.

Wannaveg. (2014). Retrieved October 10, 2014, from http://wannaveg.com

White, D. G., Zhao, S., Sudler, R., et al. (2001). The isolation of antibiotic-resistant Salmonella from retail ground meats. *N Engl J Med, 345,* 1147–1154.

Willcox, B. J., Willcox, D. C., & Suzuki, M. (2001). *The Okinawa program.* New York, NY: Clarkson Potter.

Willcox, D. C., Willcox, B. J., Todoriki, H., & Suzuki, M. (2009). The Okinawan diet: Health Implications of a low-calorie, nutrient-dense, antioxidant-rich dietary pattern low in glycemic load. *J Am Coll Nutr, 28*(Suppl 4), 500S–516S.

Willett, W. C. (2006). The Mediterranean diet: Science and practice. *Public Health Nutr, 9,* 105–110.

Wing, R. R., & Phelan S. (2005). Long-term weight loss maintenance. *Am J Clin Nutr, 82,* 222S–225S.

Winter, C. K., & Davis, S. F. (2006). Organic foods. *J Food Sci, 71,* R117–R124.

Woo, H. D., Park, K. S., Shin, A., & Kim, J. (2013). Glycemic index and glycemic load dietary patterns and the associated risk of breast cancer: A case-control study. *Asian Pac J Cancer Prev, 14,* 5193–5198.

Worthington, V. (2001). Nutritional quality of organic versus conventional fruits, vegetables, and grains. *J Altern Comp Med, 7,* 161–173.

Xu, X., Yu, E., Gao, X., Song, N., Liu, L., Wei, X., … Fu, C. (2013). Red and processed meat intake and risk of colorectal adenomas: A meta-analysis of observational studies. *Int J Cancer, 132,* 437–448.

Zhang, X., Shu, X. O., Li, H., et al. (2005). Prospective cohort study of soy food consumption and risk of bone fracture among postmenopausal women. *Arch Intern Med, 165,* 1890.

Zhao, S., McDermott, P. F., Friedman, S., et al. (2006). Antimicrobial resistance and genetic relatedness among Salmonella from retail foods of animal origin: NARMS retail meat surveillance. *Foodborne Pathog Dis, 3,* 106–117.

3

Dietary Supplements

MARY HARDY AND TIERAONA LOW DOG

CASE STUDY: A TALE OF TWO PATIENTS

PATIENT ONE

Sally had heard about the benefits of calcium and vitamin D in newspapers and from her friends, but her intake was low because she restricted dairy products in her diet due to lactose intolerance. She rightly decided that she would need to take a supplement to get enough of these two nutrients. On her first trip to the store, she was so overwhelmed by the number and variety of available products that she gave up and did nothing. During our next office visit, she raised these questions: How do I decide what supplements are right for me? How can I tell if a product is of good quality? How do I know which one to pick?

PATIENT TWO

Lisa was a young woman with a hormone-sensitive breast cancer who had developed elevated liver enzymes since she was started on tamoxifen. After questioning her more closely, her oncologist discovered that Lisa was taking dietary supplements (DSs) during active treatment—a startling revelation for the doctor! At the request of the oncologist, I saw Lisa in order to determine whether her increased liver enzymes were due to her supplements, her tamoxifen, or a combination of both. At my request, the patient brought all her medication (prescription and over-the-counter) and supplements to her first visit with me.

Lisa brought in four shopping bags of supplements, over 30 products that she faithfully took every day, firm in the belief that these would keep her cancer from returning. This was much more than what her oncologist had thought. Lisa had decided what to take after reading a wide variety of information from books and Internet sources as well as questioning friends, family, and clerks at her local health food store for their suggestions and ideas. She was so afraid of a recurrence that she grasped anything with any potentially positive information. Needless to say, she was spending hundreds of dollars a month on her supplements, as well as contributing to her elevated liver function tests.

These two, apparently very different patients, demonstrate common challenges that women using DSs face. They were using supplements as part of a self-care program, initially without involvement from their healthcare provider. An open-minded provider, well informed about issues and opportunities inherent in DS use, would be able to help women design an appropriate strategy for DS use and integrate it into their overall medical plan.

Introduction

Dietary supplements are used by most Americans; more than 70% according to some surveys (Timbo, Ross, McCarthy, & Lin, 2006). A recent review found that among those who use DSs, multivitamins (MVs) were the most commonly used supplement (71%), followed by omega-3 or fish oil (33%), calcium (32%), vitamin D (32%), and vitamin C (32%) (Dickinson, Blatman, El-Dash, & Franco, 2014). Women constitute the majority of DS users and they generally direct use for the rest of their family. To adequately counsel women using DSs, providers must understand how and why women decide to use DSs as well as how DSs are regulated in the United States and the implications for quality, safety, and efficacy. (For information regarding the use of DS for specific conditions, please refer to the appropriate chapter in this text.)

Use of Dietary Supplements by Women

Women use a variety of DSs including products specifically related to women's health, such as black cohosh (*Actaea racemosa*), or evening primrose oil, as well as others for less gender-specific uses such as glucosamine and St. John's wort (*Hypericum perforatum*) (Wold et al., 2005). These patterns of use are relatively stable year to year. Herbal medicine use is less frequent (17%–30% in most surveys) (Gardiner, Graham, et al., 2007) and more variable over time. The dietary supplement market is large and growing, with herbal product use increasing almost 8% in 2013 (Herbalgram, 2013).

Consumers of DSs frequently take multiple products and often use them for extended periods of time. For example, an elderly cohort reported taking an average of three nonvitamin, nonmineral (NVNM) DSs for more than two years (Wold et al., 2005). While vitamin and mineral preparations were the most commonly used supplements by the elders (84%), almost 60% also used a DS that was not an MV or calcium. In addition, 25% reported using herbal medications (Gordon & Schaffer 2005). Use increased over time when measured longitudinally in an elderly cohort from 5% at beginning of the study to 30% after more than 15 years (Knudtson et al., 2007).

While the typical DS user is a well-educated, middle-aged white woman with a higher socioeconomic status, DS use is also high in multiple ethnic groups and within lower socioeconomic groups, as supported by data from the Multiethnic Cohort Study that evaluated the use among African Americans, Latinos, Native Americans, Native Hawaiians, and Caucasians. On average, half of the cohort used MV or multivitamin/mineral (MVM) supplements, with highest use reported by Caucasians (57%) and lowest by Native Hawaiians (37%) (Park, Murphy, Martin, & Kolonel, 2008). In one survey, 50% of Hispanics and Asians, 41% of whites, and only 22% of African Americans reported using herbs (Kuo, Hawley, Weiss, Balkrishnan, & Volk, 2004). Despite financial constraints, indigent patients are high users of DSs. In a survey at a large urban clinic serving the indigent, 37% of the 311 responders reported using a wide variety of DSs for a broad range of medical conditions (Clay, Glaros, & Clauson, 2006).

Reasons for Using Dietary Supplements

In surveys, the reasons most often cited for supplement use were for overall health and wellness (58%) and to fill nutrient gaps in the diet (42%) (Dickinson et al., 2014). Illness prevention and symptom reduction were the most common reasons that Canadian women gave for their use of DSs (Pakzad, Boucher, Kreiger, & Cotterchio, 2007). Older adults (≥60 years) were more likely than younger adults to report condition or site-specific reasons like heart, bone and joint, and eye health (Bailey, Nisly, Zimmerman, Gryzlak, & Wallace, 2013). Some consumers take supplements to counteract the effects of negative health behaviors, such as eating junk food or smoking, or to mitigate the adverse events of sustained stress. Women might also substitute a "safe" DSs for a prescription drug with a higher perceived risk (Nichter & Thompson 2006). Dietary supplements may also be used to substitute for expensive or unavailable medical care, particularly in patients with lower socioeconomic status (Gardiner, Graham, et al., 2007).

Supplement users often cite the declining quality of the food supply and inability to get sufficient nutrition from their diet as a reason to use DSs. Interestingly, trend data for common garden crops have shown significant declines in the last half of the 20th century for vitamins A and C, thiamine, riboflavin, and niacin as well as protein, calcium, phosphorus, and iron (Davis, Epp, & Riordan, 2004). In fact, conventional growing methods yielded significantly less micronutrients and phytochemicals with higher amounts of toxins according to recent studies (Hunter et al., 2011; Johansson et al, 2014). Equally troubling is the fact that most people don't meet the goals of *Healthy People 2010*, of a minimum of two fruit and three vegetable servings daily. According to Centers for Disease Control (CDC) data, only 32.5% ate fruit two or more times per day, while 26.3% ate vegetables three or more times per day (MMWR, 2010). Sadly, this level of intake has been fundamentally unchanged since 1994 despite public health messages encouraging increased intake.

Dietary supplement use accounts for a significant portion of dietary intake of many important nutrients in the United States (Rock, 2007; Archer et al., 2005). Nutrient deficiencies do occur and vary according to ethnicity, race, age, and gender. According to the CDC's *Second National Report on Biochemical Indicators of Diet and Nutrition in the U.S. Population,* 13% of Mexican American women of childbearing age (12 to 49 years) had iron deficiency, and African Americans (31%) had the highest incidence of vitamin D deficiency. Concerning, this report also noted that women ages 20–39 have borderline iodine insufficiency, which could have significant implications during pregnancy, as iodine deficiency is associated with mental retardation (CDC, 2014b). Inadequate nutrient intake may be especially problematic for other at-risk groups including the elderly (Sebastian, Cleveland, Goldman, & Moshfegh, 2007), pregnant and lactating women (Haugen, Brantsaeter, Alexander, & Meltzer, 2008), vegetarians/vegans (Zeuschner et al., 2013), and those who have undergone obesity surgery, such as gastric bypass (Stein, Stier, Raab, & Weiner, 2014). Women taking prescription medications may be at higher risk for nutrient deficiency secondary to drug-induced nutrient depletion: proton pump inhibitors (e.g., calcium, magnesium, iron, vitamin B12), metformin (e.g., vitamin B12), angiotensin-converting enzyme inhibitors and thiazide diuretics (e.g., zinc), etc. (Heidelbaugh, 2013; Koren-Michowitz et al., 2005; Niafar, Hai, Porhomayon, & Nader, 2014).

Information Resources, Disclosure, and Decision-Making Regarding Dietary Supplement Use

Women often do not disclose their use of DS to their healthcare providers. In a survey of more than 5,457 users of DSs, only 33% of herbal and dietary supplement users reported disclosing use of herbal and dietary supplements to their conventional healthcare provider (Mehta, Gardiner, Phillips, & McCarthy, 2008). There are multiple reasons for this nondisclosure, ranging from an expectation of a negative response (Tasaki, Maskarinec, Shumay, Tatsumura, & Kakai, 2002) to the perception that providers do not have the requisite knowledge to counsel their patients about DSs (Blendon, DesRoches, Benson, Brodie, & Altman, 2001). Assessment of a cohort of healthcare practitioners taking an online herbal course supported these assertions rating providers' knowledge of herbal DSs as only moderate and noting that their communication skills in this area were poor (Kemper, Gardiner, Gobble, & Woods, 2006). This lack of knowledge may help explain that in one large survey of American adults (n = 11,956), only 23% of DS products being used by participants were based on recommendations of a healthcare provider (Bailey et al., 2013).

Clerks in health food stores frequently dispense advice regarding the use of DSs, even in customers with significant medical conditions. Eighty-nine percent of health food store clerks gave advice to researchers posing as 8-weeks pregnant women with nausea (Buckner, Chavez, Raney, & Stoehr, 2005). Although ginger, a safe and effective remedy for this indication, was recommended most frequently, less than 4% of the time did clerk recommendations agree with the medical literature either in dose or product type. Fifteen percent of the time, products were recommended that are contraindicated in pregnancy. In another study, an actor portrayed a consumer with symptoms of type 1 diabetes at eight community pharmacies and 12 health food stores in Pittsburgh, Pennsylvania, and Chapel Hill and Durham, North Carolina (Kavalieratos, Weinberger, & Rao, 2010). Six pharmacists recommended urgent physician follow-up, as did two health food store employees (HFSEs), while two HFSEs explicitly advised against a physician visit. One pharmacist recommended a product. Nine HFSEs recommended at least one product (monthly costs, range: $24.70–$209.96).

Women frequently turn to their friends and family to advise them regarding DS use (Nichter & Thompson, 2006). Many elders cite mail order information as the most common source of DS information (Wold et al., 2007). The Internet represents a major source of information for consumers about health in general and DSs in particular (Nichter & Thompson, 2006). Patients and physicians have difficulty distinguishing unbiased from biased websites (Bauer et al., 2003). The majority of websites analyzed in a recent survey (76%) were retail sites selling product and 81% of these made one or more health claim in violation of current regulations.

CONTROVERSY OVER BENEFITS OF DIETARY SUPPLEMENTS

The use of DSs for prevention of diseases, such as cancer and heart disease, in the general population is not encouraged by groups such as the US Preventative Services Taskforce (USPSTF), reportedly because a lack of convincing evidence for their efficacy (Fortmann et al., 2013; Moyer, 2014). Some medical authorities have extended their conclusions by asking for patients to stop wasting their money using ineffective and potentially dangerous dietary supplements. The message is simple: "Most supplements do not prevent chronic disease or death, their use is not justified and they should be avoided" (Guallar et al., 2013).

A more appropriate and nuanced conclusion looking at the totality of the literature is that selected dietary supplements for specific populations confer benefit and are cost-effective for the overall healthcare system (Shanahan & deLorimier, 2014). The strategic use of dietary supplements could possibly save billions of dollars related to treatment/prevention of coronary heart disease, diabetes related heart disease, age-related macular degeneration, cataracts, and osteoporosis, mainly realized through reductions in hospital use. Throughout this book, there are numerous examples of improvements in health or quality of life as the result of targeting selected supplement use to specific populations.

One exception to targeted use of DSs may be vitamin D supplementation. Vitamin D deficiency is epidemic in our population, and the effects of vitamin D in the body are protean and essential for health. Therefore, a number of authorities are recommending that it is more cost-effective to treat for vitamin D deficiency in the general population than to perform regular screening (Kopes-Kerr, 2013).

While scientific evidence is very important to healthcare providers, it appears to carry less weight with consumers. A number of negative clinical trials have been reported with respect to the use of antioxidants or MVM supplements to reduce mortality in healthy populations (Bjelakovic, Nikolova, Gluud, Simonetti, & Gluud, 2008) and the USPSTF reports no benefit for the primary prevention of cardiovascular risk or mortality from any single vitamin or combination (Moyer et al., 2014). In spite of these data, consumers are generally skeptical of scientific evidence, especially with regard to lack of efficacy (Nichter & Thompson, 2006). Belief in efficacy of DSs is so strong that almost three-quarters of current users reported that they would continue to use their herbs even if scientific studies were negative (Kuo et al., 2004).

Dietary Supplement Regulation

The regulation of DSs in the United States is unique within the global regulatory community, and many of the issues associated with DS sales in the United States are the result of the provision of this regulatory structure. Dietary supplement manufacture and sales are regulated by the Dietary Supplement Health and Education Act (DSHEA) of 1994, which was drafted by Congress in order to secure consumer access to high quality DSs. A recent survey revealed that physician knowledge of DS regulation was limited and most did not know where to report adverse events (Ashar, Rice, & Sisson, 2007; Cellini et al., 2013). Consumers also demonstrated poor knowledge when questioned about information on the DS label (Miller & Russell, 2004).

Three provisions of DSHEA engender the most concern and confusion. First, only structure function claims, for example those claims that support the normal structure or function of the body, are allowed (Wollschlaeger, 2003). Manufacturers of DSs are expressly forbidden to use "drug" claims, for example those that intend to diagnose, treat, cure, or prevent any disease. This may lead to vague terms such as "supports a healthy immune system" as opposed to "treats the common cold." This regulatory requirement creates a troublesome paradox between what can be claimed versus how products are researched by scientists and perceived by the public. Research generally does not assess structure function claims and patients are adept at "decoding" structure function claims into their disease-based counterparts (Knudtson et al., 2007).

Second, all DS ingredients sold on the market before the passage of DSHEA (October 1994) are presumed to be safe and no premarket approval is required. The Food and Drug Administration (FDA) has the right to remove any unsafe DSs from the market, but the burden of proof is on the agency (Wollschlaeger, 2003). Assessing the risk associated with DSs can be difficult, given the lack of adverse event reporting by clinicians and the fact that many DS products are multi-ingredient, complicating the picture of which ingredient might be causing harm.

Third, while regulations regarding good manufacturing processes have been required since the passage of DSHEA, they have only been recently implemented and enforced. The current good manufacturing practice (cGMP) rules put in place by the FDA in 2007 were designed to assure the identity, purity, quality, strength, and composition of DSs (Crowley & FitzGerald, 2006). All companies had to be in compliance with these guidelines by 2010.

Quick Tips for Reading Supplement Labels

- On vitamins and minerals, look carefully at the percent daily value (%DV) and the serving size. To get 100% of the daily value you might need to take one or three tablets per day. As most people prefer to take fewer pills, this can affect adherence and increase cost.
- A single nutrient may be present in a number of different supplements. Include all amounts in all supplements when assessing for adequate or excessive intake.
- Remember the %DV is a simplification of the recommended daily allowance and does not take into account age or gender. You must help your patient understand how much she needs to take.
- Some products contain nutrients for which a daily value has not been established (i.e., boron, herbs, etc.). Confirm that the amounts included make sense and are not excessive.
- Do not exceed 70%–100% of the daily value for most vitamins and minerals to avoid excessive intake.
- Discard supplements after their expiration dates have passed.
- DS products should all contain the manufacturer/distributor name and contact information.
- Products that contain quality seals on their labels from the United States Pharmacopeia (USP), National Sanitation Foundation (NSF), or Consumer Labs (CL), indicate that the manufacturer has had their product independently tested for quality and purity by a third party.

One of the most overwhelming aspects of the DS industry for patients and providers is the variety and number of available DSs. In a survey of over 26,000 multiethnic subjects in Los Angeles and Hawaii, more than 1,200 different products were used (Murphy, White, Park, & Sharma, 2007). These products represented wide variations in composition and concentration of ingredients. Variability may be highest for herbal products because of both the greater variability inherent in botanical materials and significant differences in formulation.

In one study conducted on single-ingredient herb supplements obtained from both retail and Internet outlets, variation between different batches at a single company was relatively low (Krochmal et al., 2004). However, much larger differences were seen between various products of the same herb from different companies. Instruction for use (dosage) also varied significantly between companies for the same herb as well. Therefore, it is imperative to examine the actual products the patient is taking and to avoid changing products once the clinical effect is established.

Dietary Supplement Use in Conditions of Special Interest to Women

PREGNANCY

Nutrient demands of pregnancy are high and it has been estimated that without supplementation up to 75% of pregnant women would be deficient in at least one vitamin (Kontic-Vucinic, Sulovic, & Radunovic, 2006). Recommendations for taking a prenatal vitamin are pretty strong. A systematic review of nine trials (n = 15,378) by the Cochrane Collaboration found a decrease in the number of low-birth-weight, small-for-gestational-age babies, and maternal anemia when low- or middle-income women took multivitamins most days during pregnancy (Rumbold, Middleton, & Crowther, 2005).

In some surveys, the use of prenatal vitamins is as high as 89.2% (Refuerzo et al., 2005), however, overall there has been a decline in the percentage of women of childbearing age taking DSs containing at least 400 mcg of folic acid from 40% in 2004 to 33% in 2005 (MMWR, 2005). Awareness of the benefits of folic acid before conception and during pregnancy remains low (Fehr, Fehr, & Protudjer, 2011), and even among women actively planning pregnancy; many are not taking adequate amounts of folic acid either in diet or through DSs (Hilton, 2007). Folic acid intake also varies by ethnicity. Hispanic/Latina women have the highest rate of children born with neural tube defects and lower blood folate levels than either African Americans or Caucasians. They are also less likely to consume foods fortified with folic acid or to take vitamins containing folic acid before pregnancy (CDC, 2014a).

In pregnant women, use of DSs, other than prenatal vitamins, is low at about 13%, and 75% informed their primary care provider of their use. Relief from nausea and vomiting was cited as the most common reason for use, and ginger was one of the most commonly used DS (Buckner et al., 2005; Tsui, Dennehy, & Tsourounis, 2001). There is a growing body of evidence suggesting the importance of calcium, vitamin D, and omega-3 fatty acids, particularly docosahexaenoic acid (DHA), during pregnancy, yet the intake for all three may be low in many pregnant women. For more detailed information regarding specific supplement usage in pregnancy, refer to the chapter "Pregnancy and Lactation."

MENOPAUSE

Reports regarding the risk-benefit ratio of hormone therapy (HT) have raised concerns among women and healthcare providers. It has also generated interest in the effectiveness and safety of DSs for managing menopausal symptoms. It is reported that in both the United States and United Kingdom, 80% of menopausal women use DSs, and 66% of these users believe that such supplements are helpful (Geller & Studee, 2005). The most commonly used herb for menopause is soy. A recent study reported that users cited reduction of hot flashes, improved sleep and mood, and effect on osteoporosis as the major reasons for using soy. Users were generally satisfied with the results (Girardi et al., 2014).

There are numerous mechanisms by which plants might relieve menopause-related symptoms. Those with potential estrogenic activities include red clover (*Trifolium pratense*), kudzu (*Pueraria lobata*), hops (*Humulus lupulus*), licorice (*Glycyrrhiza glabra*), rhubarb (*Rheum palmatum*), and chasteberry (*Vitex agnus castus*). Others that appear to exert progestogenic activity include red clover, hops, wild yam (*Dioscorea villosa*), and chasteberry. Antidepressant medications are increasingly being used to relieve hot flashes in women who cannot take HT. Black cohosh (*Actaea racemosa*), kudzu, kava (*Piper methysticum*), licorice, and dong quai (*Angelica sinensis*) have reported 5-hydroxytryptamine receptor 7 ligands or have been shown to inhibit serotonin reuptake (Hajirahimkhan, Dietz, & Bolton, 2013). It is very possible that these herbs singly, or in combination, may prove to be beneficial to women during this transition.

Given the potential impact on hormones, researchers must also study how these botanicals might influence hormone-driven cancers. Because women may take these products for several years, long-term safety and potential herb-drug interactions should be assessed. Although women may be inappropriately worried about soy, it is important to note that use of soy beginning in childhood has been associated with a consistent reduction in breast cancer in later years (Korde et al., 2009). See the chapter "Menopause" for more information.

An important health concern in postmenopausal women, indeed in the whole population, is obesity. Weight loss for postmenopausal women can be particularly difficult because of hormonally related sarcopenia and dieters often turn to DSs for help. However, the Federal Trade Commission, responsible for enforcing truthful advertising of DSs, routinely takes action against weight-loss DSs for misleading claims (Federal Trade Commission, 2014). There still is a role for dietary supplements in weight loss if supplements are taken in conjunction with a healthy diet and exercise. For example, achieving full vitamin D repletion (to normal serum levels) was shown in a recent trial to improve weight loss, increase lean body mass, and reduce markers of inflammation in a group of vitamin D–deficient, obese, largely postmenopausal women (Mason et al., 2014). For women desirous of losing weight, guidance for appropriate lifestyle and dietary supplement choices must be given.

OSTEOPOROSIS

Women are at higher risk and account for 75% of the ten million cases of osteoporosis in the United States. Dietary intake of calcium and vitamin D is insufficient for many Americans. Fifty-nine percent of women report eating less than two servings of dairy per day (Dawson-Hughes, Harris, Dallal, Lancaster, & Zhou, 2002), and only 40% of the participants in the National Health and Nutrition Examination Study (NHANES) survey met the minimum adequate intake levels for calcium. In addition, only 48% of the respondents reported using a calcium supplement (Ma, Johns, & Stafford, 2007). Even when the diagnosis of osteoporosis is made, use of calcium and vitamin D remains low. In a survey of elderly nursing home patients with osteoporosis, only 66% were prescribed calcium and 58% vitamin D (Kamel, 2004). In the United States, the adequate intake levels for women are 1,300 mg/day from age 9 to 18, 1,000 mg/day from age 19 to 50, and 1,200 mg/day from age 50 onward.

Vitamin D deficiency and insufficiency is common throughout North America. Obtaining sufficient amounts of vitamin D in the diet is difficult, and most women use sunscreen, significantly limiting sun absorption and subsequent manufacture of vitamin D in the skin. Vitamin D supplements are an inexpensive and reliable way to ensure adequate intake. The dietary reference intake levels are 600 IU/day for women aged 19–70 and 800 IU for women over 70 years of age. Many experts below these levels are not sufficient to maintain optimum serum levels.

It is therefore highly recommended that clinicians check a serum 25-hydroxyvitamin D level to assess sufficiency. The Endocrine Society's Clinical Practice Guideline "suggests that all adults who are vitamin D deficient be treated with 50,000 IU of vitamin D2 or D3 once a week for eight weeks or its equivalent of 6000 IU of vitamin D2 or D3 daily to achieve a blood level of 25(OH)D above 30 ng/mL (75 nmol/L), followed by a maintenance therapy of 1500–2000 IU per day" (Holick et al., 2011). However, given the very favorable risk-benefit ratios and the high likelihood of need, some experts recommend bypassing screening and treating with vitamin D. Because the dose required to ensure achievement of optimal serum vitamin D levels varies, it is still recommended to follow serum levels to monitor response.

CANCER

Use of complementary therapies may be as high as 90% during cancer treatment, with DSs representing a major proportion of all use (Moyer, 2014, Molassiotis, Ozden, & Platin, 2006; Yates, Mustian, & Morrow,

2005). Women with cancer, particularly breast and gynecological cancers, frequently use DSs. A survey of 2,596 women from Kaiser Permanente Northern California found that over half (60.2%) reported initiating a vitamin/mineral following the diagnosis of breast cancer, 46.3% discontinued a vitamin/mineral, 65.6% reported using a vitamin/mineral continuously, and only 7.2% reported not using any vitamin/mineral supplement before or after diagnosis (Greenlee et al., 2014). Women in this survey were most likely to start taking calcium (38.2%), vitamin D (32.01%), vitamin B6 (12.3%), and magnesium (11.31%) after the diagnosis. Other studies have shown that indole-3-carbinol, a compound found in cruciferous vegetables and its biologically active congener diindolylmethane (DIM) as well as vitamin D3 are commonly used by women hoping to reduce the risk of recurrence of estrogen-driven cancers (Gissel, Rejnmark, Mosekilde, & Vestergaard, 2008; Hardy, 2008; Mulvey et al., 2007).

Many oncologists are concerned about DS usage, especially antioxidants, while undergoing chemotherapy or radiation. Despite more than 20 years of research investigating the use of dietary antioxidant supplementation during conventional chemotherapy and radiation therapy, their use remains controversial (Ozben, 2014). There are data, limited in both quality and sample size, suggesting that certain antioxidant supplements may reduce adverse reactions and toxicities (Fuchs-Tarlovsky, 2013).

Utility also depends on the antioxidant being studied. A review of eight randomized controlled trials of solid tumors found that 20 mg/day of melatonin taken concurrently with chemotherapy or radiotherapy significantly improved complete and partial remission and 1-year survival and dramatically decreased radiochemotherapy-related side effects including thrombocytopenia, neurotoxicity, and fatigue (Wang et al., 2012). Frequent use of vitamin C and vitamin E in the period after breast cancer diagnosis was associated with a decreased likelihood of recurrence, whereas frequent use of combination carotenoids was associated with increased mortality in 2,264 women in the Life After Cancer Epidemiology (LACE) cohort (Greenlee et al., 2012). The majority (53%) of women being tested for genetic risk of developing breast cancer reported using DSs to decrease their risk (DiGianni et al., 2003).

Based on the controversy over antioxidants, one review published by the *Journal of the National Cancer Institute* concluded that their use should be discouraged because of the possibility of tumor protection and reduced survival (Lawanda et al., 2008). Because physicians are usually unaware of their patients' use of DSs, it is necessary to explicitly and respectfully ask about use. Communication is complicated by the lack of evidence-based guidelines to assist them when counseling high-risk women or breast cancer survivors (Velicer & Ulrich, 2008), but open dialogue must be maintained.

Safety Concerns With Dietary Supplements

Consumers generally perceive DSs as safe (Nichter & Thompson, 2006). Over half of women in a recent survey agreed in theory that DSs might have adverse effects, but 66% of them would not associate observed adverse effects with a DS (Albertazzi, Steel, Clifford, & Bottazzi, 2002).

Clinician's concerns revolve largely around issues of adverse events arising from allergy, contamination/adulteration of the DS, or interaction with conventional medications. Allergy (immediate hypersensitivity) has been reported with herbal medicines but is not commonly seen. Adulteration has been reported particularly in ethnic or imported products (Posadzki, Watson, & Ernst, 2013). Chinese patent medicines have been found to contain pharmaceutical drugs or heavy metals (Ko, 2006). Ayurvedic products have also been shown to be high in a variety of heavy metals (Saper et al., 2008). Misidentification or substitution of a more toxic herb has occurred. On rare occasions this has led to serious adverse outcomes as in the case of using *Aristolochia* species in place of the safer *Stephania* herb (Debelle, Vanherweghem, & Nortier, 2008), which led to numerous cases of acute renal failure and late onset of genitourinary cancers.

Interaction of DSs with conventional medicine is an oft-cited concern for providers. Approximately one-third (34.3%) of all US adults reported concomitant DS and prescription medication use (Farina, Austin, & Lieberman, 2014). Concurrent DS and medication use is of particular concern in the elderly, where, according to one survey, 52% of this population was taking DSs and prescriptions concurrently (Qato et al., 2008). In fact, some patients may preferentially combine herbal and prescribed medication. Respondents in a survey of multiethnic herbal medicine users reported that 40% believed that combining herbs with drugs had a synergistic effect (Kuo et al., 2004).

Authoritative information on dietary supplement-drug interaction is scarce, but concern exists for drugs that are critical or have a narrow therapeutic index (Yetley, 2007). Anticoagulant medications, especially warfarin, were the drugs most often identified as having highest risk for DS/drug interactions (Qato et al., 2008). Despite the identification of theoretical interactions, relatively few events are documented. In a 5-year retrospective chart review of elderly DS/drug users in which 142 potential interactions were noted, no specific events were identified (Wold et al., 2005). Botanicals most likely to produce clinically important herb–drug interactions are those with constituents that act as inhibitors of cytochrome P450 enzyme activity (e.g., goldenseal [*Hydrastis canadensis*], black pepper [*Piper nigrum*], schisandra [*Schisandra chinensis*]) or function as ligands for orphan nuclear receptors (e.g., St. John's wort [*Hypericum perforatum*]) (Gurley, Fifer, & Gardner, 2012).

Conclusions and Recommendations

Dietary supplement use is highly prevalent in women throughout their life spans and across a broad array of conditions and diseases. Women often don't disclose their use of DSs to the healthcare team, and therefore it is recommended that inquiries about DS use must be made at all patient encounters.

Questioning should be nonjudgmental in order to encourage full disclosure. Assessing the reasons for supplement usage and asking about information sources used by the patient allows for much clearer insight into use. Respect for a woman's worldview and support for her efforts toward health enhancement is recommended.

Due to the high degree of variability in products, it is critical to look at the actual labels in order to most accurately determine intake. One must document all products used in the medical chart and be alert for potential adverse effects and herb–drug interactions, as well as therapeutic benefit.

Avoid blanket, negative declarations about DSs. This does not discourage use, but rather damages provider credibility. However, when specific concerns about DS use arise, especially if safety is the issue, sharing this information with your patient can change behavior. Engaging women in this manner will optimize her health and well-being.

Questions That Can Help Clinicians Assess a Woman's Beliefs, Cultural Practices, and Use of Dietary Supplements

- Many women use vitamins or herbal remedies to improve their health or treat medical problems. What is your experience? Do you use DSs? If so, what are your goals and how do you think they are working?
- How did you learn about using vitamins or herbal remedies?
- Would you be willing to bring your vitamins or herbal remedies with you to your next appointment so that we could look at them together?

Helpful Resources for Dietary Supplement Evidence, Safety, and Dose

- The National Center for Complementary and Integrative Health, NCCIH (www.nccih.nih.gov)

Look for the Alerts and Advisories, treatment information, resources, and links to other organizations (FDA, AHRQ, ODS, etc.). (Free)

- Office of Dietary Supplements, ODS (ods.od.nih.gov)

Very helpful site; under Health Information you will find excellent DS fact sheets. (Free)

- National Institute's of Health Dietary Supplement Label Database (dsld.nlm.nih.gov)

The Dietary Supplement Label Database (DSLD) contains the full label contents from a sample of dietary supplement products marketed in the United States. This is an excellent resource for clinicians to review dietary supplement products and find links to clinical trials, adverse event literature, and so forth.

- Health Canada (http://www.hc-sc.gc.ca)

The Canadian government regulates natural health products in Canada, licensing products with proof of safety and efficacy. This is a very helpful site—it lists products licensed in Canada and has helpful monographs.

Other Websites

- American Botanical Council (www.herbalgram.org)

The American Botanical Council is a nonprofit, international member-based organization providing education using science-based and traditional information on herbal medicine. The website offers an excellent online bookstore and an Herb Clip service summarizing current research articles and an educational resource section offering continuing education credits for healthcare professionals.

- Natural Medicines Comprehensive Database (www.naturaldatabase.com)

Herbal Monographs include extensive information about common uses, evidence of efficacy and safety mechanisms, interactions, and dosage. Also continuing medical education (CME), listserv, and interactions information available. (Subscription available)

- Natural Standard (www.naturalstandard.com)

This is an independent collaboration of international clinicians and researchers who created a database that can be searched by complementary and alternative medicine subject or by medical condition. CME available. Quality of evidence is graded for each supplement. (Subscription available)

- Consumer Labs (www.consumerlabs.com)

Evaluates commercially available DSs for composition, purity, bioavailability, and consistency of products. Part of the website is free. More in-depth reports of product quality are available by subscription.

REFERENCES

Albertazzi, P., Steel, S. A., Clifford, E., & Bottazzi, M. (2002). Attitudes towards and use of dietary supplementation in a sample of postmenopausal women. *Climacteric, 5*, 374–382.

Archer S. L. (2005). Association of dietary supplement use with specific micronutrient intakes among middle-aged American men and women: the INTERMAP Study. *J Am Diet Assoc*, 105(7), 1106–1114.

Ashar, B. H., Rice, T. N., & Sisson, S. D. (2007). Physicians' understanding of the regulation of dietary supplements. *Arch Intern Med, 167*, 966–969.

Bailey, R. L., Gahche, J. J., Miller, P. E., et al. (2013). Why US adults use dietary supplements. *JAMA Intern Med, 173*, 355–361.

Bardia, A., Nisly, N. L., Zimmerman, M. B., Gryzlak, B. M., & Wallace, R. B. (2007). Use of herbs among adults based on evidence-based indications: Findings from the National Health Interview Survey. *Mayo Clin Proc, 82*, 561–566.

Bauer, B., Lee, M., Wahner-Roedler, D., Brown, S., Pankratz, S., & Elkin, P. (2003). A controlled trial of physicians' and patients' abilities to distinguish authoritative from misleading complementary and alternative medicine Web sites. *J Cancer Integr Med, 1*, 48–54.

Bjelakovic, G., Nikolova, D., Gluud, L. L., Simonetti, R. G., & Gluud, C. (2008). Antioxidant supplements for prevention of mortality in healthy participants and patients with various diseases. *Cochrane Database Syst Rev*, 2:CD007176.

Blendon, R. J., DesRoches, C. M., Benson, J. M., Brodie, M., & Altman, D. E. (2001). Americans' views on the use and regulation of dietary supplements. *Arch Intern Med, 161*, 805–810.

Buckner, K. D., Chavez, M. L., Raney, E. C., & Stoehr, J. D. (2005). Health food stores' recommendations for nausea and migraines during pregnancy. *Ann Pharmacother, 39*, 274–279.

CDC. Centers for Disease Control. (2014a). *Folic acid: Data and statistics*. Retrieved December 19, 2014, from http://www.cdc.gov/ncbddd/folicacid/data.html

CDC. Centers for Disease Control. (2014b). *Second national report on biochemical indicators of diet and nutrition*. Retrieved December 19, 2014, from http://www.cdc.gov/media/releases/2012/p0402_vitamins_nutrients.html

Cellini, M., Attipoe, S., Seales, P., et al. (2013). Dietary supplements: Physician knowledge and adverse event reporting. *Med Sci Sports Exerc, 45*, 23–28.

Clay, P. G., Glaros, A. G., & Clauson, K. A. (2006). Perceived efficacy, indications, and information sources for medically indigent patients and their healthcare providers regarding dietary supplements. *Ann Pharmacother, 40*, 427–432.

Crowley, R., & FitzGerald, L. H. (2006). The impact of cGMP compliance on consumer confidence in dietary supplement products. *Toxicology, 221*, 9–16.

Davis, D. R., Epp, M. D., & Riordan, H. D. (2004). Changes in USDA food composition data for 43 garden crops, 1950 to 1999. *J Am Coll Nutr, 23*, 669–682.

Dawson-Hughes, B., Harris, S. S., Dallal, G. E., Lancaster, D. R., & Zhou, Q. (2002). Calcium supplement and bone medication use in a US Medicare health maintenance organization. *Osteoporosis Int, 13*, 657–662.

Debelle, F., Vanherweghem, J. L., & Nortier, J. L. (2008). Aristolochic acid nephropathy: A worldwide problem. *Kidney Int, 74*, 158–169.

Dickinson, A., Blatman, J., El-Dash, N., & Franco, J. C. (2014). Consumer usage and reasons for using dietary supplements: Report of a series of surveys. *J Am Coll Nutr, 33*, 176–182.

DiGianni, L. M., Kim, H. T., Emmons, K., Gelman, R., Kalkbrenner, K. J., & Garber, J. E. (2003). Complementary medicine use among women enrolled in a genetic testing program. *Cancer Epidemiol Biomarkers Prev, 12*, 321–326.

Farina, E. K., Austin, K. G., & Lieberman, H. R. (2014). Concomitant dietary supplement and prescription medication use is prevalent among US adults with doctor-informed medical conditions. *J Acad Nutr Diet, 114*, 1784–1790.

Federal Trade Commission. (2014). *Weighing the claims in diet ads: Consumer information*. Retrieved December 20, 2014, from http://www.consumer.ftc.gov/articles/0061-weighing-claims-diet-ads

Fehr, K. R., Fehr, K. D., & Protudjer, J. L. (2011). Knowledge and use of folic acid in women of reproductive age. *Can J Diet Pract Res, 72*, 197–200.

Fortmann, S. P., Burda, B. U., Senger, C. A., et al. (2013). Vitamin and mineral supplements in the primary prevention of cardiovascular disease and cancer: An updated systematic evidence review for the U.S. Preventative Services Task Force. *Ann Int Med, 159*, 824–834.

Fuchs-Tarlovsky, V. (2013). Role of antioxidants in cancer therapy. *Nutrients, 29*, 15–21.

Gardiner, P., Graham, R., Legedza, A. T., Ahn, A. C., Eisenberg, D. M., & Phillips, R. S. (2007). Factors associated with herbal therapy use by adults in the United States. *Altern Ther Health Med, 13*, 22–29.

Gardiner, P., Kemper, K. J., Legedza, A., & Phillips, R. S. (2007). Factors associated with herb and dietary supplement use by young adults in the United States. *BMC Complement Altern Med, 7*, 39.

Geller, S., & Studee, L. (2005). Botanical and dietary supplement use for menopausal symptoms: What works, what does not. *J Women's Health, 14,* 634–649.

Gissel, T., Rejnmark, L., Mosekilde, L., & Vestergaard, P. (2008). Intake of vitamin D and risk of breast cancer—A meta-analysis. *J Steroid Biochem Mol Biol, 111,* 195–199.

Gordon, N. P., & Schaffer, D. M. (2005). Use of dietary supplements by female seniors in a large Northern California health plan. *BMC Geriatr, 5,* 4.

Greenlee, H., Kwan, M. L., Ergas, I. J., et al. (2014). Changes in vitamin and mineral supplement use after breast cancer diagnosis in the Pathways Study: A prospective cohort study. *BMC Cancer, 14,* 382. doi: 10.1186/1471240714-382.

Greenlee, H., Kwan, M. L., Kushi, L. H., et al. (2012). Antioxidant supplement use after breast cancer diagnosis and mortality in the Life After Cancer Epidemiology (LACE) cohort. *Cancer, 118,* 2048–2058.

Guallar, E., Stranges, S., Mulrow, C., et al. (2013). Enough is enough: Stop wasting money on vitamin and mineral supplements. *Ann Int Med, 159,* 850–851.

Gurley, B. J., Fifer, E. K., & Gardner, Z. (2012). Pharmacokinetic herb-drug interactions: Part 2. Drug interactions involving popular botanical dietary supplements and their clinical relevance. *Planta Med, 78,* 1490–1514.

Hajirahimkhan, A., Dietz, B. M., & Bolton, J. L. (2013). Botanical modulation of menopausal symptoms: Mechanisms of action? *Planta Med, 79,* 538–553.

Hardy, M. L. (2008). Dietary supplement use in cancer care: Help or harm. *Hematol Oncol Clin North Am, 22,* 581–617, vii.

Haugen, M., Brantsaeter, A. L., Alexander, J., & Meltzer, H. M. (2008). Dietary supplements contribute substantially to the total nutrient intake in pregnant Norwegian women. *Ann Nutr Metab, 52,* 272–280.

Heidelbaugh, J. J. (2013). Proton pump inhibitors and risk of vitamin and mineral deficiency: Evidence and clinical implications. *Ther Adv Drug Saf, 4,* 125–133.

Herbalgram. (2013). *2013 herb market report.* Retrieved December 21, 2014, from http://cms.herbalgram.org/press/2014/2013_Herb_Market_Report.html?ts=1419362156&signature=2c7cc121c26bbd8ce5d138bbbf30e107

Hilton, J. J. (2007). A comparison of folic acid awareness and intake among young women aged 18–24 years. *J Am Acad Nurse Pract, 19,* 516–522.

Holick, M. F., Binkley, N. C., Bischoff, H. A., et al. (2011). Evaluation, treatment and prevention of vitamin D deficiency. *Journal of Clinical Endocrinology and Metabolism, 96,* 1911–1930.

Hunter, D., Foster, M., McAuthur, J. O., et al. (2011). Evaluation of the micronutrient composition of plant foods produced by organic and conventional agricultural methods. *Crit Rev Food Sci Nutr, 51,* 57–82.

Johansson, E., Hussain, A., Kuktaite, R., et al. (2014). Contribution of organically grown crops to human health. *Int J Environ Res Public Health, 11,* 3870–3893.

Kamel, H. (2004). Underutilization of calcium and vitamin D supplements in an academic long-term care facility. *J Am Med Dir Assoc, 5,* 98–100.

Kavalieratos, D., Weinberger, M., & Rao, J. K. (2010). Recommendations of community pharmacists and health food store employees regarding undiagnosed symptoms of diabetes. *J Gen Intern Med, 25,* 799–802.

Kemper, K. J., Gardiner, P., Gobble, J., & Woods, C. (2006). Expertise about herbs and dietary supplements among diverse health professionals. *BMC Complement Altern Med*, 6, 15.

Knudtson, M. D., Klein, R., Lee, K. E., et al. (2007). A longitudinal study of nonvitamin, nonmineral supplement use: Prevalence, associations, and survival in an aging population. *Ann Epidemiol*, 17, 933–939.

Ko, R. (2006). Safety of ethnic imported herbal and dietary supplements. *Clin Toxicol (Phila)*, 44, 611–616.

Kontic-Vucinic, O., Sulovic, N., & Radunovic, N. (2006). Micronutrients in women's reproductive health: I. Vitamins. *Int J Fertil Womens Med*, 51, 106–115.

Kopes-Kerr, C. (2013). Should family physicians screen for vitamin D deficiency? *Am Fam Physician*, 87.

Korde, L. A., Wu, A. H., Fears, T., et al. (2009). Childhood soy intake and breast cancer risk in Asian American women. *Cancer Epidemiol Biomarkers Prev*, 18, 1050–1059.

Koren-Michowitz, M., Dishy, V., Zaidenstein, R., et al. (2005). The effect of losartan and losartan/hydrochlorothiazide fixed-combination on magnesium, zinc, and nitric oxide metabolism in hypertensive patients: A prospective open-label study. *Am J Hypertens*, 18, 358–363.

Krochmal, R., Hardy, M., Bowerman, S., et al. (2004). Phytochemical assays of commercial botanical dietary supplements. *Evid Based Complement Alternat Med*, 1, 305–313.

Kuo, G. M., Hawley, S. T., Weiss, L. T., Balkrishnan, R., & Volk, R. J. (2004). Factors associated with herbal use among urban multiethnic primary care patients: A cross-sectional survey. *BMC Complement Altern Med*, 4, 18.

Lawanda, B. D., Kelly, K. M., Ladas, E. J., Sagar, S. M., Vickers, A., & Blumberg, J. B. (2008). Should supplemental antioxidant administration be avoided during chemotherapy and radiation therapy? *J Natl Cancer Inst*, 100, 773–783.

Ma, J., Johns, R. A., & Stafford, R. S. (2007). Americans are not meeting current calcium recommendations. *Am J Clin Nutr*, 85, 1361–1366.

Mason, C., Xiao, L., Imayama, I., et al. (2014). Vitamin D3 supplementation during weight loss: A double-blind randomized controlled trial. *Am J Clin Nutr*, 99, 1015–1026.

Mehta, D. H., Gardiner, P. M., Phillips, R. S., & McCarthy, E. P. (2008). Herbal and dietary supplement disclosure to health care providers by individuals with chronic conditions. *J Altern Complement Med*, 14, 1263–1269.

Miller, C. K., & Russell, T. (2004). Knowledge of dietary supplement label information among female supplement users. *Patient Educ Couns*, 52, 291–296.

MMWR. (2005, September 30). Use of dietary supplements containing folic acid among women of childbearing age—United States. *Morb Mortal Wkly Rep*, 54, 955–958.

MMWR. (2007, March 16). Fruit and vegetable consumption among adults—United States, 2005. *Morb Mortal Wkly Rep*, 56, 213–217.

MMWR. (2008, January 11). Use of supplements containing folic acid among of childbearing age. *Morb Mortal Wkly Rep*, 57, 5–8.

MMWR. (2010, September 10). State-specific trends in fruit and vegetable consumption among adults—United States, 2000—2009. *Morb Mortal Wkly Rep, 59*, 1125–1130. Retrieved December 19, 2014, from http://www.cdc.gov/mmwr/preview/mmwrhtml/mm5935a1.htm

Molassiotis, A., Ozden, G., & Platin, N. (2006). Complementary and alternative medicine use in patients with head and neck cancers in Europe. *Eur J Cancer Care (Engl), 15*, 19–24.

Moyer, V. A.; U.S. Preventive Services Task Force. (2014). Vitamin, mineral, and multivitamin supplements for the primary prevention of cardiovascular disease and cancer: U.S. Preventive Services Task Force recommendation statement. *Ann Intern Med, 160*, 558–564.

Mulvey, L., Chandrasekaran, A., Liu, K., et al. (2007). Interplay of genes regulated by estrogen and diindolylmethane in breast cancer cell lines. *Mol Med, 13*, 69–78.

Murphy, S. P., White, K. K., Park, S. Y., & Sharma, S. (2007). Multivitamin-multimineral supplements' effect on total nutrient intake. *Am J Clin Nutr, 85*, 280S–284S.

Niafar, M., Hai, F., Porhomayon, J., & Nader, N. D. (2014). The role of metformin on vitamin B12 deficiency: A meta-analysis review. *Intern Emerg Med, 10*, 93–102.

Nichter, M., & Thompson, J. J. (2006). For my wellness, not just my illness: North Americans' use of dietary supplements. *Cult Med Psychiatry, 30*, 175–222.

Ozben, T. (2014, December 9). Antioxidant supplementation on cancer risk and concurrent use of antioxidants during cancer therapy: An update. *Curr Top Med Chem.* [Epub ahead of print]

Pakzad, K., Boucher, B. A., Kreiger, N., & Cotterchio, M. (2007). The use of herbal and other non-vitamin, non-mineral supplements among pre- and post-menopausal women in Ontario. *Can J Public Health, 98*, 383–388.

Park, S. Y., Murphy, S. P., Martin, C. L., & Kolonel, L. N. (2008). Nutrient intake from multivitamin/mineral supplements is similar among users from five ethnic groups: The Multiethnic Cohort Study. *J Am Diet Assoc, 108*, 529–533.

Posadzki, P., Watson, L., & Ernst, E. (2013). Contamination and adulteration of herbal medicinal products (HMPs): An overview of systematic reviews. *Eur J Clin Pharmacol, 69*, 295–307.

Qato, D. M., Alexander, G. C., Conti, R. M., Johnson, M., Schumm, P., & Lindau, S. T. (2008). Use of prescription and over-the-counter medications and dietary supplements among older adults in the United States. *JAMA, 300*, 2867–2878.

Refuerzo, J. S., Blackwell, S. C., Sokol, R. J., et al. (2005). Use of over-the-counter medications and herbal remedies in pregnancy. *Am J Perinatol, 22*, 321–324.

Rock, C. L. (2007). Multivitamin-multimineral supplements: who uses them? *Am J Clin Nutr, 85*(1), 277S–279S.

Rumbold, A., Middleton, P., & Crowther, C. A. (2005). Vitamin supplementation for preventing miscarriage. *Cochrane Database Syst Rev, 2*:CD004073.

Saper, R., Phillips, R., Sehgal, A., et al. (2008). Lead, mercury, and arsenic in US- and Indian-manufactured Ayurvedic medicines sold via the Internet. *JAMA, 300*, 915–923.

Sebastian, R. S., Cleveland, L. E., Goldman, J. D., & Moshfegh, A. J. (2007). Older adults who use vitamin/mineral supplements differ from nonusers in nutrient intake adequacy and dietary attitudes. *J Am Diet Assoc*, *107*, 1322–1332.

Shanahan, C. J., & deLorimier, R. (2014). From science to finance—A toll for deriving economic implication from the results of dietary supplement clinical studies. *J Diet Suppl*. [E-pub ahead of print]

Stein, J., Stier, C., Raab, H., & Weiner, R. (2014). Review article: The nutritional and pharmacological consequences of obesity surgery. *Aliment Pharmacol Ther*, *40*, 582–609.

Tasaki, K., Maskarinec, G., Shumay, D., Tatsumura, Y., & Kakai, H. (2002). Communication between physicians and cancer patients about complementary and alternative medicine: Exploring patients' perspective. *Psychooncology*, *11*, 212–220.

Timbo, B. B., Ross, M. P., McCarthy, P. V., & Lin, C. T. (2006). Dietary supplements in a national survey: Prevalence of use and reports of adverse events. *J Am Diet Assoc*, *106*, 1966–1974.

Tsui, B., Dennehy, C. E., & Tsourounis, C. (2001). A survey of dietary supplement use during pregnancy at an academic medical center. *Am J Obstet Gynecol*, *185*, 433–437.

Velicer, C. M., & Ulrich, C. M. (2008). Vitamin and mineral supplement use among US adults after cancer diagnosis: A systematic review. *J Clin Oncol*, *26*, 665–673.

Wang, Y. M., Jin, B. Z., Ai, F., et al. (2012). The efficacy and safety of melatonin in concurrent chemotherapy or radiotherapy for solid tumors: A meta-analysis of randomized controlled trials. *Cancer Chemother Pharmacol*, *69*, 1213–1220.

Wold, R. S., Lopez, S. T., Yau, C. L., et al. (2005). Increasing trends in elderly persons' use of nonvitamin, nonmineral dietary supplements and concurrent use of medications. *J Am Diet Assoc*, *105*, 54–63.

Wold, R. S., Wayne, S. J., Waters, D. L., & Baumgartner, R. N. (2007). Behaviors underlying the use of nonvitamin nonmineral dietary supplements in a healthy elderly cohort. *J Nutr Health Aging*, *11*, 3–7.

Wollschlaeger, B. (2003). The dietary supplement and health education act and supplements: Dietary and nutritional supplements need no more regulations. *Int J Toxicol*, *22*, 387–390.

Yates, J., Mustian, K., & Morrow, G. (2005). Prevalence of complementary and alternative medicine use in cancer patients during treatment. *Support Care Cancer*, *13*, 806–811.

Yetley, E. A. (2007). Multivitamin and multimineral dietary supplements: Definitions, characterization, bioavailability, and drug interactions. *Am J Clin Nutr*, *85*, 269S–276S.

Zeuschner, C. L., Hokin, B. D., Marsh, K. A., et al. (2013). Vitamin B12 and vegetarian diets. *Med J Aust*, *199*(Suppl 4), S27–32.

4

Physical Activity

PATRICIA LEBENSOHN

Physical Activity and Women's Health

Life is like riding a bicycle. To keep your balance you must keep moving.

—*Albert Einstein*

As the primary caregivers in most societies, women of all ages struggle to keep balance in their lives. When it comes to taking care of themselves, women often have trouble prioritizing what is good for their health and what is needed from them to care for others in their families, communities, and workplaces. In my family medicine practice, for almost 25 years I have heard the same reasons from women about why it is hard for them to be physically active: no time, too tired, hard to get motivated, physical limitations, unsafe neighborhoods, and so on.

In my late twenties, I was at the same place as most of my patients—going through medical school and residency, and starting a family prevented me from being physically active for years. Then, at age 27, I was diagnosed with thyroid cancer. This wake-up call motivated me toward a path of making physical activity a priority in my life. The primary motivation then was to be able to have a long and healthy life to be available to my family. Physical activity has given me not only the physical and mental sense of well-being I have today, but it has also allowed me to become a member of a community of physically active women and has empowered me to have a positive outlook when facing the challenges of the complex world we live in.

This chapter reviews the general recommendations for physical activity and exercise for healthy women, providing specific guidelines for those with common medical conditions. It also addresses important issues to discuss with our patients as we encourage them to get motivated to start and maintain regular physical activity as part of their lifestyle.

The Burden of Physical Inactivity in Women

Throughout their lifecycle, women are less physically active than their male counterparts. In the United States in 2011 only 17.9% of women met the muscle strengthening recommendations from Healthy People 2020 compared with 23.4% of males; 50.2% of women met the aerobic exercise recommendations compared with 53% of males. In addition, in 2012 30.8% of women reported no leisure-time physical activity compared with 28.3% of men (CDC, 2013; Healthy People 2020, n.d.).

Heart disease continues to be the leading cause of death for women (23.5%) in the United States, with 292,188 deaths in 2009 (or one in four female deaths). Cancer is the second leading cause of death (22.1%) and first for Asian/Pacific Islanders, Hispanic, and American Indian/Alaska Natives women (CDC, 2010). There is strong evidence that regular physical activity reduces rates of all-cause mortality: coronary heart disease, high blood pressure, stroke, metabolic syndrome, type 2 diabetes, breast cancer, colon cancer, depression, and falls, and that it increases cardiorespiratory and muscle fitness, promotes healthier body composition, improves bone health, and improves functional health and cognitive function. (Kochanek et al., 2011; US Department of Health and Human Services, 2008; Warburton et al., 2010; WHO, 2010) Physical activity may also decrease risk of lung, endometrial, ovarian, and other cancers (Brown et al., 2007) as well as osteoporosis (Borer, 2005; Ondrak & Morgan, 2007; Schwab & Klein, 2008). Moderate physical activity improves chronic pain syndromes such as osteoarthritis and fibromyalgia (F. Jones et al., 2005). Despite this knowledge, a large proportion of the world's population remains physically inactive. Using calculated population attributable fractions, Lee et al. (2012) quantified the effect of physical inactivity on the world's major noncommunicable diseases. They estimated that physical inactivity causes 6% of the burden of disease from coronary heart disease, 7% of type 2 diabetes, and 10% of both breast and colon cancers. Inactivity causes 9% of premature mortality, or more than 5.3 million of the 57 million deaths that occurred worldwide in 2008. If inactivity were decreased instead by 10%, more than 533,000 deaths could be averted every year; if reduced by 25%, the number of averted deaths could be more than 1.3 million per year.

The following definitions will help healthcare professionals speak a common language as they develop patient-centered recommendations (US Department of Health and Human Services, 2008).

- *Physical activity*: Bodily movement produced by the contraction of skeletal muscle that substantially increases energy expenditure above the resting level.
- *Baseline activity*: Light intensity activities of daily life such as standing, walking slowly, and lifting lightweight objects. People who do only baseline activity are considered to be inactive.
- *Health-enhancing physical activity*: Activity that when added to baseline activity produces health benefits: brisk walking, jumping rope, dancing, yoga, and so forth.
- *Physical fitness*: The ability to carry out daily tasks with vigor and alertness, without undue fatigue and with ample energy to enjoy leisure-time pursuits and meet unforeseen emergencies. Performance-related components of fitness include agility, balance, coordination, power, and speed. Health-related components of physical fitness include body composition, cardiorespiratory function, flexibility, and muscular strength/endurance.

The US Department of Health and Human Services (2008) identifies four levels of physical activity: Inactive (no activity beyond baseline); low (activity beyond baseline but fewer than 150 minutes a week), moderate (150–300 minutes a week); and high (more than 300 minutes).

One framework used to counsel patients about physical activity is to develop an exercise prescription advising the frequency, intensity, time, and type (acronym FITT) of physical activity. Age, level of fitness, medical conditions and physical limitations, ethnicity, culture, and social context also need to be addressed for the recommendation to be initiated and maintained over time (Speck & Harrell, 2003).

Recommendations

If we could give every individual the right amount of nourishment and exercise, not too little and not too much, we would have found the safest way to health.

—*Hippocrates*

The following recommendations have been adopted by the World Health Organization (WHO, 2010) and the Centers for Disease Control (CDC) (www.cdc.gov/physicalactivity/everyone/guidelines/) for women and girls throughout the lifecycle:

GIRLS AND ADOLESCENTS (5–17)

Physical activity includes play, games, sports, transportation, recreation, and physical education or planned exercise in the context of family, school, or community activities. In order to improve cardiorespiratory and muscular fitness, bone health, and metabolic health biomarkers and reduce symptoms of anxiety and depression:

1. Accumulate at least 60 minutes of moderate or vigorous activity daily.
2. Physical activity in amounts greater than 60 minutes daily will provide greater health benefits.
3. Most daily activity should be aerobic, and vigorous activity that strengthens muscle and bone should be incorporated three times a week.

WOMEN 18 TO 64 YEARS OLD

Physical activity includes recreational or leisure-time activity, transportation, occupational activity, household chores, play, games, sports, and planned exercise in the context of daily family and community activities. In order to improve cardiorespiratory and muscular fitness and bone health and to reduce the risk of noncommunicable disease and depression:

1. At least 150 minutes of moderate intensity or 75 minutes of vigorous intensity aerobic physical activity throughout the week or a combination of the two intensities.
2. Aerobic activity should be performed in bouts of at least 10 minutes' duration.
3. For additional health benefits, increase the moderate intensity aerobic physical activity to 300 minutes or engage in 150 minutes of vigorous activity.
4. Muscle strengthening activities should be done involving major muscle groups—legs, hips, back, abdomen, chest, shoulders, and arms—on two or more days a week (see Box 4.1).
5. For women who need to maintain or lose weight, the recommendation is 60–90 minutes of moderate exercise most days of the week.

Box 4.1 Glossary of Exercise Terminology

Exercise intensity:

Generally expressed as a percentage of either HR (heart rate) or VO_2 (volume of oxygen uptake). Since VO_2 is not practical to measure in the practitioner's office, heart rate is generally used.

Heart rate reserve (HRR):

Maximal heart rate (HR_{max}) observed during a symptom-limited exercise stress test minus the resting heart rate (HR_{rest}). A percentage of the HRR range is added to the HR at rest to determine a target heart rate (THR) range to be used during exercise.

Target heart rate (THR):

For most individuals 50%–85% HRR added to the HR at rest is generally recommended. For deconditioned individuals, 50% HRR may be more appropriate for beginning exercise. Physically active individuals may require higher intensities to achieve improvements in their conditioning.

Max heart rate (HR_{max}):

Can be calculated using the following formula:

Sedentary women 226 – age

Fit women 211 – (age/2)

Metabolic equivalents (METs):

Useful units when recommending exercise. By definition, one MET is the amount of oxygen consumed at rest or about 3.5 mL/kg/min. Most people walking 2 mph require two METs, and those walking 3 mph require three to four METs. Published MET tables describe many activities in terms of the estimated MET requirements (CDC, *Physical activity for everyone, 2008*: http://www.cdc.gov/physicalactivity/downloads/PA_Intensity_table_2_1.pdf)

Moderate-intensity aerobic activity:

Raises the heartbeat and leaves the person feeling warm and slightly out of breath. It increases the body's metabolism three to six times the resting level (3–6 METs). Brisk walking has an equivalent of 4.5 METs.

Vigorous-intensity aerobic activities:

Enables people to work up a sweat and become out of breath. These activities usually involve sports or exercise such as running or fast cycling, which raise the metabolism to at least six times resting level. Activities include rhythmic, repetitive physical exercise that uses large muscle groups at 70% or more of maximum heart rate for age.

Muscle strength or resistance training:

Any exercise that causes the muscles to contract against an external resistance with the expectation of increases in strength, tone, mass, and/or endurance. The external resistance can be provided by dumbbells, free weights, rubber exercise tubing, one's own body weight, bricks, bottles of water, or any other object that causes the muscles to contract. A typical recommendation is 8–15 repetitions of 10 major muscle groups.

It is recommended that a woman start with a weight with which she can do 8 repetitions and continue at that weight until she is able to do 15 repetitions. She can then advance the weight and start again with 8 repetitions, increase to 15, and so forth. Yoga, Pilates, and tai chi all include strength-training activities.

Flexibility training:

Good flexibility can help prevent injuries throughout life by enhancing the range of motion around a joint. Warm-up and cool-down stretching, as well as yoga and tai chi are examples.

6. For pregnant women without contraindications, the recommendation is to continue similar levels of physical activity as prior to pregnancy. For inactive pregnant women, it is recommended to start slow and build up to 150 minutes per week of moderate aerobic physical activity. Walking and swimming are excellent choices during pregnancy. Yoga enhances strength and flexibility training to prevent back pain, and breathing exercises could help prepare for the birthing experience. Exercises to avoid while pregnant include activities that involve lying on the back or that put women at risk of falling or abdominal injury, such as horseback riding, soccer, or basketball. It is important to counsel pregnant women to avoid overheating and dehydration when exercising.

WOMEN 65 YEARS OLD AND ABOVE

Same as above and:

1. Adults of this age with poor mobility should perform physical activity on three or more days a week to enhance balance and prevent falls.
2. When adults of this age group cannot do the recommended amount of physical activity due to health conditions, they should be as physically active as their abilities and conditions allow.

Cardiovascular Disease and Physical Activity

The increased risk for cardiovascular disease (CVD) from established modifiable risk factors: tobacco use, hypertension, diabetes mellitus, and hypercholesterolemia—is well documented. More recently, nonestablished behavioral and lifestyle risk factors—like obesity, physical inactivity, and sedentary behavior— have been studied. Based on the 2013 update from the American Heart Association, the leading cause of death for women is CVD, with 401,495 deaths in the United States in 2009. Gender differences for physical inactivity start early in life, with girls more likely to report physical inactivity than boys (17.7% vs. 10.0%). Moreover, only 17.1% of adult women met the 2008 Federal Physical Activity recommendations in 2011. Physical activity and physical inactivity have shown independent effects on CVD.

DOSE-DEPENDENT EFFECT OF PHYSICAL ACTIVITY

There is an inverse relationship between physical activity levels and CVD events in women. Reductions in CVD events in women with physical activity are in the range of 30%–50% despite the fact that changes in individual risk factors are modest; lipids are reduced 5%, blood pressure 3–5 mmHg, and hemoglobin A1C by 1% (Hu et al., 2004; Stevens et al., 2002)

Mora et al. (2007) examined the extent to which traditional and novel risk factors explain the cardioprotective benefits of physical activity. Using prospectively collected data from the Women's Health Study, which followed 27,055 initially healthy women for 11 years, they found that even moderate levels of physical activity (at least 600 kcal/week or the equivalent of just over 2 hours per week of brisk walking) were associated with 30%–40% relative risk reduction for CVD. A dose response was seen as physical activity increased in intensity and/or duration. Inflammatory and hemostatic biomarkers (high-sensitivity C-reactive protein, fibrinogen, and soluble intracellular adhesion molecule-1) provided the largest contribution to lowered risk (33%), followed by blood pressure (27%), lipids (19%), body mass index (BMI; 10%), and glucose abnormalities (9%), with minimal contribution from changes in renal function or homocysteine.

Kelley, Kelley, and Tran (2005) conducted a meta-analysis of the effects of aerobic exercise on lipids in women. They concluded that aerobic exercise was correlated with reductions of 2% for total cholesterol, 3% for LDL cholesterol, and 5% for triglycerides; in addition, they observed an increase of 3% in HDL cholesterol.

Another review confirms the multiple benefits of physical activity for women (Brown, Burton, & Rowan, 2007). Studies revealed 28%–58% risk reduction of cardiovascular disease and 14%–46% risk reduction of diabetes. The protective benefits were seen with as little as 60 minutes of moderate-intensity physical activity per week or 4 MET hours (see Table 4.1).

Table 4.1. Examples of Moderate and Vigorous Exercise for Women

Moderate Exercise (3–6 METs)	Vigorous Exercise (>6 METs)
Walking at 3–4.5 mph	Race walking 5 mph
Hiking	Jogging/running
Bicycling less than 9 mph	Bicycling more than 10 mph
Aerobic dancing	High-impact aerobics
Water aerobics	Martial arts
Yoga	Circuit training
Golfing, carrying clubs	Most competitive sports
Tennis doubles	Tennis singles
Recreational swimming	Swimming laps

In a systematic review Boone-Heinonen et al. (2009) conclude that walking is a viable intervention for sedentary populations to decrease CVD. Increasing the walking pace from 2 to 3 mph, 3 to 4 mph, to more than 4 mph decreases CVD risk by 14%, 24%, and 42%, respectively.

SEDENTARY LIFESTYLE, PHYSICAL ACTIVITY, AND RISK OF CVD

Sedentary behavior is recognized as a distinct construct beyond lack of leisure-time physical activity. Chomistek et al. (2013) analyzed data from the Women's Health Initiative Observational Prospective Study of 71,018 postmenopausal women between baseline 1993–1998 until 2010. They concluded that sitting ≥ 10 hours/day compared with ≤ 5 hours/day was associated with increased CVD risk (HR = 1.18, 95% CI 1.09, 1.29) in multivariable models including physical activity. Risk of CVD was higher in older and overweight women and women that reported lowest physical activity (less than 1.7 METs per week).

This study, as well as other recent studies on sedentary lifestyle, points to the importance of discussing with our patients the effects of hours of sitting. Recommendations for change can include alternatives such as treadmill desks or a structured workday with physical activity breaks (Tudor-Locke et al., 2014).

Social Support and Physical Activity

Fischer Aggarwal, Liao, and Mosca (2008) evaluated possible pathways through which social support may reduce CVD risk in a diverse population of women. Higher social support was positively associated with minutes of physical activity per week, number of days of physical activity per week, and with increased HDL cholesterol.

Physical Activity and Cancer

Epidemiologic studies have shown that breast cancer risk is reduced 30%–40% in highly physically active women compared with inactive women. In a population-based breast cancer case-control study in Poland conducted in 2000–2003, Peplonska et al. (2008) analyzed data on physical activity patterns in 2,176 cases of breast cancer and 2,326 controls. They concluded that moderate to vigorous physical activity levels (6–15 METs/week) during adulthood may reduce breast cancer risk. This applies to activities including recreation, outdoor chores, and occupational tasks (see Table 4.2). The protective effect of moderate/vigorous activities occurred independently of menopausal status, BMI, family history of breast cancer, and tumor features. Their study suggested that increases in activity levels when a woman is in her fifties might be particularly relevant.

Exercise is not merely safe and feasible for breast cancer patients but also is a complementary treatment for achieving physiological and psychological improvements. There is increasing evidence that regular exercise after the diagnosis of breast cancer might have a substantial positive impact on mortality,

Table 4.2. **Examples of Recreational or Occupational Physical Activity That Have Similar Energy Expenditure as Moderate and Vigorous Exercise**

Moderate Recreational or Occupational PA	Vigorous Recreational or Occupational PA
Gardening: raking, bagging leaves	Gardening: digging ditches, swinging an axe
Housework: scrubbing floors, sweeping, washing windows	Housework: pushing heavy furniture, carrying objects up the stairs
Putting groceries away: items less than 50 lb.	Grocery shopping while carrying children or carrying 25 lb. bags up the stairs
Actively playing with children	Vigorously playing with children, running
Animal care: feeding, grooming farm animals	Animal care, carrying heavy equipment
Waiting tables	Aerobic instructor
Patient care (bathing, dressing, moving patients)	Loading/unloading a truck, fire-fighting

Source: Adapted from Centers for Disease Control and Prevention: *http://www.cdc.gov/physicalactivity/downloads/PA_Intensity_table_2_1.pdf*

morbidity, prognosis, and quality of life (Eyigor & Kanyilmaz, 2014). In a systematic review, Fontein et al. (2014) concluded that there is improved overall and breast-cancer-specific survival in physically active breast cancer patients, especially older, postmenopausal women.

Physical activity and psychosocial therapies are the two main nonpharmacological modalities to treat the cancer-related fatigue syndrome that affects so many women with breast cancer. The greatest benefits are seen in programs with multiple exercise components that are individualized, more than eight weeks long, and at least partially home-based (Berger, Gerber, & Mayer, 2012).

A meta-analysis of 52 observational studies in both genders found an inverse relationship between level of physical activity and incidence of colorectal cancer (CRC). The overall relative risk was 0.76 (95% confidence interval [CI]: 0.72–0.81) (Wolin et al., 2009).

Kuiper et al. (2012) found that among 1,339 women diagnosed with CRC in the prospective study from the Women's Health Initiative, 265 (13%) deaths occurred during a median study follow-up of 11.9 years, of which 171 (65%) were attributed to CRC. Compared with women reporting no prediagnostic recreational physical activity, those reporting activity levels of $\geq$ 18 MET-hr/week had significantly lower colorectal-cancer-specific mortality (hazard ratio [HR] = 0.68; 95% CI: 0.41–1.13) and all-cause mortality (HR = 0.63; 95% CI: 0.42–0.96). Similar inverse associations were seen for postdiagnostic recreational physical activity. Neither pre- nor postdiagnostic BMI were associated with mortality after CRC diagnosis. These findings were similar to those of an earlier study by Kuiper et al. (2012) of 573 women with stage 1–3 CRC.

There is also growing evidence of the impact of physical activity on reduction of developing bladder cancer and lung cancer among smokers (Keimling et al., 2014).

For patients with gynecological cancers like ovarian and endometrial cancer, there is some evidence that physical activity is feasible but the effect on survivorship is not well documented (Gil & von Gruenigen, 2011).

Physical Activity and Depression

Both leisure time physical activity and reduction of sedentary behavior can decrease the risk for depression and potentially improve depressive disorders in women (Uffelen et al., 2013). There is clear evidence demonstrated in three systematic reviews of the potential benefits (effect size 0.80–0.86) of aerobic exercise, weight training, and walking versus no treatment for individuals with depression (Rethorst, Wipfli, & Landers, 2009; Rimer et al., 2012; Robertson et al., 2012). Exercise may be as effective in treating depression as medications or psychotherapy (Conney et al., 2013; Krogh et al., 2011). Stanton et al., (2014) recommend supervised individual or group cardiovascular exercise performed at low or moderate or self-selected intensity for 30–40 min per session, and three to four sessions a week over a period of 9 to 12 weeks may be beneficial for mood disorders including depression, postnatal depression, and bipolar disorder.

Griffiths et al. (2014) followed over 26,000 Finnish working women from 18–69 years of age over a 4-year period and found that physical activity was associated with a reduced future risk of mental ill-health independently from sociodemographic, work-related and lifestyle factors, health conditions, and BMI. Moreover there was an inverse dose-response relationship (≤14 METs – ≥60 METs/week) between physical activity and likelihood of later symptoms of mental ill-health. This effect was more evident in midlife and in older women than in younger women. This differential effect could be attributed to the positive effect of exercise on mood and sleep-related menopausal symptoms. Brown et al. (2005) followed 9,207 middle-aged Australian women over a period of 6 years and found a dose-response relationship between increased physical activity and decreasing depressive symptoms independent of preexisting physical and psychological health.

A study comparing the effects of different intensities of exercise on the mental health of 6,800 women and men in Belgium found a positive effect on mental health variables for all intensities (Azstalos & De Bourdeaudhuij, 2010). Men showed the most benefit from vigorous exercise on symptoms of depression and somatization, while women had positive association between walking and emotional well-being and moderate physical activity and symptoms of somatization.

Physical Activity and Diabetes

Exercise and weight reduction are effective tools for most women in the primary prevention of type 2 diabetes mellitus (T2DM). Exercise increases insulin sensitivity and decreases triglycerides and total cholesterol. Overall, both men and women with T2DM tend to be sedentary. However, women with T2DM typically have lower levels of recreational physical activity than men with T2DM (Nelson, Reiber, & Boyko, 2002).

Men and women with T2DM also differed in how intensely and where they wanted to exercise (Barret, Plotnikoff, Courneya, & Raine, 2007). Forbes et al. (2010) found that men preferred moderate or vigorous exercise more often than did women. Not only did women prefer low-intensity exercise to higher-intensity exercise but also they favored a scheduled session with supervision (e.g., exercise classes).

In addition to the general recommendations for regular physical activity for prevention of chronic disease, resistance and high-intensity interval training (HIIT) have emerged for prevention of T2DM related outcomes (Roberts, Little, & Thyfault, 2013). High-intensity interval training is a form of exercise that alternates anaerobic exercise intervals lasting several seconds to several minutes with low-intensity recovery periods. The total interval time usually takes less than 30 minutes including rest periods (Laursen & Jenkins, 2002).

An example of HIIT would include: approximately five minutes of warm up, by working aerobically at about 40% effort, followed by a 20- to 30-second period of intense effort, followed by a rest period of 10–30 seconds. The cycles could be repeated four to eight times. The high intensity exercise could be running, cycling, rowing or weight training or a combination of activities, and the total duration of the workout could last from 5 to up to 45 minutes (including warm up and cool down).

Anaerobic exercise is a form of exercise that uses either preformed energy (ATP) in the body or derives its energy through glycolytic-lactate forming metabolism. High-intensity interval training that uses intervals lasting less than 30 seconds is using more of the preformed ATP pathway and intervals from 30–120 seconds derive the energy more from the glycolytic-lactate forming pathway (Little et al., 2011). High-intensity interval training has been shown to be safe and beneficial for both healthy and diseased populations (peripheral artery disease, CAD, heart failure, asthma, T2DM, chronic obstructive pulmonary disease [COPD], and older adults). The benefits include improved glucose tolerance, increased fat burning, and increased aerobic capacity (VO_2 max) (Tabata et al., 1996). High-intensity interval training addresses time as a barrier and may motivate women to try higher-intensity physical activity and decrease this gender-based health disparity (Bird & Hawley, 2012).

Physical Activity and Bone Health

Recent advances in bone biology have established that exercise in the form of short, repetitive mechanical loading leads to the greatest gains in bone strength. As demonstrated by both observational and randomized exercise intervention trials, these gains are best achieved in childhood (Gunter et al., 2012) but can be maintained in adulthood with continued regular weight-bearing exercise. In the later years, there is evidence to support the implementation of balance training to decrease fall risk, especially in elderly patients with low bone mass (Borer, 2005; Ondrak & Morgan, 2007; Schwab & Klein, 2008).

Regular exercise, including resistance training and high-impact activity, contributes to the development of high peak bone mass and may reduce the risk of falls in older women (Hagey & Warren, 2008). A study of mature female athletes found that women who regularly engage in high-impact physical activity in the premenopausal years have higher bone mineral density (BMD) than nonathletic controls (Dook et al., 1997). See the chapter "Osteoporosis" for recommendations.

Physical Activity and Menopause

Although many of the chronic illnesses that increase in postmenopausal women are positively affected by physical activity, there is no definitive evidence that activity improves vasomotor symptoms. Van Poppel and Brown (2008) assessed the relationship between changes in physical activity and self-reported menopausal symptoms using data from the Australian Longitudinal Study on Women's Health. Physical activity was not associated with total menopausal symptoms, vasomotor symptoms, or psychological symptoms. Weight gain was associated with increased total, vasomotor, and somatic symptoms, while weight loss reduced total and vasomotor symptoms.

A Cochrane review found only one small trial assessing the effectiveness of exercise in the management of vasomotor menopausal symptoms (Daley et al., 2007). Exercise was not as effective as hormone therapy (HT) in this trial. They found no evidence that exercise is an effective treatment relative to other interventions or no intervention in reducing hot flashes and/or night sweats in symptomatic women. In a more recent systematic review by Cramer et al. (2012) of five randomized controlled trials on the effectiveness of yoga in menopausal symptoms, the reviewers found evidence of short-term improvements on psychological symptoms. While it is important to recommend physical activity for prevention of chronic illness, women should not be given unrealistic expectations regarding its effects on vasomotor symptoms (Hagey & Warren, 2008).

Fibromyalgia and Physical Activity

Physical activity relieves many symptoms in fibromyalgia patients; it helps women maintain general fitness, physical function, emotional well-being, and overall health; it also provides women with enhanced feelings of control over their well-being. Forty-six exercise treatment studies with a total of 3,035 subjects were reviewed, and the strongest evidence is for aerobic exercise (Jones et al., 2006). The greatest effect and lowest attrition occurred in exercise programs that were of lower intensity. Exercise that is of appropriate intensity, self-modified, and symptom-limited is most likely to be of help.

Bircan, Karasel, Akgun, El, and Alper (2008) randomized 30 women with fibromyalgia to either an aerobic exercise program or a strengthening exercise program for 8 weeks; both programs were similarly effective at improving symptoms, tender point count, fitness, depression, and quality of life. Similar findings were reported by the Ottawa panel (Brosseau et al., 2008). In a recent Cochrane review, Busch et al. (2013) concluded that the evidence suggested moderate and moderate-to high-intensity resistance training improves multidimensional function, pain, tenderness, and muscle strength in women with fibromyalgia. The evidence also suggested that 8 weeks of aerobic exercise was superior to moderate-intensity resistance training for improving pain in women with fibromyalgia.

Challenges to motivating women with fibromyalgia to exercise include that many are deconditioned due to pain and fatigue; many are overweight or obese; and some have become socially isolated. Interventions unique to patients with fibromyalgia include the following:

- Greater exercise adherence occurs when there is greater agreement between patient and physician regarding the patient's level of well-being and when the patient's pain and stress have been addressed (Rooks, 2008).
- Physical activity recommendations should be tailored to the individual patient.
- Initial discussions should concentrate around ways to increase physical activity daily; for example, adding walking tasks with or without a pedometer, parking farther away from the destination, using stairs, and engaging in gardening and house cleaning.

Enhancing Motivation

The secret of getting ahead is getting started.

—*Agatha Christie*

Strength does not come from physical capacity. It comes from an indomitable will

—*Mahatma Gandhi*

The challenge to motivate women to increase their physical activity is twofold. First is the motivation to initiate physical activity and second is the ability to maintain regular physical activity (defined as maintaining the required levels of exercise for more than six months) (Marcus et al., 1992).

Maintaining regular, long-term physical activity is critical to achieving its benefits. However, the dropout rate in clinical programs is 50% or greater within the first six months (Dishman, 1988). Variables that impact motivation were identified in a review article and include demographic, psychological, social, environmental, physiologic, health status, and physical capability (Speck & Harrell, 2003).

Demographic variables such as age are important considerations when designing studies and developing interventions. Older women exercise at lower levels and less frequently than younger women (Scharff et al., 1999). One study found differing predictors of four types of activity: sports/exercise, active living, household/caregiving, and occupational activities (Sternfeld, Ainsworth, & Quesenberry, 1999). Women with the highest levels of both sports/exercise and active living were likely to be white, better educated, younger, without young children at home, with lower BMI, higher self-efficacy, and lower perceived barriers to exercise. Women with the highest level of household/caregiving responsibilities were more likely to be Hispanic, older, married with young children in the home, and not employed. Women with the highest occupational physical activity were likely to be less educated and to be current smokers.

In analyses of a national survey, women in all three ethnic classifications—Caucasian, African American, Mexican American—had higher percentages of inactivity than men, ranging from 22% to 47% for women and 14% to 32% for men (Crespo et al., 2000). Among women, African Americans and Mexican Americans had higher percentages of inactivity than Caucasians in nearly every category of the social class indicators (education, income, occupation, poverty, employment, and marital status).

HEALTH STATUS VARIABLES

A national survey of ethnically diverse women aged 40 and over ($n = 2,912$) found the personal barrier "not in good health" to be one of 11 variables that were significant predictors of being sedentary (King et al., 2000). Heesch, Brown, and Blanton (2000) further analyzed this data and found "bad health" was identified as a frequent barrier to exercise in Caucasian, Native American, and Hispanic subjects in the precontemplation stage of physical activity, but not in African Americans. Precontemplators were defined as not currently exercising and with no plan to begin exercising in the next six months.

PSYCHOLOGICAL VARIABLES

Self-efficacy is the belief that one is capable of performing a specific behavior (Bandura 1986). Self-efficacy is consistently positively correlated with higher levels of physical activity (Piazza, Conrad, & Wilbur, 2001; Speck, 2003; Sternfeld et al., 1999). Other studies have demonstrated that self-efficacy is a predictor of initiation and early adherence to exercise but maintenance is predicted by the interaction of self-efficacy and the type of program (McAuley et al., 1994; Oman & King, 1998). When the physical activity is self-selected instead of prescribed by the study design, self-efficacy might play a bigger role in maintenance. Outcome expectation is the belief that performing a specific behavior will lead to a specific outcome and is linked to self-efficacy. Overly optimistic expectations of inexperienced exercisers may lead to disappointment and attrition (Jones et al., 2005).

PHYSICAL ACTIVITY VARIABLES

Aspects of physical activity may be important because negative experiences with a behavior can lead to suppression of the behavior and positive experiences can increase a woman's self-efficacy around that behavior (Bandura, 1986). Variables include type of activity and the number of relapses from regular physical activity.

Many studies have shown that walking is an important activity for women. For example, in an Australian survey (Booth et al., 1997), more than 60% of women identified walking as their preferred physical activity, 14% identified swimming, and all other activity choices were chosen by less than 10% of the women. Variables in the social environment include support of friends and family as well as social and environmental barriers; 19% of the women identified lack of someone to exercise with as a barrier and 35% preferred to exercise with the support of a group. Another study (Wallace, Raglin, & Jastremski, 1995) demonstrated that women had better adherence when they exercised with their spouses than alone. However, higher family support predicted lower maintenance. This paradoxical finding could mean that for working women with families, spending time with family is a higher priority than exercising.

The most frequently identified barrier to activity maintenance in women is lack of time due to work and family obligations (Booth et al., 1997; Jaffe et al., 1999). Qualitative studies of barriers to physical activity in both African American women and Caucasian women found lack of time, motivation, and social support (Nies, Vollman, & Cook, 1998, 1999). Barriers identified only by African Americans were lack of childcare, lack of space for exercise in the home, and unsafe neighborhoods. A barrier unique to Caucasian women was poor body image.

New Trend: The Benefits of "Green Exercise"

Green exercise is a term adopted in 2005 to describe the potential synergistic benefit to health that occurs when exercising in nature (Pretty et al., 2005). The decline of physical activity in the developed world parallels the decreased time in nature for individuals of all ages (Gladwell et al., 2013). There is a growing body of evidence that "green exercise" might increase enjoyment of participation, social interaction, and frequency of activity (Hug et al., 2009). It may also alter the perception of effort and, therefore, allow individuals to achieve a greater intensity of exercise and improve motivation and adherence. Green exercise has shown increased benefits in mental health outcomes compared with indoor activity (Thompson et al., 2011) as well as improvement of cardiovascular and metabolic markers related to the stress response (Li et al., 2011). The value of the experience of nature in health and well-being should guide urban planning as well as conservation of forests, countryside, mountains, and oceanside. Facilitating access to these natural resources for all could potentiate the health benefits of physical activity.

Recommendations For Clinicians

As healthcare providers, we can empower women to be physically active. We have plenty of evidence—as reviewed in this chapter—of the benefits of regular physical activity for primary and secondary prevention of chronic illnesses. As integrative providers, we have the tools to provide patient-centered care and to elicit the unique needs, preferences, and barriers women of all ages and ethnic backgrounds have around physical activity. We can communicate that even small increments in physical activity, leisure time with family, occupational, structured exercise, or alternative ways of transportation can improve health and well-being.

After my thyroidectomy, when I learned I had cancer with extensive lymph node involvement, I turned to exercise to improve my well-being. The first week, I could hardly jog for 5 minutes. Even those few minutes gave me a sense of well-being and hope and I increased the frequency, intensity, and time as I felt ready. I also added different exercises: swimming, yoga, and biking. Today, at age 55, I am still in the best athletic condition of my entire life. I am grateful to feel this way. It is my hope that you will be inspired by this chapter not only to work with your women patients to help them make activity a part of their daily routine but also to be a model for your patients and advocate in your community.

REFERENCES

American Heart Association. (2013). *Women and cardiovascular disease.* Retrieved from http://www.heart.org/idc/groups/heart-public/@wcm/@sop/@smd/documents/downloadable/ucm_319576.pdf

Asztalos, M., & De Bourdeaudhuij, I. (2010). The relationship between physical activity and mental health varies across activity intensity levels and dimensions of mental health among women and men. *Public Health Nutr, 13,* 1207–1213.

Bandura, A. (1986). *Social learning theory.* Englewood Cliffs, NJ: Prentice Hall.

Barret, J. E., Plotnikoff, R. C., Courneya, K. S., & Raine, K. D. (2007). Physical activity and type 2 diabetes: Exploring the role of gender and income. *Diabetes Educ, 33,* 128–143.

Berger, A. M., Gerber, L. H., & Mayer, D. K. (2012). Cancer-related fatigue. *Cancer, 118*(8 Suppl), 2261–2269. doi:10.1002/cncr.27475

Bircan, C., Karasel, S. A., Akgun, B., El, O., & Alper, S. (2008). Effects of muscle strengthening versus aerobic exercise program in fibromyalgia. *Rheumatol Intl, 28,* 527–532.

Bird, S. R., & Hawley, J. A. (2012). Exercise and type 2 diabetes: New prescription for an old problem. *Maturitas, 72,* 311–316.

Boone-Heinonen, J., Evenson, K. R., Taber, D. R., et al. (2009). Walking for prevention of cardiovascular disease in men and women: A systematic review of observational studies. *Obes Rev, 10,* 204–217.

Booth, M. L., Bauman, A., Owen, N., et al. (1997). Physical activity preferences, preferred sources of assistance, and perceived barriers to increased activity among physically inactive Australians. *Am J Prev Med, 26,* 131–137.

Borer, K. T. (2005). Physical activity in the prevention and amelioration of osteoporosis in women: Interaction of mechanical, hormonal and dietary factors. *Sports Med, 35,* 779–830.

Brosseau, L., Wells, G. A., Tugwell, P., et al. (2008). Ottawa Panel evidence-based clinical practice guidelines for strengthening exercises in the management of fibromyalgia: Part 2. *Phys Therapy, 88,* 873–886.

Brown, W. J., Burton, N. W., & Rowan, P. J. (2007). Updating the evidence on physical activity and health in women. *Am J Prev Med, 33,* 404–411.

Brown, W. J., Ford, J. H., Burton, N. W., et al. (2005). Prospective study of physical activity and depressive symptoms in middle-aged women. *Am J Prev Med, 29,* 265–272.

Buffart, L. M., Singh, A. S., van Loon, E. C. P., et al. (2014). Physical activity and the risk of developing lung cancer among smokers: A meta-analysis. *J Sci Med Sport*, *17*, 67–71.

Busch, A. J., Webber, S. C., Richards, R. S., et al. (2013). Resistance exercise training for fibromyalgia. *Cochrane Database Syst Rev*, *12*.

CDC. (2008). *Physical activity for everyone*. Retrieved from http://www.cdc.gov/physicalactivity/downloads/PA_Intensity_table_2_1.pdf

CDC. (2010). *Leading causes of death by race/ethnicity, all females—United States, 2010*. Retrieved from www.cdc.gov/women/lcod/2010/WomenRace_2010.pdf

CDC. (2013). *Adult Participation in Aerobic and Muscle-Strengthening Physical Activities-United States, 2011. MMWR*, *62*, 326–330.

Chomistek, A. K., Manson, J. E., Stefanick, M. L., et al. (2013). The relationship of sedentary behavior and physical activity to incident cardiovascular disease: Results from the Women's Health Initiative. *J Am Coll Cardiol*, *61*, 2346–2354.

Cooney, G. M., Dwan, K., Greig, C. A., et al. (2013). Exercise for depression. *Cochrane Database Syst Rev*, *9*.

Cramer, H., Lauche, R., Langhorst, J., et al. (2012). Effectiveness of yoga for menopausal symptoms: A systematic review and meta-analysis of randomized controlled trials. *Evidence-Based Complementary and Alternative Medicine: eCAM*, *2012*. Article ID 863905.

Crespo, C. J., Smit, E., Andersen, R. E., et al. (2000). Race/ethnicity, social class and their relation to physical inactivity during leisure time: Results from the Third National Health and Nutrition Examination Survey, 1988–1994. *Am J Prev Med*, *18*, 46–53.

Daley, A., MacArthur, C., Mutrie, N., et al. (2007). Exercise for vasomotor menopausal symptoms. *Cochrane Database Syst Rev*, *4*.

Dishman, R. K. (1988). *Exercise adherence: Its impact on public health*. Champaign, IL: Human Kinetics.

Dook, J. E., James, C., Henderson, N. K., et al. (1997). Exercise and bone mineral density in mature female athletes. *Med Sci Sports Exerc*, *29*, 291–296.

Eyigor, S., & Kanyilmaz, S. (2014). Exercise in patients coping with breast cancer: An overview. *World J Clin Oncol*, *5*, 406–411.

Fischer Aggarwal, B. A., Liao, M., & Mosca, L. (2008). Physical activity as a potential mechanism through which social support may reduce cardiovascular disease risk. *J Cardiovasc Nurs*, *23*, 90–96.

Fontein, D. B. Y., de Glas, N. A., Duijm, M., et al. (2014). Age and the effect of physical activity on breast cancer survival: A systematic review. *Cancer Treat Rev*, *39*, 958–965.

Forbes, C. C., Plotnikoff, R. C., Courneya, K. S., et al. (2010). Physical activity preferences and type 2 diabetes: Exploring demographic, cognitive, and behavioral differences. *Diabetes Educ*, *36*, 801–815.

Gil, K. M., & von Gruenigen, V. E. (2011). Physical activity and gynecologic cancer survivorship. *Recent Results Cancer Res*, *186*, 305–315.

Gladwell, V. F., Brown, D. K., Wood, C., et al. (2013). The great outdoors: How a green exercise environment can benefit all. *Extreme Physiol Med*, *2*, 3.

Griffiths, A., Kouvonen, A., Pentti, J., et al. (2014). Association of physical activity with future mental health in older, mid-life and younger women. *Eur J Public Health*, *24*, 813–818.

Gunter, K. B., Almstedt, H. C., & Janz, K. F. (2012). Physical activity in childhood may be the key to optimizing lifespan skeletal health. *Exercise Sport Sci Rev*, *40*, 13–21.

Hagey, A. R., & Warren, M. P. (2008). Role of exercise and nutrition in menopause. *Clin Obstet Gynecol*, *51*, 627–641.

Healthy People 2020. (n.d.). *Physical activity*. Retrieved from http://www.healthypeople.gov/2020/topics-objectives/topic/physical-activity

Heesch, K. C., Brown, D. R., & Blanton, C. J. (2000). Perceived barriers to exercise and stage of exercise adoption in older women of different racial/ethnic groups. *Women Health*, *30*, 61–76.

Hu, F. B., Willett, W. C., Li, T., et al. (2004). Adiposity as compared with physical activity in predicting mortality among women. *N Engl J Med*, *351*, 2694–2703.

Hug, S. M., Hartig, T., Hansmann, R., et al. (2009). Restorative qualities of indoor and outdoor exercise settings as predictors of exercise frequency. *Health Place*, *15*, 971–980.

Jaffe, L., Lutter, J. M., Rex, M., et al. (1999). Incentives and barriers to physical activity for working women. *Am J Health Promot*, *13*, 215.

Jones, F., Harris, P., Waller, H., et al. (2005). Adherence to an exercise prescription scheme: The role of expectations, self-efficacy, stage of change and psychological well-being. *Br J Health Psychol*, *10*, 359–378.

Jones, K. D., Adams, D., Winters-Stone, K., et al. (2006). A comprehensive review of 46 exercise treatment studies in fibromyalgia (1988–2005). *Health Qual Life Outcomes*, *4*, 67.

Keimling, M., Behrens, G., Schmid, D., et al. (2014). The association between physical activity and bladder cancer: Systematic review and meta-analysis. *Br J Cancer*, *110*, 1862–1870.

Kelley, G. A., Kelley, K. S., & Tran, Z. V. (2005). Aerobic exercise and lipids and lipoproteins in women: A meta-analysis of randomized controlled trials. *J Women's Health (Larchmt)*, *13*, 1148–1164. [Erratum in *J Women's Health (Larchmt)*, 14, 198.]

King, A. C., Castro, C., Wilcox, S., et al. (2000). Personal and environmental factors associated with physical inactivity among different racial-ethnic groups of U.S. middle-aged and older-aged women. *Health Psychol*, *19*, 354–364.

Kochanek, K. D., Xu, J. Q., Murphy, S. L., et al. (2011). Deaths: Final data for 2009. *National Vital Statistics Reports*, *60*.

Krogh, J., Nordentoft, M., Sterne, J. A., et al. (2011). The effect of exercise in clinically depressed adults: Systematic review and meta-analysis of randomized controlled trials. *J Clin Psychiatry*, *72*, 529–538.

Kuiper, J. G., Phipps, A. I., Neuhouser, M. L., et al. (2012). Recreational physical activity, body mass index, and survival in women with colorectal cancer. *Cancer Causes Control*, *23*, 1939–1948.

Laursen, P. B., & Jenkins, D. G. (2002). The scientific basis for high-intensity interval training. *Sports Medicine*, *32*, 53–73.

Lee, I. M., Shiroma, E. J., Lobelo, F., et al. (2012). Lancet Physical Activity Series Working Group. Effect of physical inactivity on major non-communicable diseases worldwide: An analysis of burden of disease and life expectancy. *Lancet*, 380, 219–229.

Li, Q., Otsuka, T., Kobayashi, M., et al. (2011). Acute effects of walking in forest environments on cardiovascular and metabolic parameters. *Eur J Appl Physiol*, 111, 2845–2853.

Little, J. P., Gillen, J. B., Percival, M. E., et al. (2011). Low-volume high-intensity interval training reduces hyperglycemia and increases muscle mitochondrial capacity in patients with type 2 diabetes. *J Appl Physiol*, 111, 1554–1560.

Marcus, B. H., Selby, V. C., Niaura, R. S., et al. (1992). Self-efficacy and the stages of exercise behavior change. *Res Q Exerc Sport*, 63, 60–66.

McAuley, E., Courneya, K. S., Rudolph, D. L., et al. (1994). Enhancing exercise, adherence in middle-aged males and females. *Am J Prev Med*, 23, 498–506.

Mora, S., Cook, N., Buring, J. E., et al. (2007). Activity and reduced risk of cardiovascular events: Potential mediating mechanisms. *Circulation*, 116, 2110–2118.

Nelson, K. M., Reiber, G., & Boyko, E. J. (2002). Diet and exercise among adults with type 2 diabetes: Findings from the third National Health and Nutrition Examination Survey (NHANES III) *Diabetes Care*, 25, 1722–1728.

Nies, M. A., Vollman, M., & Cook, T. (1998). Facilitators, barriers, and strategies for exercise in European American women in the community. *Public Health Nurs*, 15, 263–272.

Nies, M. A., Vollman, M., & Cook, T. (1999). African American women's experiences with physical activity in their daily lives. *Public Health Nurs*, 16, 23–31.

Oman, R. F., & King, A. C. (1998). Predicting the adoption and maintenance of exercise participation using self-efficacy and previous exercise participation rates. *Am J Health Promot*, 12, 154–161.

Ondrak, K. S., & Morgan, D. W. (2007). Physical activity, calcium intake and bone health in children and adolescents. *Sports Med*, 37, 587–600.

Peplonska, B., Lissowska, J., Hartman, T. J., et al. (2008). Adult lifetime physical activity and breast cancer. *Epidemiology*, 19, 226–236.

Piazza, J., Conrad, K., & Wilbur, J. (2001). Exercise behavior among occupational health nurses. *AAOHN J*, 49, 79–86.

Pretty, J., Peacock, J., Sellens, M., et al. (2005). The mental and physical health outcomes of green exercise. *Int J Environ Health Res*, 15, 319–337.

Rethorst, C. D., Wipfli, B. M., & Landers, D. M. (2009). The anti-depressive effects of exercise: A meta-analysis of randomized trials. *Sports Med*, 39, 491–511.

Rimer, J., Dwan, K., Lawlor, D. A., et al. (2012). Exercise for depression. *Cochrane Database Syst Rev*, 11, 7.

Roberts, C. K., Little, J. P., & Thyfault, J. P. (2013). Modification of insulin sensitivity and glycemic control by activity and exercise. *Med Sci Sports Exerc*, 45, 1868–1877.

Robertson, R., Robertson, A., Jepson, R., et al. (2012). Walking for depression or depressive symptoms: A systematic review and meta-analysis. *Ment Health Phys Act*, 5, 66–75.

Rooks, D. S. (2008). Talking to patients with fibromyalgia about physical activity and exercise. *Curr Opin Rheumatol, 20,* 208–212.

Scharff, D. P., Homan, S., Kreuter, M., et al. (1999). Factors associated with physical activity in women across the life span: Implications for program development. *Women Health, 29,* 115–134.

Schwab, P., & Klein, R. F. (2008). Nonpharmacological approaches to improve bone health and reduce osteoporosis. *Curr Opin Rheumatol, 20,* 213–217.

Speck, B. J., & Harrell, J. S. (2003). Maintaining regular physical activity in women: Evidence to date. *J Cardiovasc Nurs, 18,* 282–291; quiz 292–293.

Stanton, R., Happell, B., Hayman, M., et al. (2014). Exercise intervention for the treatment of affective disorders—Research to practice. *Front Psychiatry, 5,* 46.

Sternfeld, B. S., Ainsworth, B. E., & Quesenberry, C. P. (1999). Physical activity patterns in a diverse population of women. *Am J Prev Med, 28,* 313–323.

Stevens, J., Cai, J., Evenson, K. R., et al. (2002). Fitness and fatness as predictors of mortality from all causes and from cardiovascular disease in men and women in the lipid research clinics study. *Am J Epidemiol, 156,* 832–841.

Tabata, I., Nishimura, K., Kouzaki, M., et al. (1996). Effects of moderate-intensity endurance and high-intensity intermittent training on anaerobic capacity and VO2max. *Med Sci Sports Exerc, 28,* 1327–1330.

Thompson, C. J., Boddy, K., Stein, K., et al. (2011). Does participating in physical activity in outdoor natural environments have a greater effect on physical and mental wellbeing than physical activity indoors? A systematic review. *Environ Sci Technol, 45,* 1761–1772.

Tudor-Locke, C., Schuma, J. M., Fresman, L., et al. (2014). Changing the way we work: Elevating energy expenditure with workstation alternatives. *Int J Obes (Lond), 38,* 755–765.

van Uffelen, J. G., van Gellecum, Y. R., Burton, N. W., et al. (2013). Sitting-time, physical activity, and depressive symptoms in mid-aged women. *Am J Prev Med, 45,* 276–281.

US Department of Health and Human Services. (2008). *Physical activity guidelines for Americans.* Retrieved from www.health.gov/paguidelines/guidelines/

van Poppel, M. N., & Brown, W. J. (2008). "It's my hormones, doctor"—Does physical activity help with menopausal symptoms? *Menopause, 15,* 78–85.

Warburton, D. E., Charlesworth, S., Ivey, A., et al. (2010). A systematic review of the evidence for Canada's Physical Activity Guidelines for Adults. *Int J Behav Nutr Phys Act, 7.*

Wallace, J., Raglin, J., & Jastremski, C. (1995). Twelve month adherence of adults who joined a fitness program with a spouse vs without a spouse. *J Sports Med Phys Fitness, 35,* 206–213.

Wolin, K. Y., Yan, Y., Colditz, G. A., et al., (2009). Physical activity and colon cancer prevention: A meta-analysis. *Br J Cancer, 100,* 611–616.

World Health Organization, Geneva. (2010). Global recommendations on physical activity for health. Retrieved from http://www.who.int/dietphysicalactivity/publications/9789241599979/en/

5

Mind–Body Therapies

RITA BENN

CASE STUDY

Susan expressed her delight today at turning 60. She thought she would never live to see this day. Two years ago she was diagnosed with stage IV lung cancer after an 8-year remission from breast cancer. I first met Susan one week after she got this news. She was extremely distressed. Fear and anxiety were interrupting her ability to get anything done during the day. Feelings of anger at her husband over the divorce that occurred almost a decade ago kept resurfacing. She approached our weekly drop-in meditation program with an intention to find equanimity. Almost immediately she experienced relief. In the days that followed, she immersed herself with listening to meditation podcasts. Slowly she gained confidence that she was doing "it" right and was able to sit through a practice without any observable agitation for almost a half hour at a time. She was able to let go of the belief that meditation and yoga was a betrayal of her religion, and along with that, a few of her old church friends who met these practices with disapproval. Through chemotherapy treatment, snowy weather, retirement, and deaths of newly made friends, Susan was unwavering in her commitment to not miss one drop-in session. While she still struggles to maintain a regular sitting practice at home, she is the first to advocate to any newcomer how much these mind–body sessions sustain her. To date, Susan's scans show no evidence of cancer.

Introduction

Mind–body therapies are widely used by the public. In the 2002 Centers for Disease Control and Prevention (CDC) population-based survey of 31,000 adults, mind–body therapies, excluding prayer, was the second largest category of use of complementary therapies (Barnes et al., 2002). In the next administration of this survey, Barnes and colleagues (2008) reported that, overall, 16.6% of US adults, representing 34.1 million Americans, used at least one mind–body therapy in the past year. Deep breathing exercises were most commonly used (12.7%), followed by meditation (9.4%), yoga (6.1%), progressive muscle relaxation (2.9%), and guided imagery (2.2%), while tai chi and qigong were used by 1% and 0.3%, respectively. Use of hypnosis and biofeedback remained relatively uncommon (each 0.2%; Barnes, Bloom & Nahin, 2008). The most recent CDC report investigating complementary therapy use with 34,525 adults indicates that mind–body therapies are still widely popular, with marked regional variation (Peregoy et al., 2014). The practice of yoga with deep breathing or meditation is approximately 40% higher in the Pacific and Mountain regions than in the United States overall.

Exclusive users of mind–body medicine, in contrast to those who exclusively use nonvitamin natural products, reveal significant differences (Prasad et al., 2013). They are more likely to be women (60% vs. 49.1%), of younger age (less than 49 years), educated beyond high school (68% vs 60.9%) and from diverse multiethnic origins. From a health perspective, the statistics suggest that individuals practicing mind–body therapies are also more likely to report more mental health problems related to anxiety and depression than other users of CAM therapies.

> I was first introduced to meditation in college. In practicing meditation for the past 35 years, I have come to appreciate how this simple practice of sitting still has helped anchor me to the fullness of the present moment, allowing me to deeply experience a connection to an underlying sense of wholeness. Meditation has been, and continues to be, a repeated invitation to meet and explore the relationship of my feelings, thoughts, and reactions to the external world and regain a sense of balance, acceptance, and gratitude for all that life brings.

The purpose of this chapter is to demonstrate how mind–body practices may optimize health and reduce distress in women. There has been a tremendous increase in the number of well-controlled studies and systematic reviews published in the past several years. The chapter begins with a description of mind–body therapies and their underlying mechanisms. A discussion of the relationship between health and stress follows. Key findings from systematic reviews and meta-analyses on the effectiveness of mind–body therapies along with examples of recent randomized controlled trials (RCTs) in specific areas of women's health are presented. The chapter concludes with implications for clinical practice, suggesting how providers may use mind–body options as adjunctive treatment as well as for the promotion of health.

Description of Mind–Body Therapies

Mind–body therapies consist of a variety of techniques that have their origins in Asian healing systems, European medical practices, and Western psychological therapies. Meditation, hypnosis, and movement therapies, such as yoga and tai chi, are some examples. Mind–body therapies share a common assumption that an inner-directed experiential practice can alleviate tensions and stress originating in the mind and/or expressed in the body.

The National Center for Complementary and Alternative Medicine (NCCAM) of the National Institutes of Health (NIH) defined mind–body approaches as those "practices that focus on the interactions of the brain, mind, body and behavior, with the intent to use the mind to affect physical functioning and promote health" (NCCAM, n.d.). While conventional psychological approaches such as support groups and cognitive behavioral therapies adhere to this definition, they are not typically considered complementary from the biomedicine perspective. This chapter will focus on practices that are more typically considered in the mind–body therapeutic realm. A list of these practices, with definitions, is presented in Table 5.1.

Often clients ask what form of relaxation or meditation they should learn. I recommend that individuals use a technique that most resonates with them. Just as there are many different types of physical exercise that have aerobic benefits, there are also a range of mind–body practices. Most meditation techniques emphasize inner stillness, using an internal point of focus, such as silently repeating a mantra, following the flow of the breath or body movements, or centering on a loving phrase. Like exercise, it may not matter which technique one uses. The key is to consistently incorporate its practice into one's daily routine.

Table 5.1. Descriptions of Common Mind–Body Techniques

Mind–Body Technique	Definition
Autogenics	Use of self-guided verbal instructions directed to a specific body function (e.g., my forehead is cool, etc.) in order to alter that physiological response.
Biofeedback	External feedback of bodily measurements (e.g., brain waves, heart rate) provided from a device connected to the skin, heart, or scalp and used to modulate a physiological response. Some common biofeedback approaches are known as EMG, heartmath, or neurofeedback.
Breathwork	The active direction of attention to inhalation and exhalation of the breath, and/or its pacing or volume, to cultivate various states of awareness. Common breathing techniques include deep abdominal breathing, alternate nostril breathing, chaotic breathing, and practices known as holotropic breathwork.
Expressive writing	A structured or unstructured process of journaling used to uncover deep thoughts, feelings, and new meanings. Studied practices involve writing 15 minutes daily or several times per week on the effect and meaning of health events or symptoms.
Guided imagery	Directed verbal instructions that invoke sensory images to facilitate awareness and mastery of feelings, emotions, thoughts, and tensions. The imagery may include pleasant scenes, physiologically directed functions, mental performance, or receptive or metaphoric foci.
Healing Arts	
Art therapy	The process of using specific media and materials to stimulate awareness, relaxation, and/or resolution of feelings, emotions, and conflicts.
Dance therapy	The use of choreographed or improvised movement with music to facilitate expression of feelings, emotions, conflicts, tension release, mood alteration, and relaxation.
Music therapy	The process of listening to specific musical pieces, using one's voice, or playing instruments to create musical compositions or sounds geared to alleviate physical and psychological symptoms.
Hypnosis	Guided facilitation of ideas, suggestions, and mental imagery to induce a state of inner absorption and focused attention that allows for new perceptions and behavior changes to emerge.

(*continued*)

Table 5.1. Continued

Mind–Body Technique	Definition
Meditation	The process of intentionally directed attention to create a state of inner stillness or awareness that may be facilitated by the use and/or focus of a mantra, word, phrase, sound, image, or breath. There are hundreds of types of meditation practices. Popular forms include transcendental meditation (TM), mindfulness meditation (also known as Vipassana or insight), mindfulness-based stress reduction (MBSR), mindfulness-based cognitive therapy (MBCT), loving kindness, relaxation response, and Zen.
Movement-related meditations	
Yoga	A system of practice of various physical postures (asanas) and breathing techniques to align the body's musculoskeletal structure and emotional equilibrium. All yoga stems from hatha yoga. Different schools emphasize various dimensions according to its pre-eminent teacher. Iyengar, Vinyasa, Anusara, Ashtanga, Bikram, and Bhakti yoga are the most common forms.
Tai chi	A system of slow coordinated sequences of graceful movements that flow into one another to achieve steadiness in mind and body. Many styles exist (such as Chen, Sun, Wu, and Yang) which vary in terms of intensity and rhythm.
Qigong (internal)	A system of slow, gentle and deliberate circular movements, breathwork and meditation to improve the flow of "Qi" (life force) and emotional stability.
Progressive muscle relaxation (PMR)	The release of emotional and muscular tension through conscious attention of flexing and release of various muscle joints and groups. The term "applied relaxation" uses this technique in collaboration with breathing to achieve a conditioned response.

THEORETICAL MECHANISMS OF ACTION

All mind–body therapies focus on inducing a state of physiological relaxation and stillness. The mental and physical awareness that arises through relaxation can induce positive affective states and facilitate recognition of negative emotions and thought patterns that are held outside of everyday consciousness. Over time, individuals may gain insights that can help restore psychological and physical well-being. Mind–body therapies can be thought of as medicine as they engage physiological and psychological processes that reduce distress, facilitate well-being, and promote health (Ader, 2007; Jacobs, 2001; McEwen & Lasley, 2002; Steptoe, Wardle, & Marmot, 2005). Increasingly, psychoneuro-endocrine and immunological research is validating the interconnection of our biology with our psychology (McDonald, O'Connell, & Lutgendorf, 2013; Eisenberger & Cole, 2012; Fredrickson et al., 2013).

Stress, Positive Affect, and Health Outcomes

The role that stress plays in exacerbating illness is now well documented by epidemiological and outcome-based research. Long-term exposure to stress is demonstrated to predispose individuals to (1) increased cardiovascular risk (McEwen & Lasley, 2002), leading to strokes and heart attacks (Irribarren et al. 2000; Mittleman et al. 1995; Williams & Chesney, 1993; Wittstein et al. 2005), and (2) weakened immune functioning (McEwen & Lasley, 2002; Segerstrom & Miller, 2004), resulting in increased inflammation (Weik, Herforth, Kolb-Bachofen, & Deinzer, 2008) and greater susceptibility to colds (Cohen, Alper, Doyle, Treanor, & Turner, 2006), allergies (Hoglund et al. 2006), and a variety of other illnesses (Chandola, Brunner, & Marmot, 2006; Cohen, Janicki-Deverts, & Miller, 2007). There are increasing numbers of studies that link stress with the risk of breast, ovarian, and cervical cancers (Fang et al. 2008; Helgesson, Cabrera, Lapidus, Bengtsson, & Lissner, 2003; Lillberg et al. 2003; Thacker et al. 2006). Using animal models, researchers have shown how catecholamines, glu-cocorticoids, and other stress hormones influence the progression of cancer by altering the tumor microenvironment (Antoni et al., 2006; Lutgendorf & Sood, 2011). Advances in genomics-based research are now clarifying the molecular pathways by which psychological and social factors regulate tumor cell gene expression (Cole, 2013). Analysis of genomic transcriptions of leukocytes in patients with cancer and others diseases suggest that stress and negative affective states appear to be mapped along the same disease and inflammation pathways (Cole, 2014; Denniger, Libermann, Antoni, Irwin, & Manoj, 2014). A recent study has demonstrated that psychosocial interventions can causally influence gene expression in cancer patients, down-regulating pro-inflammatory and metastasis-related genes (Antoni et al., 2012).

In the last decade, studies have begun to demonstrate how stress can change genomic structures. In individuals overburdened by caregiving, such as moth-ers whose children have a disability (Eppel et al., 2004) and women caregiv-ers of family members with Alzheimer's (Damjanovic et al., 2007), or women exposed to trauma, such as domestic violence (Humphreys et al., 2011), genomic structures controlling cell division become permanently altered. Blood samples depict shortened telomere length, suggesting premature biological aging. New research findings suggest that it is not only chronic stress over a long duration that can have this high-risk impact. In a study of 239 postmenopausal healthy women, Puterman, Lin, Krauss, Blackburn, and Epel (2014) determined that the accumulation of life stressors in a year's time predicted telomere attrition. Furthermore, each additional life stress event accelerated the shortening of telomeres. Engaging in healthier lifestyle behaviors (as measured by physical activity, sleep quality, and diet) seemed to moderate its impact.

The accumulation of stressors that influence telomere shortening may place women at higher risk for other chronic diseases. Johansson et al. (2013) interviewed and followed 800 women in Sweden for four decades. They found that women at midlife who experienced a greater number of common life stressors, as well as those with long-standing distress, were at higher risk for developing dementia and Alzheimer's later in life. Moreover, it did not seem to matter whether a woman continued to feel "stressed out" by the event.

Experiencing purpose in life and positive affect may serve as a buffer against life challenges and help promote health (Cohen, Doyle, Turner, Alper, & Skoner, 2003; Steptoe, Demakakos, de Oliveira, & Wardle, 2012; Steptoe, Wardle, & Marmot, 2005). Danner, Snowden, and Friesen (2001) examined the journals of 180 Catholic nuns over their lifetime and found a positive relationship between expressed positive affect and longevity. A strong association between psychological well-being with reduced mortality in both healthy and diseased populations was revealed in a meta-analysis of 70 published prospective studies (Chida & Steptoe, 2008) and corroborated by several longitudinal studies (Davidson et al. 2010; Steptoe et al., 2012; Xu & Roberts, 2010). Investigations of biological correlates of well-being and gendered effects are suggesting different patterns for men and women. Steptoe et al. (2012), using a sample of close to 8,000 participants, describes that for women, well-being is related to lower levels of inflammatory markers and HDL cholesterol, independent of age, illness, wealth, and other confounders. Based on a large midlife sample, frequency of positive events measured through momentary sampling over eight days was also linked to lower inflammatory markers of interleukin-6 (IL-6) for both women and men (Sin, Graham-Engeland, & Almeida, 2014).

One of the by-products of practicing meditation and yoga is an embodied contentment during or immediately after a period of practice. As a novice, this experience may be short-lived. With continued practice, this felt sense of ease is maintained for longer and longer periods. I often recommend to patients to not have the expectation that they will always have this type of positive experience. I do feel confident to assure them that with continuing practice, they will feel this benefit more often and access it more easily in their everyday life.

THE GENDERED EXPERIENCE OF STRESS

Women report high levels of stress and unhappiness that consequently place them at increased risk for disease. A national survey ($n = $ 1,848) indicates that 82% of women perceive that stress negatively impacts their health and well-being (American Psychological Association, 2007). Women describe higher levels of stress than men in both psychological symptoms (irritability or anger, nervousness, and lacking energy) and physical symptoms (fatigue, headaches, upset stomach, muscular tension, and change in appetite). It is noteworthy that these same symptoms contribute to 60%–90% of primary care visits (Fava & Sonino, 2005).

Women describe that they experience a greater number of stressful life events and are more negatively influenced by them than men, even when their exposure rate is similar (Davis, 1999; Tolin & Foa, 2006). More women than men also indicate that they handle stress poorly (American Psychological Association, 2007). National statistics report that women at every age are more likely than their male counterparts to report unhealthy eating behaviors due to stress (American Psychological Association, 2014). Under periods of stress, more women than men give up healthy activities, such as exercise, even though they tend to perceive it as more beneficial to their sense of well-being. At work, women report feeling less valued (American Psychological Association, 2013), and as they age, they report less happiness and more dissatisfaction with their lives than do men (Plagnol & Easterlin, 2008). A higher prevalence of affective and anxiety disorders has been observed for women over their lifetime (Kessler et al., 1994).

Recent findings suggest a gender-specific neural activation model underlying the stress response. Researchers observed functional magnetic resonance imaging (fMRI) results of 32 men and women undergoing stressful tasks; the men had increased blood flow to the left orbital frontal cortex, the area presumed to activate resources for the "flight and fight" response, while in women, stress activated the limbic system, the area associated with processing of emotions (Wang et al., 2007). In a more recent study, additional gender differences were found in brain areas responsible for interpretation of interpersonal emotion (Mather, Lighthall, Nga, & Gorlick, 2010). Women under stress showed increased activity in the brain area involved with visual processing of emotions and coordination among parts of the brain that help interprets emotional faces, while men showed decreased function in both these areas.

Many studies using imaging techniques with large samples are now showing gender differences in the functional organization of the human brain (Tomasi & Volkow, 2012). Reports indicate that cortical networks show greater overall anatomical connectivity and more efficient organization in the female than the male brain. Analyses of areas of connectivity suggest that female brains are more structured to facilitate communication between analytical and intuitive processing modes than male brains (Ingalhalikar et al., 2014). Differences in the functional organization of the brain and psychological and neurobiological response to stress may have implications for the kinds of interventions that providers recommend. Mind–body interventions that access emotional and intuitive pathways may have more beneficial effects for women than those that focus on prefrontal areas that emphasize cognitive-focused solutions.

For women, group-based interventions incorporating mind–body instruction may have added benefit. A "tend-and-befriend" model has been posited to characterize women's need for relationship and support during times of stress (Taylor, 2002). Studies of female laboratory animal responses exposed to stress reveal nurturing and affiliative behavior with other animals in contrast to the aggressive or withdrawal responses evident in males (Taylor, Klein, Lewis, Gruenewald, Gurung, & Updegraff, 2000). In laboratory situations, observational experiments of men and women under stress confirm this differential pattern of response (Tomova, Dawans, Heinrichs, Silani, & Lamm, 2014). Stressed males tend to become more self-centered and less able to distinguish their own emotions and intentions from those of other people. For women, the exact opposite occurred; they offered more prosocial, empathic behaviors. Hence, providing group-based social support when learning mind–body therapies may optimize this sense of reciprocity and inclusion and enhance the value of mind–body experiences over and above one-on-one instruction.

Changes in lifestyle behaviors to incorporate daily mind–body practice may serve as an antidote to women's experience of normative daily stress and boost their capacity to resist inflammation and illness. For example, Black et al. (2013) demonstrated in a small sample ($n = 39$) of women caregivers of dementia family members that those who practiced daily kriya meditation (chanting), in contrast to those who listened to relaxing music (chanting), were able to reverse a pattern of up-regulation of pro-inflammatory signaling pathways and down-regulation of antiviral pathways. Psycho-immunological researchers are suggesting that inflammation and accelerated aging represent important predisease mechanisms that may be improved or worsened through multiple behavioral and biomedical pathways (Kiecolt-Glaser, Jaremka, Derry, & Glaser, 2013).

Several studies have begun to show significant associations between increased telomerase length and telomerase enzymatic activity in both healthy and nonhealthy individuals who commit to regular practice of meditation (Jacobs et al., 2011; Ornish et al., 2013). A meta-analysis of four RCTs ($n = 190$) examining the impact of mindfulness meditation found a medium size effect on increasing telomerase activity (Schutte & Malouff, 2014). Hoge et al. (2013) reported that long-term practice of loving kindness along with mindfulness-based meditation was significantly associated with increased telomere length, only, however, for women. Given the different physiological make-up and gendered experience of stress, it may be that mind–body practices that focus on opening the heart to oneself and others, offer greater comfort and resilience for women than men.

> Susan is a great example of how a stress-management group in which women learn mind–body practices can be of enormous benefit. Within the safe context of a group, a woman may feel empowered to look at herself and respond to physical or mental health challenges in new ways. By experimenting with mind–body practices, women can discover an inner voice that reveals a very deep place of knowing. In listening generously to one another, the sense of acceptance grows and women feel their own sense of agency, emboldened to move forward with their lives.

Mind–Body Therapies on Health Conditions: Evidence

In 2003, Astin, Shapiro, Eisenberg, and Forys examined 28 systematic reviews (N = 46,045) of studies on various mind–body therapies. The authors concluded that the strength of mind–body research compared favorably with other areas of medical research. To date, an update using this broad lens has not been replicated. In the last decade, many systematic reviews have examined the effectiveness of mind–body interventions on pain management, stress, and symptoms specific to or comorbid with various diseases such as cancer, fibromyalgia, and cardiovascular disease (Chen et al., 2012; Chiesa & Serretti, 2011a; Emani & Binkley, 2010; Goyal et al., 2014; Langhorst, Klose, Dobos, Bernardy, & Häuser, 2013; Lee, Kim, Ha, Boddy, & Ernst, 2009; Mayden, 2012; Mist et al., 2013). Small to medium changes in effect size have been shown for the inflammatory markers Il-6 and C-reactive protein (CRP), with a very small effect change on tumor necrosis factor (TNF) (Morgan, Irwin, Chung, & Wang, 2014). Evidence for some improvement in regard to general pain, anxiety, or depression symptoms as a result of mind–body practice is found in these reviews.

Investigation of the effectiveness of individual mind–body therapies on specific heath conditions has also proliferated. *CAM on Pubmed* lists more than 600 clinical trials on yoga, meditation, and tai chi effects on health outcomes that have been published in the period 2010–2015. An abundant number of systematic reviews on these and other mind–body practices (biofeedback, hypnosis, qigong, guided imagery, expressive arts, writing, and music therapies) summarize the various adaptations in which they have been delivered with different populations and studied (see for example, Bardt, Dileo, Grocke, & Magill, 2011; Bernardy, Füber, Klose, & Häuser, 2011; Boehm, Cramer, Staroszynski, & Ostermann, 2014; Cepeda et al., 2006; Chiesa & Serretti, 2011b; Cramer, Lange, Klose, Paul, & Dobos, 2012; Cramer, Lauche, Langhorst, & Dobos, 2013; Cramer et al., 2104a; Cramer et al., 2104b; Hackney & Wolf, 2014; Hartley, Flowers, Lee, Ernst, & Rees, 2014; Jahnke et al., 2010; Keng, Smoski, & Robins, 2011; Lauche, Cramer, Dobos, Langhorst, & Schmidt, 2013; McCall, Ward, Roberts, & Heneghan, 2013; Montgomery, Schnur, & Kravits, 2013; Musial, Büssing, Heusser, Choi, & Ostermann, 2011; Nightingale, Rodriguez, & Carnaby, 2013; Orme-Johnson & Barnes, 2014; Schaefert, Klose, Moser, & Häuser, 2014; Schoenberg & David, 2014; Wang et al. 2013; J. Wang, Xiong, & Liu, 2013; Jahnke, Larkey, Rogers, Etnier, & Lin, 2010; Zeng, Luo, Xie, Huang, & Cheng, 2014). Only a very small number of these reviews use meta-analyses to provide pooled estimates of data, and even fewer isolate or discuss the relationship of gender to specific health effects. The lack of attention to this subgroup analysis may inflate or deflate the strength of the findings and hinder drawing firm conclusions.

Overall, findings have suggested that mind–body therapies do provide relief from emotional distress in the short term. Mindfulness meditation, in particular, has shown small to moderate size effects for alleviation of anxiety, depression, and pain (Carlson, 2012; Chen et al., 2012; Goyal et al., 2014; Khoury et al., 2013). When considering long-term effects or improvements on disease-specific biological markers, the results are not as impressive. The heterogeneity in outcome measures, implementation of the investigated therapy, types of controls, and sample sizes, make it challenging to make recommendations with confidence for the use of one mind–body therapy over another. These issues are also reflected when examining the research on the effects for women's health.

DYSMENORRHEA, PREGNANCY, AND FERTILITY

For patients with primary and secondary dysmenorrhea, a Cochrane systematic review (Proctor, Murphy, Pattison, Suckling, & Farquhar, 2009) of five trials ($N = 213$) found progressive muscle relaxation (PMR), with or without imagery, to be helpful for spasmodic pain. No other published studies examining the effect of mind–body therapies for this condition have been published.

Systematic reviews examining the effects of relaxation and mind–body therapies during pregnancy suffer from severe methodological limitations (Beddoe & Lee, 2008; Khianman, Pattanittum, Thinkhamrop, & Lumbiganon, 2012).

Based on three RCTs (with $n = 110$; 58; 31) that evaluated the effect of a specific mind–body therapy (applied relaxation, guided imagery, or mindfulness meditation) on anxiety using the same measurement tool (Bastani, Hidarnia, Kazemnejad, Vafaei, & Kashanian, 2005; Teixeira et al., 2005; Vietin & Astin, 2008), significant pre–post reductions were demonstrated for each of these therapies. Two of the studies used 5- to 8-week group-based classes of mind–body techniques, while the other provided only a single experiential session. A Cochrane review that included 556 participants from eight RCTs (two of which were included above) investigating the effectiveness of mind–body interventions (autogenics, imagery, yoga, PMR, and tai chi) on anxiety in pregnancy also found significant improvement (Marc et al., 2011).

Mindfulness-based stress reduction (MBSR) is an 8-week group-based meditation program that is widely available in hospitals and communities to assist patients in coping more effectively with stress and chronic pain in their lives. Since its inception, many MBSR programs have been adapted to focus on unique issues in different populations. For expectant parents, two mindfulness programs have been piloted (CALM, Coping with Anxiety through Living Mindfully, and MIL, Mindfulness in Labor) with small samples, and preliminary results show significant positive effects on coping with anxiety from pre- to post testing (Duncan & Bardacke, 2010; Goodman et al., 2014). In comparison with a control group, MIL participants had significantly lower depressive symptoms post program, and this difference grew in magnitude post partum (Duncan et al., 2014).

Despite the popularity of yoga among women in North America, its impact during pregnancy, labor, and delivery has not been well studied (Babbar, Parks-Savage, & Chauhan, 2012; Curtis, Weinrib, & Katz, 2012). Systematic reviews have reported five trials with control groups and sizable samples, all of which were conducted outside the United States and Canada. Significant differences on at least one of the measured outcomes, including anxiety, were observed, and no adverse events reported for maternal or fetal variables. Subsequent to this review, an RCT investigating the impact of yoga with 68 high-risk pregnant women was published that demonstrated significantly fewer pregnancy complications (i.e., pregnancy-induced hypertension, preeclampsia, gestational diabetes, and intrauterine growth restriction), as well as fewer babies born small for gestational age or with lower Apgar scores (Rakhshani et al., 2012).

Two additional Cochrane reviews investigated the effect of relaxation and mind–body therapies on preterm labor and birth. One identified 11 randomized studies ($N = 833$) and also found no evidence of benefits or harm for these therapies or supportive counseling (Khianman et al., 2012). Another examined the effects of self-hypnosis in seven RCTs ($n = 1,213$) and found no differences in terms of spontaneous birth, patient satisfaction, and use of analgesics for pharmacological relief (Madden, Middleton, Cyna, Matthewson, & Jones, 2012).

Despite the clinical observation and support in the research literature of the link between stress and fertility (Boivin, Griffiths, & Venetis, 2011; Greil, 1997), there has been little research exploring the influence of mind–body therapies on fertility. Alice Domar and her colleagues (Domar, Clapp, Slawsby, Dusek, et al., 2000; Domar, Clapp, Slawsby, Kessel, et al., 2000) used a RCT to compare the efficacy of a 5-year, 3-arm group-based intervention (10 weeks of a 2-hour cognitive-behavioral program, 10 weeks of a 2-hour social support group, and treatment as usual) with 184 women who had experienced 2 years of infertility. The cognitive-behavioral program included autogenics, relaxation response meditation, PMR, imagery, and cognitive restructuring. All three groups suffered some attrition, with the control group impacted the most heavily. At 12 months, both treatment arms showed significantly lower levels of psychological distress and higher conception rates than the control; and the cognitive-behavioral group showed greater reduction in distress than the social support group. The conception rate in both treatment groups was remarkably similar, 55% and 54%, as compared with 20% for the control.

Domar et al. (2011) subsequently examined whether this same mind–body program could be effective in facilitating fertility in patients undergoing in vitro fertilization (IVF). In a randomized trial of 143 patients, they found higher conception rates after women participated in several of the mind–body sessions than women in the control group: 52% versus 20%. Mind–body practices may help alleviate the intensity of distress that is linked with lower IVF success rates (Boivin et al., 2011). Another controlled study with 90 IVF patients demonstrated that a program of mindfulness was able to relieve distress in the IVF patients, and that these effects appear to be sustained at a 6-month follow-up (Galhardo, Cunha, & Pinto-Gouveia, 2013). Valoriani et al. (2014) demonstrated that a program in yoga was similarly successful only in a subset of highly stressed IVF patients.

MENOPAUSE

Two systematic reviews investigated the influence of mind–body therapies on menopausal symptoms based on clinical trials published before 2009 (Innes, Selfe, & Vishnu, 2010; Lee et al., 2009). Improvements in vasomotor symptoms were noted for these therapies, ranging from 16% to 84% reduction in overall symptoms. A recent Cochrane review investigating the effect of relaxation training on perimenopausal and postmenopausal symptoms included four studies (N = 281) in their analysis and did not find any differences in hot flash severity (Saensak, Vutyavanich, Somboonporn, & Srisurapanont, 2014). Recently, two RCTs with control arms have explored the influence of yoga on the reduction of vasomotor systems and hot flashes in healthy menopausal women (Avis, Legault, Russell, Weaver, & Danhauer, 2014; Newton et al., 2013). Both confirm reduction in hot flash severity and frequency, with no advantage for the yoga arm compared with an exercise or a wellness education treatment arm. Reed et al. (2014) found a modest effect on overall quality of life scale in favor of the yoga intervention group.

Slow breathing is a by-product of the relaxation response invoked through mind–body practices and integral to yoga and meditation. Early research showed that slow deep breathing (paced respiration) seemed effective for decreasing the intensity and/or frequency of hot flashes (Freedman & Woodard 1992, 1995; Irvin, Domar, Clark, Zuttermeister, & Friedman, 1996). Two large randomized trials (Carpenter et al., 2013; Sood et al., 2013) evaluated the effectiveness on hot flash reduction and severity of a paced breathing method, slow abdominal breathing for six to eight breaths per minute, when compared with a normal breathing practice, 14 breaths per minute, or a faster shallow breathing practice. Participants in these groups were instructed to use these methods when triggered as well as to implement a 15-minute practice period once or twice a day. No superiority or difference in reducing hot flash severity was observed in either study. Results from an RCT trial examining the impact of applied relaxation (which includes PMR in this treatment approach) in 60 women found significant reductions in hot flashes as well as changes in vasomotor symptoms on a menopausal quality of life scale (Lindh-Astrand & Nedstrand, 2013).

Elkins, Fisher, Johnson, Carpenter, and Keith (2013) examined the impact of a five-session hypnosis program in 187 postmenopausal women using a RCT design with an attention-control comparison. Results showed significantly greater reductions in hot flashes in the hypnosis over the control group; hot flash frequency was reduced by 64%, compared with a 9% reduction in the control group upon program completion and at week 12, 75%, compared with a 17% reduction.

BREAST CANCER

Various mind–body practices have been offered to breast cancer patients to assist them with their anxiety during and after their treatments, as well as with the ensuing symptoms of pain, fatigue, and nausea. In the last decade, studies have been conducted with more rigor. Few have evaluated the use of hypnosis in cancer care (Montgomery, Schnur, & Kravits, 2013). One unblinded RCT of 200 women scheduled to undergo breast biopsy or lumpectomy illustrated the benefits of short-term hypnotic induction for alleviation of procedural pain and distress (Montgomery et al., 2007). In this study, investigators compared a 15-minute hypnotic intervention to nondirected empathetic listening and measured the use of analgesia and sedatives as well as self-reported pain, nausea, fatigue, and distress. Patients in the hypnosis group required significantly less anesthesia and reported less surgical pain and other measured side effects; there was no difference in the number of recovery room medications.

Many psychosocial interventions have been developed for breast cancer patients and include guided imagery, hypnosis, or relaxation practices as a component (e.g., Andersen, Farrar, et al. 2007; Andersen, Shelby, & Golden-Kreutz, 2007; Gaston-Johansson, 2013). Untangling the benefit of these practices from other treatment aspects has rarely been the focus of research. Faller et al. (2013) examined the impact of 46 trials ($N = 3159$) of relaxation training (defined by stand-alone treatment of relaxation and imagery techniques) in a meta-analysis of 198 studies of psycho-oncology intervention with cancer patients. Small, short-term effects were observed for distress or quality of life independent of the type of cancer. In a study of 227 women with stage II breast cancer receiving cognitive stress reduction with PMR as relaxation adjuvant cancer treatment, patients reported that this relaxation component was the most satisfying aspects of their weekly treatment program (Andersen, Farrar, et al., 2007; Andersen, Shelby, & Golden-Kreutz, 2007).

Research using guided imagery and expressive writing in patients with cancer showed early promise in reducing emotional distress (Low, Stanton, & Danoff-Burg, 2006; Roffe, Schmidt, & Ernst, 2005; Stanton, Danoff-Burg, & Sworowski, 2002). Findings for the benefit of guided imagery have largely been drawn from studies that did not have control groups and were not well designed methodologically. In one of the few RCTs using guided imagery with 80 women undergoing chemotherapy treatment for locally advanced breast cancer, increased immune protection (higher levels of T cell activation) in comparison with usual care was observed (Eremin et al., 2009). A 2006 meta-analysis of the effects of expressive writing showed significant and multiple health benefits for physically healthy individuals as well as those with chronic disease, irrespective of gender (Frattaroli, 2006). Of late, research with larger samples of breast cancer patients has consistently found mixed or null findings regarding its impact whether during or after cancer treatment (Gellaitry, Peters, Bloomfield, & Horne, 2010; Jensen-Johansen et al., 2012).

A substantial body of evidence has emerged with regard to the effectiveness of meditation and yoga in relieving distress and improving fatigue, sleep, and immune function indices. Cramer et al. (2012) reviewed the effect of yoga in women with cancer on psychological health and quality of life in twelve RCTs ($N = 742$ patients). Anxiety, depression, and distress were reduced significantly more for those patients who practiced yoga during active cancer treatment as opposed to after completion of treatment. Another systematic review evaluated cancer fatigue effects in breast cancer survivors. Based on analysis of 10 studies ($N = 583$), the investigators tentatively concluded that yoga interventions had beneficial impact (Sadja & Mills, 2013).

Two subsequent well-designed RCTs add more evidence for this conclusion. Kiecolt-Glaser et al. (2014) studied the impact of a 3-month biweekly yoga program with 200 breast cancer survivors: at 3-month follow-up, significant improvement on fatigue, vitality and inflammatory markers (i.e., IL-6, IL-1B, TNF-α) in comparison with a waitlist control. Surprisingly, no differences on measures of depression emerged. In another multicenter RCT utilizing a biweekly month-long yoga program with 400 cancer survivors (3/4 of whom had been diagnosed with breast cancer), better sleep quality was reported from pre- to postintervention compared with a standard usual arm on both subjective scale and actigraphy measures (Mustian et al., 2013). In addition, investigators reported a significant reduction in sleep medication use for those practicing yoga.

Several reviews have investigated the effects of MBSR-like programs with breast cancer patients (Mayden, 2012; Musial et al., 2011; Zainal, Booth, & Huppert, 2013). In a meta-analysis based on nine trials, MBSR showed significant impact on improving women's mental health, with medium to large effect sizes noted. Since these reviews, additional RCTs have been published with large samples. Two studies following 229 and 336 survivors diagnosed with stages 0 to III breast cancer (Hoffman et al., 2012; Wurtzen et al., 2013) found statistically significant improvements on measures of depression and anxiety immediately post MBSR, as compared with usual care, with sustained benefit observed 12 months later (Hoffman et al., 2012). In another RCT that followed 172 participants with early stage breast cancer over 2 years, immediate positive effects of MBSR on mental health occurred but dissipated over time (Henderson et al., 2012).

Carlson and Speca (2011) adapted MBSR for cancer recovery (mindfulness-based cancer recovery, or MBCR). In their study of 271 breast cancer patients, they found MBCR to be superior in reducing stress and improving quality of life when compared with two active control interventions: a weekly supportive expressive group therapy and a 1-day stress management program (Carlson et al., 2013). Both supportive therapy and MBCR also reduced mood disturbance in contrast to the 1-day intervention. An online modification of this program (Zernicke et al., 2014) found these same positive benefits using a smaller sample of cancer patients (75% were female, but only one-third had breast cancer). Monti et al. (2013) incorporated expressive art with mindfulness-based stress reduction (MBAT) and randomized 191 breast cancer patients of varying ethnicities to either this MBAT 8-week group program or an educational support program. Results showed positive gains for both arms on quality life and symptom stress scales; differences between arms were only significant for the MBAT group among the subgroup identified as highly stressed at baseline.

A few studies have also analyzed the impact of length of practice on outcomes in this population. Hoffman et al. (2012) found a significant relationship between the number of hours of formal mindfulness and home-based practice and improvements on quality of life and mood scores immediately post intervention and at 1-month follow-up. Kiecolt-Glaser et al. (2014) similarly found that more frequent yoga practice produced larger changes on fatigue and vitality scores as well as immune markers. The relationship between increased self-care practice and better outcomes was also observed in Andersen's trial that included PMR; the more frequently women practiced relaxation, the greater the reduction in observed symptoms (Andersen, Farrar, et al. 2007; Andersen, Shelby, & Golden-Kreutz, 2007). Engaging in more frequent home practice with meditation, yoga, or relaxation during and after participation in a formal mind–body intervention appears to have positive sequelae in patients coping with breast cancer.

Implications for Clinical Practice

As shown above, an extensive body of literature has been published and supports the use of a variety of mind–body therapies for women's health. Most mind–body therapies offer positive benefits from psychological distress and in some situations, relief from physical discomfort and pain. Practice guidelines from several professional organizations and societies now include recommendations for mind–body therapies. The American College of Cardiology (Vogel et al., 2005), the American Sleep Association (Morgenthaler et al., 2006), the American College of Physicians (Chou & Huffman, 2007), the American Pain Society (Chou & Huffman, 2007), the American Headache Society (Silberstein, 2000), the American Academy of Neurology (Silberstein, 2000) and most recently, the North American Menopause Society and American Society for Clinical Oncology (Bower et al., 2014) all provide mind–body practice recommendations.

To help women make informed choices, providers need to be able to explain the differences in mind–body techniques and suggest ways to learn them. Many excellent and cost-effective educational CDs and DVDs as well as mobile apps are available. Nonetheless, it is also important to guide women to local resources and teachers. Having the support of a group and experienced teacher cannot be underemphasized. Developing a regular mind–body practice, like any new habit, takes time, motivation, patience, and perseverance. For some women, coaching and regular follow-up will help reinforce their efforts. The more regular patients become in their practice, the more likely they will feel the benefits. There is no harm from increased practice in these therapies. Some women may need monitoring in reducing their dosages of sleep, pain, or hypertension medications as a result of engaging in these practices. For example, Dusek et al. (2008) found that 80 of 122 patients (both male and female) with elevated hypertension were able to reduce their medications after 16 weeks of practicing mindfulness meditation and relaxation techniques.

Since mind–body therapies may be equally effective in alleviating emotional distress or pain, it is important that provider recommendations reflect treatment cost and availability, as well as patient lifestyle, preference, and personality. More physically active patients may find tai chi and yoga easier to adopt as a regular routine than a sitting mindfulness practice. Highly anxious patients or patients challenged by sensory overload can benefit from either a moving meditation practice or a mindfulness or mantra-based sitting meditation practice. By learning to be still over time, patients find they are able to work through their anxiety. Mindfulness-based cognitive therapy (MBCT) can also be of use to patients with more severe clinical depression and anxiety.

Healthcare providers may want to consider developing their own personal mind–body practice. Studies demonstrate that physicians are more likely to recommend a mind–body practice if they themselves have some personal experience (Astin, Goddard, & Forys, 2005; Astin, Soeken, Sierpina, & Clarridge, 2006). Primary care physicians participating in MBSR programs report feeling less depressed and burned out (Fortney, Luchterhand, Zakletskaia, Zgierska, & Rakel, 2013; Krasner et al., 2009), and are better able to listen more deeply and respond more effectively to their patients concerns (Beckman et al., 2012). Research is beginning to demonstrate an association between physician mindfulness and improved patient communication and patient satisfaction (Beach et al., 2013). In a study of psychotherapists in training, psychiatric patients reported greater satisfaction with the course of their therapy and showed less distress if their providers had practiced Zen meditation prior to their sessions (Grepmair, Mitterlehner, Loew, Bachler, et al., 2007; Grepmair, Mitterlehner, Loew, & Nickel, 2007).

I often suggest that practitioners develop a brief ritual in between seeing their patients in order to help them re-engage and be present with each new person they see. Before knocking on the door of the next patient, providers can pause and slowly take several deep breaths. Or they can silently repeat the name of the patient they are about to see and direct a simple four-phrase loving-kindness meditation: "May you live in safety. May you be happy. May you be healthy, May you live with ease." Alternatively, thoughts of gratitude after seeing each patient may be brought to awareness. Practitioners can also actively use the hand-washing process as a deliberate point of focus for clearing their mind, paying attention to the flow of the water and sensations touching each finger. Any of these strategies may help providers replenish themselves, refocus, and re-engage with their own healing presence so they can truly be present to each patient.

Summary

Stress is a condition of life that can adversely affect the health and well-being of women. Research demonstrates that mind–body therapies can mitigate symptoms of emotional distress and facilitate positive well-being. With some mind–body therapies, such as meditation, the evidence is strong for improving anxiety and distress in healthy people, as well as in individuals struggling with chronic disease. Both mindfulness stress reduction and transcendental meditation approaches have been shown to be efficacious. Other than anxiety, there are no consistent reports of benefit for use of mind–body therapies during pregnancy, or for symptoms related to women's hormonal fluctuations (dysmenorrhea, hot flashes). Evidence for reducing inflammatory markers and improving immune function is accumulating for women with breast cancer from yoga practice; yoga may help serve a protective function in healthy people as well as those with illness. At the present time, healthcare providers can feel comfortable that there is sufficient evidence to recommend a mind–body practice to women for both health promotion and disease prevention.

REFERENCES

Ader, R. (Ed.). (2007). *Psychoneuroimmunology* (Vols. 1–2, 4th ed.). New York: Elsevier Academic Press.

American Psychological Association. (2007). *Stress in America*. Retrieved October 24, 2007, from http://apahelpcenter.mediaroom.com/file.php/138/Stress+in+America+REPORT+FINAL.doc

American Psychological Association. (2013). *2013 work and well-being survey*. Retrieved June 10, 2013, from http://c.ymcdn.com/sites/www.newonline.org/resource/resmgr/research/2013-work-and-wellbeing-surv.pdf

American Psychological Association. (2014). *2014 stress in America: Are teens adopting adults' stress habits?* Retrieved April 15, 2014, from http://www.apa.org/news/press/releases/stress/2013/stress-report.pdf

Andersen, B. L., Farrar, W. B., Golden-Kreutz, D., Emery, C. F., Glaser, R., Crespin, T., & Carson, W. E. (2007). Distress reduction from a psychological intervention contributes to improved health for cancer patients. *Brain Behav Immun, 21,* 953–961.

Andersen, B. L., Shelby, R. A., & Golden-Kreutz, D. M. (2007). RCT of a psychological intervention for patients with cancer: I. Mechanisms of change. *J Consult Clin Psychol, 75,* 927–938.

Antoni, M. H., Lutgendorf, S. K., Cole, S. W., et al. (2006). The influence of bio-behavioural factors on tumour biology: Pathways and mechanisms. *Nat Rev Cancer, 6,* 240–248.

Antoni, M. H., Lutgendorf, S. K., Blomberg, B., Carver, C. S., Lechner, S., Diaz, A., ... Cole, S. W. (2012). Cognitive-behavioral stress management reverses anxiety-related leukocyte transcriptional dynamics. *Biol Psychiatr, 71,* 366–372.

Astin, J. A., Goddard, T. G., & Forys, K. L. (2005). Barriers to the integration of mind-body medicine: Perceptions of physicians, residents, and medical students. *Explore, 1,* 278–283.

Astin, J. A., Shapiro, S. L., Eisenberg, D. M., & Forys, K. L. (2003). Mind-body medicine: State of the science, implications for practice. *J Am Brd Fam Prac, 16,* 131–147.

Astin, J. A., Soeken, K., Sierpina, V. S., & Clarridge, B. R. (2006). Barriers to the integration of psychosocial factors in medicine: Results of a national survey of physicians. *J Am Board Fam Med, 19,* 557–565.

Avis, N., Legault, C., Russell, G., Weaver, K., & Danhauer, S. (2014). A pilot study of integral yoga for menopausal hot flashes. *Menopause, 21,* 846–854.

Babbar, S., Parks-Savage, A. C., & Chauhan, S. P. (2012). Yoga during pregnancy: A review. *Am J Perinatol, 29,* 459–464.

Barnes, P. M., Powell-Griner, E., McFann, K., & Nahin, R. L. (2004). Complementary and alternative medicine use among adults: United States, 2002. *Adv Data* May 27(343), 1–19.

Bastani, F., Hidarnia, A., Kazemnejad, A., Vafaei, M., & Kashanian, M. (2005). A randomized controlled trial of the effects of applied relaxation training on reducing anxiety and perceived stress in pregnant women. *J Midwifery Womens Health, 50,* e36–e40.

Barnes, P. M., Bloom, B., & Nahin, R. CDC National Health Statistics Report #12. Complementary and Alternative Medicine Use Among Adults and Children: United States, 2007. December 10, 2008.

Beach, M. C., Roter, D., Korthuis, P. T., Epstein, R. M., Sharp, V., Ratanawongsa, N., ... Saha, S. (2013). A multicenter study of physician mindfulness and health care quality. *Ann Fam Med, 11,* 421–428.

Beckman, H. B., Wendland, M., Mooney, C., Krasner, M. S., Quill, T. E., Suchman, A. L., & Epstein, R. M. (2012). The impact of a program in mindful communication on primary care physicians. *Acad Med*, *87*, 815–819.

Beddoe, A. E., & Lee, K. A. (2008). Mind-body interventions during pregnancy. *J Obstet Gynecol Neonatal Nurs*, *37*, 165–175.

Bernardy, K., Füber, N., Klose, P., & Häuser, W. (2011). Efficacy of hypnosis/guided imagery in fibromyalgia syndrome—A systematic review and meta-analysis of controlled trials. *BMC Musculoskelet Disord*, *12*, 133.

Black, D. S., Cole, S. W., Irwin, M. R., Breen, E., St Cyr, N. M., Nazarian, N., … Lavretsky, H. (2013). Yogic meditation reverses NF-ΐ°B and IRF-related transcriptome dynamics in leukocytes of family dementia caregivers in a randomized controlled trial. *Psychoneuroendocrino*, *38*, 348.

Boehm, K., Cramer, H., Staroszynski, T., & Ostermann, T. (2014). Arts therapies for anxiety, depression, and quality of life in breast cancer patients: A systematic review and meta-analysis. *Evid Based Complement Alternat Med*, *2014*, 103297.

Boivin, J, Griffiths, E., & Venetis, C. A. (2011). Emotional distress in infertile women and failure of assisted reproductive technologies: Meta-analysis of prospective psychosocial studies. *BMJ*, *23*, 342.

Bower, J. E., Bak, K., Berger, A., Breitbart, W., Escalante, C. P., Ganz, P. A., … Jacobsen, P. B (2014). Screening, assessment, and management of fatigue in adult survivors of cancer: An American Society of Clinical Oncology clinical practice guideline adaptation. *J Clin Oncol*, *32*, 1840–1850.

Bradt, J., Dileo, C., Grocke, D., & Magill, L. (2011). Music interventions for improving psychological and physical outcomes in cancer patients. *Cochrane Database Syst Rev*, 8:CD006911. doi: 10.1002/14651858.CD006911.pub2

CAM on PubMed. Available from http://nccam.nih.gov/research/camonpubmed

Carlson, L. E. (2012). Mindfulness-based interventions for physical conditions: A narrative review evaluating levels of evidence. *ISRN Psychiatry*, *2012*, 651583.

Carlson, L. E., & Speca, M. (2011). *Mindfulness-based cancer recovery: A step-by-step MBSR approach to help you cope with treatment and reclaim your life.* Oakland CA: New Harbinger.

Carlson, L. E., Doll, R., Stephen, J., Faris, P., Tamagawa, R., Drysdale, E., & Speca, M. (2013). Randomized controlled trial of mindfulness-based cancer recovery versus supportive expressive group therapy for distressed survivors of breast cancer (MINDSET). *J Clin Oncol*, *31*, 3119–3127.

Carpenter, J. S., Burns, D. S., Wu, J., Otte, J. L., Schneider, B., Ryker, K., … Yu, M. (2013). Paced respiration for vasomotor and other menopausal symptoms: A randomized, controlled trial. *J Gen Intern Med*, *28*, 193–200.

Cepeda, M. S., Carr, D. B., Lau, J., & Alvarez, H. (2006). Music for pain relief. *Cochrane Database Sys Rev*, 2:CD004843.

Chandola, T., Brunner, E., & Marmot, M. (2006). Chronic stress at work and metabolic syndrome. *Brit Med J*, *332*, 521–525.

Chen, K. W., Berger, C. C., Manheimer, E., Forde, D., Magidson, J., Dachman, L., & Lejuez, C. W. (2012). Meditative therapies for reducing anxiety: A systematic review and meta-analysis of randomized controlled trials. *Depress Anxiety, 29,* 545–562.

Chida, Y., & Steptoe, A. (2008). Positive psychological well-being and mortality: A quantitative review of prospective observational studies. *Psychosomatic Med, 70,* 741–756.

Chiesa, A., & Serretti, A. (2011a). Mindfulness-based interventions for chronic pain: A systematic review of the evidence. *J Altern Complement Med, 17,* 83–93.

Chiesa, A., & Serretti, A. (2011b). Mindfulness-based cognitive therapy for psychiatric disorders: A systematic review and meta-analysis. *Psychiatry Res, 187,* 441–453.

Chou, R., & Huffman, L. H. (2007). Nonpharmacologic therapies for acute and chronic low back pain: A review of the evidence for an American Pain Society/American College of Physicians clinical practice guideline. Ann Intern Med, *147,* 492–504.

Cohen, S., Alper, C. M., Doyle, W. J., Treanor, J. J., & Turner, R. B. (2006). Positive emotional style predicts resistance to illness after experimental exposure to rhinovirus or influenza a virus. *Psychosom Med, 68,* 809–815.

Cohen, S., Doyle, W. J., Turner, R. B., Alper, C. M., & Skoner, D. P. (2003). Emotional style and susceptibility to the common cold. *Psychosomat Med, 65,* 652–657.

Cohen, S., Janicki-Deverts, D., & Miller, G. E. (2007). Psychological stress and disease. *JAMA, 298,* 1685–1687.

Cole, S. W. (2013). Nervous system regulation of the cancer genome. *Brain Behav Immun, 30,* S10–S18.

Cole, S. W. (2014). *Social and psychological influences on gene expression.* Plenary Presentation at the International Research Congress on Integrative Medicine and Health 2014. Retrieved from http://webcast.ircimh.org/console/player/24012?medi aType=slideVideo

Cramer, H., Haller, H., Lauche, R., Steckhan, N., Michalsen, A., & Dobos, G. (2014). A systematic review and meta-analysis of yoga for hypertension. *Amer J Hypertens, 27,* 1146–1151.

Cramer, H., Lange, S., Klose, P., Paul, A., & Dobos, G. (2012). Yoga for breast cancer patients and survivors: A systematic review and meta-analysis. *BMC Cancer, 12,* 412.

Cramer, H., Lauche, R., Haller, H., Steckhan, N., Michalsen, A., & Dobos, G. (2014). Effects of yoga on cardiovascular disease risk factors: A systematic review and meta-analysis. *Int J Cardiol, 173,* 170–183.

Cramer, H., Lauche, R., Langhorst, J., & Dobos, G. (2013). Yoga for depression: A systematic review and meta-analysis. *Depress Anxiety, 30,* 1068–1083.

Curtis, K., Weinrib, A., & Katz, J. (2012). Systematic review of yoga for pregnant women: Current status and future directions. *Evid Based Complement Alternat Med, 2012,* 715942.

Damjanovic, A. K., Yang, Y., Glaser, R., et al. (2007). Accelerated telomere erosion is associated with a declining immune function of caregivers of Alzheimer's disease patients. *J Immunol, 179,* 4249–4254.

Danner, D. D., Snowden, D. A., & Friesen, W. V. (2001). Positive emotions in early life and longevity: Findings from the nun study. *J Pers Soc Psychol, 80,* 804–813.

Davidson, K. W., Mostofsky, E., & Whang, W. (2010). Don't worry, be happy: Positive affect and reduced 10-year incident coronary heart disease: The Canadian Nova Scotia Health Survey. *Eur Heart J*, *31*, 1065–1070.

Davis, M. (1999). Is life more difficult on Mars or Venus? A meta-analytic review of sex differences in major and minor life events. *Soc Behav Med*, *21*, 83–97.

Denniger, J., Libermann, T., Antoni, M., Irwin, M., & Manoj, B. (2014). *Transforming the understanding of mind-body interventions: The genomics of stress and resiliency*. Symposium presentation at the International Research Congress on Integrative Medicine and Health.

Domar, A. D., Clapp, D., Slawsby, E. A., Dusek, J., Kessel, B., & Freizinger, M. (2000). Impact of group psychological interventions on pregnancy rates in infertile women. *Fertil Steril*, *73*, 805–811.

Domar, A. D., Clapp, D., Slawsby, E., Kessel, B., Orav, J., & Freizinger, M. (2000). The impact of group psychological interventions on distress in infertile women. *Health Psychol*, *19*, 568–575.

Domar, A. D., Rooney, K. L., Wiegand, B., Orav, E. J., Alper, M. M., Berger, B. M., & Nikolovski, J. (2011). Impact of a group mind/body intervention on pregnancy rates in IVF patients. *Fertil Steril*, *95*, 2269–2273.

Duncan, L. G., & Bardacke, N. (2010). Mindfulness-based childbirth and parenting education: Promoting family mindfulness during the perinatal period. *J Child Fam Stud*, *19*, 190–202.

Duncan, L. G., Cohn, M., Chao, M., Cook, J, Ricccobono, J., & Bardacke, N. (2014). Mind in labor: Effects of mind/body training on childbirth appraisals and pain medication use during labor. *J Altern Complement Med*, *20*, A17.

Dusek, J. A., Hibberd, P. L., Buczynski, B., et al. (2008). Stress management versus lifestyle modification on systolic hypertension and medication elimination: A randomized trial. *J Altern Complement Med*, *14*, 129–138.

Eisenberger, N. I., & Cole, S. W. (2012). Social neuroscience and health: Neurophysiological mechanisms linking social ties with physical health. *Nat Neurosci*, *15*, 669–674.

Elkins, G., Fisher, W., Johnson, A., Carpenter, J., & Keith, T. (2013). Clinical hypnosis in the treatment of postmenopausal hot flashes: A randomized controlled trial. *Menopause*, *20*, 291–298.

Emani, S., & Binkley, P. F. (2010). Advances in heart failure mind-body medicine in chronic heart failure: A translational science challenge. *Circ Heart Fail*, *3*, 715–725.

Eppel, E. S., Blackburn, E. H., Lin, J., et al. (2004). Accelerated telomere shortening in response to life stress. *Proc Natl Acad Sci U S A*, *101*, 17312–1735.

Eremin, O., Walker, M. B., Simpson, E., Heys, S. D., Ah-See, A. K., Hutcheon, A. W., & Walker, L. G. (2009). Immuno-modulatory effects of relaxation training and guided imagery in women with locally advanced breast cancer undergoing multimodality therapy: A randomized control trial. *Breast*, *18*, 17–25.

Faller, H., Schuler, M., Richard, M., Heckl, U., Weis, J., & Kuffner, R. (2013). Effects of psycho-oncologic interventions on emotional distress and quality of life in adult patients with cancer: Systematic review and meta-analysis. *Clin Oncol*, *31*, 782–793.

Fang, C. Y., Miller, S. M., Bovbjerg, D. H., et al. (2008). Perceived stress is associated with impaired T-cell response to HPV16 in women with cervical dysplasia. *Ann Behav Med*, *35*, 87–96.

Fava, G. A., & Sonino, N. (2005). The clinical domains of psychosomatic medicine. *J Clin Psychiatry*, *66*, 849–858.

Fortney, L., Luchterhand, C., Zakletskaia, L., Zgierska, A., & Rakel, D. (2013). Abbreviated mindfulness intervention for job satisfaction, quality of life, and compassion in primary care clinicians: A pilot study. *Ann Fam Med*, *11*, 412–420.

Frattaroli, J. (2006). Experimental disclosure and its moderators: A meta-analysis. *Psychol Bull*, *132*, 823–865.

Fredrickson, B. L., Grewen, K. M., Coffey, K. A., Algoe, S. B., Firestine, A. M., Arevalo, J. M. G., Ma J,… Cole, S. W. (2013). A functional genomic perspective on human well-being. *Proc Natl Acad Sci U S A*, *110*(33), 13684–13689.

Freedman, R. R., & Woodward, S. (1992). Behavioral treatment of menopausal hot flushes: Evaluation by ambulatory monitoring. *Am J Obstet Gynecol*, *167*, 436–439.

Freedman, R. R., & Woodard, S. (1995). Biochemical and thermoregulatory effects of behavioral treatment for menopausal hot flashes. *Menopause*, *2*, 211–218.

Galhardo, A., Cunha, M., & Pinto-Gouveia, J. (2013). Mindfulness-based program for infertility: Efficacy study. *Fertil Steril*, *100*, 1059–1067.

Gaston-Johansson, F., Fall-Dickson, J. M., Nanda, J. P., Sarenmalm, E. K., Browall, M., & Goldstein, N. (2013). Long-term effect of the self-management comprehensive coping strategy program on quality of life in patients with breast cancer treated with high-dose chemotherapy. *Psychooncology*, *22*, 530–539.

Gellaitry, G., Peters, K., Bloomfield, D., & Horne, R. (2010). Narrowing the gap: The effects of an expressive writing intervention on perceptions of actual and ideal emotional support in women who have completed treatment for early stage breast cancer. *Psycho-Oncology*, *19*, 77–84.

Goodman, J. H., Guarino, A., Chenausky, K., Klein, L., Prager, J., Petersen, R., … Freeman, M. (2014). CALM pregnancy: Results of a pilot study of mindfulness-based cognitive therapy for perinatal anxiety. *Arch Womens Ment Health*. doi: 10.1007/s00737-013-0402-7

Goyal, M., Singh, S., Sibinga, E. M., Gould, N. F., Rowland-Seymour, A., Sharma, R., … Haythornthwaite, J. A. (2014). Meditation programs for psychological stress and well-being: A systematic review and meta-analysis. *JAMA Intern Med*, *174*, 357–368.

Greil, A. L. (1997). Infertility and psychological distress: A critical review of the literature. *Soc Sci Med*, *45*, 1679–1704.

Grepmair, L., Mitterlehner, F., Loew, T., Bachler, E., Rother, W., & Nickel, M. (2007). Promoting mindfulness in psychotherapists in training influences the treatment results of their patients: A randomized, double-blind, controlled study. *Psychother Psychosom*, *76*, 332–338.

Grepmair, L., Mitterlehner, F., Loew, T., & Nickel, M. (2007). Promotion of mindfulness in psychotherapists in training: Preliminary study. *Eur Psychiatry*, *22*, 485–489.

Hackney, M. E., & Wolf, S. L. (2014). Impact of Tai Chi Chu'an practice on balance and mobility in older adults: An integrative review of 20 years of research. *J Geriatr Phys Ther*, *37*, 127–135.

Hartley, L., Flowers, N., Lee, M. S., Ernst, E., & Rees, K. (2014). Tai chi for primary prevention of cardiovascular disease. *Cochrane Database Syst Rev*, 4:CD010366. doi: 10.1002/14651858.CD010366.pub2

Helgesson, O., Cabrera, C., Lapidus, L., Bengtsson, C., & Lissner, L. (2003). Self-reported stress levels predict subsequent breast cancer in a cohort of Swedish women. *Eur J Cancer Prev*, *12*, 377–381.

Henderson, V. P., Clemow, L., Massion, A. O., Hurley, T., Druker, S., & Hebert, J. (2012). The effects of mindfulness-based stress reduction practices on psychosocial outcomes and quality of life in early-stage breast cancer patients: A randomized trial. *Breast Cancer Res Treat*, *131*, 99–109.

Hoffman, C. J., Ersser, S. J., Hopkinson, J. B., Nichols, P. G., Harrington, J. E., & Thomas, P. E. (2012). Effectiveness of mindfulness-based stress reduction in mood, breast- and endocrine-related quality of life, and well-being in stage 0 to III breast cancer: A randomized, controlled trial. *J Clin Oncol*, *30*, 1335–1342.

Hoge, E., Chen, M. M., Orr, E., Metcalf, C. A., Fischer, L. E., Pollack, M., ... Simon, N. M. (2013). Loving-kindness meditation practice associated with longer telomeres in women. *Brain Behav Immun*, *32*, 159–163.

Hoglund, C. O., Axen, J., Kemi, C., et al. (2006). Changes in immune regulation in response to examination stress in atopic and healthy individuals. *Clin Exp Allergy*, *36*, 982–992.

Humphreys, J., Epel, E. S., Cooper, B. A., Lin, J., Blackburn, E. H., & Lee, K. A. (2011). Telomere shortening in formerly abused and never abused women. *Biol Res Nurs*, *14*, 115–123.

Ingalhalikar, M., Smith, A., Parker, D., Satterthwaite, T. D., Elliott, M. A., Ruparel, K., Hakonarson, H., ... Verma, R. (2014). Sex differences in the structural connectome of the human brain. *Proc Natl Acad Sci U S A*, *111*, 823–828.

Innes, K. E., Selfe, T. K., & Vishnu, A. (2010). Mind-body therapies for menopausal symptoms: A systematic review. *Maturitas*, *66*, 135–149.

Irribarren, C., Sidney, S., Bild, D. E., et al. (2000). Association of hostility with coronary artery calcification in young adults: The CARDIA study; Coronary artery risk development in young adults. *JAMA*, *283*, 2546–2551.

Irvin, J. H., Domar, A. D., Clark, C., Zuttermeister, P. C., & Friedman, R. (1996). The effects of relaxation response training on menopausal symptoms. *J Psychosom Obstet Gynaecol*, *17*, 202–207.

Jacobs, G. D. (2001). The physiology of mind-body interactions: The stress response and the relaxation response. *J Altern Complement Med*, *7*(Suppl 1): S83–S92.

Jacobs, T. L., Epel, E. S., Lin, J., Blackburn, E. H., Wolkowitz, O. M., Bridwell, D. A., ... Saron, C. D. (2011). Intensive meditation training, immune cell telomerase activity and psychological mediators. *Psychoneuroendocrino*, *36*, 664–681.

Jahnke, R., Larkey, L., Rogers, R., Etnier, J., & Lin, F. A comprehensive review of health benefits of Qigong and Tai Chi. *Am J Health Promot 24*(6):e1–e25.

Jensen-Johansen, M. B., Christensen, S., Valdimarsdottir, H., Zakowski, S., Jensen, A. B., Bovbjerg, D. H., & Zachariae, R. (2012). Effects of an expressive writing intervention on cancer-related distress in Danish breast cancer survivors—Results from a nationwide randomized clinical trial. *Psychooncology, 22,* 1492–1500.

Johansson, L., Guo, X., Hällström, T., Norton, M. C., Waern, M., Östling, S., … Skoog, I. (2013). Common psychosocial stressors in middle-aged women related to long-standing distress and increased risk of Alzheimer's disease: A 38-year longitudinal population study. *BMJ Open, 3,* e003142.

Keng, S. L., Smoski, M. J., & Robins, C. J. (2011). Effects of mindfulness on psychological health: A review of empirical studies. *Clin Psychol Rev, 31,* 1041–1056.

Kessler, R. C., McGonagle, K. A., Zhao, S., Nelson, C. B., Hughes, M., Eshleman, S., … Kendler, K. S. (1994). Lifetime and 12-month prevalence of DSM-III-R psychiatric disorders in the United States: Results from the National Comorbidity Survey. *Arch Gen Psychiatry, 51,* 8–19.

Khianman, B., Pattanittum, P., Thinkhamrop, J., & Lumbiganon, P. (2012). Relaxation therapy for preventing and treating preterm labour. *Cochrane Database of Systematic Reviews, 8:* CD007426.

Khoury, B., Lecomte, T., Fortin, G., Masse, M., Therien, P., Bouchard, V., … Hofmann, S. G. (2013). Mindfulness-based therapy: A comprehensive meta-analysis. *Clin Psychol Rev, 33,* 763–771.

Kiecolt-Glaser, J. K., Bennett, J. M., Andridge, R., Peng, J., Shapiro, C. L., Malarkey, W. B., … Glaser, R. (2014). Yoga's impact on inflammation, mood, and fatigue in breast cancer survivors: A randomized controlled trial. *J Clin Oncol, 32,* 1040–1049.

Krasner, M. S., Epstein, R. M., Beckman, H., Suchman, A. L., Chapman, B., Mooney, C. J., & Quill, T. E. (2009). Association of an educational program in mindful communication with burnout, empathy, and attitudes among primary care physicians. *JAMA, 302,* 1284–1293.

Langhorst, J., Klose, P., Dobos, G. J., Bernardy, K., & Häuser, W. (2013). Efficacy and safety of meditative movement therapies in fibromyalgia syndrome: A systematic review and meta-analysis of randomized controlled trials. *Rheumatol Int, 33,* 193–220.

Lauche, R., Cramer, H., Dobos, G., Langhorst, J., & Schmidt, S. (2013). A systematic review and meta-analysis of mindfulness-based stress reduction for the fibromyalgia syndrome. *J Psychosom Res, 75,* 500–510.

Lee, M. S., Kim, J. I., Ha, J. Y., Boddy, K., & Ernst, E. (2009). Yoga for menopausal symptoms: A systematic review. *Menopause, 16,* 602–608.

Lillberg, K., Verkasalo, P. K., Kaprio, J., Teppo, L., Helenius, H., & Koskenvuo, M. (2003). Stressful life events and risk of breast cancer in 10,808 women: A cohort study. *Am J Epidemiol, 157,* 415–423.

Lindh-Åstrand, L., & Nedstrand, E. (2013). Effects of applied relaxation on vasomotor symptoms in postmenopausal women: A randomized controlled trial. *Menopause, 20,* 401–408.

Low, C. A., Stanton, A. L., & Danoff-Burg, S. (2006). Expressive disclosure and benefit finding among breast cancer patients: Mechanisms for positive health effects. *Health Psychol, 25,* 181–189.

Lutgendorf, S. K., & Sood, A. K. (2011). Biobehavioral factors and cancer progression: Physiological pathways and mechanisms. *Psychosom Med, 73*, 724–730.

Madden, K., Middleton, P., Cyna, A. M., Matthewson, M., & Jones, L. (2012). Hypnosis for pain management during labour and childbirth. *Cochrane Database of Systematic Reviews*, 11: CD009356.

Marc, I., Toureche, N., Ernst, E., Hodnett, E. D., Blanchet, C., Dodin, S., & Njoya, M. M. (2011). Mind-body interventions during pregnancy for preventing or treating women's anxiety. *Cochrane Database of Systematic Reviews*, 7:CD007559.

McDonald PG, O'Connell M, Lutgendorf SK. (2013). Psychoneuroimmunology and cancer: A decade of discovery, paradigm shifts, and methodological innovations. *Brain Behav Immun. 2013; 30(0)*: S1–S9.

Mather, M., Lighthall, N. R., Nga, L., & Gorlick, M. A. (2010). Sex differences in how stress affects brain activity during face viewing. *NeuroReport, 21*, 933–937.

Mayden, K. D. (2012). Mind-body therapies: Evidence and implications in advanced oncology practice. *J Adv Pract Oncol, 3*, 357–373.

McCall, M. C., Ward, A., Roberts, N. W., & Heneghan, C. (2013). Overview of systematic reviews: Yoga as a therapeutic intervention for adults with acute and chronic health conditions. *Evid Based Complement Alternat Med, 2013*, 945895.

McEwen, B. S., & Lasley, E. N. (2002). *The end of stress as we know it*. Washington, DC: Joseph Henry Press.

Mist, S. D., Firestone, K. A., & Jones, K. D. (2013). Complementary and alternative exercise for fibromyalgia: A meta-analysis. *J Pain Res, 6*, 247–260.

Mittleman, M. A., Maclure, M., Sherwood, J. B., et al. (1995). Triggering of acute myocardial infarction onset by episodes of anger: Determinants of Myocardial InfaRCTion Onset Study Investigators. *Circulation, 92*, 1720–1725.

Montgomery, G. H., Bovbjerg, D. H., Schnur, J. B., et al. (2007). A randomized clinical trial of a brief hypnosis intervention to control side effects in breast surgery patients. *J Natl Cancer Inst, 99*, 1304–1312.

Montgomery, G. H., Schnur, J. B., & Kravits, K. (2013). Hypnosis for Cancer Care: 200 years young. *CA Cancer J Clin, 63*, 31–44.

Monti, D. A., Kash, K. M., Kunkel, E. J., Moss, A., Mathews, M., Brainard, G., ... Newberg, A. B. (2013). Psychosocial benefits of a novel mindfulness intervention versus standard support in distressed women with breast cancer. *Psychooncology, 22*, 2565–2575.

Morgan, N., Irwin, M. R., Chung, M., & Wang, C. (2014). The effects of mind-body therapies on the immune system: Meta-analysis. *PLoS One, 9*, e100903. doi:10.1371/journal.pone.0100903

Morgenthaler, T., Kramer, M., Alessi, C., et al. (2006). Practice parameters for the psychological and behavioral treatment of insomnia: An update; An American academy of sleep medicine report. *Sleep, 29*, 1415–1419.

Musial, F., Büssing, A., Heusser, P., Choi, K. E., & Ostermann, T. (2011). Mindfulness-based stress reduction for integrative cancer care: A summary of evidence. *Forsch Komplementmed, 18*, 192–202.

Mustian, K. M., Sprod, L. K., Janelsins, M., Peppone, L. J., Palesh, O. G., Chandwani, K., ... Morrow, G. R. (2013). Multicenter, randomized controlled trial of yoga for sleep quality among cancer survivors. *J Clin Oncol*, *31*, 3233–3241.

National Center for Complementary and Alternative Medicine. (n.d.). *Backgrounder: Mind-body medicine: An overview.* Retrieved September 24, 2008, from http://nccam.nih.gov/health/backgrounds/mindbody.htm

Nightingale, C. L., Rodriguez, C., & Carnaby, G. (2013). The impact of music interventions on anxiety for adult cancer patients: A meta-analysis and systematic review. *Integr Cancer Ther*, *12*, 393–403.

Newton, K. M., Reed, S. D., Guthrie, K. A., Sherman, K. J., Booth-LaForce, C., Caan, B., ... LaCroix, A. Z. (2013). Efficacy of yoga for vasomotor symptoms: A randomized controlled trial. *Menopause*, *21*, 339–346.

North American Menopause Society. (2012). *The menopause guidebook* (7th ed.). Cleveland, OH: Author.

Orme-Johnson, D., & Barnes V. (2014). Effects of the transcendental meditation technique on trait anxiety: A meta-analysis of randomized controlled trials. *J Altern Complement Med*, *2014*, 330–341.

Ornish, D., Lin, J., Chan, J. M., Epel, E., Kemp, C., Weidner, G., ... Blackburn, E. H. (2013). Effect of comprehensive lifestyle changes on telomerase activity and telomere length in men with biopsy-proven low-risk prostate cancer: 5-year follow-up of a descriptive pilot study. *Lancet Oncol*, *14*, 1112–1120.

Peregoy, J. A., Clarke, T. C., Jones, L. I., et al. (2014). *Regional variation in use of complementary health approaches by US adults.* NCHS data brief, no 146. Hyattsville, MD: National Center for Health Statistics.

Plagnol, A., & Easterlin, R. (2008). Aspirations, attainments, and satisfaction: Life cycle differences between American woman and men. *J Happiness Stud*. doi: 10.1007/s10902–008-9106–5

Prasad, K., Ziegenfuss, J. Y., Cha, S. S., et al. (2013). Characteristics of exclusive users of mind-body medicine, vs. other alternative medicine approaches in the United States. *Explore*, *9*, 219–225.

Proctor, M., Murphy, P. A., Pattison, H. M., Suckling, J. A., & Farquhar, C. (2007). Behavioural interventions for dysmenorrhoea. *Cochrane Database of Systematic Reviews*, *3*: CD002248. doi: 10.1002/14651858.CD002248.pub3. Updated 2009.

Puterman, P. E., Lin, J., Krauss, J., Blackburn, E. H., & Epel, E. S. (2014). Determinants of telomere attrition over 1 year in healthy older women: Stress and health behaviors matter. *Mol Psychiatr*, *71*, 921–923.

Rakhshani, A., Nagarathna, R., Mhaskar, R., Mhaskar, A., Thomas, A., & Gunasheela, S. (2012). The effects of yoga in prevention of pregnancy complications in high-risk pregnancies: A randomized controlled trial. *Prev Med*, *55*, 333–340.

Reed, S., Guthrie, K. A., Newton, K. M., Anderson, G. L., Booth-LaForce, C., Caan B, ... LaCroix, A. Z. (2014). Menopausal quality of life: RCT of yoga, exercise, and omega-3 supplements. *Am J Obstet Gynecol*, *210*, 244.e1–e11.

Roffe, L., Schmidt, K., & Ernst, E. (2005). A systematic review of guided imagery as an adjuvant cancer therapy. *Psychooncology*, *14*, 607–617.

Sadja, M. S., & Mills, P. J. (2013). Effects of yoga interventions on fatigue in cancer patients and survivors: A systematic review of randomized controlled trials. *Explore, 94*, 232–243.

Saensak, S., Vutyavanich, T., Somboonporn, W., & Srisurapanont, M. (2014). Relaxation for perimenopausal and postmenopausal symptoms. *Cochrane Database Syst Rev,* 7:CD008582. doi: 10.1002/14651858.CD008582.pub2

Schaefert, R., Klose, P., Moser, G., & Häuser, W. (2014). Efficacy, tolerability, and safety of hypnosis in adult irritable bowel syndrome: Systematic review and meta-analysis. *Psychosom Med, 76*, 389–398.

Schoenberg, P. L., & David, A. S. (2014). Biofeedback for psychiatric disorders: A systematic review. *Appl Psychophysiol Biofeedback, 39*, 109–135.

Schutte, N. S., & Malouff, J. M. (2014). A meta-analytic review of the effects of mindfulness meditation on telomerase activity. *Psychoneuroendocrino, 42*, 45–48.

Segerstrom, S. C., & Miller, G. E. (2004). Psychological stress and the human immune system: A meta-analytic study of 30 years of inquiry. *Psychol Bull, 130*, 601–630.

Silberstein, S. D. (2000). Practice parameter: Evidence-based guidelines for migraine headache (an evidence-based review): Report of the Quality Standards Subcommittee of the American Academy of Neurology. *Neurology, 55*, 754–762. http://www.neurology.org/cgi/content/full/neurology56/1/142-a

Sin, N. L., Graham-Engeland, J. E., & Almeida, D. M. (2014). Daily positive events and inflammation: Findings from the National Study of Daily Experiences. *Brain, Behav Immun*. doi: 10.1016/j.bbi.2014.07.015

Sood, R., Sood, A., Wolf, S. L., Linquist, B. M., Liu, H., Sloan, J. A., … Barton, D. L. (2013). Paced breathing compared with usual breathing for hot flashes. *Menopause, 20*, 179–184.

Stanton, A. L., Danoff-Burg, S., & Sworowski, L. A. (2002). Randomized, controlled trial of written emotional expression and benefit finding in breast cancer patients. *J Clin Oncol, 20*, 4160–4168.

Steptoe, A., Demakakos, P., de Oliveira, C., & Wardle, J. (2012). Distinctive biological correlates of positive psychological well-being in older men and women. *Psychosom Med, 74*, 501–508.

Steptoe, A., Wardle, J., & Marmot, M. (2005). Positive affect and health-related neuroendocrine, cardiovascular, and inflammatory processes. *Proc Natl Acad Sci, 102*, 6508–6512.

Taylor, S. E. (2002). *The tending instinct: How nurturing is essential to who we are and how we live.* New York, NY: Holt.

Taylor, S. E., Klein, L. C., Lewis, B. P., Gruenewald, T. L., Gurung, R. A., & Updegraff, J. A. (2000). Biobehavioral responses to stress in females: Tend-and-befriend, not fight-or-flight. *Psychol Rev, 107*, 411–429.

Teixeira, J., Martin, D., Prendiville, O., & Glover, V. (2005). The effects of acute relaxation on indices of anxiety during pregnancy. *J Psychosom Obstet Gynaecol, 26*, 271–276.

Thacker, P. H., Han, L. Y., Kamat, A. A., et al. (2006). Chronic stress promotes tumor growth and angiogenesis in a mouse model of ovarian carcinoma. *Nat Med, 12*, 939–944.

Tolin, D. F., & Foa, E. B. (2006). Sex differences in trauma and posttraumatic stress disorder: A quantitative review of 25 years of research. *Psychol Bull, 132,* 959–992.

Tomasi, D., & Volkow, N. D. (2012). Gender differences in brain functional connectivity density. *Hum Brain Mapp, 33,* 849–860.

Tomova, L., Dawans, B. V., Heinrichs, M., Silani, G., & Lamm, C. (2014). Is stress affecting our ability to tune into others? Evidence for gender differences in the effects of stress on self-other distinction. *Psychoneuroendocrino, 43,* 95.

Valoriani, V., Lotti, F., Vanni, C., Noci, M. C., Fontanarosa, N., Ferrari, G., … Noci, I. (2014). Hatha-yoga as a psychological adjuvant for women undergoing IVF: A pilot study. *Eur J Obstet Gynecol Reprod Biol, 176,* 158–162.

Vieten, C., & Astin, J. (2008). Effects of a mindfulness-based intervention during pregnancy on prenatal stress and mood: Results of a pilot study. *Arch Womens Ment Health, 11,* 67–74.

Vogel, J. H. K., Bolling, S. F., Costello, R. B., et al. (2005). Integrating complementary medicine into cardiovascular medicine: A report of the American College of Cardiology Foundation Task Force on Clinical Expert Consensus Documents (Writing Committee to Develop an Expert Consensus Document on Complementary and Integrative Medicine). *J Am Col Cardio, 46,* 184–221.

Wang, F., Lee, E. K., Wu, T., Benson, H., Fricchione, G., Wang, W., & Yeung, A. S. (2013). The effects of tai chi on depression, anxiety, and psychological well-being: A systematic review and meta-analysis. *Int J Behav Med, 21,* 605–617.

Wang, J., Korczykowski, M., Rao, H., et al. (2007). Gender difference in neural response to psychological stress. *Soc Cogn Affect Neurosci, 2,* 227–239.

Wang, J., Xiong, X., & Liu, W. (2013). Yoga for essential hypertension: A systematic review. *PloS One, 8,* e76357.

Weik, U., Herforth, A., Kolb-Bachofen, V., & Deinzer, R. (2008). Acute stress induces proinflammatory signaling at chronic inflammation sites. *Psychosom Med, 70,* 906–912.

Williams, R. B., & Chesney, M. A. (1993). Psychosocial factors and prognosis in established coronary artery disease: The need for research on interventions. *JAMA, 270,* 1860–1861.

Wittstein, I. S., Thiemann, D. R., Lima, J. A. C., et al. (2005). Neurohumoral features of myocardial stunning due to sudden emotional stress. *N Engl J Med, 352,* 539–548.

Wurtzen, H., Dalton, S. O., Elsass, P., Sumbundu, A. D., Steding-Jensen, M., Karlsen, R. V., … Johansen, C. (2013). Mindfulness significantly reduces self-reported levels of anxiety and depression: Results of a randomized controlled trail among 336 Danish women treated for stage 1-III breast cancer. *Eur J Can, 49,* 1365–1373.

Xu, J., & Roberts, R. E. (2010). The power of positive emotions: It's a matter of life or death—Subjective well-being and longevity over 28 years in a general population. *Health Psychol, 29,* 9–19.

Zainal, N. Z., Booth, S., & Huppert, F. A. (2013). The efficacy of mindfulness-based stress reduction on mental health of breast cancer patients: A meta-analysis. *Psychooncology, 22,* 1457–1465.

Zeng, Y., Luo, T., Xie, H., Huang, M., & Cheng, A. (2014). Health benefits of qigong or tai chi for cancer patients: A systematic review and meta-analyses. *Complement Ther Med, 22,* 173–186.

Zernicke, K. A., Campbell, T. S., Speca, M., McCabe-Ruff, K., Flowers, S., & Carlson, L. E. (2014). A randomized wait-list controlled trial of feasibility and efficacy of an online mindfulness-based cancer recovery program for underserved distressed cancer survivors: The eCALM trial. *Psychosom Med, 76,* 257–267.

6

Healthy Aging

ELIZABETH R. MACKENZIE AND BIRGIT RAKEL

Age has its own glory, beauty, and wisdom that belong to it. Peace, love, joy, beauty, happiness, wisdom, goodwill, and understanding are qualities that never grow old or die.

—Joseph Murphy

Introduction

Aging is not a disease. Growing old is a natural process, the denouement in the narrative of a woman's life. The purpose of this chapter is to emphasize the potential for *healthy aging*. We know that our bodies change with age. Skin loses its elasticity, wrinkles emerge, bones may become more brittle, muscle tone diminishes, and we gain weight more readily. Chronic conditions that have been forming for years may manifest as full-blown symptoms claiming our attention. Our energy levels may be lower, almost as though our vital force is leaking away. Still, there is potential for vibrant health if these challenges are approached with the proper perspective and if we are equipped with the best of integrative medicine. When thinking about how to support patients in their efforts to age healthfully, it is important for health professionals to move away from the perception of aging as a problem to be solved. As Andrew Weil, MD, has noted, a crucial component of the healthy aging paradigm is to reconfigure the concept of aging.

I'm interested in the areas of our experience in which we value aging. I want to consider old trees, cheese, wine, whiskey, and steak. What are the qualities that we appreciate in aged things? I think they include roundedness and smoothness as opposed to angularity and a kind of deep strength combined with mellowness. (Weil, 2001)

A key to healthy aging is the understanding that achieving good health does not necessarily mean having *perfect* health. It is possible to live fully while managing a chronic condition or coping with a disability. Wholeness does not require a perfect body, free from all flaws and disorders. However, the healthier we can be, the stronger we will feel in our bodies, and the more fully our lives can unfold. What we are after here is excellent energy, strong bodies, flexible forms, calm minds, and joyful spirits.

Women age differently, based on genetics, lifestyle, life events, social support, mental outlook, and other factors, both known and unknown. The life force is an important but often mysterious ally for health professionals. Most of us have met older women who are thriving despite a lifetime of smoking, drinking, and sedentary living, while others, conscientious about their health, are beset with illness. We can influence, but not control, health. The idea is to guide patients toward activities and interventions that will increase the probability of good health.

This is decidedly not an "anti-aging" chapter, and we will not refer to "turning back the hands of time" or use similar metaphors. Actually, "anti-aging" is a strange term, as we begin to age at birth. Being born sets the aging process in motion and only death can stop it. Our goals, as health professionals, should be to extend life while enhancing quality of life by preventing disease when possible, and otherwise by managing it optimally.

The Conventional Approach to Aging

Conventional approaches to aging have strengths. Medicine is very good at screening and early detection, the treatment of acute illness, and dealing with advanced disease states. Cancer, for example, is no longer the "death sentence" it once was, and long-term survival rates for certain forms of cancer are quite high. However, it should be noted that *screening* is not a good substitute for *prevention* and conventional medicine has not had a good track record on the health promotion side of the equation.

The biggest failing of conventional medicine with regard to aging, though, is its tendency to view aging as pathology, rather than a natural stage in the life cycle. An obvious recent example is the conventional approach to menopause. For decades, hormone therapy (HT) was the standard response to changing hormonal levels in middle-aged women. At least two generations of American women were strongly encouraged to replace their hormones as they were tapering off during menopause. Then, the Women's Health Initiative (WHI) trial was stopped early when researchers realized that the risks of cardiovascular disease (CVD, from conjugated equine estrogen) and breast cancer (from conjugated equine estrogen plus medroxyprogesterone acetate) associated with HT were greater than its benefits (Heiss et al., 2008). This finding was confirmed when national breast cancer rates fell after a widespread cessation of HT in response to media coverage (Heiss et al., 2008).

Nutrition and Aging

Eating fresh fruits and vegetables and whole grains and avoiding overly processed foods is a central part of establishing a healthy diet. Specific considerations related to healthy aging include vegetarianism, adequate protein, and the need for supplementation.

VEGETARIANISM

Some evidence suggests that vegetarianism promotes longevity. Singh et al. report, "Current prospective cohort data from adults in North America and Europe raise the possibility that a lifestyle pattern that includes a very low meat intake is associated with greater longevity" (Singh, Sabaté, & Fraser, 2003). However, other large-scale European studies suggest that it may not be eschewing meat that is the critical factor, but adhering to a diet high in whole grains, vegetables, and fruit (Ginter, 2008; Sabate, 2003). Vegetarians do seem to have less incidence of ischemic heart disease, lower prevalence of obesity, and higher consumption of antioxidants (Ginter, 2008).

One study of 45 Korean vegetarians found that long-term vegetarianism (15+ years) was associated with lower levels of oxidative stress, body fat, and cholesterol (Kim, Cho, & Park, 2012). A US study that examined the relationship between cancer incidence (n = 2,939) and vegetarianism found that vegetarians had lower risk of cancer overall and of female-specific cancers (Tantamango-Bartley, Jaceldo-Siegl, Fan, & Fraser, 2013). Vegetarian diets appear to be associated with lower rates of many chronic diseases (especially coronary heart disease, hypertension, and diabetes mellitus) (Fraser, 2009).

While these studies do not constitute a total indictment of meat consumption, they do point to the health benefits of reducing—but not necessarily eliminating—meat consumption, and focusing the diet on whole grains, vegetable, and fruits. Patients who choose to adhere to a strict vegetarian diet should make sure they are not deficient in essential nutrients. Lacto-ova vegetarians have an easier time getting enough protein and B vitamins than vegans. Most vegans will need to supplement their diet with sublingual B12 vitamins or use Brewer's yeast.

Sufficient protein is also an important consideration with aging. A recent study analyzed data from 6,381 men and women over the age of 50 in the United States. They found that from age 50–65 those who ate a diet high in animal protein (defined as 20% or more of daily calories from protein) had a 74% increase in overall mortality and a fourfold increased risk of dying from cancer. In contrast, those over the age of 65 who ate a high animal protein diet had a 28% reduced all-cause mortality (Levine et al, 2014). In particular, higher protein intake may be important after age 65 to prevent frailty. Most Americans consume more protein than the recommended daily allowance (RDA) of 0.8g/kg/day, and perhaps this is becoming even truer with the popularity of paleo diets. While the RDA for seniors has not been altered for seniors, some recommend protein intake of 1.5 g/kg/day (Wolfe, Miller, & Miller, 2008).

Detoxification: Key to Preventing Disease or Expensive Hoax?

Although we may not like to reflect on this, we are surrounded by varying levels of potentially dangerous chemicals in the air, water, soil, and in our own bodies. "Different toxins accumulate in different tissues with many toxins being stored in lipid deposits where they can persist over the lifespan. It is possible that these toxins contribute to the development of cancers of the breast, prostate and leukemia, which all originate in fatty tissues" (Cohen, 2007).

Many proponents of various detox programs believe that fasting, special diets, juices, colonics, saunas, sweat lodges, chelation therapy, and so on can be used to help detoxify the body. There is little scientific evidence to support the effectiveness of detoxification programs (Cohen, 2007). However, as women may be exploring these options on their own, physicians should be aware of these practices.

DIETARY SUPPLEMENTS

Although it is optimal to receive all necessary vitamins and minerals through food, many older adults may need to supplement their diets. Here a few of the most popular supplements for older women.

Calcium

Calcium's main role as a supplement is in the prevention and treatment of osteoporosis. Dietary sources are calcium rich foods such as dairy, dark green leafy vegetable, and beans. Calcium supplementation in the elderly and postmenopausal women helps reduce bone loss (Devine et al., 1997; Napoli, Thomson, Civitelli, & Armamento Villareal, 2007; Reid et al., 1993) Some studies have found that calcium may also lower blood pressure (Conlin et al., 2000; Wang, Manson, Lee, & Sesso, 2008). Calcium supplementation is safe when used orally, but some patients might experience GI symptoms such as nausea, constipation, and abdominal pain. Although there is controversy surrounding the use of calcium supplements and potential correlation for an increase in CVD, the guidelines regarding use of calcium for osteoporosis have not changed in recent years (Chrysant & Chrysant, 2014; Paik et al., 2014; US Preventive Services Taskforce [USPSTF], 2013). The RDA for women over the age of 50 years is 1,200 mg/day. Clinicians should calculate dietary intake and supplement the difference.

Vitamin D

Vitamin D plays a critical role in providing protection from osteoporosis (Deane et al., 2007) and from cancer (Lappe et al., 2007; Schumann & Ewigman, 2007). Vitamin D supplementation may promote longevity in general (Autier & Gandini, 2007). Populations who may be at a high risk for vitamin D deficiencies include obese individuals, dark-skinned individuals, the elderly, and those who have limited sun exposure. The USPSTF concluded that vitamin D supplementation is effective in preventing falls in community-dwelling adults age 65 and older who are at risk for falls. Low vitamin D levels are implicated in the progression of dementia in the elderly. Although it is not recommended that vitamin D levels be used as diagnostic or prognostic indicators of dementia, supplementation is recommended (Annweiler, Durson, et al, 2014; Annweiler, Karras, Anagnostis, & Beauchet, 2014; USPSTF, 2013).

Omega-3 Fatty Acids (Fish Oils)

Epidemiologic studies and randomized controlled trials have shown that taking recommended amounts of docosahexaenoic acid (DHA) and eicosapentaenoic acid (EPA) in the form of dietary fish or fish oil supplements lowers triglycerides and reduces the risk of death, heart attack, abnormal heart rhythms, and strokes in people with known CVD; slows atherosclerotic plaques; and lowers blood pressure (Kris-Etherton, Harris, & Appel, 2003). The American Heart Association recommends that fish should be included in the diet for all individuals and fish oil supplements in those with a history of CVD. Omega-3 fatty acids may be beneficial for reducing the risk of age-related macular degeneration (SanGiovanni et al., 2008). Studies generally show a protective association between omega-3 levels, fish consumption, and cognitive decline, though omega-3 has not been demonstrated to be effective in the treatment of Alzheimer's disease (Robinson, Ijioma, & Harris, 2010),

Glucosamine

Glucosamine is an aminomonosaccharide naturally produced in humans. It is believed to play a role in cartilage formation and repair, and thus useful in the treatment of arthritis (Reginster et al., 2001). Many studies, though not all, show glucosamine sulfate to be an effective intervention for relieving the symptoms of osteoarthritis (Vangsness, Spiker, & Erickson, 2009). Long-term studies (6 months to 3 years) confirm the safety of glucosamine sulfate and also suggest that it may delay joint structure changes (Bruyere et al., 2014). Typical dosage is 1,500 mg/day, although obese patients may require larger dosages (derMarderosian & Briggs, 2006).

Ginkgo

Ginkgo (*Ginkgo biloba*) is widely used for its potential benefits on memory and cognition. However, when looking at the totality of the data, the evidence that ginkgo has predictable and clinically significant benefit for people with dementia or cognitive impairment is inconsistent and unreliable (Birks & Grimley Evans, 2009). Because many of the ginkgo studies were small in size and short in duration, the National Institutes of Health–funded the Ginkgo Evaluation of Memory (GEM) study followed more than 3,000 participants for an average of six years. This study found that *G. biloba* at 120 mg twice a day of standardized extract was not effective in reducing either the overall incidence rate of dementia or Alzheimer's dementia in individuals 75 years and older with normal cognition or those with mild cognitive impairment (DeKosky et al., 2008). Though an increased risk of bleeding has been widely publicized, *G. biloba* appears to be safe in use with no excess side effects compared with placebo (Birks & Grimley Evans, 2009). Most of the research seems to indicate limited or no statistically significant benefit of ginkgo over placebo or current treatment in the progression of Alzheimer's disease. However, given it's excellent safety profile, its use is not discouraged (Vellas et al., 2012; Natascia et al., 2013).

Adaptogens

Perhaps the most useful herbs to support older women's overall health belong to the class entitled "adaptogens." These are generally considered to be those that have a modulating effect on the neuroendocrine system, particularly during periods of stress. Primary botanicals in this class are ashwagandha (*Withania somnifera*), ginseng (*Panax ginseng*), rhodiola (*Rhodiola rosea*), schisandra (*Schisandra chinensis*), and codonopsis (*Codonopsis pilosula*) as well as the reishi mushroom (*Ganoderma lucidum*). Since many of these plants/mushrooms are native to Asia and the Indian subcontinent, they have only recently come to the attention of Western researchers. A useful primer on this class of herbs is *Adaptogens: Herbs for Strength, Stamina, and Stress Relief* (Winston & Maimes, 2007).

Manual Medicine: The Importance of Alignment and Touch

Manual therapies can be an important part of the care of aging women. Massage, chiropractic, and more esoteric practices such as Alexander Technique, Feldenkrais Method, Bowen Work, and so on, may be useful allies in promoting healthy aging. For example, massage can alleviate insomnia; ease pain associated with misalignments, arthritis, and tense muscles; speed recovery from surgery; improve blood and lymphatic circulation; and encourage deep relaxation (Kennedy & Chapman, 2006). Because many older women are both touch deprived and coping with chronic pain, bodywork modalities should not be overlooked by physicians who care for them. Ideally, practitioners who are experienced with working with older clients are recommended.

Exercise

PHYSICAL ACTIVITY

Exercise has consistently been shown to support healthy aging. Our bodies are made for motion and suffer when we do not use them. Exercise is among the best-known methods to prevent disability and addresses many different aspects of healthy aging from preventing osteoporosis (Kemmler, von Stengel, Engelke, Häberle, & Kalender, 2010) to protecting against cognitive decline (Behrman & Ebmeier, 2014; Best, Nagamatsu, & Liu-Ambrose, 2014). Exercise can also decrease the risks of falls by reversing sarcopenia, as demonstrated in the SEFIP study (Aagaard et al., 2010; Kennis et al., 2013; Melow et al., 2007). Furthermore, regular aerobic exercise decreases CVD risk factors (Lee, Kim, & Seo, 2014). There is even data to support that taking up physical exercise later in life will result in overall improved health, so it is never too late to incorporate an age-appropriate exercise regimen (Hamer, Lavoie, & Bacon, 2014).

Mind–Body Practices: Yoga, Tai Chi, Qigong, and Meditation

Many therapies are available to help women stay physically fit, emotionally balanced, and spiritually connected. A few practices address all three dimensions and receive special mention here: yoga, tai chi, qigong, and meditation. These are all activities that can be begun late in life and have the added bonus of helping women learn to accept and love their bodies while enhancing flexibility, balance, strength, cognitive function, and immunity. Health professionals and patients alike can benefit from the regular practice of these activities. Moreover, mind–body practices such as yoga, tai chi, and qigong may reduce insulin resistance and metabolic syndrome in postmenopausal women, and thus may help to prevent CVD, the leading cause of death for US women (Innes, Selfe, & Taylor, 2008).

YOGA

"It might surprise you to learn that traditionally, the ideal age to begin the practice of yoga was said to be fifty-three, the age marking one's passage into a new stage of life, one of contemplation and self-discovery" (Alice Christensen, in Butera, 2006, p. 199). The word *yoga* means "yoke" or "union" in Sanskrit, referring to the integration of mind, body, and spirit. Yoga can be practiced solely as a physical exercise, though this was not the traditional intent. There are eight "limbs" of yoga, and only one of them refers to the physical poses or *asanas*. The other seven are restraint (*yama*), observances (*niyamas*), breath control (*pranayama*), sensory withdrawal (*pratyahara*), and finally concentration, meditation, and perfect concentration.

In the United States, most yoga classes focus on the *asanas* with some inclusion of *pranayama*. Many individuals prefer to work with instructors who understand the deeper dimensions of the practice, and can help them cultivate *prana* (the Sanskrit term for life force), while others are more comfortable approaching yoga as more of a physical exercise. The many different forms of yoga available today in the United States helps to ensure that older adults can find a style that works for them. Interviewing yoga instructors about their approach to teaching and the rigors of the class will help patients choose an appropriate style and level.

Yoga promotes health on many levels and is one of the most frequently studied mind–body practices. A comprehensive review of all scientific findings on its health benefits is not possible here. Among the conditions associated with aging, small studies of yoga have found beneficial effects in coronary artery disease (Hartley et al., 2014), musculoskeletal disorders, and hypertension (Butera, 2006).

Yoga has also been found to increase levels of psychological well-being in a cohort of 211 women ages 45–80 (Moliver, Mika, Chartrand, Haussmann, & Khalsa, 2013). And a three-arm randomized controlled study of 72 women experiencing distress found those who practiced Iyengar yoga weekly had improvements in levels of perceived stress, trait anxiety, depression, quality of life, and bodily complaints (e.g., back pain) (Michalsen et al., 2012). Cheung, Wyman, Resnick, and Savik (2014) found that a weekly yoga practice reduced pain and stiffness in a cohort of 36 older women with osteoarthritis of the knee.

TAI CHI AND QIGONG

Like yoga, qigong is a practice that promotes a healthy body, mind, and spirit. Both qigong and tai chi are ancient practices rooted in the Chinese philosophy of balancing energies within the body itself and between the body and the environment. Both practices help the practitioner cultivate and circulate qi to support vibrant health. "Qigong" is the broader term; tai chi is actually a form of qigong. Both use slow, precise movements to encourage the flow of qi. Some forms of qigong emphasize breathing practices and movement, while others focus more on meditative activities.

The potential health benefits from the regular practice of qigong are numerous and include stress reduction, prevention of stroke, decreased hypertension, and treatment of arthritis (Chen, Mackenzie, & Hou, 2006). While many of these studies were conducted in China, US studies are beginning to explore the health benefits of qigong, especially for aging populations. For example, a recent review of clinical trials found that qigong and tai chi "may help older adults improve physical function and reduce blood pressure, fall risk, and depression and anxiety" (Rogers, Larkey, & Keller, 2009).

MEDITATION

With regular practice, meditation may both reduce the risk of developing CVD (Schneider, Walton, Salerno, & Nidich, 2006) and improve immunity (Davidson et al., 2003). From a mind–body perspective, this is not surprising. We would expect the quieting of the mind to help people better cope with stressors and thus improve their physical health. Even more importantly, meditation assists people in accessing their core spiritual support, allowing them to draw on inner reserves in times of stress and loss. Numerous studies have found that meditation improves physical, psychological, and spiritual well-being (Yuen & Baime, 2006).

There are several forms of meditation practice common in the United States. One of the best known is transcendental meditation (TM). Introduced to Americans by the Maharishi Mahesh Yogi in the 1960s, TM is closely tied to the Indian Vedic tradition (Yuen & Baime, 2006). Practitioners are given a mantra (a syllable, word, or phrase) to chant as a tool to achieve a transcendent state of consciousness. Another increasingly popular form of meditation is mindfulness meditation (or mindfulness-based stress reduction [MBSR]). This form of meditation grew out of the Buddhist tradition, and was shaped by Jon Kabat-Zinn, PhD, for use by health professionals and their patients. Mindfulness-based stress reduction has been extensively studied and has been shown to reduce depression and anxiety, decrease perception of pain, reduce use of medication, improve adherence to medical treatments, and increase motivation to make lifestyle changes (Ludwig & Kabat-Zinn, 2008).

Several recent studies highlight the potential for mindfulness practice to support healthy aging. De Frias and Whyne (2015) report that trait mindfulness is associated with mental health in older adults (ages 50–85) and that negative effects of stress were ameliorated for those with higher levels of mindfulness. Mindfulness may slow the rate of cellular aging (Epel, Daubenmier, Moskowitz, Folkman, & Blackburn, 2009). A systematic review of twelve studies suggests that mindfulness practice can prevent or ameliorate age-related cognitive decline (Gard, Hölzel, & Lazar, 2014).

Yoga, qigong, and meditation are holistic self-care practices that enhance the well-being of body, mind, and spirit. Aging women can integrate these practices into their lives to promote both mental and physical health, and because these are *self-care* practices, successfully initiating a regular practice has the added benefit of cultivating a subjective sense of empowerment.

Healthy Aging and Social Connection

It is hard to overestimate the importance of social connection for older adults. Giving and receiving social support may be one of the most important factors in maintaining health in old age (Giles, Glonek, Luszcz, & Andrews, 2005; McReynolds & Rossen, 2004).

In a groundbreaking study, Taylor et al. (2000) found that women responded to stress differently from men. Specifically, females' stress responses were characterized by "tend and befriend" activities, rather than "fight of flight" patterns (Taylor et al., 2000). The study found that during times of stress, women were likely to engage in nurturing activities (called "tending" by the authors of the study) that "promote safety and reduce distress." They define "befriending" as the "creation and maintenance of social networks that may aid in this process" (Taylor et al., 2000). The researchers speculate that endorphins and oxytocin play roles in establishing the nurturing activity, while factors like learning and socialization reinforce the behavior. Both oxytocin and endorphins may also contribute to the formation and maintenance of social networks. Social connection may turn out to be a crucial part of our stress-buffering mechanism and healthy immune system functioning and not just an important factor in psychological health.

These findings, coupled with decades of data on social support and health, suggest that social connection may be an important component of health promotion among older adults (Dupertuis, Aldwin, & Bosse, 2001; Fiori, Antonucci, & Cortina, 2006; Lyyra & Heikkinen, 2006). Older adults are often isolated from their friends and families and must make a great effort to connect with others. In the same way that they encourage exercise, health professionals can support older patients by recommending that they seek out social connection. This may be especially important for single, widowed, and divorced women.

Spirituality and Health

Older adults experience loss on many levels: loss of physical functions; of energy and stamina; of career, status, and identity; of independence, and of loved ones. Many older women suffer as they lose their conventionally defined physical attractiveness, or their powerful social roles as mothers, homemakers, or professionals. A great number of older women outlive their husbands/partners and must cope with the loss of their marriage, and some witness the death of beloved adult children. As the popular saying has it, "Old age is not for sissies." Loss in the outer world offers us the opportunity to turn inward and start soul searching. A solid connection to one's spirituality is a proven psychological coping mechanism for dealing with loss (Pargament, 1997).

> Compared with younger populations, the aged often face negative stressors that are difficult to control.... The aged have a strong need to learn how to accept or to cope with pain, dependency, and their own mortality, while simultaneously enjoying what life still has to offer. For many persons, an acute awareness of the ephemeral nature of life can actually increase one's sense of joy. (Ai & Mackenzie, 2006)

From this perspective, the negative stressors associated with aging become catalysts for a journey of spiritual growth. Reframing their experience in this way can be enormously helpful to older adults coping with loss, and health professionals should not be reticent to discuss patients' spiritual lives. Although some women may not be open to discussing their spirituality with health professionals, studies indicate that the majority of patients welcome the opportunity (Ehman, Ott, Short, Ciampa, & Hansen-Flaschen, 1999; McCord et al., 2004).

There is no standard algorithm for addressing the spiritual concerns of patients, and there are as many ways to encourage spiritual exploration as there are people. Patients with ties to traditional religions may just need some encouragement to participate more fully in their congregations. Others can be helped in their journey through meditation, yoga, tai chi, or qigong, all of which are in essence spiritual disciplines. Gently inquiring into the kinds of activities that help your patient feel more at peace (e.g., walking in nature, gardening, caring for grandchildren) may provide important clues about where her spiritual home is located. The important thing is to acknowledge the connection between health and spirituality and to let patients know that their moral, metaphysical, and spiritual concerns are an important dimension of their overall well-being. As Larry Dossey, MD, wrote, "We find ourselves in society that is spiritually malnourished and hungry for meaning" (Dossey, 2005). Health professionals seeking to care for whole persons have an obligation to respond to this hunger.

Table 6.1.   The Whole Woman Approach to Healthy Aging: A Clinician's Guide

1. One mind–body practice: meditation, yoga, tai chi, or qigong (daily)

2. Feasible and appropriate exercise routine (6 days per week)

3. Establish or maintain social network (weekly)

4. Regular bodywork (monthly)

5. A nutrition/supplement plan tailored to the individual

6. Address spiritual concerns as appropriate

Conclusion

One of the most important things health professionals can do is to introduce their older patients to the idea that they can accept aging as a natural part of the life cycle without resigning themselves to pain, dysfunction, or decrepitude. Coaching patients to adopt lifestyle changes can set the stage for healthy aging while maximizing vitality, wholeness, and quality of life. It is appropriate to exhort older women to find ways to restore their vitality while acknowledging the health challenges inherent in becoming old (Table 6.1).

REFERENCES

Aagaard, P., Suetta, C., Caserotti, P., et al. (2010). Role of the nervous system in sarcopenia and muscle atrophy with aging: Strength training as a countermeasure. *Scand J Med Sci Sports, 20,* 49–64.

Ai, A., & Mackenzie, E. R. (2006). Spiritual well-being the care of older adults. In: E. R. Mackenzie & B. Rakel (Eds.), *Complementary and alternative medicine for older adults* (pp. 276–xxx). New York, NY: Springer.

Annweiler, C., Dursun, E., Féron, F., et al. (2014). Vitamin D and cognition in older adults: Updated international recommendations. *J Intern Med, 277,* 45–57.

Annweiler, C., Karras, S. N., Anagnostis, P., & Beauchet, O. (2014). Vitamin D supplements: A novel therapeutic approach for Alzheimer patients. *Front Pharmacol, 5,* 1–4.

Autier, P., & Gandini, S. (2007). Vitamin D supplementation and total mortality: A meta-analysis of randomized controlled trials. *Arch Intern Med, 167,* 1730–1737.

Behrman, S., & Ebmeier, K. P. (2014). Can exercise prevent cognitive decline? *Practitioner, 258,* 17–21.

Best, J. R., Nagamatsu, L. S., & Liu-Ambrose, T. (2014). Improvements to executive functions during exercise training predict maintenance of physical activity over the following year. *Front Human Neurosci, 8,* 353.

Birks, J., & Grimley Evans, J. (2009). Ginkgo biloba for cognitive impairment and dementia. *Cochrane Database Syst Rev,* CD003120.

Brondino, N., De Silvestri, A., Re, S., et al. (2013). A systematic review and meta-analysis of ginkgo biloba in neuropsychiatric disorders: From ancient tradition to modern-day medicine. *J Evid Based Complementary Altern Med, 2013*.

Bruyere, O., Cooper, C., Pelletier, J. P., et al. (2014). An algorithm recommendation for the management of knee osteoarthritis in Europe and internationally: A report from a task force of the European Society for Clinical and Economic Aspects of Osteoporosis and Osteoarthritis (ESCEO). *Semin Arthritis Rheum, 44*, 253–263.

Butera, R. (2006). Yoga: An introduction. In E. R. Mackenzie & B. Rakel (Eds.), *Complementary and alternative medicine for older adults* (pp. 199–213). New York, NY: Springer.

Chen, K., Mackenzie, E. R., & Hou, F. (2006). The benefits of qigong. In E. R. Mackenzie & B. Rakel (Eds.), *Complementary and alternative medicine for older adults* (pp. 175–198). New York, NY: Springer.

Cheung, C., Wyman, J. F., Resnick, B., & Savik, K. (2014). Yoga for managing knee osteoarthritis in older women: A pilot randomized controlled trial. *BMC Compl Altern Med, 14*, 1–11.

Chrysant, S. G., & Chrysant, G. S. (2014). Controversy regarding the association of high calcium intake and increased risk for cardiovascular disease. *J Clin Hypertens, 16*(8), 545–550.

Cohen, K. (1997). *The way of qigong: The art and science of Chinese energy healing.* New York, NY: Ballantine Books.

Cohen, M. (2007). "Detox": Science or sales pitch? *Aust Fam Physician, 36*, 1009–1010.

Conlin, P. R., Chow, D., Miller, E. R., 3rd, et al. (2000). The effect of dietary patterns on blood pressure control in hypertensive patients: Results from the Dietary Approaches to Stop Hypertension (DASH) trial. *Am J Hypertens, 13*, 949–955.

Davidson, R. J., Kabat-Zinn, J., Schumacher, J., et al. (2003). Alterations in brain and immune function produced by mindfulness meditation. *Psychosomatic Med, 65*, 564–570.

Deane, A., Constancio, L., Fogelman, I., et al. (2007). The impact of vitamin D status on changes in bone mineral density during treatment with bisphosphonates and after discontinuation following long-term use in post-menopausal osteoporosis. *BMC Musculoskelet Disord, 8*, 3.

DeKosky, S. T., Williamson, J. D., Fitzpatrick, A. L., et al. (2008). Ginkgo biloba for prevention of dementia: A randomized controlled trial. *JAMA, 300*, 2253–2262.

de Frias, C. M., & Whyne, E. (2015). Stress on health-related quality of life in older adults: the protective nature of mindfulness. *Aging Mental Health, 19*(3), 201–206.

derMarderosian, A., & Briggs, M. (2006). Supplements and herbs. In E. R. Mackenzie & B. Rakel (Eds.), *Complementary and alternative medicine for older adults* (pp. 31–78). New York, NY: Springer.

Devine, A., Dick, I. M., Heal, S. J., et al. (1997). A 4-year follow-up study of the effects of calcium supplementation on bone density in elderly postmenopausal women. *Osteoporos Int, 7*, 23–28.

Dossey, L. (2005). What does illness mean? In M. Schlitz, T. Amorok, & M. Micozzi, (Eds.), *Consciousness and healing: Integral approaches to mind-body medicine* (pp. 151–xxx). St. Louis MO: Elsevier/Churchill Livingstone.

Dupertuis, L. L., Aldwin, C. M., & Bosse, R. (2001). Does the source of support matter for different health outcomes? *J Aging Health, 13,* 494–510.

Ehman, J. W., Ott, B. B., Short, T. H., Ciampa, R. C., & Hansen-Flaschen, J. (1999). Do patients want physicians to inquire about their spiritual or religious beliefs if they become gravely ill? *Arch Intern Med, 159,* 1803–1806.

Epel, E., Daubenmier, J., Moskowitz, J. T., Folkman, S., & Blackburn, E. (2009). Can meditation slow rate of cellular aging? Cognitive stress, mindfulness, and telomeres. *Annals of the New York Academy of Sciences, 1172,* 34–53.

Fiori, K. L., Antonucci, T. C., & Cortina, K. S. (2006). Social network typologies and mental health among older adults. *J Gerontol: Series, B, 61,* P25–P32.

Fraser, G. E. (2009). Vegetarian diets: What do we know of their effects on common chronic diseases? *Amer J Clin Nutr, 89,* 1607S–1612S.

Gard, T., Hölzel, B. K., & Lazar, S. W. (2014). The potential effects of meditation on age-related cognitive decline: A systematic review. *Ann NY Acad Sci, 1307,* 89–103.

Giles, L. C., Glonek, G. F., Luszcz, M. A., & Andrews, G. R. (2005). Effect of social networks on 10 year survival in very old Australians. *J Epidemiol Community Health, 59,* 574–579.

Ginter, E. (2008). Vegetarian diets, chronic diseases and longevity. *Bratislavske Lekarske Listy, 109,* 463–466.

Hamer, M., Lavoie, K. L., & Bacon, S. L. (2014). Taking up physical activity later in life and healthy aging: The English longitudinal study of aging. *Br J Sports Med, 48,* 239–243

Hartley, L., Dyakova, M., Holmes, J., Clarke, A., Lee, M. S., Ernst, E., & Rees K. (2014).Yoga for the primary prevention of cardiovascular disease. *Cochrane Database Syst Rev,* 5:CD010072. doi: 10.1002/14651858.CD010072.pub2

Heiss, G., Wallace, R., Anderson, G. L., et al. (2008). Health risks and benefits 3 years after stopping randomized treatment with estrogen and progestin. *JAMA, 299,* 1036–1045.

Holloszy, J. O., & Fontana, L. (2007). Caloric restriction in humans. *Exp Gerontol, 42,* 709–712.

Innes, K. E., Selfe, T. K., & Taylor, A. G. (2008). Menopause, the metabolic syndrome, and mind-body therapies. *Menopause (New York, NY), 15,* 1005–1013.

Kemmler, W., von Stengel, S., Engelke, K., Häberle, L.,& Kalender, W. A. (2010). Exercise effects on bone mineral density, falls, and health care costs in older women: The Randomized Controlled Senior Fitness and Prevention Study (SEFIP), *Arch Intern Med, 170*(2), 179–185.

Kennedy, E., & Chapman, C. (2006). Massage therapy and older adults. In E. R. Mackenzie & B. Rakel (Eds.), *Complementary and alternative medicine for older adults* (pp. 138–139). New York, NY: Springer.

Kennis, E., Verschueren, S., Bogaerts A., et al. (2013). Long-term impact of strength training on muscle strength characteristics in older adults. *Arch Phys Med Rehab, 94,* 2054–2060.

Kim, M. K., Cho, S. W., & Park, Y. K. (2012). Long-term vegetarians have low oxidative stress, body fat, and cholesterol levels. *Nutr Res Prac, 6*, 155–161.

Kris-Etherton, P. M., Harris, W. S., & Appel, L. J. (2003). Fish consumption, fish oil, omega-3 fatty acids, and cardiovascular disease. *Arterioscler Thromb Vasc Biol, 23*, e20–e30.

Lappe, J. M., Travers-Gustafson, D., Davies, K. M., et al. (2007). Vitamin D and calcium supplementation reduces cancer risk: Results of a randomized trial. *Am J Clin Nutr, 85*, 1586–1591.

Lee, J. S., Kim, C. G., & Seo, T. B. (2014). Effects of 8 week combined training on body composition, isokinetic strength, and cardiovascular disease in older women. *Aging Clin Exp Res, 27*(2), 179–186.

Levine, M. E., Suarez, J. A., Brandhorst, S., et al. (2014). Low protein intake is associated with a major reduction in IGF-1, cancer, and overall mortality in the 65 and younger but not older population. *Cell Metabol, 19*, 407–417.

Ludwig, D. S., & Kabat-Zinn, J. (2008). Mindfulness in medicine. *JAMA, 300*, 1350–1352.

Lyyra, T. M., & Heikkinen, R. L. (2006). Perceived social support and mortality in older people. *J Gerontol: Series, B, 61*, S147–S152.

McCord, G., Gilchrist, V. J., & Grossman, S. D., et al. (2004). Discussing spirituality with patients: A rational and ethical approach. *Ann Fam Med, 2*, 356–361.

McReynolds, J. L., & Rossen, E. K. (2004). Importance of physical activity, nutrition and social support for optimal aging. *Clin Nurse Spec, 18*, 200–206.

Melow, S., Tarnopolsky M. et al. (2007). Resistance exercise reverses aging in human skeletal muscle. *PLoS ONE, 2*, e465.

Michalsen, A., Jeitler, M., Brunnhuber, S., Lüdtke, R., Büssing, A., Musial, F., & Kessler, C. (2012). Iyengar yoga for distressed women: A 3-armed randomized controlled trial. *J Evid Based Complementary Altern Med, 2012*, 408727.

Moliver, N., Mika, E. M., Chartrand, M. S., Haussmann, R. E., & Khalsa, S. B. S. (2013). Yoga experience as a predictor of psychological wellness in women over 45 years. *Internat J Yoga, 6*, 11–19.

Morris, M. C., Sacks, F., & Rosner, B. (1993). Does fish oil lower blood pressure? A meta-analysis of controlled trials. *Circulation, 88*, 523–533.

Moyer, V. A. (2013). Vitamin D and calcium supplementation to prevent fractures in adults: US Preventive Services Task Force recommendation statement. *Ann Intern Med, 158*, 691–696.

Murphy, J. (2000/1963). *The power of your subconscious mind.* New York, NY: Bantam Books.

Napoli, N., Thomson, J., Civitelli, R., & Armamento Villareal, R. C. (2007). Effects of dietary calcium compared with calcium supplements on estrogen metabolism and bone mineral density. *Am J Clin Nutr, 85*, 1428–1433.

Paik, J. M., Curhan, G. C., Sun, Q., Rexrode, K. M., Manson, J. E., Rimm, E. B., & Taylor, E. N. (2014). Calcium supplement intake and risk of cardiovascular disease in women. *Osteoporosis International, 25*(8), 2047–2056.

Pargament, K. I. (1997). *The psychology of religion and coping.* New York, NY: Guilford Press.

Reginster, J. Y., Deroisy, R., Rovati, L. C., et al. (2001). Long-term effects of glucos-amine sulphate on osteoarthritis progression: A randomised, placebo-controlled clinical trial. *Lancet, 357*, 251–256.

Reid, I., Ames, R. W., Evans, M. C., et al. (1993). Effect of calcium supplementation on bone loss in postmenopausal women. *N Engl J Med, 328*, 460–464.

Robinson, J. G., Ijioma, N., & Harris, W. (2010). Omega-3 fatty acids and cognitive function in women. *Women's Health (Lond Eng), 6*, 119–134.

Rogers, C. E., Larkey, L. K., & Keller, C. (2009). A review of clinical trials of tai chi and qigong in older adults. *West J Nurs Res, 31*, 245–279.

Sabate, J. (2003). The contribution of vegetarian diets to human health. *Forum Nutr, 56*, 218–220.

SanGiovanni, J. P., Chew, E. Y., Agrón, E., et al. (2008). The relationship of dietary omega-3 long-chain polyunsaturated fatty acid intake with incident age-related macular degeneration: AREDS report no. 23. *Arch Ophthalmol, 126*, 1274–1279.

Schneider, R. H., Walton, K. G., Salerno, J. W., & Nidich, S. I. (2006). Cardiovascular disease prevention and health promotion with the TM program. *Ethn Dis, 16*(Suppl 4), 15–26.

Schumann, S. A., & Ewigman, B. (2007). Double-dose vitamin D lowers cancer risk in women over 55. *J Fam Pract, 56*, 907–910.

Singh, P. N., Sabaté, J., & Fraser, G. E. (2003). Does low meat consumption increase life expectancy in humans? *Am J Clin Nutr, 78*(3 Suppl), 526S–532S.

Tantamango-Bartley, Y., Jaceldo-Siegl, K., Fan, J., & Fraser, G. (2013). Vegetarian diets and the incidence of cancer in a low-risk population. *Cancer Epidemiol Biomarkers Prev, 22*, 286–294.

Taylor, S. E., et al. (2000). Biobehavioral responses to stress in females: Tend-and-befriend not fight-or-flight *Psychol Rev, 107*, 411–429.

US Preventive Services Taskforce. (2013). *Vitamin D and calcium to prevent fractures: Preventive medication.* Retrieved December 31, 2014, from http://www.uspreventiveservicestaskforce.org/uspstf/uspsvitd.htm

Vangsness, C. T., Jr., Spiker, W., & Erickson, J. (2009). A review of evidence-based medicine for glucosamine and chondroitin sulfate use in knee osteoarthritis. *Arthroscopy, 25*, 86–94.

Vellas, B., Coley, N., Ousset, P. J., et al. (2012). Long-term use of standardised Ginkgo biloba extract for the prevention of Alzheimer's disease (GuidAge): A randomized placebo-controlled trial. *Lancet Neurol, 11*, 851–859.

Wang, L., Manson, J. E., Lee, I. M., & Sesso, H. D. (2008). Dietary intake of dairy products and vitamin D and the risk of hypertension in middle-aged and older women. *Hypertension, 51*, 1073–1079.

Weil, A. (2001). On integrative medicine and the nature of reality (Interview with Bonnie Horrigan). *Altern Ther Health Med, 7*, 103.

Willcox, B. J., Willcox, D. C., Todoriki, H., et al. (2007). Caloric restriction, the traditional Okinawan diet, and healthy aging: The diet of the world's longest-lived people and its potential impact on morbidity and life span. *Ann N Y Acad Sci, 1114*, 434–455.

Winston, D., & Maimes, S. (2007). *Adaptogens: Herbs for strength, stamina, and stress relief*. Rochester, VT: Healing Arts Press.

Wolfe, R. R., Miller, S. L., & Miller, K. B. (2008). Optimal protein intake in the elderly. *Clin Nutr, 27*, 675–684.

Yuen, E., & Baime, M. (2006). Meditation and healthy aging. In E. R. Mackenzie & B. Rakel (Eds.), *Complementary and alternative medicine for older adults* (pp. 233–2703). New York, NY: Springer.

PART II

Systems and Modalities

7

Traditional Chinese Medicine

LESLIE MCGEE

CASE STUDY

Sally M. was 36 years old and a veteran of 6 years of intrauterine inseminations (IUIs) and seven failed in vitro fertilizations
(IVFs), with not a single pregnancy in her quest to have a child.
She arrived in my office about one month before the eighth IVF
was scheduled. She told me that her uterine lining was never
more than 6 mm thick for the embryo transfer (a minimum of
8 mm thickness is best for embryo implantation). Sally also told
me that she always had a very short and scant 3-day menstrual
period and never remembers having any noticeable midcycle
egg-white quality cervical mucus.

Chinese medicine developed theories describing women's
physiology many centuries ago. Long before modern science
identified hormones and the hypothalamic-pituitary-ovarian
axis, Chinese medicine provided care for women from menarche beyond menopause and provided insight into the mechanisms of health and disease. Chinese medicine proposes an
elaborate theory of women's physiology, which continues to
attract modern practitioners and patients with its capacity to
restore balance in women's lives.

Acupuncture is the best-known modality of Chinese medicine, but is just one aspect of the full range of treatment options
within this system. Women's health issues are usually considered internal medicine conditions, and for these, Chinese herbs,
typically in complex and individualized formulations, are used.

In addition, Chinese medicine practitioners promote lifestyle and diet changes as being fundamental to long-term wellness (Flaws, 1997; Maciocia, 1998).

Fundamental Theories

Chinese medicine developed over 2000 years ago. Its theories and ideas link human beings and our health with natural phenomenon: heaven and earth, cycles of growth and decline, the seasons, movement and stillness, and every observable process seen in our world, both animate and inanimate. One of the fundamental ideas of Chinese medicine is the theory of yin and yang. Yin represents form, substance, stillness, moisture, darkness, the interior, and coolness. Yang represents energy, activity, transformation, heat, the exterior, brightness, and dryness. Yin and yang are opposite qualities, and as such, they are mutually consumptive. For example, yin's moisture can extinguish yang's heat. Or yang's activity can transform yin's stillness and inertia. These qualities translate into the body: Our form and substance are yin; the body's metabolic processes are yang. The inside of the uterus is yin. The moment the egg is released from the ovary is yang. Any bodily process or substance can be analyzed in this way.

Paradoxically, it is said that yin and yang are mutually transformative. Extreme yin can transform into yang, and vice versa. For example, the follicular phase in a woman's cycle is considered the yin phase. As yin maximizes there is a sudden transformation to the yang activity of ovulation. In other words, yin and yang can destroy each other, yet they can also become each other. They are opposed, inseparable yet, mutually transformative (Maciocia, 2005).

Another fundamental theory of Chinese medicine is the concept of the vital substances. The most significant of these are known as the "three treasures," qi ("chee"), blood, and essence. Qi roughly translates as vital energy and has a yang nature in its functions of moving, warming, and transforming. Blood is dark and fluid thus, more yin and serves as the substantial nourishment of both body and mind. Essence is a fundamental, highly refined substance, with both yin and yang qualities. It governs growth and reproduction, and declines with age. The body functions and lives through the presence and activities of these substances.

Chinese medicine also theorizes that a complex web of meridians or channels traverses the body. Acupuncture points along those meridians are used to adjust the function and balance of the body, using the fine needles of acupuncture or manual stimulation of acupressure.

Over 2000 years ago in the medical classic *Su Wen–Simple Questions*, Chinese doctors remarked on the stages of life affecting women. Women's lives are governed by the slow maturation and decline of essence in 7-year cycles. They wrote, "The Tian Gui [the heavenly water or menstrual blood] arrives at age 14 (2 × 7) if the Ren vessel is free-flowing and the Chong vessel is exuberant. The menstruation descends periodically, and one can have children.... At 7 × 7, 49 years, the Ren vessel is vacuous and the Chong vessel is debilitated and scanty. The Tian Gui, heavenly water, is exhausted and the pathways are not free-flowing. Thus the body is decrepit and there are no children" (Ting-Liang, 1995). Fortunately, decrepitude is not the destiny of every 49-year-old modern woman, but the onset of menopause remains still, on average, at age 49. Imagine if more women saw their menstrual blood as a form of heavenly water!

It is the complex interplay of the three vital substances that governs women's physiology. To be healthy, fertile, and energetic, women need not only an adequate quantity of qi, blood, and essence but also their proper cyclic movements. The maturation of essence leads to menarche. The ability of qi to properly move the blood in a monthly fashion, filling and then emptying meridians and the uterus, creates the menstrual cycle. Adequate essence maintains the ovaries and fertility.

The relationship and harmony of yin and yang underscores every aspect of women's health: the balance between energy and restfulness, the proper biphasic curve of the monthly basal body temperature chart, and the ground for an easy and predictable monthly cycle. Chinese medicine, without the modern concepts of hormones and biochemistry, describes women's health with clarity and logical consistency.

Pathology in women is analyzed according to the theory of Chinese medicine. Any discomfort unique to women is discussed in the Chinese gynecological literature, both ancient and modern. Treatment is determined not by the disease but by the pattern of disharmony underlying the disease. Thus, for example, there is no single acupuncture or herbal prescription for dysmenorrhea. The pattern underlying the pain must be determined first and then correct treatment chosen.

To take this example further, a careful analysis of the mechanisms of dysmenorrhea and the woman's unique presentation will lead the practitioner to the correct pattern differentiation. From there treatment flows, including acupuncture points, herbal therapies, and lifestyle recommendations. *A Handbook of Menstrual Diseases in Chinese Medicine* (Flaws, 1997) lists eight different patterns possible in dysmenorrhea, and each pattern has its unique herbal and acupuncture prescriptions.

Women are often surprised by the inquisitive nature of a good Chinese gynecological assessment. All aspects of the cycle are scrutinized. Regularity, quantity, and quality of blood flow (is it pink, red, purple, brown, thin, thick, clotted?); any cyclic discomforts—both emotional and physical; any pain anywhere in the body that seems linked to the period; and for the menstrual pain itself: does it occur before, during, or after the menses and what is its quality (dull, sharp, fixed, mobile?). Other aspects of a woman's life are also explored such as sleep quality, energy, and digestion. All these questions are asked and their answers ascertained.

Women's health issues treated by Chinese medicine include premenstrual syndrome, irregular cycles, polycystic ovarian syndrome, dysmenorrhea, endometriosis, vaginal infections, frequent miscarriage, infertility, menopause, and many others. Regular acupuncture and herbal medicine may be needed for many weeks to effect lasting change. Or in some cases, a monthly acupuncture session or herbal formula is adequate. For others, diet and lifestyle recommendations alone can empower them and restore health.

> In Chinese medicine, ideas about connections between different parts of the body are common. For instance, we say the feet are a reflection of the kidney and the kidney is closely associated with the uterus. Thus, keeping the feet warm is a strategy for keeping the uterus warm and protecting a pregnancy. I often find that infertile women have cold feet, and this informs my diagnosis of their Chinese pattern—cold feet equals deficiency of kidney yang, or the fundamental fire of the body. In modern medicine, cold feet can be associated with hypothyroid function, and optimal thyroid function supports fertility and pregnancy (Poppe, Velkeniers, & Glinoer, 2008). The global nature of these insights was brought home when I asked a Mexican American client who was hoping to get pregnant to please keep her feet warm, and she told me that her mother had told her to stop walking barefoot on the tile floors once her period started or the cold would enter her uterus and cause menstrual cramps.

Modern Research

In China, a vast literature exists describing the treatment of women with Chinese medicine. Each year, hundreds of Chinese medical journals are published. On the whole, the research methodologies used are often unsophisticated, leaving the reader with piqued interest and unanswered questions. In spite of this failing, the research suggests avenues that merit further exploration.

One example of research done in China combining Western and Chinese medicine involved 110 infertile women who were divided into two groups. The treatment group received clomiphene and complex Chinese herb formulas adjusted to each of four weeks of their cycle. One formula was used for the menstrual period week, another formula for the postmenstrual week, a third formula for midcycle, and a fourth formula for the premenstrual/postinsemination week. The control group received just clomiphene.

Outcome measures included endometrial thickness, cervical mucus, and conception rate. The treatment group had thicker uterine lining, better quality cervical mucus, and a conception rate of 41%. The control group's conception rate was 22% (Flaws, 2008).

Western research of Chinese medicine has advanced in the past decade and some of the findings are perplexing. In an effort to create a valid control, various sham acupuncture methods have been used. These controls range from needle insertion at nonacupuncture points to methods in which the patient believes a needle has been inserted when it has not. In several studies the sham acupuncture control performed almost as well as the "real" acupuncture. Meng, Xu, and Lao (2011) reviewed multiple randomized controlled trials and found that inserting needles in sham acupuncture points was inferior to non-insertion sham acupuncture as a control. In addition, the evidence indicated that acupuncture outperformed wait-list or usual biomedical care in many trials. In reviewing the findings, Langevin et al. (2011) explore these paradoxes and suggest avenues for further research.

Studies to determine the exact mechanism of acupuncture's effects are also being conducted. Meridians and acupuncture points demonstrate unique biophysical characteristics, including electrical, acoustic, thermal, vascular, and myoelectric properties (Li et al., 2012; Liu et al., 2013). Another area of research involves using functional magnetic resonance imaging (fMRI) during acupuncture needling. Huang reviewed English as well as Chinese, Korean, and Japanese databases and concluded that acupuncture can modulate brain activity. The effects on the brain were complex, and in some cases corresponded with the traditional view of the point's actions (Huang et al., 2012).

One of the strengths of Chinese medicine is the individualized nature of treatment. Researchers are exploring methods that allow treatment to be tailored while also meeting standards of research design and reproducibility (Schnyer & Allen, 2002). Some researchers are using a "whole-systems" research design that attempts to evaluate individualized care using the whole range of modalities available in Chinese medicine (acupuncture, herbs, massage, lifestyle) (Elder et al., 2012; Hullender Rubin et al., 2014; Ritenbaugh et al., 2012). These studies more accurately reflect how Chinese medicine is practiced in the clinical setting.

Most of the research on women's health using Chinese medicine in the West has been done on acupuncture and less often on Chinese herbal interventions.

The quality of this research varies considerably. A review of controlled trials of acupuncture for women's reproductive healthcare concluded that design flaws excluded many studies from their review, but acupuncture for dysmenorrhea and infertility provided the most promising outcomes (White, 2003). Electro-acupuncture to induce ovulation in women with polycystic ovarian syndrome may be effective, with several studies exploring this in the West and in China (Cochrane, Smith, Possamai-Inesedy, & Bensoussan, 2014). Acupuncture was shown to be effective for pregnant women with depression, demonstrating both symptom reduction comparable to standard depression treatment and safety during pregnancy (Manber et al., 2010). In one meta-analysis acupuncture improved hot flash frequency and severity, as well as quality of life, in women in natural menopause (Chiu et al., 2015). Another study found that acupuncture relieved hot flashes in women getting tamoxifen therapy for breast cancer (Hervik & Mjaland, 2009).

Acupuncture for IVF has been the most researched gynecological topic in Western settings. Starting with Paulus in 2002, several randomized clinical trials using acupuncture during IVF cycles have been completed. Data from those trials have been mixed, with some studies showing benefit and others showing none (Manheimer et al., 2013). These studies all used acupuncture 1 to 3 days around the day of embryo transfer (ET), and many acupuncturists believe that a 1-day intervention of acupuncture is simply not an adequate dose. Several acupuncture treatments in the weeks leading up to IVF may be more beneficial, as reported by Magarelli et al. Their protocol provided nine acupuncture sessions in the four weeks prior to IVF plus acupuncture on the day of ET. Significant changes in serum cortisol and prolactin were measured in the acupuncture group as well as improvement in clinical pregnancy rate and live births (Magarelli, 2009). Hullender Rubin et al. performed a retrospective cohort study of 1,069 IVF patients and compared live birth rates for women among three different groups (Hullender Rubin et al., 2014). One group received an average of 12 sessions of "whole-systems" traditional Chinese medicine (TCM), including acupuncture, Chinese herbs, and dietary and/or lifestyle advice. The second group had acupuncture on the day of embryo transfer, using a typical day-of-ET acupuncture protocol (Hullender Rubin, Opsahl, Taylor Swanson, & Ackerman, 2013). The third group had the usual IVF care with no known additional therapies. The group of women using whole-systems TCM had a significantly higher live birth rate. The live birth rates for the ET-day acupuncture group and the group that had usual IVF care were not significantly different, in keeping with the mixed results previously seen (Hullender Rubin et al., 2014).

Another interesting element of acupuncture practice is that it is far from homogeneous in point-selection strategies. Several unique acupuncture traditions exist, and each has its very different point-selection processes and conclusions. The most commonly practiced acupuncture style in the West is TCM. Other styles include Japanese meridian therapy (Manaka, 1995), classical Chinese style (Van Nghi, Viet Dzung, & Recours-Nguyen, 2005, 2006), five-element style (Connelly, 1992), and various microsystem styles such as Master Tong's method (Tan, 1996), Dr. Zhu's scalp acupuncture system (Dharmananda & Vickers, 2000), and auricular therapy (Oleson, 2014). Point selection and needling technique are quite varied between these different styles. Recent research is beginning to reflect this diversity. For example, Japanese style acupuncture was used to treat endometriosis-related pelvic pain in adolescents, with significant pain relief in the treatment group (Wayne et al., 2008).

There is more agreement and uniformity in the selection of Chinese herbs for women than among point selections. Chinese herbal medicine's framework is well defined by TCM. Pattern differentiation and herb selection have been extensively documented in the Chinese literature and translated into many languages (Sionneau & Gang, 1996–2000). Many, if not most, gynecological complaints are treated with complex herb formulas in China and other Asian countries. Thirty-nine trials of Chinese herbs for the treatment of dysmenorrhea were reviewed from Chinese literature (Zhu, Proctor, Bensoussan, Smith, & Wu, 2007). Many of these trials had methodological problems, but the reviewers found that Chinese herbs were generally effective against dysmenorrhea and in some cases rapidly effective. Most of the formulas used in these trials were typical multiherb, individually tailored prescriptions. Western physicians were advised to seek the expertise of fully trained practitioners of Chinese medicine in order to properly select herbal formulas for individual women.

Research on complex, multiherb formulas continues to be rare in Western settings, but is much more common in Asia. A search of clinicaltrials.gov revealed over 200 trials in progress or completed using Chinese herbs to treat a variety of conditions, including menopause, endometriosis, myelodysplastic disorders, type II diabetes, and osteoporosis. Many of these studies are being done at academic medical centers in China (clinicaltrials.gov, 2014).

Based on my Chinese medicine assessment, I concluded that Sally's TCM pattern was a combination of yin and blood deficiency, with some blood stasis. Because Sally was receiving extensive pharmaceutical ovarian management and stimulation, she elected to use only acupuncture, and not herbs, to support her chance for pregnancy. Seven acupuncture treatments were given prior to this IVF transfer.

Ultrasound revealed her lining to have improved to a thickness of 8 mm with a decent trilaminar appearance. The day of the embryo transfer, a complex acupuncture protocol was utilized. A single embryo/fetal sac was seen on ultrasound with an uneventful progression until Sally had a miscarriage at 11 weeks. Devastated after this event, Sally decided that she would take a break from the Western approach to her infertility and give Chinese herbs a try. For 2 months, Sally used whole Chinese herbs and consumed them as a cooked decoction. The formula contained herbs to nourish her yin, blood, and essence, and secondarily to rectify the qi and blood.

After about a month on the herbs she returned to her reproductive endocrinologist (RE) and on ultrasound examination he noticed that her uterus looked unusually plump. A month later, when Sally had not resumed ovulating, she decided to do another IVF. The herbs were discontinued while her doctor stimulated her ovaries and recovered a number of eggs. At this time, acupuncture was resumed to support her lining and nourish her yin. The RE followed her uterus on ultrasound and found that its plump condition was maintained and the lining at transfer time was unusually thick for her. Three embryos were transferred and pregnancy occurred. The surprise was that three fetal sacs were seen at the first ultrasound. Somehow her uterine lining had become far more hospitable for her embryos! Fortunately, over the next few weeks, first one and then the other embryo faded, and Sally was pregnant with one fetus with a strong heartbeat. Acupuncture was administered every week during the first trimester to support the pregnancy and then tapered to every 3 or 4 weeks for the duration of the pregnancy. Sally had a healthy baby girl at 37 weeks by C-section. When the baby was 8 months old, Sally came in for acupuncture for seasonal allergies and reported that her period resumed at about 4 months and it had changed considerably. She now has a 5-day moderate flow of bright red blood, and fairly abundant, midcycle cervical mucus. She is hopeful that she and her husband might be able to conceive without assisted reproductive technology and have a second child.

Conclusion

The language of Chinese medicine gynecology, with its references to yin and yang, essence and heavenly water, may seem quaint and poetic. Chinese medicine proposes that every human being is connected to the universe and our health is affected by climate, season, cycles of day and night, and all natural phenomenon. Dr. Ngyuen Van Nghi, one of the greatest classical Chinese acupuncturists and translator of ancient Chinese texts (Van Nghi et al., 2005, 2006), has stated: "Woman is little nature, a child of heaven and earth, a product of cosmic forces" (Garbacz, 2008). This statement captures the essence of Chinese insight into women's health. Chinese medicine recognizes that women, with monthly expression of these natural cycles, are indeed human displays of cosmic forces. The physical, emotional, biochemical, and hormonal reality of a woman's life is connected to heaven and earth, yin and yang, and the ebb and flow of tides and moons. The wisdom of Chinese medicine, using unique concepts and therapies, has a wealth of history behind it and invites further research to explore its reputation as an effective system to enhance women's health.

REFERENCES

Chiu, H. Y., Pan, C. H., et al. (2015). Effects of acupuncture on menopause-related symptoms and quality of life in women on natural menopause: A meta-analysis of randomized controlled trials. *Menopause, 22.* [E-pub ahead of print]

clinicaltrials.gov. (2014). National Institutes of Health, Bethesda, MD.

Cochrane, S., Smith, C., Possamai-Inesedy, A., & Bensoussan, A. (2014). Acupuncture and women's health: An overview of the role of acupuncture and its clinical management in women's reproductive health. *Int J Women's Health, 6,* 313–325.

Connelly, D. (1992). *Traditional acupuncture: The law of the five elements* (5th ed.). Columbia, MD: Centre for Traditional Acupuncture.

Dharmananda, S., & Vickers, E. (2000). *Synopsis of scalp acupuncture.* Portland, OR: Institute for Traditional Medicine.

Elder, C., Ritenbaugh, C., Aickin, M., et al. (2012). Reductions in pain medication use associated with traditional Chinese medicine for chronic pain. *Perm J, 16,* 18–23.

Flaws, B. (1997). *A handbook of menstrual diseases in Chinese medicine.* Boulder, CO: Blue Poppy Press.

Flaws, B. (2008, Feb). A four-step protocol for improving the effects of clomiphene in patients with ovulatory dysfunction infertility. *Acupuncture Today, 9*(2).

Garbacz, E. (2008, May). Quoting a lecture by Dr. Ngyuen Van Nghi, reported in The Acupuncture Energetics of the Normal Female Reproductive System seminar. Tucson, AZ.

Hervik, J., & Mjaland, O. (2009). Acupuncture for the treatment of hot flashes in breast cancer patients, a randomized, controlled trial. *Breast Cancer Res Treat, 116,* 311–316.

Huang, W., Pach, D.,& Napadow, V., et al. (2012). Characterizing acupuncture stimuli using brain imaging with fMRI: A systematic review and meta-analysis of the literature. *PLoS ONE, 7,* e32960. doi:10.1371/journal.pone.0032960

Hullender Rubin, L. H., Opsahl, M. S., Taylor Swanson, L., & Ackerman, D. L. (2013). Acupuncture and in vitro fertilization: A retrospective chart review. *J Alt Complement Med, 19,* 637–643.

Hullender Rubin, L., Opsahl, M. S., Wiemer, K., et al. (2014). The effects of adjuvant whole-systems traditional Chinese medicine on in vitro fertilization live births: A retrospective cohort study [Abstract]. *J Alt Complement Med, 20,* A12–A13.

Langevin, H., Wayne, P. M.,Macpherson, H., et al. (2011). Paradoxes in acupuncture research: Strategies for moving forward. *Evid B Compl Alt Med, 2011.* Article ID 180805. doi.10.1155/2011/180805

Li, J., Wang, Q., Liang, H., et al. (2012). Biophysical characteristics of meridians and acu-points: A systemic review. *Evid B Compl Alt Med, 2012.* Article ID 793841. doi:10.1155/2012/793841

Liu, C., Xiaohu, W., Hua, X., et al. (2013). X-ray phase-contrast CT imaging of the acu-points based on synchrotron radiation. *Journal of Electron Spectroscopy and Related Phenomena, 196,* 80–84.

Maciocia, G. (1998). *Obstetrics and gynecology in Chinese medicine.* London, UK: Churchill Livingstone.

Maciocia, G. (2005). *The foundations of Chinese medicine* (2nd ed.). London, UK: Churchill Livingstone.

Magarelli, P. C., Cridennda, D. K., Cohen, M. (2009). Changes in serum cortisol and prolactin associated with acupuncture during controlled ovarian hyperstimulation in women undergoing in vitro fertilization-embryo transfer treatment. *Fertil Steril*, 92, 1870–1879.

Manaka, Y. (1995). *Chasing the dragon's tail*. Brookline, MA: Paradigm.

Manber, R., Schnyer, R., Lyell, D., et al. (2010). Acupuncture for depression during pregnancy: A randomized controlled trial. *Am Col Obstr Gyn*, 115, 511–520.

Manheimer, E., van der Windt, D., Cheng, K., et al. (2013). The effects of acupuncture on rates of clinical pregnancy among women undergoing in vitro fertilization: A systemic review and meta-analysis. *Human Reproductive Update*, 19, 696–713.

Meng, X., Xu, S., & Lao, L. (2011). Clinical acupuncture research in the west. *Front Med*, 5, 134–140.

Oleson, T. (2014). *Auricular therapy manual: Chinese and western systems of ear acupuncture* (4th ed.). London UK: Churchill Livingstone.

Paulus, W. E., Zhang, M., Strehler, E., El-Danasouri, I., & Sterzik, K. (2002). Influence of acupuncture on the pregnancy rate in patients who undergo assisted reproductive therapy. *Fertil Steril*, 77, 721–724.

Poppe, K., Velkeniers, B., & Glinoer, D. (2008). The role of thyroid auto-immunity in fertility and pregnancy. *Nat Clin Pract Endocrinol Metab*, 4, 394–405.

Ritenbaugh, C., Hammerschlag, R.,Dworkin, S. F., et al. (2012). Comparative effectiveness of traditional Chinese medicine and psychosocial care in the treatment of TMD-associated chronic facial pain. *J Pain*, 13, 1075–1089.

Schnyer, R., & Allen, J. (2002). Bridging the gap in complementary and alternative medicine research: Manualization as a means of promoting standardization and flexibility of treatment in clinical trials of acupuncture. *J Altern Complement Med*, 8, 623–634.

Sionneau, P., & Gang, L. (1996–2000). *The treatment of disease in TCM* (Vols. 1–7). Boulder, CO: Blue Poppy Press.

Tan, R. (1996). *Twelve and twelve in acupuncture* (2nd ed.). San Diego, CA: Author.

Ting-Liang, Z. (1995). A Handbook of Traditional Chinese Gynecology (4th ed). Boulder, CO: Blue Poppy Press.

Van Nghi, N., Viet Dzung, T., & Recours-Nguyen, C. (2005). *Huangdi Neijing Lingshu*. (Vol. 1). Sugar Grove, NC: Jung Tao.

Van Nghi, N., Viet Dzung, T., & Recours-Nguyen, C. (2006). *Huangdi Neijing Lingshu*. (Vol 2.). Sugar Grove, NC: Jung Tao.

Wayne, P., Kerr, C., Schnyer, R., et al. (2008). Japanese-style acupuncture for endometriosis-related pelvic pain in adolescents and young women: Results of a randomized sham-controlled trial. *J Pediatr Adolesc Gynecol*, 21, 247–257.

White, A. R. (2003). A review of controlled trials of acupuncture for women's reproductive health care. *J Fam Plann Reprod Health Care*, 29, 233–236.

Zhu, X., Proctor, M., Bensoussan, A., Smith, C. A., & Wu, E. (2007). Chinese herbal medicine for dysmenorrhea. *Cochrane Database Syst Rev*, 4:CD005288.

8

Ayurveda

PREMAL PATEL

CASE STUDY

Amy is a 52-year-old financial consultant. She is single, travels 4 days a week for her job, and often gives up sleep for work. Amy skips breakfast, eats a salad for lunch, and dinner at restaurants. She jogs three times a week. She thrives on competition at work but is facing some insecurity about retirement. She has constipation and flatulence. She is postmenopausal and has been experiencing hot flashes and insomnia. She has been treating her osteoarthritis with ibuprofen as needed.

PHYSICAL EXAMINATION FINDINGS INCLUDE THE FOLLOWING

Prakruti: Pitta predominant, Vata secondary
Vikruti: Vata and Pitta imbalanced
Tongue: Light, white coating (ama) on the back of the tongue

RECOMMENDATIONS

Diet

- Eat a warm, sweet breakfast (like oatmeal).
- Eat the biggest meal at lunch—warm, cooked, not dry.
- Choose soups instead of raw salad.

Sleep

- Set a sleep and wake time, with 7 to 8 hours of sleep.
- Take a warm bath before bed.
- Massage soles of feet with warm sunflower oil before bed.

Routine

- On weekends at home, perform self-massage with warm oil before shower.
- Try swimming and brisk walking instead of jogging.
- On weekends, join a yoga class doing restorative poses and pranayama.

Supplements

- Take 2 tablespoons of aloe vera gel three times a day.
- Take ½ teaspoon of triphala with warm water every night.

Introduction

Ayurveda is translated as the "science or knowledge of life." Life, according to Ayurveda, is the inseparable and integral union of mind, body, and spirit. The key in this union is balance. A healthy life is not just one without disease. Health involves a balanced state of the three doshas, the seven bodily tissues, the wastes created by the body, and the digestive fire; it also involves a joyful and content state of the senses, mind, and spirit; and finally, true health exists when one is centered in his or her true self (Lad, 1984). This chapter provides a brief overview of this healing system, with special attention given to the health of women.

The Five Elements and Three Doshas

Space, air, fire, water, and earth are the classical five elements discussed in Ayurveda. They are different from the elements found in the periodic table. Rather, each is a combination of qualities that represent archetypal patterns of behavior. These patterns manifest in human beings with the further aid of three fundamental principles: *vata, pitta, and kapha*—the three *doshas*. It is critical to have some understanding of the relationships between doshas and elements in order to understand health and pathology from an Ayurvedic perspective.

Vata is associated with the space and air elements and governs movement of all kinds. It is required for functions such as physical motion, nerve impulses, thinking, respiration, circulation, ingestion, peristalsis, elimination of wastes, menstruation, and childbirth.

Pitta is associated with fire and water and governs transformation. It is key for any processing to occur in the body, including metabolism, digestion, maintenance of body temperature, comprehension, appetite, and thirst.

Kapha is associated with water and earth, and represents structure and stability. It is essential for growth and nourishment in the body, including physical (bone and muscle) structure, lipid structure, repair and regeneration, lubrication, stamina, sleep, water and electrolyte balance, and memory.

Qualities of Doshas		
Vata: Space and Air	Pitta: Fire and Water	Kapha: Earth and Water
Dry	Sharp	Heavy
Light	Penetrating	Cold
Cold	Hot	Dull
Rough	Light	Oily
Subtle	Liquid	Liquid
Mobile	Mobile	Smooth
Clear	Oily	Dense
		Soft
		Static
		Cloudy
		Hard
		Gross

Source: Lad (2002).

All three doshas exist in all people; what varies is the extent to which they are present and whether or not they are balanced.

Balance and Imbalance of the Three Doshas

The balanced state, called prakruti, is the individual's constitution, which is a unique combination of doshas determined for each person at conception and which remains unchanged throughout life. A person's prakruti may be

Table 8.1. Vata: Space and Air

General Traits	Imbalanced
Thin	Osteoporosis
Delicate	Osteoarthritis
Narrow eyes–narrow lips	Scoliosis
Variable appetite	Insomnia
Light sleep	Constipation
Creative	Difficulty with attention and concentration
Flexible	

dominant in one dosha, two doshas, or all three doshas (though, again, everyone has all three). As long as one maintains this unique balance, he or she remains healthy and vibrant; this person "ages gracefully." Prakruti also determines a person's experience of the world. For example, when faced with a challenge such as losing a job and finding a new one, a vata-predominant person may respond with creativity or fear and anxiety; a pitta-predominant person may respond with confidence or anger and judgment. And a kapha-predominant person may respond with steadiness or despondency.

While there are advantages and challenges associated with each dosha, no dosha is inherently better or worse. Individuals may make choices that preserve balance as dictated by their prakruti. These choices include diet, daily practices, forms of exercise, emotional digestion, and so on. If these choices exacerbate any of the doshas, pathology begins. When the doshas become increased or decreased, an imbalanced state, called vikruti, comes into existence. It is this imbalance that brings ill health (See Tables 8.1, 8.2, and 8.3, and Lad, 2002, 2006). The goal of healing is to bring one back to his or her unique prakruti. For example, a person with a kapha-predominant prakruti will already have a larger frame, but when that large frame accumulates excess

Table 8.2. Pitta: Fire and Water

General Traits	Imbalanced
Medium frame	Hyperacidity
Bright eyes	Skin rashes
Sharp hunger	Inflammation
Passionate	Ulcers
Sharp, probing intellect	Uncontrolled anger/judgment/criticism
	Heat intolerance

Table 8.3. Kapha: Earth and Water

General Traits	Imbalanced
Large frame	Obesity
Strong	High cholesterol
Large eyes	Excess mucus
Thick, smooth skin	Tumors
Steady appetite	Stubborn
Good memory	Possessive
Strong faith	
Compassionate	
Patient	

weight, then kapha is increased. However, to return the person to balance, the goal is to return him or her to the healthy large frame, not a thin frame that is more natural for a vata individual.

Agni: The Digestive Fire

Digestion is the root of all health in Ayurveda, and agni is the fire responsible for digestion (Caldecott, 2006). Food is one part of nourishment, but the sounds, sights, smells, tastes, and textures we experience also create an impact. It is then crucial how we digest these experiences. Witnessing a tragic accident can create a similar sense of unease, indigestion, and difficulty sleeping as ingesting a bad piece of meat can. It is agni's job to transform all food and experiences. If agni is healthy and what is ingested is of good quality, agni can transform it into nourishment for the body, mind, and spirit. If what is ingested is of poor quality, healthy agni can transform it into a form the body can safely expel. When agni is unhealthy, food and experience are not properly transformed. This results in toxic buildup, or *ama*. Ama creates blockages, and tissues can no longer function optimally. Ama is at the root of many imbalances and disease. Physically, ama can manifest in a multitude of ways: sluggish metabolism, lethargy and fatigue, indigestion, odorous breath or wastes (stool, urine, sweat), bodily aches, and lack of mental clarity. A heavy coating on the tongue is one clear physical sign that indicates the presence of systemic ama (Lad, 1998).

The key to balancing agni is to protect it and not make it work harder than is required.

BASIC PRACTICAL TIPS

1. Drink warm or at least room temperature liquids—avoid cold and ice.
2. Follow nature—agni is highest when the sun (nature's agni) is highest; eat the heaviest foods/largest meal in the afternoon.
3. Assist the internal fire. If food is cooked and thoroughly chewed, that is less work required of the internal agni.
4. Use warming spices (black pepper, ginger, cinnamon, cardamom, etc.) with foods that are heavier and difficult to digest. To boost agni and decrease ama, try one to two thin 1-inch slices of ginger with lime juice and a hint of salt.
5. Do not douse the agni with large amounts of liquids around mealtimes. For lubrication, drink only occasional sips of warm water with meals.
6. Eat only when hunger is present, and do not overeat.
7. Consume all six tastes in the diet (sweet, sour, salty, pungent, bitter, astringent), favoring those appropriate to any imbalanced dosha.
8. Eat with awareness—do not multitask while eating. Even if the time for a meal is short, give full attention for these few minutes. If the television is on during a mealtime, then agni must multitask in digesting the food as well as processing the images and sounds from the television and it cannot give full attention to creating optimal nourishment from food.

One is bound to have some exposure to behavior or experiences (through diet, lifestyle, environmental toxins, etc.) that lead to ama formation. Ayurveda calls for cleansing processes to clear this. Daily, the predominant outlet to release ama (and excess doshas) is the gastrointestinal (GI) tract, and regular, healthy bowel movements are considered of utmost importance. This can be achieved naturally or with the help of herbal remedies such as triphala, starting with 1/2 tsp daily at bedtime (or two tablets), and then titrating up or down as needed.

Seasonally, one may consider a complete cleanse. Panchakarma is the predominant method.

Panchakarma

Though this process should be done with a trained professional (as there are indications and contraindications), it is introduced here. It refers to five procedures, each of which predominantly works on specific dosha(s). Traditionally, the five procedures are emesis for kapha imbalances, purgation and blood-letting for pitta imbalances, therapeutic enemas for vata imbalances, and the nasal administration of substances for all three doshas. Other procedures may be added as needed, and, specific to women's health, vaginal administration of herbal preparations, called uttara basti, can also be used. Preparation is done for panchakarma using oils (external massage and internal ingestion) and steam. Following the cleanse, rejuvenation is normally required. While this phase is very case-dependent, in general, it includes rebuilding agni, a slow resumption of a full diet appropriate to the person's constitution, daily routine practices appropriate for the person's constitution (yoga, pranayama, meditation, etc.), herbs appropriate to any continuing imbalance as well as to tonify/rejuvenate the weaker tissues, slow resumption of appropriate activities (such as work, daily responsibilities, etc.) and exercise, proper sleep health, and stress management (Lad, 1984).

The Golden Rule in Creating Balance

The key principle in balancing doshas is to first remove the root cause and then remedy lingering imbalances with the opposite (Lad, 1998). Consider the qualities that are imbalanced and return them to balance using the opposite qualities. If there is an excess of kapha and/or ama, and the heavy, cold, gross, dense, wet, and static qualities are present, one may present with disorders such as obesity and fibroid tumors. Choose foods and spices that have the opposite qualities: light, warm, subtle, dry, and kindling of agni. Choose activities that help move the stagnation, such as stimulating massage. Choose yoga poses or pranayama (breathing techniques) that stimulate agni and improve metabolism. And choose herbs that also kindle agni and provide what Ayurveda calls "a scraping action," which removes ama.

The Toolbox

Ayurveda has a number of modalities to reestablish balance. Examples include diet, lifestyle, herbs, sense therapies (such as aromatherapy, visualization, music, etc.), meditation, marma (energy points), and detoxification treatments such as panchakarma. Ayurveda also draws on the healing capacities of its sister sciences, such as yoga (beyond just physical postures, and including pranayama), and jyotisha (the study of astronomy and astrology).

While balancing each dosha requires a case-specific regimen, there are some general guidelines that one can follow using the principle of treating with the opposite qualities (Lad, 1984; Miller, 1999).

TO BALANCE VATA

1. Routine and rest are crucial. As irregularity and movement are inherent to vata, it must be grounded. Have set sleep and wake times, mealtimes, and so on.
2. Avoid cold, windy, dry weather.
3. Prefer warm, cooked, soft, and easy-to-digest foods. Include oils in diet, though not as deep fried foods. Also include warming spices.
4. Prefer gentler exercises, including flowing yoga poses that are grounding and strengthen one's core and swimming in warm water.
5. Prefer naturally sweet, sour, and salty tastes in moderation.
6. Prefer sweet, warm scents like orange, cinnamon, and holy basil; warm colors like deep red, orange, yellow, and green; and gentle, grounding music.

TO BALANCE PITTA

1. Prefer naturally cooling, soothing foods. Avoid spicy or fermented foods and excess oil. Use cooling spices and condiments such as mint, cilantro, cumin, fennel, and coconut.
2. Prefer naturally sweet, bitter, and astringent tastes.
3. Avoid hot, intense weather.
4. Prefer calming activities, including soothing exercise.
5. Surrender to the moment and avoid unnecessary competition.
6. Prefer sweet, cool scents like mint, rose, and sandalwood; soothing colors like blue and purple; and sweet music.

TO BALANCE KAPHA

1. Prefer warm, light foods and hot liquids. Use warming spices.
2. Prefer pungent, bitter, and astringent tastes.
3. Avoid oversleeping and daytime naps.
4. Avoid cold, damp weather.

5. Get things moving. Prefer vigorous (but not excessive) exercise, including yoga poses and pranayama.
6. Prefer warm scents like eucalyptus and clove; avoid blue; and prefer active music.

Effects of the Six Tastes on Doshas

	Vata	Pitta	Kapha
Sweet	↓	↓	↑
Sour	↓	↑	↑
Salty	↓	↑	↑
Pungent	↑	↑	↓
Bitter	↑	↓	↓
Astringent	↑	↓	↓

Source: Lad (2002).

ABHYANGA (MASSAGE)

One technique for balancing all three doshas is a daily self-massage, or abhyanga. Assuming there is not a lot of ama, this is traditionally done with warm oil specific to the dosha, such as sesame oil (heating) for vata and kapha, or sunflower oil (cooling) for pitta. Oil carries significant benefits in Ayurveda, including strengthening and toning the tissues and calming the nervous system. In general, use circular motions on the scalp, head, trunk, and joints, and long strokes on the extremities and flanks. This decreases stagnation in the tissues and is also an opportunity for self-nurturing, as the same word (snehan) represents oil and love in Sanskrit.

Topics Specific to Women

PREGNANCY

In an analogy comparing the conception and growth of a child with the germination of a plant from a seed, Ayurveda lists four factors necessary for a healthy pregnancy (Lad, 1995):

1. Rtu: "Season." This refers to various timings, including a woman's fertile time of life and of the month and the effect of the seasons. It also includes the proper time for having sex, which is said to be between 9 and 11, pm, as it is thought that daytime sex weakens the kidney, midnight sex weakens the liver, and sex at dawn weakens the colon.

2. Kshetra: "Field." This is the body of the woman, and specifically the health of the reproductive organs and the womb.

3. Ambu: "Water." This refers to the woman's ova, proper hormonal balance, and the nutrition the fetus receives. The condition of a woman's egg affects the growth and development of her fetus. Provided her eggs are healthy, the next concern is nutrition. For the mother, a diet rich in fresh, cooked, building foods is recommended, including milk, ghee (clarified butter), wheat, and proteins (assuming the mother can digest these). In conjunction with these foods, the mother should also maintain a diet appropriate to her doshic balance. A fetus is also nourished by everything the mother experiences and feels (Slattery, 2008).

4. Bija: "Seed." This refers to the health of the sperm. Ovum and sperm carry the doshic balances and imbalances of mother and father. Therefore, Ayurveda recommends that people desiring to become parents should receive cleansing procedures like panchakarma prior to conception.

After birth, the mother is susceptible to vata imbalances in particular and should be given preventative treatments, including massage, abdominal binding, and a nourishing diet. Breast milk is also affected by the doshas. The qualities of the foods that the mother eats, as well as her balanced and imbalanced doshas, affect her milk's qualities. This in combination with the child's own prakruti and vikruti can account for many digestive issues faced by newborns. A simple diet that is appropriate for mother and baby's constitution is best. In other words, if the mother or baby have a vata imbalance, and the mother consumes a vata-aggravating diet (raw, dry, cold foods), the breast milk will have a vata quality, and could cause more indigestion for the baby. In general, breastfeeding mothers should consume foods that are warm, moist, and nutritious. Examples include ghee, milk, almond milk, rice pudding with almonds and pistachios, sweet potato or yam, pumpkin, dates, tapioca, and mung dal. Of course, this list is general and is recommended with the assumption that it should be followed only if both the mother and baby do not show any intolerance to these foods. The most popular herb for enhancing breast milk production is shatavari (Lad, 1995).

THE MENSTRUAL CYCLE

The Vedic tradition, in which Ayurveda is rooted, honors the feminine energy, which brings creativity to fruition. Mother nature works in cycles; it is only natural that the feminine energy also has a cycle that allows for a proliferative, creative phase and a reflective, cleansing phase. Most of the ancient texts of Ayurveda prescribe routines that are appropriate for a healthy menses (Murthy, 2005; Sharma, 2003, 2004; Tewari, 1996), but the gist of all these routines is an inward retreat. It is a monthly reminder to let go of the past and start afresh in the present.

Physically, menses is a taxing experience for the body, as is any cleansing process, and requires rest. However, it is not inherently a painful or disgruntling process. The symptoms of discomfort reflect imbalanced dosha(s), which can be addressed, even with simple measures as discussed above.

Premenstrual Syndrome

While there are over 200 symptoms that have been linked to premenstrual syndrome (PMS) (Dickerson, Mazyck, & Hunter, 2003), Ayurveda views the symptoms as one, two, or three imbalanced doshas (Jadhav & Bhutani, 2005; Lad, 2006).

- Imbalanced vata creates irregularity in cycles, scanty flow, low back pain, cramps, constipation, anxiety, difficulty concentrating, and insomnia.
- Imbalanced pitta manifests as heavy flow, cramps, small clots, irritability, acne, inflammatory conditions, migraines, diarrhea, intense or sharp hunger, excess heat, anger, and judgmental or competitive behavior.
- Imbalanced kapha generates a mucus-like consistency to the menstrual flow, big clots, cramps, water retention and edema, dull aches and cramps, a sense of heaviness, lethargy, desire for "comfort foods," excess sleep, and a depressed mood.

Generally, more than one dosha is involved, often along with ama, and regularity in following the appropriate recommendations is key.

Menopause

The "change of life" is a mind, body, and spirit phenomenon, an evolution into a new stage (Atreya, 1999).

The three doshas rule different ages in life. Childhood is dominated by kapha. The child is growing and forming his or her physical and emotional being. Pitta is predominant in early adulthood. This stage is marked by extroverted efforts to establish career and family. Vata prevails in later adulthood, including menopause and beyond. Balanced vata brings creativity, clarity, communication, intuition, and joy. Vata governs elimination, and this is the time to rid oneself of all the old baggage one has accumulated over a lifetime (Svoboda, 2000).

Corresponding to this shift in roles, the body also transitions. But menopause does not occur overnight (Grady, 2006). If one has arrived at this stage with balanced doshas, one can experience a smooth transition. If one's life experiences thus far have fostered an imbalance in doshas, then the change in hormones is like the loss of a security blanket. One may then feel the intensity of the imbalanced doshas. Vata brings osteoporosis and fractures, osteoarthritis, vaginal dryness, memory loss, and insecurity. Pitta brings sweating, and irritability. Kapha brings weight gain, high cholesterol, and tumors. Certain conditions, such as heart disease, involve multiple doshas, as kapha is necessary for plaque formation, pitta for inflammation, and vata for plaque eruption/movement. Hot flashes can also be related to the heat of pitta and/or the extreme fluctuations of vata.

The intensity of these imbalances is a way for nature to send loud messages. If a woman has not given herself the time and nurturing that she showers on the rest of society, now is the time. And the solution is within reach—rebalance the doshas.

Reintroducing Amy

Now back to Amy again. Her prakruti and vikruti can be determined by interview and physical examination, including pulse examination. Pitta being predominant in her prakruti, she has always been driven, often sacrificing health for work. Her lifestyle and diet all point to one word: irregularity. This aggravates vata dosha, which is composed primarily of space and air and is increased by qualities that match these elements. She travels frequently: Movement increases the mobile and light qualities (especially travel by airplane, which goes against gravity and also affects the subtle quality); and being on the go impacts the rough quality (as different roads, vehicles, hotels are "rough" on

Table 8.4. Ayurvedic Herbs Commonly Used in Women's Health (Available in the West)

Latin	Sanskrit/English	Dosha Effect[**]	Traditional Uses in Women's Health	Comments
Aloe indica/vera/barbadensis	Kumari/Aloe vera	Gel: VPK = Powder: V+ P− K−	Regulates menses (especially excess flow), cleanses blood, soothes hot flashes	May inhibit prostaglandins
Asparagus racemosus	Shatavari	V− P− K+	Tones FRO[*], regulates menses, helps menopausal symptoms, increases breast milk	
Cyperus rotundus	Musta	V+ P− K−	Regulates menses (especially amenorrhea), improves PMS symptoms (especially bloating, pain, depression), relieves dysmenorrhea	Contains phytoestrogen substance
Glycyrrhiza glabra	Yashti Madhu/Licorice	V− P− K−/+ in excess	Strengthens FRO[*], improves vaginal dryness (improves secretions), can be used in vaginal douche	Avoid in hypertension and electrolyte imbalances
Pueraria tuberosa	Vidari	V− P− K+	Improves quality of FRO[*], fertility, increases breast milk production, building/nourishing—good post partum	
Saraca indica	Ashoka	V+ P− K−	Regulate menses (especially excess flow and congestion), uterine tonic, relieves dysmenorrhea	
Withania somnifera	Ashwagandha	V− P+ K−	Improves sexual (and general) debility, muscle tone, calms stress, and nervous system	Traditionally used to stabilize fetus, but excess may cause abortion

[*]FRO, Female reproductive organs/artava dhatu.

[**]Symbols for Dosha effect.

(−) Decreases or pacifies.

(+) Increases or aggravates.

(=) Balances all three doshas.

Sources: Frawley and Lad (2001), Pole (2006), Simon and Chopra (2000), Williamson (2002).

the body). Her diet does not help ground vata: Skipping meals aggravates the light quality; and salads and raw food worsen the rough, dry, cold qualities. Her habits also add to the imbalanced vata: Not sleeping because of work aggravates the light quality, and jogging regularly is also rough and drying for joints. And becoming engulfed in the competition at work activates the intensity of pitta. Arriving at a transitional point in her life with imbalanced vata and pitta, she is feeling the results of the imbalance more than ever before: insomnia, flatulence, constipation, osteoarthritis, hot flashes, and insecurity. Her challenge is to ground vata primarily, and secondarily soothe pitta. Routine is key for vata: regular, warm meals; oil massages to ground and calm the nervous system; and less stressful exercise. Eating her largest meal at lunch and choosing warm, cooked foods will also protect her agni, so that she can derive optimal nourishment. Aloe will help pitta and can be a support for the menopausal changes, including hormonal changes and hot flashes. And triphala, per Ayurveda, will help cleanse the built-up toxins, relieve constipation, and support the immune system. Amy can begin by implementing one recommendation at a time (Table 8.4), and even a few simple changes can create a lasting impact on her well-being.

REFERENCES

Atreya. (1999). *Ayurvedic healing for women*. York Beach, ME: Samuel Weiser.

Caldecott, T. (2006). *Ayurveda: The divine science of life*. New York, NY: Mosby Elsevier.

Dickerson, L., Mazyck, P., & Hunter, M. (2003). Premenstrual syndrome. *Am Fam Phys, 67*, 1743–1752.

Frawley, D., & Lad, V. (2001). *The yoga of herbs: An Ayurvedic guide to herbal medicine* (2nd ed.). Twin Lakes, WI: Lotus Press.

Grady, D. (2006). Management of menopausal symptoms. *N Engl J Med, 355*, 338–2347.

Jadhav, A., & Bhutani, K. K. (2005). Ayurveda and gynecological disorders. *J Ethnopharmacol, 97*, 151–159.

Lad, V. (1984). *Ayurveda: The science of self-healing*. Twin Lakes, WI: Lotus Press.

Lad, V. (1995). Pregnancy and infant care. *Ayurveda Today, 8*(3), 1–6.

Lad, V. (1998). *The complete book of Ayurvedic home remedies*. New York, NY: Three Rivers Press.

Lad, V. (2002). *Textbook of Ayurveda: Fundamental principles*. Albuquerque, NM: Ayurvedic Press.

Lad, V. (2006a). Female health issues: Part one. *Ayurveda Today, 18*(3), 1–6.

Lad, V. (2006b). Female health issues: Part two. *Ayurveda Today, 18*(4), 1–5.

Lad, V. (2006c). *Textbook of Ayurveda: A complete guide to clinical assessment*. Albuquerque, NM: Ayurvedic Press.

Miller, L. (1999). *Ayurvedic remedies for the whole family*. Twin Lakes, WI: Lotus Press.

Murthy, S. (Trans.). (2005). *Astanga Samgraha of Vagbhata*. Varanasi, India: Chaukhambha Orientalia.

Pole, S. (2006). *Ayurvedic medicine: The principles of traditional practice*. Philadelphia, PA: Churchill Livingstone Elsevier.

Sharma, P. V. (Ed., Trans.). (2003). *Caraka Samhita*. Varanasi, India: Chaukhambha Orientalia.

Sharma, P. V. (Ed., Trans.). (2004). *Susruta-Samhita*. Varanasi, India: Chaukhambha Visvabharati.

Simon, D., & Chopra, D. (2000). *The Chopra Center herbal handbook: Forty natural prescriptions for perfect health*. New York, NY: Three Rivers Press.

Slattery, D. A., & Neumann, I. D. (2008). No stress please! Mechanisms of stress hypo-responsiveness of the maternal brain. *J Physiol, 586*, 377–385.

Svoboda, R. E. (2000). *Ayurveda for Women: A Guide to Vitality and Health*. Rochester, NY: Healing Arts Press.

Tewari, P. V. (Ed., Trans., Comment.). (1996). *Kasyapa-Samhita*. Varanasi, India: Chaukhambha Visvabharati.

Williamson, E. M. (Ed.). (2002). *Major herbs of Ayurveda*. Philadelphia, PA: Churchill Livingstone.

9

Energy Medicine

ANN MARIE CHIASSON

CASE STUDY

An 80-year-old woman came to my office with severe itching in her lower legs. She was also experiencing grief and worry from a difficult emotional situation with her daughters. Physical examination revealed mild edema and severe excoriations of her lower limbs, with longitudinal scabs and areas of hypertrophic skin. She had tried multiple therapies prescribed by her general physician and dermatologist, including diuretics and topical steroids, with no benefit. My diagnosis was neurodermatitis, secondary either to edema from venous stasis or to the stress of her family situation. I prescribed 5 minutes daily of toe tapping, a form of qigong that moves the energy in the legs, promotes relaxation, and increases lymphatic flow in the lower limbs. I also prescribed 5 minutes of a heart-centered meditation daily. This meditation stimulates energy in the heart chakra and will often help with emotional difficulty and reactivity. One month later the patient returned with resolution of her symptoms and an improved physical examination. She also felt much more settled about her daughters. The patient continued to meditate and toe tap for 5 minutes each morning and by her 2-month follow-up appointment, her lower legs were normal and there was no scarring. Two-and-one-half years later, the itching had returned. I suggested she resume the toe tapping, and again her symptoms quickly resolved.

This is a dramatic example of healing, and certainly not all patients have remarkable results like this patient. I attribute her success, in part, to her willingness and ability to complete the prescribed exercise and meditation daily (Figures 9.1 and 9.2).

Toe tapping is a qigong exercise from the Dahn tradition. The patient lies on the floor with legs apart at a comfortable distance. The hips and legs rotate first externally then internally; the toes meet ("tap") at the first toe and metatarsal. It is best done very quickly; playing fast rhythmic music is helpful. It is important that the movement comes from rotation of the hips rather than adducting the legs or ankle alone. Relaxation of the legs and better rotation of the hips will alleviate most difficulties with the technique. Patients with back problems may do this while lying in bed. Pregnant women should not do this exercise until after their pregnancy is over.

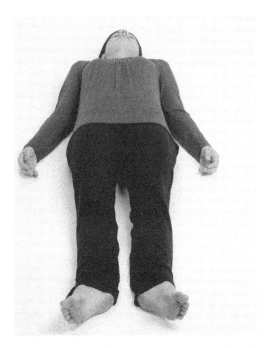

FIGURE 9.1. Toe tapping. Legs and feet first rotate outward from the hip.
Source: Reprinted from Chiasson (2013).Used with permission from Sounds True.

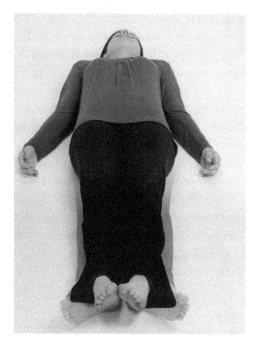

FIGURE 9.2. Toe tapping. Legs and feet then rotate inward from the hips, toes tap together.
Source: Reprinted from Chiasson (2013). Used with permission from Sounds True.

Definition and Prevalence of Energy Medicine Use in the United States

*E*nergy medicine (EM) is a relatively modern term that describes those practices that use energy fields to promote health. The National Center for Complementary and Alternative Medicine (NCCAM) acknowledges that the "concept that human beings are infused with a subtle form of energy" has been around for 2000 years, and has many names, "such as Qi in traditional Chinese medicine (TCM), ki in the Japanese Kampo system, doshas in Ayurvedic medicine, and elsewhere as prana, etheric energy, fohat, orgone, odic force, mana, and homeopathic resonance" (National Center for Complementary and Alternative Medicine [NCCAM], 2003). How the energy body and the physical body interact is described differently depending on the tradition, but there is general agreement that the energy system, called the energy body, biofield, or subtle body, is housed within the physical body and is fundamental to the functioning of the physical body.

From a historical perspective, EM may be seen as a resurgence of the concept of "vital-ism" or the belief that an underlying vital force exists and is central to health. This concept predates Hippocrates, who espoused that the vital force was dependent on the balance of four humors. This underlying theory of vital energy lost some of its prominence when medicine shifted its focus to organ-based systems and diagnosis. I think this resurgence is actually an integration of prior views of health and healing with conventional medicine. Energy medicine has the potential to augment our views of health and how we treat illness.

Energy medicine deals with both measureable and nonmeasurable ener-gies. NCCAM recognizes two types of energy fields, veritable and putative. The veritable energies are those that are measurable (through wavelengths and frequencies) and "employ mechanical vibrations (such as sound) and electro-magnetic forces, including visible light, magnetism, monochromatic radiation (such as laser beams), and rays from other parts of the electromagnetic spec-trum" (NCCAM, 2003). Many medical interventions employ electromagnetic fields including magnetic resonance imaging, cardiac pacemakers, radiation therapy, ultraviolet light for psoriasis, and laser keratoplasty (NCCAM, 2003).

Putative energy fields, according to NCCAM, are those that "have defied measurement to date by reproducible methods. Therapists claim that they can work with this subtle energy, see it with their own eyes, and use it to effect changes in the physical body and influence health" (NCCAM, 2003). When practitioners and researchers discuss EM, most are referring to therapies that work with the putative field.

Ninety-four cultures have a documented concept that describes the under-lying energy of the body (Di Nucci, 2005); work with this energy is alternately characterized as spiritual healing or EM, and includes aspects of traditional Chinese medicine (TCM), mind–body medicine, and some manual medicine therapies. Nurses tend to use EM, both in their usual work and as a sepa-rate modality. Healing touch was developed by a nurse, for use by nurses, as an adjunct therapy for hospitalized patients. Many nurses are also trained in Reiki.

Defining the scope of EM is controversial. Since many EM practitioners postulate that everything is energy, one can place much of complementary and alternative medicine (CAM) within the EM paradigm. This chapter focuses on EM modalities that address the subtle body and do not fall under other CAM paradigms. These modalities include therapeutic touch (TT), healing touch, reiki, craniosacral therapy, joh rei, sound healing, zero balancing, jin shin jytsu, quantum touch, Barbara Brennan's work, and Rosalyn Bruyere's healing. Acupuncture and movement therapies such as yoga, qigong, and tai chi also work with the energy flow in the body. Spiritual healing, natural healing, and shamanic healing are not addressed in this chapter (Table 9.1).

Until a method is devised to measure the body's subtle field, confusion about the definition and scope of EM will continue. Currently, gas discharge visualization (GDV), which measures biophoton emissions; superconducting quantum interference devices (SQUID); and low-frequency pulsed electromagnetic fields (PEMFs) are being researched to measure the electromagnetic field of the body (Di Nucci, 2005; Korotkov, Matravers, Orlov, & Williams, 2010).

Despite the definitional uncertainty, EM modalities are regularly used in the United States. The 2007 National Health Interview Survey revealed that

Table 9.1. A List of Common Energy Medicine Techniques

Technique	Theory
Acupuncture	Uses needles to stimulate energy flow at meridian points on the body.
Craniosacral therapy	Transfers energy by laying the hands onto the body to affect the cerebrospinal fluid; based on cranial osteopathy.
Healing touch	Transfers energy by laying hands onto the body; based on the chakra system
Joh rei	Detoxifies the energy body by sending universal energy to the patient from the healer's hands across a short distance.
Polarity therapy	A touch therapy that balances positive and negative energy flows in the body.
Qigong	Uses movement and laying on of hands to cultivate balanced energy flow throughout the body.
Reiki	Channels universal energy into the patient's body through the hands of the healer.
Sound and light therapies	Uses vibration through sound or light to affect the energetic body of the patient.
Tai chi	A series of movements and postures to stimulate and increase energy flow.
Therapeutic touch	Transfers energy by placing the hands into the patients' electromagnetic field around the body.
Yoga	Philosophy, poses, and breathing techniques to promote energy flow and balanced energy.
Zero balancing	A gentle touch and movement therapy that balances energy at the zero-point field of the body.

Source: Adapted from Baggott (1999).

approximately 0.5% of adults in the United States use reiki or another form of EM (Korotkov et al., 2010). When acupuncture, yoga, tai chi and qigong are included, the percentage of adults in the United States who ever used an energy modality rises to 9.3% (CDC, 2008). An even larger percentage (45%–50%) of people with chronic pain and chronic illness use EM (CDC, 2008). Overall, women use EM modalities more than men. Most patients used EM as an adjunct for symptom relief rather than cure (Rao, 1999). As of 2014, 76 hospitals and clinics in the United States provide some form of EM as an adjunctive therapy, and new forms of EM techniques and schools are popping up each year (Center for Reiki Research, 2014).

Anatomy, Illness, and Healing Within the Paradigm of Energy Medicine

The anatomy of the underlying energy field varies according to the tradition. Traditional Chinese medicine describes three dan tiens, or major energy centers, with superficial energy channels throughout the body described as meridians; the Hindu tradition introduced the chakra system with seven energy centers and a radiant energy that exudes from the body called an aura; and multiple indigenous cultures describe a matrix of energy that flows within the body.

Conceptually the relationship between these anatomies can be seen as layers. At the deepest layer are the dan tiens, the next layer houses the seven chakras, next is the matrix, and finally, at the interface with the organs, are the meridians. A simple map of these layers is presented in Figure 9.3.

Different EM techniques are thought to work on different layers of the biofield. For example, healing touch works at the chakra layer, while TCM works at the core energy centers and most superficial layer. Healers tend to perceive the energy field of the system they trained in, although some are able to perceive and work in multiple systems and layers (Chiasson, 2013).

In the natural history of a disease, it is thought that first the energetic field is blocked or goes out of balance, then pathology develops, and finally symptoms appear. Major cellular pathology appears years after a block in the natural flow of energy, although pain, which is considered a form of blocked energy, can occur right away. Factors that contribute to, or cause a block, include outside insults, genetic or hereditary causes, and physical or emotional trauma. Treatment is based on transferring energy to remove blocks and restore normal energy flow. It is believed that keeping the energy field clear and the energy flowing promotes health and healing (Chiasson, 2013).

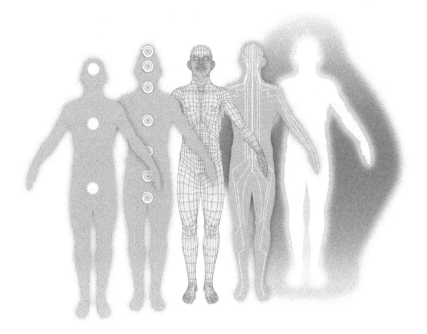

FIGURE 9.3 A summary of energy healing anatomy. At the deepest layer are the dan tiens, moving outward are the chakras, then the matrix, and finally the meridians. The aura extends off the body.
Source: Reprinted from Chiasson (2013). Used with permission from Sounds True.

Energy medicine therapies are believed to shift or change the underlying energy field of the body. The most common technique involves laying the hands on, or over, the patient's body. Other techniques employ vibration, light, sound, movement, magnets, or direct current. Movement is extremely important, as it promotes energy flow. The patient can continue to "work on themselves" through movement or self-administered EM techniques, thus reducing the frequency of visits with an EM practitioner (Chiasson, 2013).

Research on Energy Medicine

While there is a paucity of well-done studies on EM, data are emerging. Research on veritable energy fields includes studies on magnet therapy, millimeter wave therapy, sound energy therapy, and light therapy. Unfortunately, the studies on putative energy fields is scant and of poor quality (NCCAM, 2003).

Most studies have focused on TT, developed by Delores Krieger in the 1970s; Reiki, a Japanese form of healing; and healing touch. Claims for EM modalities include decreased pain, anxiety, and healing times.

In the 1970s, Dr. Herbert Benson's research demonstrated the effect of relaxation on the body. He documented shifts in blood pressure, heart rate, and brain wave activity as well as improvements in immune system, peristalsis, and kidney function (Benson, 1976). Similar physiological changes have been found in studies of EM treatments. For example, two studies demonstrated significant increases in hemoglobin and hematocrit levels in healthy persons learning Reiki (Miles, 2003; Movaffaghi et al., 2006). Wardell illustrated significant decreases in anxiety and blood pressure, increased salivary immunoglobulin A (IgA), increased skin temperature, and decreased electromyographic (EMG) activity during a Reiki treatment (Wardell & Engebretson, 2001). Similar findings were demonstrated by Manville with healing touch; he reported statistically significant decreases in post-treatment systolic and diastolic blood pressure, heart rate, skin conductance level, EMG activity, and trait anxiety when compared with pretreatment measurements (Manville, Bowen, & Benham, 2008).

Placebo effects, relaxation, the effects of human touch, and the healer/patient relationship are all potentially important factors in EM treatments. Energy medicine sessions, which are usually an hour long, can help patients cope more effectively with their illness. Noticeably, the patient's breath shifts during a healing session to slower, deeper, abdominal breathing. Zero balancing teaches that this breath shift is indicative that the healing is effective.

Systematic reviews of EM in various settings reveal a broad range of rigor. In 2009, Jain et al. reviewed 66 studies on biofield therapies and concluded that many of the studies were of medium and adequate quality. They found strong evidence (level 1) for decreased pain in studies that used a visual analog scale. In studies that used more comprehensive assessment tools that included functional status, they found conflicting evidence about benefit of EM therapies (evidence level 4). They also concluded that there is moderate evidence (level 2) that EM therapies decrease acute pain in the hospital setting, including postoperative pain (Jain & Milla, 2010).

In 2003, Jonas published a review of 19 randomized controlled trials, most of which were on TT; they found 11 out of 19 studies showed statistically significant treatment effects with a mean effect of reduction in symptoms of 0.60. The authors concluded that the evidence for EM modalities for relieving pain and anxiety was "level B," or poor to fair (Jonas, Wayne, & Crawford, 2003). Astin et al. reported the mean effect of TT was 0.63 in a systematic review of 11 TT studies; this review found 7 of the 11 studies showed a positive effect on at least one outcome. When all healing trials (including prayer and distant healing) were reviewed, the mean effect size was 0.40. The mean effect score for distant healing, which included Reiki, was 0.38. Reiki studies showed greater effects than TT and healing touch. Two of the five studies evaluating analgesic usage supported the claim that these therapies reduced analgesic usage (Astin, Harkness, & Ernst, 2000).

Energy medicine may be useful in osteoarthritis. In a review by Ernst, magnet therapy, as measured by PEMF, was examined in 75 patients with knee osteoarthritis. While there was no difference overall between the experimental and control group, magnet therapy showed an increase in quality of life secondary measures in the intervention group (Ernst, 2002). Gordon demonstrated that TT statistically decreased pain and improved function in patients receiving TT versus mock TT, although there was no difference in the functional disability index (Gordon, Merenstein, D'Amico, & Hudgens, 1998). Energy medicine has also been used as an adjunct to cancer treatment to help alleviate side effects for over 20 years (Stephen, Mackenzie, Sample, & Macdonald, 2007).

Research on women's health and EM is limited. A Canadian study of a convenience sample of menopausal women found 21% of women had received Reiki or TT for menopausal symptoms and 66% of these women reported it was beneficial (Lunny & Fraser, 2010). In addition, qualitative evidence suggests that EM works well with postpartum women and in specific cultural groups such as Hawaiian women (Kiernan, 2002; Starn, 1998). Brewitt examined five patients with chronic illness (MS, lupus, fibromyalgia, and goiter) who were given 11 Reiki treatments. They reported a decrease in skin resistance over acupuncture meridians, and the patients reported decreased pain and anxiety (Brewitt, Hartwell, & Vittetoe, 1997).

For fibromyalgia, findings have been negative; a systematic review of 25 randomized controlled trials on nonpharmacological interventions for fibromyalgia syndrome failed to find evidence of benefit for EM (Sim, & Nicola, 2002). Sutherland et al. published positive findings in a qualitative trial of chronic headaches at Kaiser Permanente. They found that 11 out of 13 patients had profound shifts in multiple subjective healing aspects of their lives; this effect lasted from 24 hours to 6 months. The authors concluded that EM is better researched using qualitative methods (Sutherland, Ritenbaugh, Kiley, Vuckovic, & Elder, 2009). While difficult to research, the patient–healer relationship may also have contributed to the treatment effect along with the EM technique. Interestingly, Kerr et al. examined sensory experiences of patients with sham acupuncture in an effort to differentiate how the placebo effect may be interacting with energy therapies. They hypothesized that energy therapies may stimulate an attentional filtering of tactile sensations and brain sensory activity in the ritual of the therapy, as the actual effect on the brain for the healing tool (Kerr et al., 2011).

Properly used, EM has minimal negative effects. Practitioners report there may be an increase in pain after the first few treatments. This is understood by practitioners to represent the release of blocked energies and is expected to diminish and dissipate with subsequent treatments. Another finding reported by practitioners is that diabetic patients may experience a drop in their blood glucose levels during a session or immediately after. This effect is negligible in all but very brittle diabetic patients. For these patients, practitioners recommend checking a finger stick blood sugar level after a session. While these observations are not rigorously researched, these "side effects" are considered standard knowledge in the field of energy healing and are taught as such in healing touch training as well as in other modalities.

Consideration for Referral

Patients who are seeking adjunctive therapies for symptoms of pain, menopause, cancer, and anxiety and who have openness, or cultural alignment to EM, may be appropriate for referral. Matching the patients' belief system to the specific available energy modalities is useful. Energy medicine can be a valuable adjunct to their medical management, with few side effects. If a patient does not experience positive physical or mental effects within a few visits, it may be more appropriate for the patients to use their resources on another modality. Chronic pain patients may be advised that if their symptoms continue to flair after a series of treatments, they should consider spacing sessions further apart or consider a cessation of treatment.

For most EM modalities, there are websites with certification guidelines and lists of practitioners, for example, www.iarp.org, www.healingtouchinternational.org, www.barbarabrennan.com, and www.zerobalancing.com.

> When choosing a practitioner for referral, I have a few considerations. I choose practitioners that do not "hex" or put down conventional medicine. I tend to choose practitioners that have more experience, preferably over three years. Experience is not equal to expertise, yet I find healers who have been doing it longer are, as a group, better. I try to visit the healer myself prior to referring. I will often do this anonymously, so I may have a "standard" session to see what my patients will experience.

Conclusion

Energy medicine is based on an ancient concept of a vital force within the body and is found across healing paradigms in different cultures throughout the world. While research is limited, emerging evidence suggests that EM is most helpful for decreasing chronic pain and postoperative pain. In addition, women may find benefit from symptoms of menopause, anxiety, and the side effects of cancer therapies. The therapeutic aspect of the practitioner–client relationship is also beneficial for healing and improved outcomes.

REFERENCES

Astin, J., Harkness, E., & Ernst, E. (2000). The efficacy of "Distant Healing": A systematic review of randomized trials. *Ann Intern Med, 132*, 903–910.

Baggott, A. (1999). *The encyclopedia of energy healing.* New York, NY: Sterling Publishing.

Benson, H. (1976). *The relaxation response.* New York, NY: Harper Collins.

Brewitt, B., Hartwell, B., & Vittetoe, T. (1997). The efficacy of Reiki: Improvements in spleen and nervous system function as qualified by electro-dermal screening. *Alter Ther, 3*, 89–97.

CDC. (2008). *Complementary and alternative medicine use among adults and children: United States, 2007.* National Health Statistics Report, No. 12.

Center for Reiki Research. (2014). *List of hospitals and clinic settings.* http://www.centerforreikiresearch.org/

Chiasson, A. M. (2013). *Energy healing: The essentials of self-care.* Boulder CO: Sounds True.

Di Nucci, E. M. (2005). Energy healing: A complementary treatment for orthopaedic and other conditions. *Orthopaedic Nursing, 24*, 259–269.

Ernst, E. (2002). Complementary and alternative medicine in rheumatology. *Bailliere's Clin Rheumatol, 14*, 731–749.

Gordon, A., Merenstein, J. H., D'Amico, F., & Hudgens, D. (1998). The effects of therapeutic touch on patients with osteoarthritis of the knee. *J Fam Pract, 47*, 271–277.

Jain, S., & Milla, P. J. (2010). Biofield therapies: Helpful or full of hype? A best evidence synthesis. *Int J Behav Med, 17*, 1–16.

Jonas, M. D., Wayne, B., & Crawford, C. C. (2003). Science and spiritual healing: A critical review of spiritual healing, "energy" medicine, and intentionality. *Alternat Therap, 9*, 56–61.

Kerr, C. E., Shaw, J. R., Conboy, L. A., Kelley, J. M., Jacobson, E, & Kaputchuk, T. J. (2011). Placebo acupuncture as a form of ritual touch healing: A neurophenomological model. *Conscious Cogn, 20*, 784–791.

Kiernan, J. (2002). The experience of therapeutic touch in the lives of five postpartum women. *MCN Am J Matern Child Nurs, 27*, 47–53.

Korotkov, K. G., Matravers, P., Orlov, D. V., & Williams, B. O. (2010). Application of electrophoton capture (EPC) analysis based on gas discharge visualization (GDV) technique in medicine: A systematic review. *J Altern Complement Med, 16,* 13–25.

Lunny, C. A., & Fraser, S. N. (2010). The use of complementary and alternative medicines among a sample of Canadian menopausal-aged women. *J Midwifery Women's Health, 55,* 335–343.

Manville, J. A., Bowen, J. E., & Benham, G. (2008). Effect of healing touch on stress perception and biological correlates. *Holistic Nurs Pract, 22,* 103–110.

Miles, P. (2003). Reiki: Review of biofield therapy, history, theory, practice and research. *Alternat Therap, 9,* 62–72.

Movaffaghi, Z., Hsanpoor, M., Farsi, M., et al. (2006). Effects of therapeutic touch on blood hemoglobin and hematocrit level. *J Holist Nurs, 24,* 41–48.

National Center for Complementary and Alternative Medicine (NCCAM). (2003). *Energy medicine: An overview.* Backgrounder, National Institute for Health.

Rao, J. K. (1999). Use of complementary therapies for arthritis among patients of rheumatologists. *Ann Intern Med, 131,* 409–416.

Sim, J., & Nicola, A. (2002). Systematic review of randomized controlled trials of non-pharmacological interventions for fibromyalgia. *Clin J Pain, 18,* 324–336.

Starn, J. R. (1998). Energy healing with women and children. *J Obstet Gynecol Neonatal Nurs, 27,* 576–584.

Stephen, J. E., Mackenzie, G., Sample, S., & Macdonald, J. (2007). Twenty years of therapeutic touch in a Canadian cancer agency: Lessons learned from a case study of integrative oncology patients. *Supp Care Cancer, 15,* 993–998.

Sutherland, E. G., Ritenbaugh, C., Kiley, S. J., Vuckovic, N., & Elder, C. (2009). An HMO based prospective pilot study of energy medicine for chronic headaches: Whole-person outcomes point to the need for new instrumentation. *J Altern Complement Med, 15,* 819–826.

Wardell, D. W., & Engebretson, J. (2001). Biological correlates of Reiki Touch healing. *J Adv Nurs, 33,* 439–445.

10

Homeopathy

PAMELA A. PAPPAS AND IRIS R. BELL

CASE STUDY

A 32-year-old woman with history of recurrent genital herpes was 37 weeks into her third pregnancy. Her outbreaks had been mostly controlled with medications over the years, but they would always last for 7 days when they occurred. Presenting with a genital herpes outbreak in the last 24 hours, she had been told by her obstetrician that a C-section would be needed unless this cleared in 48 hours. She did not want a C-section and sought alternatives.

During her first trimester, she had experienced severe nausea and vomiting; recurrent hemorrhoids marked her second trimester. In addition, she described a recurring, intermittent "bearing down" sensation throughout the pregnancy, along with frequent sinus infections. Currently, she experienced labial burning and eruptions similar to her previous outbreaks. She was also quite irritable, having a particular aversion to her husband throughout her pregnancy.

Homeopathic study of the case included the following descriptive rubrics from the *Complete 2008 Repertory* (van Zandvoort, 2008):

FEMALE: Eruptions, Herpetic
STOMACH: Vomiting, Pregnancy in
RECTUM: Hemorrhoids, Pregnancy, in
MIND: Irritability, Pregnancy in

MIND: Husband; Aversion to
FEMALE: Pain; Bearing down

After case analysis, the patient was given one dose of the homeopathic remedy *Sepia*, 200C. Within 8 hours, all signs of herpes resolved. Her obstetrician repeated the culture, which was negative. The patient went on to have a full-term pregnancy with normal delivery, and the child did well. This case (courtesy of Todd Rowe, MD, MD(H), CCH) demonstrates how a remedy prescribed to match the patient's clinical symptoms stimulated her healing responses enough to eliminate a herpes outbreak.

Homeopathic *Sepia* is made from the ink of the common cuttlefish, a sea creature belonging to the Cephalopod family such as octopuses and squid. Like its relatives, the cuttlefish can change both the color and texture of its skin and can escape danger by squirting ink into the water while jetting away in the opposite direction. This remedy has a repertory rubric found nowhere else:

MIND: Dreams; Pursued of being, run backwards, must. (van Zandvoort, 2008)

Sometimes remedies that heal are found through odd correspondences between patient characteristics and remedy source like this. *Sepia* is known to help many conditions experienced by women, including vaginitis, menopausal hot flashes, depression, and nausea and vomiting in pregnancy. Women responding to *Sepia* for chronic conditions often note irritability, sarcasm followed by remorse, and feeling overwhelmed especially with family responsibilities (Morrison, 1993).

Introduction and Background

Classical homeopathy is a controversial 200-year-old system of medicine founded by the German physician Samuel Hahnemann, MD (Lansky, 2003; Merrell & Shalts, 2002). It is also one of the most popular forms of complementary and alternative medicine in the UK and elsewhere (Hunt & Ernst, 2010). Like other whole systems of care such as traditional Chinese medicine (TCM) and Ayurveda, homeopathy differs from conventional Western medicine in theoretical foundations, diagnostic approaches,

Table 10.1. Comparison of Homeopathy and Conventional Medical Models of Disease, Treatment, and Outcome

Feature	Homeopathic Model	Conventional Medical Model
Implicit scientific world view	Holism	Reductionism
Focus of diagnosis	Patient as a unique indivisible dynamical individual	Specific disease entity
Likely mechanism of action for medicines	Unknown, probably dependent on endogenous adaptive pathways in the body. May include electromagnetic, optical, or epitaxic structural signals from the individually salient medicine (remedy) as a source and/or source-doped silica nanoparticle to the cell stress-related signaling pathways. The complex biological networks of the person as an integrated system then amplify the impact of the small danger signal endogenously, resulting in global and local changes in gene expression and function. A macro-entanglement hypothesis has also been proposed.	Probably involving specific biochemical ligand–receptor interactions
Goals of treatment	Cure of person's tendency toward disease at any level of organizational scale, mental, emotional, physical	Suppression of expression of disease in each local body part as dysfunctions or lesions develop
Clinical strengths	Chronic diseases with multiple comorbidities involving dysfunction	Life-threatening emergencies, acute illnesses, and injury/physical trauma
Clinical limitations	Minimal effects on established structural changes	Significant safety risks of side effects and drug–drug interactions

Source: From Bell and Pappas (2008); Bell, Sarter, et al. (2013).

treatments, and outcome assessment (Bell & Koithan, 2006; Koithan, Bell, Niemeyer, & Pincus, 2012; Verhoef et al., 2005; see Table 10.1). Based on the idea that healing is a concerted effort of the entire organism rather than any isolated part, it uses medicines corresponding precisely to the symptoms experienced in order to stimulate this healing process. Holistic approaches like homeopathy may be particularly useful for women seeking whole-person interventions. Especially when patients present with complex biopsychosocial diagnoses across multiple systems, homeopathy can offer a safe, gentle, and comprehensive approach (Bell & Pappas, 2008).

Use of Homeopathy

Homeopathy is one of the most popular forms of complementary and alternative medicine (CAM) in the world, especially in Great Britain, where more than 40% of physicians refer their patients to homeopaths; in France, where 30%–40% of physicians prescribe homeopathic medicines; and in Germany, where 20% of physicians follow this practice (Ullman, 2008). Also very popular in Latin America and India, homeopathy leads the list of therapies for 59% of CAM-provider MDs, followed by acupuncture and botanical therapy (WHO, 2002).

Use of homeopathy has been limited in the United States (use assessed at 3.7% in 1997; Barnes, Powel-Griner, McFann, & Nahin, 2004; Eisenberg et al., 1998), due at least partially to the Flexner report in the early 1900s and the rise of pharmaceutical care. Yet this use still increased fivefold between Eisenberg's two CAM surveys, with 82% (or 5.5 million) of users self-prescribing rather than consulting homeopathic practitioners (Eisenberg et al., 1998). A 1999 survey found that 17% of Americans were using homeopathy for self-care (Roper Starch Worldwide, 1999).

Types of Homeopathic Prescribing

Homeopathy may be used in a variety of ways. This chapter focuses on "classical" homeopathy, which uses one homeopathic medicine ("remedy") at a time, selected for its similarity to the symptoms and state experienced by the patient and prescribed in the minimum dose necessary to elicit a healing response (Ullman, 2008). Thousands of homeopathic remedies are available, many having had clinical "provings" to determine their medicinal and curative properties. "Provings" test the effects of unknown homeopathic remedies on healthy people, similar to Phase 1 drug trials, but are often double-blinded (Mollinger, Schneider et al., 2009). Although Dr. Hahnemann briefly experimented with using multiple remedies simultaneously, this single "proven" remedy approach was the one he strongly recommended (Hahnemann, 1996/1843).

Despite Dr. Hahnemann's preferences, there have long been practitioners and pharmacies combining multiple homeopathic remedies in "complexes" or "formulas" to give to a wide variety of people seeking to have the same disease. This is called "complex homeopathy" because multiple remedies, often in different strengths, are contained in the same preparation (Carlston, 2003). These prepackaged mixtures are labeled according to condition treated, such as "headaches," "teething," or "menstrual cramps." Although they do not follow the principles of classical homeopathy, there is a research base for their use (de Oliveira et al., 2008; Oberbaum et al., 2001; Weiser, Strosser, & Klein, 1998), suggesting that they provide relief for some people. Combination remedies might be reasonable choices when one cannot figure out which single remedy to give or when the indicated single remedy is unavailable in the health food store or pharmacy. The needed remedy might be contained in an available "complex," and be a better option than no treatment (Ullman, 2008).

While these mixtures have their applications, most experienced homeopaths believe that the symptom relief they afford is usually temporary and that a complete, deep cure is unlikely to be accomplished through them. If a complaint is recurrent, chronic, or keeps returning after the combination or single acute remedy wears off, more in-depth case-taking with a professional homeopath is needed. Some homeopaths also believe that combination remedies may even worsen chronic illnesses if used longer than 10 to 14 days (Shalts, 2004). These complex mixture products in the United States are typically labeled for self-care in time-limited acute conditions.

Professional homeopathic care for chronic conditions usually focuses on "constitutional" treatment: prescribing a homeopathic medicine ("remedy") based on a woman's genetic inheritance, past health history and medical treatment, plus totality of physical, emotional, and mental/spiritual symptoms (Ullman, 2008). This broad assessment is necessary, as the same basic disturbance is expressed on multiple levels. The correct "constitutional" remedy can stimulate healing from chronic diseases, reduce the influence of hereditary diseases, strengthen a woman's emotional and mental state, and reduce the frequency and severity of acute ailments. If acute illness does arise, a dose of one's constitutional remedy may stimulate complete cure.

Unlike herbal or nutritional products, homeopathic remedies are recognized as over-the-counter drugs and undergo regulatory oversight by the Food and Drug Administration (FDA) through the *Homeopathic Pharmacopoeia of the United States,* which standardizes their preparation (Bell & Pappas, 2008). This requires homeopathic manufacturers to state the specific condition the homeopathic remedy is indicated to treat—another difference from dietary supplements, for which the FDA does not allow specific disease indications. Homeopathic remedies have many actions on multiple levels, but the FDA-required label might list only one indication. Consumers need to understand this as a feature of FDA regulation rather than the remedies themselves; homeopaths may use a remedy for more complex indications than its label shows.

Women, Healing, and Homeopathy

With a rich tradition in many forms of healing (Achterberg, 1990), women have been especially strong proponents of homeopathy (Kirschmann, 2004; Ullman, 2007). The first woman homeopath was Melanie Hahnemann (Dr. Samuel Hahnemann's second wife) in the 1800s (Winston, 1999). Since then, many women have come to homeopathy as patients, to prescribe for their families, and as professional homeopaths.

Historians estimate that two-thirds of homeopathic patients in the nineteenth century were women, possibly seeking safer care than the bleeding, arsenic, and mercury treatments conventional physicians favored (Kirschmann, 2004). Other reasons may have been homeopathy's success in treating infectious epidemics such as cholera, typhoid, yellow fever, scarlet fever, and others (Ullman, 2007).

"Ladies' Physiological Societies" sprang up in the 1840s and 1850s to teach women hygiene principles, including homeopathy; out of these grew the first medical colleges for women (Winston, 1999). The women's suffrage movement in the 1840s encouraged this, although it took many years for women to gain admission to male-dominated medical schools. Still, women spread homeopathy's popularity in their communities. At the 1869 meeting of the American Institute of Homeopathy (AIH), one [male] homeopathic physician observed: "Many a woman, armed with her little stack of remedies, had converted an entire community to homeopathy" (Winston, 1999, p. 141). The AIH finally opened membership to women in 1870, 5 years before the American Medical Association did.

Beyond treating physical concerns, homeopathy also offered women a way to understand and treat emotional and mental issues. Thus, it was "holistic" before this term ever came into vogue. When suffering a nervous breakdown from Crimean War traumas, the famous nursing pioneer Florence Nightingale (1820–1910) sought care from homeopathic physician Dr. James Gully (Ullman, 2007); she referred to him as "a genius" (Jenkins, 1972).

Applying Homeopathy in Women's Health

Classical homeopathy has applications in many women's conditions (Steinberg & Beal, 2003), including those in pregnancy such as morning sickness, breech presentation, retained placenta (Castro, 1993; Moskowitz, 1992), and labor induction (Kistin & Newman, 2007). Other uses include repeated miscarriage, infertility, postpartum depression (Reichenberg-Ullman, 2000), premenstrual syndromes (Jones, 2003; Yakir et al., 2001), breast problems including mastitis and nursing issues (Chernin, 2006), fibromyalgia (Bell, Lewis, Brooks, et al., 2004; Bell, Lewis, Lewis, et al., 2004), and menopausal symptoms (Bordet, Marijnen, Masson, & Trichard, 2008; Jacobs, Herman, Heron, Olsen, & Vaughters, 2005; Relton & Weatherly-Jones, 2005). Homeopathy also has applications in psychiatric conditions frequent in women, such as anxiety and mood disorders (Bell & Pappas, 2007, 2008), and the aftermath of child sexual abuse (Coll, 2002).

Despite these many uses, a big difference exists between prescribing homeopathic remedies for an "acute" or "first aid" condition and for chronic illness (Shalts, 2004). Homeopaths distinguish carefully between these types of treatment. The term "first aid" applies to those conditions that are emergent and might be treated with whatever materials are at hand, such as traumatic injury including emotional shock. A true "acute" illness is one that is new, never experienced before, and self-limited. Someone with a single urinary tract infection or episode of diarrhea might meet this definition. However, someone with symptoms that recur monthly or that never really remit has a chronic condition. Successfully prescribing for chronic or repeated illnesses requires much more in-depth interviewing and research through the 4,000 to 5,000 existing homeopathic remedies for the one that best fits the woman's total state. By comparison, acute illnesses may present more dramatically, have clearer symptom pictures, and respond more readily to the lower potency single remedies available to beginning prescribers. Also as discussed earlier, combination ("complex homeopathy") remedies or mixtures may be helpful for acute conditions as long as their limitations are recognized.

Several women's conditions amenable to homeopathic treatment are explored in further detail in what follows.

MENOPAUSE AND HOMEOPATHY

Menopause can be a challenging transition for many women, bringing uncomfortable symptoms such as poor sleep, hot flashes, and fatigue. When closely tailored to the complete person (in-depth constitutional prescribing), classical homeopathy can offer both lasting relief and improvement in overall health.

An audit of 102 women treated with single remedy, "constitutional" classical homeopathy through a National Health Service menopause clinic (Relton & Weatherly-Jones, 2005) found 83 had improvement in their symptoms, including hot flashes, tiredness, anxiety, mood swings, crying, sleep difficulties, headaches, and joint and muscle pains. Bordet et al. (2008) also published an observational study involving 438 patients (average age 55) and 99 homeopathic physicians in 8 countries. Treatment focused on hot flashes, selected through in-depth "constitutional" classical homeopathy, and the most commonly prescribed remedies were *Lachesis, Belladonna, Sepia, Sulphur,* and *Sanguinaria.* Ninety percent of the women reported disappearance or lessening of their symptoms, usually within 15 days of starting homeopathic treatment.

Homeopathic treatment for menopausal symptoms has also been explored in breast cancer survivors. However, results have so far been equivocal. One randomized, double-blind, placebo-controlled study evaluated menopausal symptoms in 57 breast cancer survivors (Thompson, Oxon, Montgomery, Douglas, & Reilly, 2005; Thompson & Reilly, 2003) who showed improvements in symptom scores over the study period. Although 90% of women rated their satisfaction with treatment as 7 or above on a 10-point scale, the study did not clearly show a specific effect of the homeopathic remedy.

Another study (Jacobs et al., 2005) examined the effectiveness of two types of homeopathy for the treatment of breast cancer survivors with menopausal symptoms. Here, 83 such women who had completed all surgery, chemotherapy, and radiation treatment—and who averaged at least three hot flashes per day for the previous month—were randomized to receive an individualized ("constitutional") homeopathic single remedy, a homeopathic combination medicine, or placebo. Seen by homeopathic providers every 2 months for a year, they were evaluated for hot flash frequency and severity, Kupperman Menopausal Index, and a quality of life questionnaire. No statistically significant difference in outcome measure was found, but there was a positive trend in the single-remedy group during the first 3 months of the study. Also researchers noted a statistically significant improvement in general health for the single-remedy-treated patients. Alarmingly, evidence of a homeopathic "drug proving" in the subjects receiving the combination homeopathic medicine was also found. A homeopathic drug proving occurs when, after taking a remedy, the patient experiences symptoms that are completely new, or existing symptoms become extremely aggravated. In this case, the suspected symptoms were increased hot flash frequency and severity plus new headaches. The combination medicine contained three remedies, two of which (*Amyl nitrate* and *Sanguinaria*) were in relatively strong crude doses—and the women took these three times daily for a year. Women receiving the combination medicine who had not taken tamoxifen were more likely to experience this intensification of symptoms, but even they noted improved general health test scores compared with the placebo group.

Homeopathic remedies are most effectively prescribed according to the woman's total state rather than to eliminate single symptoms like hot flashes. Remedies such as *Lachesis* (from the Bushmaster snake), *Pulsatilla* (from the wind flower), and *Natrum muriaticum* (from table salt) derive from different kingdoms (animal, plant, and mineral, respectively), have different overall symptom pictures, and yet may all be indicated for menopausal complaints.

PREMENSTRUAL SYNDROMES

Menstrual pain is common in women, often interrupting their work and other life activities. Well-chosen homeopathic remedies can provide rapid relief from pain arising out of acute premenstrual syndrome (PMS). With some study in basic homeopathy courses offered at many homeopathic schools, women can often treat themselves (self-treatment) at least in limited fashion. Even so, they should recognize that while some symptoms may be ameliorated, the remedy selected may not be their overall constitutional one. If symptoms persist after one or two "acute" remedy trials or are recurrent, consultation with a professional homeopath is advised.

One controlled, double-blind study (Yakir, Kreitler, Brzesinski, Vithoulkas, & Bentwich, 2006) followed 96 women in a university outpatient clinic who were randomized to individualized homeopathic treatment or placebo for menstrual distress. After 3 months, 44% of actively treated women versus 34% of placebo controls perceived themselves as suffering less; 47% versus 22% felt they needed no further treatment. Psychological suggestibility was not correlated with outcomes for either the verum (active remedy) or placebo groups. Jones (2003) also described successfully using remedies such as *Lac caninum* (made from dog milk) and *Natrum muriaticum* to treat women with premenstrual symptoms.

MORNING SICKNESS IN PREGNANCY

As a consultation-liaison psychiatrist before homeopathic training, one of us (PP) was frequently asked to see pregnant women with severe nausea and vomiting (hyperemesis gravidarum; Kemker & Gamboa, 2006). Often these women did not respond to standard antiemetics. One extremely difficult case involved a 22-year-old single

African American woman, in her fifth month of pregnancy. She had been admitted multiple times for intractable vomiting, inability to eat, and dehydration. She would stay on the Ob-Gyn unit just long enough for IV rehydration and fetal monitoring, before being discharged to home, where her abusive boyfriend and mother waited. They never visited her in the hospital. It was a revolving door, and the Maternal-Fetal Medicine team was at its wit's end.

Each time she returned I would see her. She always lay in the dark—irritable and moaning about her belly cramps and headache. The slightest smell of food would evoke new surges of nausea and vomiting, which gave no relief. Crowding her bedside were paper cups filled with the profuse saliva she spat out constantly; seeing me, she would yell, "Get the hell out of here! All you do is torture me!" None of my medicines or manner helped; I also withheld analytic ideas about "oral attempts at abortion" (Chertok, 1972) because they seemed both impractical and punitive. In short, my presence was useless.

How enlightening years later to learn about the homeopathic remedy *Ipecacuanha*, which in material doses is a conventional medicine used to induce vomiting (*Ipecac*). Symptoms for which *Ipecacuanha* is known include terrible nausea unrelieved by vomiting, migraine headache, extreme irritability, and profuse salivation with drooling and spitting. Patients are weak and frequently need admission for IV hydration. Were it possible to go back in time, I would have offered this woman a few pellets of *Ipecacuanha* 30C.

Other useful remedies for pregnancy-associated nausea and vomiting (each having a slightly different symptom picture) include *Cocculus, Tabacum, Sepia,* and *Kreosotum* (Reichenberg-Ullman, 2000).

OTHER PREGNANCY-RELATED ISSUES

Appropriately prescribed homeopathic remedies can be helpful for aches and pains during pregnancy. Common ones include *Arnica montana* (from leopard's bane) whenever there are symptoms of bruising and swelling of muscles, and *Bellis perennis* (from common daisy) especially when the uterus and abdominal wall are sore and uncomfortable (Brennan, 1999). Breech presentation responds to the remedy *Pulsatilla* up to 40% of the time (Moskowitz, 1992). Premature labor can respond to remedies such as *Aconite* (from monkshood); labor can sometimes be induced with the remedy *Caulophyllum* (from blue cohosh; Brennan, 1999; Kistin & Newman, 2007). As shown by the case study at the start of this chapter, resolution of infections such as herpes in pregnancy is possible as well through homeopathic treatment.

SOMATOFORM AND OTHER PSYCHIATRIC DISORDERS

Fibromyalgia is an idiopathic, chronic nonarticular pain syndrome defined by widespread musculoskeletal pain and generalized tender points. Accompanied by sleep disturbances, fatigue, headache, morning stiffness, depression, and anxiety, it is also approximately 10 times more common in women than men (Chakrabarty & Zoorob, 2007). Bell published a 2004 paper in *Rheumatology* describing a double-blind, placebo-controlled trial with 62 fibromyalgia patients randomized to receive an oral daily dose of an individually chosen homeopathic medicine or placebo. Evaluating patients at baseline, 2 months, and 4 months, researchers found that 50% of those given the homeopathic medicine experienced a 25% or greater improvement in tender joint pain, compared with only 15% of those given placebo. After 4 months, the homeopathic patients rated the "helpfulness of treatment" significantly greater than those given placebo (Bell, Lewis, Brooks, et al., 2004).

Another feature of Bell's study involved administering the first dose by olfaction (smell) as Hahnemann described in his *Organon* (Hahnemann, 1996/1843) with both groups being monitored by an electroencephalogram (EEG). Patients given the "real" homeopathic medicine showed a significant and identifiable difference in EEG patterns compared with those given placebo (Bell, Lewis, Lewis, et al., 2004). Combined evidence of clinical improvement with an objective physiological response makes this trial unique. Remedies used included *Rhus toxicodendron* (poison ivy), *Bryonia* (white bryony, from the gourd family), and *Kalmia* (mountain laurel). A subsequent study confirmed that repeatedly sniffing an individually salient homeopathic remedy can produce significant EEG changes even after controlling for placebo sniffs (Bell, Brooks, Howerter, Jackson, & Schwartz, 2013).

Mood and anxiety disorders are approximately twice as common in women as men (Robinson, 2006). Mental and emotional symptoms indicate deeper dysfunction of the vital force than physical symptoms alone (Vithoulkas, 1980). Mood and anxiety complaints are often less specifically described than physical symptoms; this can make finding appropriate homeopathic remedies challenging. Dr. Rajan Sankaran has advanced homeopathic case-taking and prescribing by using such complaints as a starting point and then allowing patients to progressively describe their experiences. Eventually conversations reach a level deep enough to encompass all mental, emotional, physical, and spiritual symptoms—and the single required remedy can be found (Sankaran, 2004, 2007). A correctly prescribed remedy catalyzes the self-healing process; consciousness itself shifts to a more free and peaceful state (Sankaran, 2007). Bell and Pappas provide extensive reviews of homeopathy's use in psychiatric conditions (Bell & Pappas, 2007, 2008).

Childhood sexual abuse, estimated to be present in 25% of adult women in the United States, often leads to the combined physical, emotional, mental, and spiritual symptoms that classical homeopathy excels in treating. Clinical syndromes may include dissociation, depression, extreme rage and anxiety, chronic pain, and so on. The best remedy is determined through case-based research by an experienced homeopath (Chappel, 2008; Coll, 2002).

ADVERSE EFFECTS OF HOMEOPATHY

Reported rates of adverse effects with homeopathy in large observational studies range from 2% to 5% (Bell & Pappas, 2008). Not only new unexpected adverse symptoms are included in these rates but also transient "aggravations" (temporary increases in existing symptoms that occur early in treatment and resolve spontaneously). Aggravation rates are reported as up to 24% in the first 2 months of treatment (Thompson, Barron, & Spence, 2004). Only a small fraction (0.4%) of patients report prolonged aggravations (Sevar, 2005). There are no reports of mortality from unadulterated, properly prepared and prescribed homeopathic medicines in the clinical literature. However, overuse of low potency [less than 12C or 24X] remedies made from toxic substances such as Arsenicum and Aconite, may risk material dose exposure with potentially toxic responses in some patients (Posadzki, Alotaibi, & Ernst, 2012). Such low potencies may be more common in "complex" combinations sold in health food stores than in remedies prescribed by professionally trained homeopaths.

Summary and Recommendations

Despite skeptics who consider it sham or placebo (Lancet, 2005), classical homeopathy has a long history of safety and clinical benefits in women's health. Differentiating it from other leading forms of CAM involving natural products, homeopathy has a manufacturing process for its remedies that is standardized and regulated by the Food and Drug Administration (FDA). Basic science, animal, and psychophysiological research (Bell & Pappas, 2008; Bigagli et al., 2014; Bornhoft & Matthiessen, 2011; Endler et al., 2010; Frenkel et al., 2010) suggests that homeopathically prepared remedies have biological and behavioral effects beyond those of placebo. More research remains to be done.

Qualified homeopathic clinicians can be found through several professional organizations, including the American Institute of Homeopathy (www.homeopathyusa.org) for MDs and DOs, the Homeopathic Academy of Naturopathic Physicians (www.hanp.net) for NDs, the North American Society of Homeopaths (www.homeopathy.org) for professional but medically unlicensed homeopaths, and the National Center for Homeopathy (www. nationalcenterforhomeopathy.org), which is a mixed lay and professional group. For physicians wishing to learn homeopathic prescribing, courses such as those offered through American Medical College of Homeopathy (www. amcofh.org) are helpful. Effective prescribing for first aid and acute illnesses may be learned with 40–50 hours of training and accompanying study, but treating patients with chronic illness is not recommended without full homeopathic training and supervision. Classical homeopathy offers safe, gentle, and effective treatment for many women presenting with complex illnesses.

REFERENCES

Achterberg, J. (1990). *Woman as healer: A panoramic survey of the healing activities of women from prehistoric times to the present.* Boston, MA: Shambhala.

Barnes, P. M., Powel-Griner, E., McFann, K., & Nahin, R. L. (2004). Complementary and alternative medicine use among adults: United States, 2002. In Centers for Disease Control, *Advance Data from Vital and Health Statistics.* Hyattsville, MD. National Center for Health Statistics.

Bell, I. R., Brooks, A. J., Howerter, A., Jackson, N., & Schwartz, G. E. (2013). Acute electroencephalographic effects from repeated olfactory administration of homeopathic remedies in individuals with self-reported chemical sensitivity. *Alternative Therapies in Health and Medicine, 19,* 46–57.

Bell, I. R., & Koithan, M. (2006). Models for the study of whole systems. *Integr Cancer Ther, 5,* 294–307.

Bell, I. R., Lewis, D. A. I., Brooks, A. J., et al. (2004). Improved clinical status in fibromyalgia patients treated with individualized homeopathic remedies versus placebo. *Rheumatology, 43,* 577–582.

Bell, I. R., Lewis, D. A. I., Lewis, S. E., et al. (2004). EEG alpha sensitization in individualized homeopathic treatment of fibromyalgia. *Int J Neurosci, 114,* 1195–1220.

Bell, I. R., & Pappas, P. A. (2007). Homeopathy. In: J. H. Lake & D. Spiegel (Eds.), *Complementary and alternative treatments in mental health care* (pp. 195–224). Arlington, VA: American Psychiatric.

Bell, I. R., & Pappas, P. A. (2008). Homeopathy and its applications in psychiatry. In D. Mischoulon & J. Rosenbaum, J. (Eds.), *Natural medications for psychiatric disorders* (2nd ed., pp. 303–321) Philadelphia, PA: Lippincott Williams & Wilkins:.

Bell, I. R., Sarter, B., Koithan, M., Standish, L. J., Banerji, P., &. Banerji, P. (2013). Nonlinear response amplification mechanisms for low doses of natural product nanomedicines: Dynamical interactions with the recipient complex adaptive system. *J Nanomed Nanotechnol, 4,* 179.

Bigagli, E., Luceri, C., Bernardini, S., Dei, A., Filippini, A., & Dolara, P. (2014). Exploring the effects of homeopathic *Apis mellifica* preparations on human gene expression profiles. *Homeopathy, 103,* 127–132.

Bordet, M. F., Marijnen, P., Masson, J., & Trichard, M. (2008). Treating hot flushes in menopausal women with homeopathic treatment—Results of an observational study. *Homeopathy, 97,* 10–15.

Bornhoft, G., & Matthiessen, P. F. (2011). *Homeopathy in healthcare—Effectiveness, appropriateness, safety, costs.* Berlin, Germany: Springer-Verlag.

Brennan, P. (1999). Homeopathic remedies in prenatal care. *J Nurse Midwifery, 44,* 291–299.

Carlston, M. (2003). *Classical homeopathy.* Medical Guides to Complementary and Alternative Medicine. Philadelphia, PA: Churchill Livingstone.

Castro, M. (1993). *Homeopathy for pregnancy, birth, and your baby's first year.* New York, NY: St. Martin's Press.

CDC. (2007). Unintentional poisoning deaths—United States 1999-2004. *MMWR Weekly, 56,* 93–95.

Chakrabarty, S., &. Zoorob, R. (2007). Fibromyalgia. *Am Fam Physician, 76,* 247–254.

Chappell, P. (2008). Post-traumatic stress disorder and the vital sensation. *Homeopathic Links, 21,* 12–15.

Chernin, D. (2006). *The complete homeopathic resource for common illnesses.* Berkeley, CA: North Atlantic Books.

Chertok, L. (1972). The psychopathology of vomiting of pregnancy. In J. G. Howells (Ed.), *Modern perspectives in psycho-obstetrics* (pp. 283–289). New York, NY: Brunner/Mazel.

Coll, L. (2002) Homeopathy in survivors of childhood sexual abuse. *Homeopathy, 91,* 3–9.

de Oliveira, C. C., de Oliveira, S. M., Goes, V. M., Probst, C. M., Krieger, M. A., & Buchi Dde, F. (2008). Gene expression profiling of macrophages following mice treatment with an immunomodulator medication. *J Cell Biochem, 104,* 1364–1377.

Eisenberg, D., Davis, R. B., Ettner, S. L., et al. (1998). Trends in alternative medicine use in the United States, 1990–1997: Results of a follow-up national survey. *JAMA, 280,* 1569–1575.

Endler, P., Thieves, K., Reich, C., Matthiessen, P., Bonamin, L., Scherr, C., & Baumgartner, S. (2010). Repetitions of fundamental research models for homeopathically prepared dilutions beyond 10(-23): A bibliometric study. *Homeopathy, 99,* 25–36.

Frenkel, M., Mishra, B. M., Sen, S., Yang, P., Pawlus, A., Vence, L., … Banerji, P. (2010). Cytotoxic effects of ultra-diluted remedies on breast cancer cells. *Int J Oncol, 36,* 395–403.

Hahnemann, S. (1996/1843). *Organon of the medical art* (W. B. O'Reilly, Ed.) (6th ed.). Redmond,WA: Birdcage Books.

Hunt, K., & Ernst, E. (2010). Patients' use of CAM: Results from the Health Survey for England 2005. *Focus Altern Complement Ther, 15,* 101–103.

Jacobs, J., Herman, P., Heron, K., Olsen, S., & Vaughters, L. (2005). Homeopathy for menopausal symptoms in breast cancer survivors: A preliminary randomized controlled trial. *J Alt Comp Med*, *11*, 21–27.

Jenkins, E. (1972). *Dr. Gulley's Story*. New York, NY: Coward, McCann & Geoghegan.

Jones, A. (2003). Homeopathic treatment for premenstrual symptoms. *J Fam Plann Reprod Health Care*, *29*, 25–28.

Kemker, K., & Gamboa, M. (2006). Pregnancy. In M. Blumenfield & J. J., Strain (Eds.), *Psychosomatic medicine*. Philadelphia, PA: Lippincott Williams & Wilkins.

Kirschmann, A. T. (2004). *A vital force: Women in American homeopathy*. Piscataway, NJ: Rutgers University Press.

Kistin, S. J., & Newman, A. D. (2007). Induction of labor with homeopathy: A case report. *J Midwifery Womens Health*, *52*, 303–307.

Koithan, M., Bell, I. R., Niemeyer, K., & Pincus, D. (2012). A complex systems science perspective for whole systems of CAM research. *Forschende Komplementarmedizin und Klassische Naturheilkunde*, *19*(Suppl 1), 7–14.

Lancet. (2005). The end of homoeopathy [Editorial]. *Lancet*, *366*, 690.

Lansky, A. L. (2003). *Impossible cure: The promise of homeopathy*. Portola Valley, CA: R.L. Ranch Press.

Merrell, W. C., & Shalts, E. (2002). Homeopathy. *Med Clin North Am*, *86*, 47–62.

Mollinger, H., Schneider, R., & Walach, H. (2009). Homeopathic pathogenetic trials produce specific symptoms different from placebo. *Forsch Komplementmed*, *16*, 105–110.

Morrison, R. (1993). *Desktop guide to keynotes and confirmatory symptoms*. Nevada City, CA: Hahnemann Clinic.

Moskowitz, R. (1992). *Homeopathic medicines for pregnancy and childbirth*. Berkeley, CA: North Atlantic Books and Homeopathic Educational Services.

Oberbaum, M., Yaniv, I., Ben-Gal, Y., et al. (2001). A randomized, controlled clinical trial of the homeopathic medication TRAUMEEL S in the treatment of chemotherapy-induced stomatitis in children undergoing stem cell transplantation. *Cancer*, *92*, 684–690.

Posadzki, P., Alotaibi, A., & Ernst, E. (2012). Adverse effects of homeopathy: A systematic review of published case reports and case series. *Int J Clin Pract*, *66*, 1178–1188.

Reichenberg-Ullman, J. (2000). *Whole woman homeopathy*. Roseville, CA: Prima.

Relton, C., & Weatherly-Jones, E. (2005). Homeopathy service in a National Health Service community menopause clinic: Audit of clinical outcomes. *J British Menopause Soc*, *11*, 72–73.

Robinson, G. E. (2006). Gender differences in depression and anxiety disorders. In S. E. Romans & M. V. Seeman (Eds.), *Women's mental health: A life-cycle approach*. Philadelphia, PA: Lippincott Williams & Wilkins.

Roper Starch Worldwide. (1999). *The growing self-care movement*. Washington, DC: Food Marketing Institute.

Sankaran, R. (2004). *The sensation in homeopathy*. Mumbai, India: Homeopathic Medical.

Sankaran, R. (2007). *Sensation refined*. Mumbai, India: Homeopathic Medical.

Sevar, R. (2005). Audit of outcome in 455 consecutive patients treatment with homeo-pathic medicines. *Homeopathy, 94*, 215–221.

Shalts, E. (2004). Homeopathy. In B. Kligler & R. Lee, (Eds.), *Integrative medicine: Principles for practice*. New York, NY: McGraw-Hill.

Steinberg, D., & Beal, M. W. (2003). Homeopathy and women's health care. *J Obstet Gynecol Neonatal Nurs, 32*, 207–214.

Thompson, E., Barron, S., & Spence, D. (2004). A preliminary audit investigating remedy reactions including adverse events in routine homeopathic practice. *J Am Inst Homeopath, 93*, 203–209.

Thompson, E., Oxon, B. A., Montgomery, A., Douglas, D., & Reilly, D. (2005). A pilot, randomized, double-blinded, placebo-controlled trial of individualized homeopathy for symptoms of estrogen withdrawal in breast-cancer survivors. *J Alt Comp Med, 11*, 13–20.

Thompson, E., & Reilly, D. (2003). The homeopathic approach to the treatment of symptoms of oestrogen withdrawal in breast cancer patients: A prospective observational study. *Homeopathy, 92*, 131–134.

Ullman, D. (2007). *The homeopathic revolution: Why famous people and cultural heroes choose homeopathy*. Berkeley, CA: North Atlantic Books.

Ullman, D. (2008). *Homeopathic family medicine: Connecting research to quality homeopathic care*. Berkeley, CA: Homeopathic Educational Services.

Van Zandvoort, R. (2008). *Complete 2008 repertory*. Kent Homeopathic Associates. http://www.kenthomeopathic.com/macrepertory.html#Roger-van-Zandvoort

Verhoef, M. J., Lewith, G., Ritenbaugh, C., Boon, H., Fleishman, S., & Leis, A. (2005). Complementary and alternative medicine whole systems research: Beyond identification of inadequacies of the RCT. *Complement Ther Med, 13*, 206–212.

Vithoulkas, G. (1980). *The science of homeopathy*. New York, NY: Grove Press.

Weiser, M., Strosser, W., & Klein, P. (1998). Homeopathic vs conventional treatment of vertigo: A randomized double-blind controlled clinical study. *Arch Otolaryngol Head Neck Surg, 124*, 879–885.

WHO. (2002). *The WHO strategy for traditional medicine: Review of the global situation and strategy implementation in the eastern Mediterranean region health and human security*. Cairo, Egypt.

Winston, J. (1999). *The faces of homoeopathy: An illustrated history of the first 200 years*. Wellington, New Zealand: Great Auk.

Yakir, M., Kreitler, M., Brzesinski, A., Vithoulkas, G., & Bentwich, P. (2006). Women with premenstrual syndrome under homeopathic treatment: Improvements in health and quality of life. In P. Darnell, M. Pinder, & K. Treacy (Eds.). *Searching for evidence: Complementary therapies research* (pp. 14–15). London, England: Prince of Wales Foundation for Integrated Health.

Yakir, M., Kreitler, S., Brzezinski, A., Vithoulkas, G., Oberbaum, M., & Bentwich, Z. (2001). Effects of homeopathic treatment in women with premenstrual syndrome: A pilot study. *Br Homeopath J, 90*, 148–153.

11

Manual Medicine

CHERYL HAWK AND RAHELEH KHORSAN

Although I had been a chiropractor for many years, my first acquaintance with the effects of manipulation on chronic pelvic pain (CPP) was not through a patient but was shared with me by a friend. Ellen had suffered from CPP since her early twenties. Her gynecological exams were negative, and she was prescribed antidepressants and analgesics, which did not completely manage her symptoms. Her CPP was incapacitating at times. She had been very active in sports in high school and college and had suffered a number of injuries including sprains and strains of her lower back and knees. She had been relatively inactive since college, when her symptoms began.

Her CPP symptoms were accompanied by lower back pain (LBP), and during a flare of especially bad LBP when she was 31 years old, she went to a chiropractor. The chiropractor manipulated her lower back, sacrum, pelvis, and femur heads, and she was astounded to find that her CPP was gone—permanently! It never came back in the 10 years since that first adjustment.

"You need to do research on this," she told me, since I had just completed my PhD in preventive medicine and had begun a career in clinical research. So I did as she suggested, and although I did not find another "miracle cure" like Ellen's, I found manipulation, especially the low-force flexion-distraction technique using a specially designed table, to be a promising conservative approach, often giving a great deal of relief to the women suffering from this complex condition.

Introduction and Background

Spinal manipulation is among the oldest healing methods, and references to its use are recorded in many ancient cultures. In fact, Hippocrates practiced manipulation (Gatterman, 2004). For centuries, "bonesetting" was a type of traditional medicine learned through apprenticeship and observation of functional movement of the human body (Meeker & Haldeman, 2002). Interestingly, one of the most famous bonesetters in eighteenth century England was a woman, Sarah Mapp, who was so popular that a play was written about her (Gatterman, 2004). Osteopathy and chiropractic arose as distinct professions in the late 19th century, and both incorporated the tradition of bonesetting as well as the concept of vitalism or life force that was popular in the 1890s.

Today, "chiropractic" is often considered to be synonymous with "spinal manipulation." However, although chiropractors perform approximately 94% of spinal manipulation in the United States, chiropractic is a profession, not a procedure, and chiropractors provide a broad array of conservative therapies in addition to spinal manipulative therapy (SMT), including soft tissue treatment and counseling on physical activity and other lifestyle factors (Meeker & Haldeman, 2002). Some osteopaths, physical therapists, massage therapists, and, in Europe, manual therapists also provide SMT.

"Spinal manipulation" refers to the application of biomechanical force to a spinal joint for the purpose of correcting joint dysfunction. It is believed in both osteopathic and chiropractic theory that such correction enhances function and promotes the body's self-healing capacity (Handoll, 2004; Hawk, 2007).

Spinal manipulative therapy has a substantial body of evidence for its effectiveness in relieving musculoskeletal complaints, especially pain that is spine related (Bronfort et al., 2008; Hurwitz, Morgenstern, Vassilaki, & Chiang, 2008). There is much less evidence for its effects on nonmusculoskeletal complaints (Hawk, 2007). This chapter reviews the evidence on the safety and effectiveness of SMT on conditions commonly experienced by women, both musculoskeletal and nonmusculoskeletal, in order to assist clinicians and their patients in making decisions about appropriate care. This chapter also reviews the evidence for the effects of massage on these conditions, since massage is among the most commonly used manual procedures and is often combined with SMT (Barnes, Bloom, & Nahin, 2008).

Spinal Manipulation and Common Conditions

The conditions addressed in this chapter are those specific to women, or those that affect women predominantly, for which there is evidence that SMT and/ or massage may have clinical benefit. Conditions are only included if there is at least some published evidence, ranging from high-level evidence such as systematic reviews and randomized controlled trials (RCTs), to low level, such as case series. If the only available evidence comes from case reports and/or expert opinion articles on theory or technique, the condition is not included. Box 11.1 lists the conditions addressed in this chapter.

BACK PAIN DURING PREGNANCY

There is substantial evidence that SMT is helpful for both acute and chronic LBP in the general adult population (Bronfort, Haas, et al., 2008; Clar et al., 2014). However, because of the physiological, hormonal, and biomechanical changes during pregnancy—as well as the "baby on board"—clinicians need to see evidence that these effects may safely be extrapolated to pregnant women.

Although relatively few clinical studies have been conducted among this population, four systematic reviews found that there was limited, but

---

Box 11.1 Women's Health Conditions for Which Spinal Manipulation May Be of Clinical Benefit

Women's Health Conditions

Conditions related to pregnancy

- Back pain during pregnancy
- Pain during labor and delivery
- Breech presentation

Disorders of the menstrual cycle

- Dysmenorrhea
- Premenstrual syndrome (PMS)

Chronic pelvic pain
Depression
Fibromyalgia
Migraine and tension headache
Multiple sclerosis (MS)

promising, evidence that SMT by chiropractors or osteopaths was of clinical benefit for LBP during pregnancy (Clar et al., 2014; Khorsan, Hawk, Lisi, & Kizhakkeveettil, 2009; Pennick & Liddle, 2013; Stuber & Smith, 2008). Both chiropractic and osteopathic education include training on appropriate ways to modify manipulative techniques for pregnant patients and contraindications to manipulation (Borggren, 2007; King et al., 2003). Manipulative techniques should be modified to minimize discomfort and the risk of adverse effects. These modifications include avoidance of prone postures and high-force manipulative maneuvers (Borggren, 2007). Because of the relaxing of ligaments during pregnancy, the sacroiliac joints become more mobile; thus, manipulation is often indicated for not only the lumbar vertebrae but also the sacroiliac area and pelvis (King et al., 2003).

None of the six published case series, two case-control studies, or one small experimental study reported any adverse effects on patients during their pregnancy or subsequent deliveries. However, one case report described an extremely rare case of a pathological cervical fracture after manipulation performed by a manual therapist in Germany (Schmitz, Lutterbey, von Engelhardt, von Falkenhausen, & Stoffel, 2005). This illustrates the importance of avoiding high-force manipulation during pregnancy, when routine diagnostic imaging is avoided, and using appropriately modified manipulative techniques.

PAIN DURING LABOR AND DELIVERY

There is much less evidence on the effect of manipulation on back pain during labor than during pregnancy (Clar et al., 2014). This may be partially explained by the fact that few chiropractors have hospital access to be able to conduct such research, and while osteopaths do have hospital access, the number who perform manipulation is relatively small. A 1982 osteopathic study investigated the effect of lumbar pressure applied by the woman's husband, coach, or nurse during labor (Guthrie & Martin, 1982). They found that requests for pain medication from women during labor were significantly less frequent than from control group women who did not receive the intervention or received a placebo intervention (pressure applied to the thoracic area). Since this is a very low-risk procedure, and one that can be taught to the birth coach, it is worth a consideration, even though the evidence is sparse.

There is somewhat more evidence on possible beneficial effects on labor and delivery from manipulation done as part of prenatal care, but not at the actual time of delivery (Diakow et al., 1991; King et al., 2003; Phillips & Meyer, 1995). Again, no adverse events during the pregnancy or during labor and delivery were reported related to manipulation. There is also some evidence that massage therapy may reduce pain for women in labor, although more research is needed (Chaillet et al., 2014; Jones et al., 2012; Smith, Levett, Collins, & Jones, 2012).

BREECH PRESENTATION CORRECTION

Although breech presentation occurs in a small proportion of singleton pregnancies, nearly 90% of these babies are delivered by Caesarean section (C-section) (Tiran, 2004). The usual medical alternative to a C-section is external cephalic version (ECV), but it has a relatively low success rate (Hutton & Hofmeyr, 2006). Since many women and their providers prefer a vaginal birth, there is growing interest in complementary and alternative medicine techniques to correct breech presentations (Tiran, 2004).

The Webster technique is a manipulative procedure developed by a chiropractor to correct musculoskeletal imbalances believed to contribute to uterine constraint that may result in breech presentation (Ohm, 2001; Pistolese, 2002). It does not involve an attempt to reposition the fetus as is done in ECV. Instead, it uses a low-force manipulation of the sacrum, followed by very light (3–6 ounces of pressure) manual trigger-point therapy to musculature of the lower abdomen (Kunau, 1998; Pistolese, 2002).

Only one case series on the Webster technique was identified. It described five cases of successful correction of the breech presentation with no adverse events, which was verified by the women's medical physicians (Kunau, 1998). All patients were Amish, a population who generally prefer natural approaches to health care. In a survey of 1,047 chiropractors, out of 187 respondents, 112 reported using the Webster technique, and 102 met with success. No adverse events were reported (Pistolese, 2002).

For a woman who desires to avoid a C-section, it may be worthwhile for her provider to locate a chiropractor who is trained and experienced in the Webster technique and who can evaluate the musculoskeletal factors amenable to correction.

DISORDERS OF THE MENSTRUAL CYCLE

Dysmenorrhea

A 2006 Cochrane review of SMT for dysmenorrhea concluded that "there is no evidence to suggest that spinal manipulation is effective for the treatment of primary or secondary dysmenorrhea," but that the risk of adverse effects from SMT are no greater than they are for sham manipulation (Proctor, Hing, Johnson, & Murphy, 2006). However, two of the four trials analyzed used sham manipulations that were very similar to the high-velocity, low-amplitude (HVLA) manipulation in the active groups. (The sham differed in the amount of biomechanical force delivered—and there were decreases in pain in both groups.) Because many chiropractors and osteopaths use low-force treatments, a maneuver that delivers a lesser amount of biomechanical force is not necessarily "inactive" or a "sham." In fact, the real-world applicability of using a manual placebo or sham procedure has been called into question because there is as yet no definitive evidence on a threshold at which biomechanical force has no effect (Hawk, Long, Rowell, Gudavalli, & Jedlicka, 2005).

An interesting finding in one well-designed RCT (Hondras, Long, & Brennan, 1999) was that while immediate treatment effects were not significant, patients showed a tendency to improve over three menstrual cycles. A 2007 systematic review concluded that the evidence was equivocal for chiropractic care for dysmenorrhea, that the most appropriate level of biomechanical force is unclear, but that care extended over at least three menstrual cycles is more likely to be of clinical benefit (Hawk, 2007).

Thus, since adverse effects appear minimal, patients with dysmenorrhea who are interested in a therapeutic trial of SMT may benefit, if they are willing to remain under care for several menstrual cycles.

Premenstrual Syndrome

Few studies have investigated the effect of manipulation on premenstrual syndrome (PMS). One systematic review (Stevinson & Ernst, 2001) found evidence insufficient, and another (Hawk, Khorsan, Lisi, Ferrance, & Evans, 2007) found evidence equivocal for the utility of SMT for PMS. It is more likely that SMT would help patients with dysmenorrhea than with PMS symptoms not related to pain.

CHRONIC PELVIC PAIN

Chronic pelvic pain (CPP), usually defined as acyclic pain in the pelvis occurring for at least 6 months, is a common reason for gynecological visits, 40% of laparoscopies, and 10% to 15% of hysterectomies (Tettambel, 2005). The majority of women with CPP also experience LBP, and involvement of the musculoskeletal system as a contributor to this complex condition is becoming increasingly accepted (Tettambel, 2005; Montenegro, Vasconcelos, Candido Dos Reis,

Nogueira, Poli-Neto, 2008). Case reports and case series have described the utility of both chiropractic and osteopathic manipulation in managing CPP (Browning, 1988, 1989; Tettambel, 2005). A single group intervention with 18 women in which chiropractic manipulation, using flexion-distraction technique (a low-force approach not involving rotation of the vertebrae) and manual trigger-point therapy, showed significant improvement in CPP after 4 weeks of care (Gay et al., 2005; Hawk, Long, & Azad, 1997). A 2014 systematic review found favorable but inconclusive evidence for the effects of SMT on CPP (Clar et al., 2014). Another systematic review reported on a small study ($n = 6$) in which Thiele massage (a transvaginal massage technique) was helpful for CPP. However, there is no evidence that traditional massage therapy affects CPP symptoms (Carinci, Pathak, Young, & Christo, 2013).

Integrative approaches to CPP are often advocated and usually include physical therapy (Chou et al., 2007), however, the 2005 Canadian consensus guidelines for management of CPP specifically recommend correction of myofascial dysfunction, postural abnormalities, and immobility of the sacrum (Chou et al., 2007). The addition of SMT, especially the use of the low-force techniques of osteopathic muscle energy and counterstrain or the chiropractic technique of flexion-distraction—all of which are unlikely to cause adverse effects—into integrative medical management seems a reasonable approach to care of women with CPP.

DEPRESSION

A 2007 systematic review took an innovative approach to investigating a possible role for SMT in treatment of depression (Williams et al., 2007). This review examined RCTs of SMT for treating back or neck pain that included a measurement of psychological outcomes, such as the mental health subscale of the SF-36 or SF-12, or a depression questionnaire.

In these trials, chiropractors, osteopaths, and physical therapists performed spinal manipulation or mobilization. Although only 12 of 129 RCTs had psychological outcomes that could be analyzed, it did appear that SMT had a modest clinical benefit. Whether this was attributable to pain relief, the positive effect of touch, or the caring effect of the therapist is not clear. For individuals who are interested in an integrative approach to depression and who have spine-related pain, the combination of established approaches like cognitive-behavioral therapy with SMT may be beneficial.

FIBROMYALGIA

Several small controlled studies have been published on both osteopathic and chiropractic manipulation for fibromyalgia (FM), providing some support for a role for SMT in the treatment of this complex condition (Blunt, Rajwani, & Guerriero 1997; Gamber, Shores, Russo, Jimenez, & Rubin, 2002; Hains & Hains, 2000). Spinal manipulative therapy was combined with soft tissue treatments that included myofascial release, and both low-force manipulation and HVLA manipulation were used in different studies.

Spinal manipulative therapy, when combined with appropriate soft-tissue treatment, may provide added value above other physical treatments such as exercise or stretching (Gamber et al., 2002). A 2009 systematic review found that there was limited evidence supporting SMT and moderate evidence supporting massage for FM (Schneider, Vernon, Ko, Lawson, & Perera, 2009), while a 2014 systematic review and meta-analysis also found that massage therapy was beneficial for FM symptoms (Li, Wang, Feng, Yang, & Sun, 2014). Because of the complexity and individual variation of FM symptoms, it is especially important that if SMT or massage is recommended by the clinician, the provider be experienced in a variety of manual techniques and be highly responsive to patient needs and preferences.

MIGRAINE AND TENSION HEADACHES

Tension headaches often accompany migraines and therefore these are often considered together in clinical studies. A 2004 Cochrane review of noninvasive treatments for headache identified 22 studies with 2,628 patients (Bronfort et al., 2004). The authors concluded that SMT may be effective for prophylaxis of migraines, having a similar short-term effect to amitriptyline. However, amitriptyline appears to be more effective than SMT for prophylaxis of chronic tension-type headaches. A 2010 systematic review found that for migraine, the evidence is positive for SMT and favorable but inconclusive for massage (Bronfort et al., 2010). The same review found the evidence is inconclusive for tension headaches for both SMT and massage (Bronfort et al., 2010). There is little risk of adverse effects for either type of headache (Bronfort et al., 2004). Patients who prefer to avoid medications may, therefore, find comparable benefit in a course of SMT and/or massage without significant risk of harm.

MULTIPLE SCLEROSIS

Only one small pilot study (seven women with multiple sclerosis [MS]) investigated the effect of SMT on MS (Yates, Vardy, Kuchera, Ripley, & Johnson, 2002). By the end of the 12-week study, there was significant improvement in the strength of the patients and the distance that they were able to walk and there was no increase in fatigue. Although there was no comparison group, these findings are encouraging, especially as no adverse events were noted. Because maintaining functional ability is essential to management of MS, it may be helpful to recommend a course of SMT for patients with low to medium levels of impairment.

SAFETY OF SPINAL MANIPULATION

Serious adverse events caused by SMT are rare, and therefore, it is difficult to estimate risks precisely; serious complications of manipulation of the lumbar spine are estimated to be one case per 100 million manipulations (Meeker & Haldeman, 2002).

The most severe complication of lumbar spine manipulation is cauda equina syndrome. For cervical spine manipulation, cerebrovascular artery dissection that leads to stroke is the most serious adverse event. This topic has been the subject of a great deal of controversy; estimates of the risk of stroke range from one per 400,000 to three to six per 10 million manipulations. However, all these estimates were based on case reports and unsubstantiated provider surveys (Meeker & Haldeman, 2002).

In 2008, a well-designed population-based case-control and case-crossover study found no increased risk of vertebrobasilar artery (VBA) stroke for chiropractic patients when compared with patients of primary care medical physicians (Cassidy et al., 2008). Patients may seek care for headaches and neck pain in the early stages of the VBA dissection; which produced an increased association with visits to all healthcare providers, not solely chiropractors (Cassidy et al., 2008).

Mild-to-moderate, transient side effects of manipulation are common; they include muscle soreness, stiffness, and increased neck or back pain (Hurwitz et al., 2005). Modifying the manipulative technique—such as using mobilization, which involves slower rotation of the spinal joints than manipulation—may reduce adverse effects (Hurwitz et al., 2005). Use of rotation-type manipulation is a predictor of adverse events—primarily increased headache or neck pain—as is more than 30 days of neck pain in the past year (Rubinstein et al., 2008).

For patients who are considered at risk for an adverse event by the clinician, or who are apprehensive about manipulation, there are many low-force manipulative techniques that do not involve rotation of the spinal joints and do not employ the high-velocity, low-amplitude (HVLA) maneuver, traditionally associated with the term "manipulation." It is important that clinicians become acquainted with local providers who use manipulation so that they know those providers who are skilled at using a variety of manipulative techniques, which they can then tailor to each patient's individual clinical presentation and personal preferences.

Summary and Conclusions

Spinal manipulative therapy has a substantial body of evidence for its utility for musculoskeletal complaints, especially back and neck pain. A growing body of evidence on massage for a variety of health concerns is also developing (Bronfort et al., 2010; Clar et al., 2014). However, less evidence is available to support the application of SMT and/or massage to special populations like pregnant women or women with nonmusculoskeletal conditions such as MS or FM. Therefore, it is important that these women be referred to a manual therapist who has had success with the specific condition and with whom the referring clinician has a relationship of mutual trust and communication.

REFERENCES

Barnes, P. M., Bloom, B., & Nahin, R. L. (2008). Complementary and alternative medicine use among adults and children: United States, 2007. *Natl Health Stat Report*, 1–23.

Blunt, K. L., Rajwani, M. H., & Guerriero, R. C. (1997). The effectiveness of chiropractic management of fibromyalgia patients: A pilot study. *J Manipulative Physiol Ther*, 20, 389–399.

Borggren, C. L. (2007). Pregnancy and chiropractic: A narrative review of the literature. *J Chiropr Med*, 6, 70–74.

Bronfort, G., Haas, M., et al. (2008). Evidence-informed management of chronic low back pain with spinal manipulation and mobilization. *Spine J*, 8, 213–225.

Bronfort, G., Haas, M., Haas, M., Evans, R., Goldsmith, C. H., Assendelft, W. J., & Bouter, L. M. (2010). Effectiveness of manual therapies: The UK evidence report. *Chiropr Osteopat*, 18, 3.

Bronfort, G., Nilsson, N., et al. (2004). Non-invasive physical treatments for chronic/recurrent headache. *Cochrane Database Syst Rev*, 3:CD001878.

Browning, J. E. (1988). Chiropractic distractive decompression in the treatment of pelvic pain and organic dysfunction in patients with evidence of lower sacral nerve root compression. *J Manipulative Physiol Ther, 11*, 426–432.

Browning, J. E. (1989). Chiropractic distractive decompression in treating pelvic pain and multiple system pelvic organic dysfunction. *J Manipulative Physiol Ther, 12*, 265–274.

Carinci, A. J., Pathak, R., Young, M., & Christo, P. J. (2013). Complementary and alternative treatments for chronic pelvic pain. *Curr Pain Headache Rep, 17*, 316.

Cassidy, J. D., Boyle, E., Côté, P., et al. (2008). Risk of vertebrobasilar stroke and chiropractic care: Results of a population-based case-control and case-crossover study. *Spine (Phila Pa 1976), 33*(4 Suppl), S176–S183.

Chaillet, N., Belaid, L., Crochetière, C. et al. (2014). Nonpharmacologic approaches for pain management during labor compared with usual care: A meta-analysis. *Birth, 41*, 122–137.

Chou, R., Qaseem, A., Snow, V., et al. (2007). Diagnosis and treatment of low back pain: A joint clinical practice guideline from the American College of Physicians and the American Pain Society. *Ann Intern Med, 147*, 478–491.

Clar, C., Tsertsvadze, A., Court, R., Hundt, G. L., Clarke, A., & Sutcliffe, P. (2014). Clinical effectiveness of manual therapy for the management of musculoskeletal and non-musculoskeletal conditions: Systematic review and update of UK evidence report. *Chiropr Man Therap, 22*, 12.

Diakow, P. R., Gadsby, T. A., Gadsby, J. B., Gleddie, J. G., Leprich, D. J., & Scales, A. M. (1991). Back pain during pregnancy and labor. *J Manipulative Physiol Ther, 14*, 116–118.

Gamber, R. G., Shores, J. H., Russo, D. P., Jimenez, C., & Rubin, B. R. (2002). Osteopathic manipulative treatment in conjunction with medication relieves pain associated with fibromyalgia syndrome: Results of a randomized clinical pilot project. *J Am Osteopath Assoc, 102*, 321–325.

Gatterman, M. I. (2004). *Chiropractic management of spine related disorders* (2nd ed.). Baltimore, MD, Lippincott Williams & Wilkins.

Gay, R. E., Bronfort, G., et al. (2005). Distraction manipulation of the lumbar spine: A review of the literature. *J Manipulative Physiol Ther, 28*, 266–273.

Guthrie, R. A., & Martin, R. H., (1982). Effect of pressure applied to the upper thoracic (placebo) versus lumbar areas (osteopathic manipulative treatment) for inhibition of lumbar myalgia during labor. *J Am Osteopath Assoc, 82*, 247–251.

Hains, G., & Hains, F. (2000). A combined ischemic compression and spinal manipulation in the treatment of fibromyalgia: A preliminary estimate of dose and efficacy. *J Manipulative Physiol Ther, 23*, 225–230.

Handoll, N. (2004). Energy medicine: An osteopath's personal view. *J Altern Complement Med, 10*, 87–89.

Hawk, C. (2007). Are we asking the right questions? *Chiropr J Australia, 37*, 15–18.

Hawk, C., Khorsan, R., Lisi, A. J., Ferrance, R. J., & Evans, M. W. (2007). Chiropractic care for nonmusculoskeletal conditions: A systematic review with implications for whole systems research. *J Altern Complement Med, 13*, 491–512.

Hawk, C., Long, C. R., & Azad, A. (1997). Chiropractic care for women with chronic pelvic pain: A prospective single-group intervention study. *J Manipulative Physiol Ther*, *20*, 73–79.

Hawk, C., Long, C. R., Rowell, R. M., Gudavalli, M. R., & Jedlicka, J. (2005). A randomized trial investigating a chiropractic manual placebo: A novel design using standardized forces in the delivery of active and control treatments. *J Altern Complement Med*, *11*, 109–117.

Hondras, M. A., Long, C. R., & Brennan, P. C. (1999). Spinal manipulative therapy versus a low force mimic maneuver for women with primary dysmenorrhea: A randomized, observer-blinded, clinical trial. *Pain*, *81*, 105–114.

Hurwitz, E. L., Carragee, E. J., van der Velde, G., et al. (2008). Treatment of neck pain: Noninvasive interventions: Results of the Bone and Joint Decade 2000–2010 Task Force on Neck Pain and Its Associated Disorders. *Spine (Phila Pa 1976)*, *33*(4 Suppl), S123–152.

Hurwitz, E. L., Morgenstern, H., Vassilaki, M., & Chiang, L. M. (2005). Frequency and clinical predictors of adverse reactions to chiropractic care in the UCLA neck pain study. *Spine (Phila Pa 1976)*, *30*, 1477–1484.

Hutton, E. K., & Hofmeyr, G. J., (2006). External cephalic version for breech presentation before term. *Cochrane Database Syst Rev*,1: CD000084.

Jones, L., Othman, M., Dowswell, T., et al. (2012). Pain management for women in labour: An overview of systematic reviews. *Cochrane Database Syst Rev*, 3:CD009234.

Khorsan, R., Hawk, C., Lisi, A. J., & Kizhakkeveettil, A. (2009). Manipulative therapy for pregnancy and related conditions: A systematic review. *Obstet Gynecol Surv*, *64*, 416–427.

King, H. H., Tettambel, M. A., Lockwood, M. D., Johnson, K. H., Arsenault, D. A., & Quist, R. (2003). Osteopathic manipulative treatment in prenatal care: A retrospective case control design study. *J Am Osteopath Assoc*, *103*, 577–582.

Kunau, P. (1998). Application of the Webster in-utero constraint technique: A case series. *J Chiropr Clin Pediatr*, *3*, 211–216.

Li, Y. H., Wang, F. Y., Feng, C. Q., Yang, X. F., & Sun, Y. H. (2014). Massage therapy for fibromyalgia: A systematic review and meta-analysis of randomized controlled trials. *PLoS One*, *9*, e89304.

Meeker, W. C., & Haldeman, S. (2002). Chiropractic: A profession at the crossroads of mainstream and alternative medicine. *Ann Intern Med*, *136*, 216–227.

Montenegro, M. L., Vasconcelos, E. C., Candido Dos Reis, F. J., Nogueira, A. A., Poli-Neto, O. B. (2008). Physical therapy in the management of women with chronic pelvic pain. *Int J Clin Pract*, *62*, 263–269.

Ohm, J. (2001). Chiropractors and midwives: A look at the Webster technique. *Midwifery Today Int Midwife*, *42*.

Pennick, V., & Liddle, S. D., (2013). Interventions for preventing and treating pelvic and back pain in pregnancy. *Cochrane Database Syst Rev*, 8:CD001139.

Phillips, J. C. J., & Meyer, J. (1995). Chiropractic care, including craniosacral therapy, during pregnancy: A static-group comparison of obstetric interventions during labor and delivery. *J Manipulative Physiol Ther*, *18*, 525–529.

Pistolese, R. A. (2002). The Webster technique: A chiropractic technique with obstetric implications. *J Manipulative Physiol Ther*, *25*, E1–E9.

Proctor, M. L., Hing, W., Johnson, T. C., & Murphy, P. A. (2006). Spinal manipulation for primary and secondary dysmenorrhoea. *Cochrane Database Syst Rev*,3: CD002119.

Rubinstein, S. M., Leboeuf-Yde, C., Knol, D. L., de Koekkoek, T. E., Pfeifle, C. E., & van Tulder, M. W. (2008). Predictors of adverse events following chiropractic care for patients with neck pain. *J Manipulative Physiol Ther*, *31*, 94–103.

Schmitz, A., Lutterbey, G., von Engelhardt, L., von Falkenhausen, M., & Stoffel, M. (2005). Pathological cervical fracture after spinal manipulation in a pregnant patient. *J Manipulative Physiol Ther*, *28*, 633–636.

Schneider, M., Vernon, H., Ko, G., Lawson, G., & Perera, J. (2009). Chiropractic management of fibromyalgia syndrome: A systematic review of the literature. *J Manipulative Physiol Ther*, *32*, 25–40.

Smith, C. A., Levett, K. M., Collins, C. T., & Jones, L. (2012). Massage, reflexology and other manual methods for pain management in labour. *Cochrane Database Syst Rev*, 2:CD009290.

Stevinson, C., & Ernst, E., (2001). Complementary/alternative therapies for premenstrual syndrome: A systematic review of randomized controlled trials. *Am J Obstet Gynecol*, *185*, 227–235.

Stuber, K. J., & Smith, D. L., (2008). Chiropractic treatment of pregnancy-related low back pain: A systematic review of the evidence. *J Manipulative Physiol Ther*, *31*, 447–454.

Tettambel, M. A. (2005). An osteopathic approach to treating women with chronic pelvic pain. *J Am Osteopath Assoc*, *105*(9 Suppl 4), S20–S22.

Tiran, D. (2004). Breech presentation: Increasing maternal choice. *Complement Ther Nurs Midwifery*, *10*, 233–238.

Williams, N. H., Hendry, M., Lewis, R.,Russell, I.,Westmoreland, A.,& Wilkinson, C. (2007). Psychological response in spinal manipulation (PRISM): A systematic review of psychological outcomes in randomised controlled trials. *Complement Ther Med*, *15*, 271–283.

Yates, H. A., Vardy, T. C., Kuchera, M. L., Ripley, B. D., & Johnson, J. C. (2002). Effects of osteopathic manipulative treatment and concentric and eccentric maximal-effort exercise on women with multiple sclerosis: A pilot study. *J Am Osteopath Assoc*, *102*, 267–275.

PART III

Reproductive Health

12

Premenstrual Syndrome

DAPHNE MILLER

CASE STUDY

Every month before my period I get terrible cramping, breast tenderness, and mood swings. It's now to the point where I don't want to go to work and I snarl at my family. My last doctor did not have much to offer me—her only suggestion was that I could start birth control pills or antidepressants. I want to feel better but I don't want to take these medications for a problem that only bothers me for three to four days each month. Plus I am very sensitive to all medication. I have taken different birth control pills in the past and they all give me headaches and make me even more depressed.

—Marie M., age 29

Introduction

Almost every woman of reproductive age experiences some amount of physical or psychological discomfort in the week preceding her menstrual period (Freeman, 2003; Halbreich et al., 2007; Johnson, 2004). Premenstrual symptoms (Box 12.1), when they are present to a degree that they affect quality of life, social engagements, and/or work performance are identified as a "syndrome" (premenstrual syndrome, or PMS) or, if more stringent criteria are met, a "disorder" (premenstrual dysphoric disorder, or PMDD). The inclusion criteria for these two diagnoses continue to be debated; yet, it is clear that those premenstrual symptoms, PMS, and PMDD represent

Box 12.1 Premenstrual Symptoms

Emotional symptoms	Depressed, sad, down, or blue
	Anxious, tense, on edge, or keyed up
	Angry or irritable
Physical symptoms	Breast tenderness
	Muscle or joint aches
	Stomach bloating or diarrhea
	Carbohydrate craving or increased appetite

a continuum of the same entity. In the end, these specific definitions have little relevance for the clinical practitioner (Halbreich et al., 2007). What is important is the degree and nature of symptoms reported by each individual woman and how her experience impacts her quality of life. Therefore, although the term PMS is used throughout this chapter and the research presented primarily includes women with a formal diagnosis of PMS or PMDD, the following recommendations will be applicable to anyone wishing to address negative premenstrual symptoms.

Theories abound on the potential causes of PMS, but after 40 years of clinical and epidemiological research, the exact etiology remains unclear. For most women, their symptoms are likely to be a complex interplay of physiological, psychological, and environmental factors. Available pharmacologic and surgical treatments are often considered unacceptable treatments for PMS, as they frequently offer disproportionately more side effects than perceived benefits. Community-based studies suggest that over 70% of women seeking to alleviate symptoms first turn to alternative (nonpharmaceutical or nonsurgical) strategies (Pullon, Reinken, & Sparrow, 1989). Taking into consideration the heterogeneous nature of PMS, the lack of a single highly effective and widely accepted conventional treatment, and a general preference for alternative therapies, PMS lends itself perfectly to an integrative medical approach.

The Personal and Social Burden of Premenstrual Syndrome

Most women in developed countries have about 400 to 500 menstrual cycles in their reproductive years, and it is conceivable that a woman could spend 12% of her life suffering from premenstrual symptoms. Severe premenstrual symptoms result in a similar burden of illness (disability-adjusted life years, DALYs) as major dysphoric disorders such as major depression (Halbreich, 2002). Compared with women with mild or no premenstrual symptoms, women who suffer moderate to severe PMS miss significantly greater workdays, report lower productivity because of their symptoms, and feel that their personal relationships (especially with spouses) are negatively impacted (Dean & Borenstein, 2004; Robinson & Swindle, 2000). In one study, women with moderate or worse symptoms had more visits to ambulatory healthcare providers and incurred higher annual healthcare costs as compared with women with mild or no PMS (Borenstein, Dean, Leifke, Korner, & Yonkers, 2007). It is also likely that PMS heightens the symptoms of other chronic pain syndromes such as irritable bowel syndrome (IBS), fibromyalgia, and chronic fatigue.

Who Gets Premenstrual Syndrome?

Accurate prevalence rates are difficult to establish; however, it is estimated that 80% to 90% of women of reproductive age experience at least mild symptoms with each menstrual cycle. Although only 2% to 3% of women have physical and psychological discomfort that is severe enough to meet the criteria for PMDD, over 20% of women have monthly experiences that are so distressing that they warrant treatment (Sternfeld, Swindle, Chawla, Long, & Kennedy, 2002). There are few identified social or biological risk factors for PMS, although prevalence studies indicate that younger women tend to have a greater intensity and variety of symptoms (Freeman, Rickels, Schweizer, & Ting, 1995; Wood, Mortola, Chan, Moossazadeh, & Yen, 1992). Women of all ethnicities experience premenstrual symptoms, and the negative symptoms related to the premenstrual period appear to transcend sociocultural divides (Robinson & Swindle, 2000; Sternfeld et al., 2002). It is interesting to note that women interviewed in areas as different as China and Australia have reported roughly the same constellation of symptoms, with irritability and depression emerging as the most frequent complaint in both regions (Gotts, Morse, & Dennerstein, 1995; Zhao, Wang, & Qu, 1998).

Women are much more likely to underreport premenstrual symptoms if they have the perception that it is not a real health problem or that they should be more stoic (Robinson & Swindle, 2000). Therefore, at each clinic visit, remember to ask detailed questions about their symptoms and validate their experience.

Diagnosing Premenstrual Syndrome

Before diagnosing PMS, it is important to undertake a complete clinical evaluation. One goal of this initial assessment is to rule out other conditions that can be confused with PMS (Table 12.1). A detailed history should include specific questions about PMS symptoms (Box 12.1) and their significance in a woman's life.

Allowing a woman to explain her symptoms and receive validation can be one of the first steps in treatment. In addition, certain interventions have been shown to be more effective against a particular set of symptoms such as depression, breast pain, or bloating, and therefore, a history can help tailor the intervention. Recording specific symptoms and their severity on a 1 to 10 scale can also help assess effectiveness of treatment. In general, a 50% decrease in symptoms translates into a noticeably improved quality of life for women with PMS (Borenstein et al., 2007).

Diagnosing PMS

The specific diagnosis of PMS or PMDD requires that women use diaries to record symptoms for two consecutive menstrual cycles. Studies show that less than 20% of physicians use this type of symptom monitoring to diagnose PMS (Craner, Sigmon, & McGillicuddy, 2014). Although diaries can be useful for women who are uncertain about the timing or severity of their symptoms, asking them a general question followed by a more detailed inquiry is often the best approach. The following is an example of the general type of question that I ask to assess for PMS-type symptoms: "Thinking specifically of the week before your period starts, would you describe the level of your symptoms as mild, moderate, strong or severe?"

Table 12.1. Differential Diagnoses of PMS

Psychological Disorders	Medical Conditions
Chronic depression	Dysmenorrhea
Major depressive episode	Endometriosis
Bipolar disorder	Hypothyroidism
Generalized anxiety disorder	Polycystic ovary syndrome
Panic disorder	Migraines
Somatoform disorder	Allergies
Substance abuse	Irritable bowel syndrome
	Perimenopausal symptoms
	Adrenal insufficiency

As part of the initial assessment, every woman should also receive a complete history, physical and pelvic exam. Laboratory tests to assess for anemia, hypothyroidism, hyperprolactinemia, and cortisol imbalances should be considered.

Approaches to Treating PMS

CONVENTIONAL TREATMENT

In the past 40 years, PMS and PMDD have been the subject of intense biological and epidemiological research in an attempt to identify causes and develop effective treatments. These efforts have uncovered many potentially relevant physiological and environmental explanations including ovarian hormonal dysfunction, abnormal regulation of aldosterone, defects in immunologic response, nutritional deficiencies, and emotional stress. However, there is no consistent link between any of these factors and PMS (Backstrom et al., 2003; Muse, 1992).

Conventional treatment strategies have focused on identifying a drug that will interfere with one of these specific processes, be it hormonal, neurohumoral, or inflammatory. This has resulted in the use of a diverse armamentarium of pharmaceuticals including serotonergic antidepressants (selective serotonin reuptake inhibitors, or SSRIs), nonsteroidal anti-inflammatory drugs (NSAIDS), anxiolytics, spironalactone, and hormones (especially birth control pills). Despite the popularity of these drugs among healthcare professionals, SSRIs are the only conventional treatment whose efficacy for PMS has been well supported by clinical trials. The SSRIs, although exceedingly helpful for a select group of women, have a rather large side-effect profile and subsequently a high rate of discontinuation (Rapkin, 2005). Unlike the approach to the treatment of depression, serotonergic antidepressants need not be given daily, but can be effective when used cyclically, only in the luteal phase, or even limited to the duration of the monthly symptoms (Rapkin & Lewis, 2013). Hormones, including birth control pills, have less compelling evidence and actually seem to exacerbate PMS symptoms in some women. The NSAIDS have their own potential side effects; most significant are gastric ulceration and renal dysfunction (see Box 12.2). Given the paucity of data as to the benefits of conventional treatments for PMS coupled with a high discontinuation rate due to side effects, first-line treatment with drugs should be reserved for women with severe symptoms (Jarvis, Lynch, & Morin, 2008).

> ### Box 12.2 Pharmacological Treatments for PMS
>
> Antidepressants (SSRIs and SNRIs)
> Oral contraceptives
> Progesterone
> Anxiolytics
> GnRH analogs
> Diuretics

INTEGRATIVE MODEL FOR PMS TREATMENT

A health practitioner who adopts an integrative approach for treating PMS will focus on the experience of each individual woman and acknowledge that there is likely to be a complex explanation for her symptoms encompassing biophysical, environmental, and/or psychological factors. In addition, the integrative practitioner approaches premenstrual symptoms less as a disorder and more as part of a normal woman's cycle. Treatment plans will therefore be multimodal, actively involving the patient and with each recommendation closely matched to her preferences. In each instance, she will begin to address her symptoms with a range of resources, be they internal (visualization and biofeedback) or external (herbs, diet, pharmaceuticals), with the goal of giving her the most benefit with the least amount of side effects.

Since pharmaceuticals are discussed in other publications, this chapter focuses principally on alternative treatments. Due to methodological challenges, many of these treatments are not supported by rigorous randomized controlled trials (RCTs). Nonetheless, all the following interventions have data promising enough to warrant their inclusion. Furthermore, virtually all of these have a wide therapeutic margin and low cost and have been shown to be very acceptable to women with PMS.

Premenstrual Syndrome Research Challenges

Challenges to assessing the effectiveness of all PMS treatments—both conventional and alternative—include variability in syndrome definition and outcome measures, small sample sizes, problems with blinding, and short treatment periods. In addition, all PMS treatments seem to have a significant placebo effect: A finding that suggests the important role that psychological factors play in PMS symptomatology

(Freeman & Rickels, 1999; Stevinson & Ernst, 2001). Alternative treatments pose their own research challenges because these modalities often rely on a personalized or individualized approach that is harder to replicate using the randomized, placebo-controlled double-blinded research model.

Nutrition and PMS

I heard that dietary supplements could make a difference in my symptoms. Can you tell me which ones are most likely to help? I also feel these intense cravings for carbs in the week before each period and find myself binging on cookies and bread. It drives me crazy and I think that is what has led to my slow weight gain.

—Marie

Most nutrition studies related to PMS have focused on the effects of nutritional supplements. Nonetheless, there is a mounting body of evidence that dietary choices may contribute to PMS symptoms.

Caffeine

In several observational studies, luteal phase consumption of caffeinated beverages including sodas and coffee has been positively correlated with severity of premenstrual symptoms (Cross, Marley, Miles, & Willson, 2001; Rossignol & Bonnlander, 1990). Caffeine could theoretically exacerbate PMS symptoms by increasing anxiety. To date, however, there has not been an intervention trial to help determine whether these eating patterns are a result of PMS food cravings or whether limiting these foods might actually *improve* PMS symptoms. Furthermore, it is not clear whether it is the caffeine itself or other additives that are also found in caffeinated foods.

Caffeine Holiday

Given the potential benefits and limited risk, I have found that it is worth recommending that women eliminate highly caffeinated foods such as coffee and sodas for two consecutive menstrual cycles in order to see whether this offers them a noticeable improvement.

Carbohydrate Cravings

Women with PMS have been observed to boost their consumption of carbohydrates during the premenstrual phase. One explanation proposed by scientists is that some women are exquisitely sensitive to the natural dips in the neurotransmitter serotonin that occur in the luteal phase. Consequently, they are trying to self-medicate with carbohydrates, which happen to be a rich source of the serotonin precursor tryptophan (Sayegh et al., 1995; Wurtman, 1990). Another explanation is that sensitivity to sweetness increases in this phase, thus making carbohydrates more attractive (Farage, Osborn, & Maclean, 2008). Recognizing this cyclical preference for carbohydrates, it is important to counsel women in their selection of starches and steer them toward lower calorie, lower glycemic, more nutritious choices such as tubers, whole grains, and legumes rather than sweets or refined flour products.

Diet, Microbiome, and Estrogen Excess

Many women report that diets high in unrefined grains and fermented foods and low in animal fats can alleviate PMS symptoms. Interestingly, there is a biological mechanism to support this observation, as estrogen, which is eliminated in the feces in a conjugated form, can be reabsorbed in the distal gut via the enterohepatic circulation when it is deconjugated by certain fecal bacteria. There is preliminary evidence to suggest that these particular bacterial populations are present in higher concentration in women who have a diet high in animal fat and refined carbohydrates (Adlercreutz, Pulkkinen, Hamalainen, & Korpela, 1984; Flores et al., 2012; Orme & Back, 1990; Winter & Bokkenheuser, 1987). In the Study of Women's Health Across the Nation (SWAN), fat intake was negatively associated with craving and bloating; fiber intake was positively correlated with breast pain, while alcohol was positively associated with premenstrual anxiety, mood changes, and headaches (Gold et al., 2007). While much remains to be discovered about the connections between diet, intestinal microbial communities, and estrogen excess, the existing science suggests that an unrefined carbohydrate, low animal fat diet could be beneficial.

Weight Gain and PMS

A subset of women with PMS do consume an excessive amount of energy in the form of fats and carbohydrates in the premenstrual phase which, over time, leads to weight gain (Cross et al., 2001). This, in turn, may further exacerbate depression, bloating, and other negative symptoms of PMS. Therefore, when I discuss diet and weight issues with women, I often focus on premenstrual symptoms and their relationship to eating habits. This can help women pay more attention to food consumption specifically in the luteal phase.

Soy Foods

Soy consumption, both in the form of soy extracts and as whole foods, may play a role in controlling PMS symptoms. It has been hypothesized that the isoflavones in soy (namely, genistein and daidzein) have mixed agonist antagonist effects on estrogen and progesterone receptors. Their role is thought to vary throughout the menstrual cycle, depending on the levels of circulating endogenous hormones (Kurzer, 2002; Lu, Anderson, Grady, & Nagamani, 2001). Transnational epidemiologic studies have shown that women in Asia, where more whole soy foods are consumed, have lower rates of PMS than women in the United States (Takeda, Tasaka, Sakata, & Murata, 2006). One recent cross-sectional study of 84 Korean women living in the United States showed that dietary soy intake was inversely correlated with PMS symptoms (Kim, Kwon, Kim, & Reame, 2006). Another crossover placebo trial in a diverse group of PMS sufferers reported that 68 mg soy isoflavones had positive effect on PMS-related bloating (Bryant et al., 2005).

Thoughts on Soy

I am most impressed by recent studies suggesting that whole soy foods have a modulating effect on estrogen levels whereas soy extracts have a stronger stimulatory effect (Trock, Hilakivi-Clarke, & Clarke, 2006). Whole soy foods (miso, edamame, tempeh, tofu, soy milk, etc.) therefore offer a wider range of nutrients than their more processed counterparts (soy protein extracts, power bars, fake meats, ice creams, etc.), I encourage women with PMS to avoid processed soy products but to include a daily serving of a whole soy food in their diet.

DIETARY SUPPLEMENTS

Many vitamin supplements are promoted for treating PMS symptoms, although few have methodologically sound research trials that substantiate their benefits. The exception to this are calcium (as citrate or carbonate) and pyridoxine (vitamin B6), both of which have a number of well-designed RCTs

Table 12.2. Nutritional Supplementation for PMS

Vitamin/Mineral	Dose	Level of Evidence
Calcium citrate or carbonate	600 mg twice a day in the luteal phase or daily	b
Vitamin B6	50–100 mg daily	b
Magnesium citrate	400 mg daily	c
Vitamin D	800–1,200 IU/day	c

to suggest that they offer a relatively low-risk, high-reward intervention for women with PMS symptoms (see Table 12.2).

Calcium

Calcium is believed to work by modulating the effect of estrogen and other hormones. In one randomized, multicenter trial, 720 women were given 1,200 mg/day of calcium carbonate versus placebo in the week preceding three menstrual cycles. By using a daily standardized PMS rating scale, the study group reported a 48% reduction ($p < 0.001$) in symptoms (Thys-Jacobs, 2000; Thys-Jacobs, Starkey, Bernstein, & Tian, 1998). Because calcium is better absorbed when given in smaller doses, it is best to prescribe calcium carbonate or citrate as 600 mg twice daily to be taken either in the luteal phase or for the entire cycle.

Vitamin B6

Vitamin B6, or pyridoxine, is thought to have positive effects on neurotransmitters such as serotonin, norepinephrine, and dopamine (Ebadi, Gessert, & Al-Sayegh, 1982). This has borne out in clinical trials in which pyridoxine has helped to improve the negative mood symptoms associated with PMS (Kashanian, Mazinani, & Jalalmanesh, 2007). A 1999 review of nine RCTs studying vitamin B6 as a treatment for PMS concluded that a dose of 50 to 100 mg/day was likely to benefit women both in terms of breast pain and depressive symptoms (Wyatt, Dimmock, Jones, & Shaughn O'Brien,, 1999). Because vitamin B6 in excessive doses can cause nerve toxicity resulting in ataxia or neuropathy, the daily dose should not exceed 100 mg/day.

Vitamin D and Magnesium

There are several observational studies linking low serum and/or urine levels of vitamin D and magnesium to PMS symptoms. Furthermore, there are plausible mechanisms for how both of these nutrients could be beneficial in treating PMS, as they serve as hormone modulators, smooth muscle relaxants, and inhibitors of prostaglandin synthesis. Unfortunately, to date, there is little evidence that supplementing with either vitamin D or magnesium is truly beneficial as a treatment for premenstrual symptoms (Bertone-Johnson et al., 2005; Girman, Lee, & Kligler, 2003; Rosenstein, Elin, Hosseini, Grover, & Rubinow, 1994; Shamberger, 2003). One small, short-term RCT did show that 200 mg of magnesium per day was better than placebo at alleviating the bloating symptoms of PMS (Walker et al., 1998). Two other trials found that magnesium 200 mg plus vitamin B6 50 mg compared favorably to magnesium alone for treating the anxiety symptoms associated with the syndrome (De Souza, Walker, Robinson, & Bolland, 2000; Fathizadeh, Ebrahimi, & Yar, 2010).

Despite the paucity of research, it should be acknowledged that low concentrations of these two nutrients are associated with a myriad of other women's health problems and that they can be safely supplemented at physiologic levels (200 to 400 mg/day magnesium and 800 to 1,200 IU/day vitamin D). Therefore, as part of a comprehensive PMS treatment plan, one worthwhile approach would be to recommend supplementation of magnesium and vitamin D to all women with moderate to severe symptoms.

EXERCISE

Elite athletes often develop amenorrhea, and they rarely experience PMS symptoms. One explanation for this phenomenon is that extreme exercise leads to suppression of steroid hormone levels. It has not been demonstrated whether moderate exercise can also reduce hormonal levels. Nonetheless, 30 min/day of moderate intensity exercise does seem to help in improving the mood and overall sense of well-being in women with PMS (Stoddard, Dent, Shames, & Bernstein, 2007). Like the dietary interventions, a half-hour daily exercise of moderate intensity has so many other proven benefits that it should be considered a first-line treatment for all women with PMS (Steege & Blumenthal, 1993).

SMOKING CESSATION

In one observational study of women with PMS, those who smoked experienced increased cramps and required more pain medication and time off from work (Kritz-Silverstein, Wingard, & Garland, 1999). Smoking correlates with depression and other pain syndromes and therefore, for many women, its link with severe PMS symptoms may be an indirect one. Nonetheless, nicotine has been noted to have a toxic effect directly on the ovaries and eliminating its use may improve symptoms. Smoking cessation is another helpful first-line intervention for women with PMS.

BOTANICALS

Growing, up, my grandmother used to give me teas and herbs when I did not feel well. I remember how well they worked. Thanks to the herbs, I really never needed to take stronger medicines. Are there any safe herbs that I can try for my PMS symptoms?

—Marie

Chasteberry

There are at least a dozen botanical supplements that researchers have studied for their potential benefit in treating premenstrual symptoms, and many of these are included in proprietary herbal formulations for women. To date, however, only chasteberry (*Vitex agnus-castus*) has enough scientific evidence to support its use for treatment of negative symptoms associated with menstruation, and in Germany, the herb is used as a first-line treatment for PMS, mastodynia, and menstrual irregularity. In a systematic review of clinical trials for premenstrual syndrome, seven of eight trials found chaste tree extracts to be superior to placebo, pyridoxine, and magnesium oxide. In premenstrual dysphoric disorder, one study reported Vitex to be equivalent to fluoxetine, while in the other, fluoxetine outperformed Vitex (van Die, Burger, Teede, & Bone, 2013)

Chasteberry or Vitex, which literally translates as "chaste lamb" in recognition of its presumed libido-lowering effects, has a number of potentially active ingredients. In the berry itself are iridoid glycosides and flavonoids, whereas the leaves and flowers contain compounds similar to sex hormones. Chasteberry decreases estrogen and prolactin secretion and raises progesterone levels (Roemheld-Hamm, 2005). In addition, it may have some mild analgesic effects, as methanol extracts of the plant have been noted to activate the mu-opiate receptor (Webster, Mortola, Chan, Moossazadeh, & Yen, 2006).

One large randomized controlled trial ($n = 170$) of chasteberry reported that after three menstrual cycles, the treatment group had significantly fewer negative premenstrual symptoms than the placebo group ($p < .001$). In the active group, 50% of women experienced at least a 50% reduction in symptoms whereas only 7 out of 86 discontinued for side effects (Schellenberg, 2001). Another randomized, double-blind, placebo-controlled trial compared chasteberry to fluoxetine as treatments for PMS. The researchers found that both interventions were equally beneficial and significantly better than placebo. Interestingly, the fluoxetine showed a slight advantage in improving psychological symptoms, whereas the chasteberry had a more positive effect on physical symptoms (Atmaca, Kumru, & Tezcan, 2003). A third chasteberry trial, which was focused specifically on treating PMS-related mastalgia, also noted a significant improvement in the chasteberry group. However, by the end of the third cycle, this significance had disappeared because of an increasingly positive response noted by the placebo group (Halaska, Beles, Gorkow, & Sieder, 1999). In summary, chasteberry seems to be a tolerable and effective treatment for PMS.

Caution: Safety of chasteberry in pregnancy is unknown and, due to its inhibitory effect on prolactin, it should not be used while breastfeeding. In higher doses, chasteberry might also have dopamine agonist activities and could theoretically increase the effects of other dopamine antagonists such as bromocriptine or metoclopramide (Daniele, Thompson Coon, Pittler, & Ernst, 2005).

Chasteberry and Libido

Because of its name, some women worry that chasteberry will cause them to lose their libido. This is not a frequently reported phenomenon when the herb is given in low doses. In fact, many women report to me that the herb has the opposite effect, probably because it helps treat other overwhelming PMS symptoms that can lower sexual drive.

Other Botanicals

Three other botanicals warrant mention in this section mainly because they are frequently used for PMS symptoms and may be useful for some women. The first is black cohosh (*Actaea racemosa; Cimicifuga racemosa*), which may modulate luteinizing and follicle-stimulating hormones and also act as a mild serotonin reuptake inhibitor. Black cohosh is widely accepted as a treatment for the negative effects of menopause including mood swing, hot flashes, and sleep disturbances. Given its mild SSRI properties, it may have its greatest efficacy as a treatment for negative mood or depression associated with PMS (Low Dog, 2001). Newer research indicates it binds serotonin and opiate receptors, which suggests it may also be useful for PMS and explains why it may have some benefit in thermoregulation during the menopausal transition (Farnsworth & Mahady, 2009).

St John's Wort (*Hypericum perforatum*), an herb that is widely used for treatment of depression, also has some promising pilot data to support its use in treating the depressive symptoms of PMS (Stevinson & Ernst, 2000). The standard dose for treatment of mild depression is 300 mg St. John's Wort three times a day, standardized to 0.3% hypericin and/or 3% to 5% hyperforin.

Evening primrose oil (*Oenothera biennis*), or EPO, is another popular herbal treatment for PMS symptoms. The seed oil contains essential fatty acids that are necessary to form the anti-inflammatory prostaglandin PGE1. Theoretically, supplementing this oil can help women who are deficient in the enzyme that is needed to endogenously synthesize these prostaglandins. Unfortunately, none of the small trials showed a difference between EPO and placebo, and a systematic review concluded that EPO has little value in treating PMS (Budeiri, Li Wan Po, & Dornan, 1996; Collins, Cerin, Coleman, & Landgren, 1993; Khoo, Munro, & Battistutta, 1990) (see Table 12.3).

Natural Progesterone

Progesterone in the form of pills, pessaries, troches, and creams is a popular treatment for PMS. Its use is based on the theory that women with PMS are experiencing a deficiency in progesterone relative to estrogen and that their symptoms

Table 12.3. Herbal Treatment for PMS

Herb	Dose
Chasteberry (*Vitex agnus castus*)	400–500 mg once a day
Black cohosh (*Actaea racemosa, Cimicifuga racemosa*)	40–80 mg standardized extract twice a day
St. John's Wort (*Hypericum perforatum*)	300 mg 3 times a day of St. John's Wort standardized to 0.3% hypericin and/or 3%–5% hyperforin
Evening primrose oil	2–3 g/day

are a result of estrogen dominance. As far back as the 1950s, the British physician Katherine Dalton used high-dose progesterone suppositories (800 mg/day) to treat PMS (Dalton, 1990). Although a large portion of her patients reported improvement with this intervention, it appears that her selection criteria would have excluded most women who are currently diagnosed with PMS. Furthermore, there is no laboratory evidence to substantiate this progesterone hypothesis.

A meta-analysis by the Cochrane collaboration of trials of progesterone for PMS identified 2 of 17 studies that merited inclusion in their review. Both studies administered progesterone or placebo from day 14 of the menstrual cycle until the onset of menstruation. One study, using 300 mg oral and 200 mg suppository, concluded that progesterone worked no better than placebo, whereas the other, using 400 mg BID of progesterone suppositories, suggested that it may be beneficial for a small subgroup of PMS sufferers. Unfortunately, the study paper did not offer criteria to help identify these women. Although progesterone seemed to be a safe therapy, both studies were of limited duration (the longer of the two lasting only four cycles) and had high attrition rates (Ford, Lethaby, Mol, & Roberts, 2006; Magill, 1995; Vaneslow, Dennerstein, Greenwood, & de Lignieres, 1996). Side effects of progesterone therapy overlap with many of the symptoms associated with PMS including headache, irregular menses, mood changes, and hypersomnia. Progesterone may also increase fertility, and therefore, women should be advised to use appropriate birth control.

Many alternative practitioners promote "natural," over-the-counter, or compounded progesterone creams as a safer and more physiologic option to prescription formulations of progesterone or progesterone derivatives (progestins) such as medroxyprogesterone and norethindrone. In truth, "natural" may be a misnomer. Although Mexican yams and soy beans are the source of the diosgenin and stigmasterol, the final products are synthesized in a laboratory and are no more natural than oral micronized progesterone. Furthermore, concentrations of progesterone vary widely even within the same product formulation, and most do not seem to achieve a physiologic dose. None of these over-the counter creams have supportive data that has been published in a peer reviewed journal (Boothby & Doering, 2008; Cirigliano, 2007).

Progesterone therapy may offer symptomatic relief to a subset of women with PMS and might be an appropriate next step when nonpharmacological approaches do not suffice. Given the variability in concentration of over-the-counter creams, it is best to prescribe oral micronized progesterone or progesterone suppositories 200–800 mg/day to be administered at the lowest effective dose from day 14 of the menstrual cycle until the first day of menstrual flow. Long-term safety data for high-dose progesterone therapy is not known.

MIND–BODY

A variety of mind–body techniques have been effective in treating PMS symptoms. These include meditation, breathing, progressive muscle relaxation, yoga, guided imagery, biofeedback, cognitive-behavioral therapy, and positive reframing. All of these techniques are described in greater detail in other places in this text. Because these are interventions that are tailored for each individual patient, they are difficult to study using conventional methodologies. Nonetheless, a growing body of research suggests that when women are given psychological support as well as self-regulatory techniques for dealing with their PMS symptoms, their quality of life and symptom severity improves significantly (Goodale, Domar, & Benson, 1990; Rapkin, 2005). A review of meditation studies found that there was strong evidence for its benefit in improving the symptoms of PMS (Arias, Steinberg, Banga, & Trestman, 2006).

In one interesting study, women were taught to use guided imagery as a means to regulate vaginal temperature and subsequently control PMS symptoms. Those women, who managed to raise their vaginal temperature, indicating a rise in progesterone, also experienced an improvement in PMS symptoms (Van Zak, 1994). Other forms of guided imagery such as directing women to *fill their pelvis with soft, warm light* or to imagine themselves *floating gently on water* are likely to be just as successful.

Choosing the Most Appropriate Mind–Body Techniques

I usually include a recommendation for at least one kind of mind–body therapy in any PMS treatment plan. These are relatively easy practices that women can do independently without taking a medication or supplement. Because there is insufficient evidence to recommend one treatment over another, I work with each individual woman to decide what best suits her preferences and skills. For example, Marie had some experience with yoga and meditation, and therefore I started with a prescription for deep belly breathing and gave her a restorative yoga pose called viparita kirani (lying on your back with your legs up the wall). I encouraged her to practice the technique as needed for the duration of her symptoms and to consider incorporating the practice daily throughout the month.

GROUP INTERVENTIONS

Group interventions or group medical visits are a promising and cost-effective way for practitioners to offer women an integrative approach to PMS treatment.

In one small study (n = 28), women with PMS attended four 2-hour sessions where they learned about the biological, environmental, and psychological causes of PMS as well as nutrition, exercise, and stress-reduction tools for treating their symptoms. At the end of the study, attendees reported significant improvement on a PMS symptom rating scale (Morse, 1999).

Traditional Chinese Medicine

Traditional Chinese medicine and other oriental medicine systems view PMS primarily as an imbalance of *qi*, or life force, and the principle goal in treatment is to remove the blockage, deficiency, stagnation, or imbalance of qi. Studies using traditional Chinese herbs, acupuncture, acupressure, or external qigong therapy have all been designed to treat specific disharmonies that have led to the imbalance (Chou & Morse, 2005). Taking into consideration the heterogeneity of diagnoses and treatments, these studies hardly lend themselves to a randomized controlled design. However, if you look at the literature in its entirety, it suggests that these forms of medicine can have a strong beneficial effect for women with PMS (Chou, Morse, & Xu, 2008; Jang & Lee, 2004; Kimura et al., 2007; Yu, Liu, Liu, & Robinson, 2005).

Manipulative Medicine

One small study with 24 women suffering from PMDD demonstrated that women receiving massage in the later part of the luteal phase experienced fewer symptoms than those assigned to relaxation therapy (Hernandez-Reif et al., 2000). In another study, women with PMS were assigned to real or sham reflexology and those experiencing the true treatment had an improvement in their symptoms score (Oleson & Flocco, 1993). One crossover trial to study the benefits of chiropractic manipulation randomized women with PMS to a real treatment or to a placebo. This study showed no difference in benefit for the women who had first experienced the placebo (Walsh & Polus, 1999).

Homeopathy

A pilot RCT (n = 20) showed that individualized homeopathic therapy offers some benefit for women with PMS symptoms. In this study, 90% of the active treatment group reported more than 30% improvement in symptoms whereas only 37.5% of the controls felt they had experienced this degree of benefit $p = .048$ (Yakir et al., 2001). In a case series, individualized homeopathy significantly decreased PMS symptoms scores in 23 women followed over a 3- to 6-month period. *Folliculinum* (87%) was the most frequently prescribed homeopathic treatment followed by *Lachesis mutus* (52.2%) (Danno, Colas, Terzan, & Bordet, 2013). Further research is needed to test the effectiveness of homeopathy as a PMS treatment.

> Marie adopted a number of changes at once. She eliminated coffee and sodas from her diet, cut down on animal fats, increased her consumption of vegetables, and started substituting whole grains for more processed ones. She started a daily breathing practice and tried to take a brisk 30-minute walk on most days. She started taking a number of supplements: A multivitamin, additional calcium, vitamin D, and chasteberry. She also saw an acupuncturist every other week. I saw her again 2 months after her first visit, and she reported that her bloating and depressive symptoms had been much better during the previous two cycles. Six months later, she returned and told me that she was only going to the acupuncturist once a month, and although some months were better than others, overall her PMS symptoms were relatively mild, and she felt she had the tools to manage things when they got off track.

Conclusion

Premenstrual syndrome is a syndrome with many possible etiologies and a variety of manifestations. The integrative approach to PMS takes into account the individual experience of each woman and seeks to treat her symptoms using a range of modalities that will offer her the maximum amount of relief with a minimum of side effects (Box 12.3). Taking into consideration the wide therapeutic safety and high tolerability of alternative treatments ranging from lifestyle changes to mind–body treatments, these are usually used as first-line therapies by integrative practitioners. In general, conventional treatments such as pharmaceuticals carry a high degree of side effects and therefore are reserved for women who have received no relief with the initial approach or are greatly incapacitated by their PMS symptoms.

Box 12.3 Integrative Check-List for Treating PMS

Nutrition	Whole grains, high fiber
	Whole soy
	Limit caffeine
	Limit red meat
Exercise	30 minutes daily moderate intensity
Smoking cessation	
Nutritional supplements	Vitamins B6 and D, calcium, magnesium
Herbals	Chasteberry, Black Cohosh, St. John's Wort
Mind–body	Cognitive-behavioral therapy, group therapy, biofeedback, breathing, yoga
Energy medicine	Acupuncture and qigong
Homeopathy	Individual treatment plans
Pharmaceutical	Assess the need for prescription pharmaceutical when the above modalities do not provide relief or symptoms are very severe

REFERENCES

Adlercreutz, H., Pulkkinen, M. O., Hamalainen, E. K., & Korpela, J. T. (1984). Studies on the role of intestinal bacteria in metabolism of synthetic and natural steroid hormones. *J Steroid Biochem, 20,* 217–229.

Arias, A. J., Steinberg, K., Banga, A., & Trestman, R. L. (2006). Systematic review of the efficacy of meditation techniques as treatments for medical illness. *J Altern Complement Med, 12,* 817–832.

Atmaca, M., Kumru, S., & Tezcan, E. (2003). Fluoxetine versus *Vitex agnus castus* extract in the treatment of premenstrual dysphoric disorder. *Hum Psychopharmacol, 18,* 191–195.

Backstrom, B., Andreen, L., Birzniece, V., et al. (2003). The role of hormones and hormonal treatments in premenstrual syndrome. *CNS Drugs, 17,* 325–342.

Berger, D., Schaffner, W., Schrader, E., Meier, B., & Brattstrom, A. (2000). Efficacy of *Vitex agnus castus* L. extract Ze 440 in patients with pre-menstrual syndrome (PMS). *Arch Gynecol Obstet, 264,* 150–153.

Bertone-Johnson, E. R., Hankinson, S. E., Bendich, A., Johnson, S. R., Willett, W. C., & Manson, J. E. (2005). Calcium and vitamin D intake and risk of incident premenstrual syndrome. *Arch Intern Med, 165,* 1246–1252.

Boothby, L. A., & Doering, P. L. (2008). Bioidentical hormone therapy: A panacea that lacks supportive evidence. *Curr Opin Obstet Gynecol, 20*, 400–407.

Borenstein, J. E., Dean, B. B., Leifke, E., Korner, P., & Yonkers, K. A. (2007). Differences in symptom scores and health outcomes in premenstrual syndrome. *J Women's Health, 16*, 1139–1144.

Bryant, M., Cassidy, A., Hill, C., Powell, J., Talbot, D., & Dye, L. (2005). Effect of consumption of soy isoflavones on behavioural, somatic and affective symptoms in women with premenstrual syndrome. *Br J Nutr, 93*, 731–739.

Bryant, M., Truesdale, K. P., & Dye, L. (2006). Modest changes in dietary intake across the menstrual cycle: Implications for food intake research. *Br J Nutr, 96*, 888–894.

Budeiri, D., Li Wan Po, A., & Dornan, J. C. (1996). Is evening primrose oil of value in the treatment of premenstrual syndrome? *Control Clin Trials, 17*, 60–68.

Craner, J. R., Sigmon, S. T., & McGillicuddy, M. L. (2014). Does a disconnect occur between research and practice for premenstrual dysphoric disorder (PMDD) diagnostic procedures? *Women and Health, 54*, 232–244. doi:10.1080/03630242.2014.883658

Chou, P., & Morse, C. A. (2005). Understanding premenstrual syndrome from a Chinese medicine perspective. *J Altern Complemen Med, 11*, 355–361.

Chou, P. B., Morse, C. A., & Xu, H. (2008). A controlled trial of Chinese herbal medicine for premenstrual syndrome. *J Psychosom Obstet Gynaecol 29*(3), 185–192.

Cirigliano, M. (2007). Bioidentical hormone therapy: A review of the evidence. *J Women's Health, 16*, 600–631.

Collins, A., Cerin, A., Coleman, G., & Landgren, B. M. (1993). Essential fatty acids in the treatment of premenstrual syndrome. *Obstet Gynecol, 81*, 93–98.

Cross, G. B., Marley, J., Miles, H., & Willson, K. (2001). Changes in nutrient intake during the menstrual cycle of overweight women with premenstrual syndrome. *Br J Nutr, 85*, 475–482.

Dalton, K. (1990). The aetiology of premenstrual syndrome is the progesterone receptors. *Med Hypothesis, 31*, 323–327.

Danno, K., Colas, A., Terzan, L., & Bordet, M.-F. (2013). Homeopathic treatment of premenstrual syndrome: A case series. *Homeopathy: The Journal of the Faculty of Homeopathy, 102*, 59–65. doi:10.1016/j.homp.2012.10.004

Daniele, C., Thompson Coon, J., Pittler, M. H., & Ernst, E. (2005). *Vitex agnus castus*: A systematic review of adverse events. *Drug Saf, 28*, 319–332.

De Souza, M. C., Walker, A. F., Robinson, P. A., & Bolland, K. (2000). A synergistic effect of a daily supplement for 1 month of 200 mg magnesium plus 50 mg vitamin B6 for the relief of anxiety-related premenstrual symptoms: A randomized, double-blind, crossover study. *J Womens Health Gend Based Med, 9*, 131–139.

Dean, B. B., & Borenstein, J. E. (2004). A prospective assessment investigating the relationship between work productivity and impairment with premenstrual syndrome. *J Occup Environ Med, 46*, 649–656.

Ebadi, M., Gessert, C. F., & Al-Sayegh, A. (1982). Drug-pyridoxal phosphate interactions. *Q Rev Drug Metab Drug Interact, 4*, 289–331.

Farage, M. A., Osborn, T. W., & Maclean, A. B. (2008). Cognitive, sensory, and emotional changes associated with the menstrual cycle: A review. *Arch Gynecol Obstet*, *278*, 299–307.

Farnsworth, N. R., & Mahady, G. B. (2009). Research highlights from the UIC/NIH Center for Botanical Dietary Supplements Research for Women's Health: Black cohosh from the field to the clinic. *Pharm Biol*, *47*, 755–760

Fathizadeh, N., Ebrahimi, E., & Yar, M. H. (2010). Evaluating the effect of magnesium and magnesium plus vitamin B6 supplement on the severity of premenstrual syndrome [Abstract]. *Iran J Nurse Midwifery*, *15*, 401–405.

Flores, R., Shi, J., Fuhrman, B., Xu, X., Veenstra, T. D., Gail, M. H., Goedert, J. J. (2012). Fecal microbial determinants of fecal and systemic estrogens and estrogen metabolites: A cross-sectional study. *Journal of Translational Medicine*, *10*, 253. doi:10.1186/1479-5876-10-253

Ford, O., Lethaby, A., Mol, B., & Roberts, H. (2006). Progesterone for premenstrual syndrome. *Cochrane Database Syst Rev*, 4:CD003415.

Freeman, E. W. (2003). Premenstrual syndrome and premenstrual dysphoric disorder: Definitions and diagnosis. *Psychoneuroendocrinology*, *28*(Suppl 3), 325–337.

Freeman, E. W., & Rickels, K. (1999). Characteristics of placebo responses in medical treatment of premenstrual syndrome. *Am J Psychiatry*, *156*, 1403–1408.

Freeman, E. W., Rickels, K., Schweizer, E., & Ting, T. (1995). Relationships between age and symptom severity among women seeking medical treatment for premenstrual symptoms. *Psychol Med*, *25*, 309–315.

Girman, A., Lee, R., & Kligler, B. (2003). An integrative medicine approach to premenstrual syndrome. *Am J Obstet Gynecol*, *188*(5 Suppl), S56–65.

Gold, E. B., Bair, Y., Block, G., et al. (2007). Diet and lifestyle factors associated with premenstrual symptoms in a racially diverse community sample: Study of Women's Health Across the Nation (SWAN). *J Women's Health*, *16*, 641–656.

Goodale, I. L., Domar, A. D., & Benson, H. (1990). Alleviation of premenstrual syndrome symptoms with the relaxation response. *Obstet Gynecol*, *75*, 649–655.

Gotts, G., Morse, C. A., & Dennerstein, L. (1995). Premenstrual complaints: An idiosyncratic syndrome. *J Psychosom Obstet Gynaecol*, *16*, 29–35.

Halaska, M., Beles, P., Gorkow, C., & Sieder, C. (1999). Treatment of cyclical mastalgia with a solution containing a *Vitex agnus castus* extract: Results of a placebo-controlled double-blind study. *Breast*, *8*, 175–181.

Halbreich, U. (2002). The pathophysiologic background for current treatments of premenstrual syndromes. *Curr Psychiatry Rep*, *4*, 429–434.

Halbreich, U., Backstrom, T., Eriksson, E., et al. (2007). Clinical diagnostic criteria for premenstrual syndrome and guidelines for their quantification for research studies. *Gynecol Endocrinol*, *23*, 123–130.

Hardy, M. L. (2000). Herbs of special interest to women. *J Am Pharm Assoc (Wash)*, *40*, 234–242; quiz 327–329.

Hernandez-Reif, M., Martinez, A., Field, T., Quintero, O., Hart, S., & Burman, I. (2000). Premenstrual symptoms are relieved by massage therapy. *J Psychosom Obstet Gynaecol*, *21*, 9–15.

Jang, H. S., & Lee, M. S. (2004). Effects of qi therapy (external qigong) on premenstrual syndrome: A randomized placebo-controlled study. *J Altern Complemen Med, 10,* 456–462.

Jarvis, C. I., Lynch, A. M., & Morin, A. K. (2008). Management strategies for premenstrual syndrome/premenstrual dysphoric disorder. *Ann Pharmacother, 42,* 967–978.

Johnson, S. R. (2004). Premenstrual syndrome, premenstrual dysphoric disorder, and beyond: A clinical primer for practitioners. *Obstet Gynecol, 104,* 845–859.

Kashanian, M., Mazinani, R., & Jalalmanesh, S. (2007). Pyridoxine (vitamin B6) therapy for premenstrual syndrome. *Int J Gynaecol Obstet, 96,* 43–44.

Khoo, S. K., Munro, C., & Battistutta, D. (1990). Evening primrose oil and treatment of premenstrual syndrome. *Med J Aust, 153,* 189–192.

Kim, H. W., Kwon, M. K., Kim, N. S., & Reame, N. E. (2006). Intake of dietary soy isoflavones in relation to perimenstrual symptoms of Korean women living in the USA. *Nurs Health Sci, 8,* 108–113.

Kimura, Y., Takamatsu, K., Fujii, A., et al. (2007). Kampo therapy for premenstrual syndrome: Efficacy of Kamishoyosan quantified using the second derivative of the fingertip photoplethysmogram. *J Obstet Gynaecol Res, 33,* 325–332.

Kritz-Silverstein, D., Wingard, D. L., & Garland, F. C. (1999). The association of behavior and lifestyle factors with menstrual symptoms. *J Womens Health Gend Based Med, 8,* 1185–1193.

Kurzer, M. S. (2002). Hormonal effects of soy in premenopausal women and men. *J Nutr, 132,* 570S–573S.

Low Dog, T. (2001). Integrative treatments for premenstrual syndrome. *Altern Ther Health Med, 7,* 32–39; quiz 40, 139.

Lu, L. J., Anderson, K. E., Grady, J. J., & Nagamani, M. (2001). Effects of an isoflavone-free soy diet on ovarian hormones in premenopausal women. *J Clin Endocrinol Metab, 86,* 3045–3052.

Magill, P. J. (1995). Investigation of the efficacy of progesterone pessaries in the relief of symptoms of premenstrual syndrome. *Br J Gen Pract, 45,* 589–593.

Martorano, J. T., Ahlgrimm, M., & Colbert, T. (1998). Differentiating between natural progesterone and synthetic progestins: Clinical implications for premenstrual syndrome and perimenopause management. *Compr Ther, 24,* 336–339.

Morse, G. (1999). Positively reframing perceptions of the menstrual cycle among women with premenstrual syndrome. *J Obstet Gynecol Neonatal Nurs, 28,* 165–174.

Muse, K. (1992). Hormonal manipulation in the treatment of premenstrual syndrome. *Clin Obstet Gynecol, 35,* 658–666.

Oleson, T., & Flocco, W. (1993). Randomized controlled study of premenstrual symptoms treated with ear, hand, and foot reflexology. *Obstet Gynecol, 82,* 906–911.

Orme, M. L., & Back, D. J. (1990). Factors affecting the enterohepatic circulation of oral contraceptive steroids. *Am J Obstet Gynecol, 163*(6 Pt 2), 2146–2152.

Pullon, S. R., Reinken, J. A., & Sparrow, M. J. (1989). Treatment of premenstrual symptoms in Wellington women. *N Z Med J, 102,* 72–74.

Rapkin, A. J. (2005). New treatment approaches for premenstrual disorders. *Am J Manag Care, 11*(16 Suppl), S480–S491.

Rapkin, A. J., & Lewis, E. (2013). Treatment of premenstrual dysphoric disorder. *Women's Health* Nov, *9*, 537–556.

Robinson, R. L., & Swindle, R. W. (2000). Premenstrual symptom severity: Impact on social functioning and treatment-seeking behaviors. *J Womens Health Gend Based Med*, *9*, 757–768.

Roemheld-Hamm, B. (2005). Chasteberry. *Am Fam Physician*, *72*, 821–824.

Rosenstein, D. L., Elin, R. J., Hosseini, J. M., Grover, G., & Rubinow, D. R. (1994). Magnesium measures across the menstrual cycle in premenstrual syndrome. *Biol Psychiatry*, *35*, 557–561.

Rossignol, A. M., & Bonnlander, H. (1990). Caffeine-containing beverages, total fluid consumption, and premenstrual syndrome. *Am J Public Health*, *80*, 1106–1110.

Sayegh, R., Schiff, I., Wurtman, J., Spiers, P., McDermott, J., & Wurtman, R. (1995). The effect of a carbohydrate-rich beverage on mood, appetite, and cognitive function in women with premenstrual syndrome. *Obstet Gynecol*, *86*(4 Pt 1), 520–528.

Schellenberg, R. (2001). Treatment for the premenstrual syndrome with agnus castus fruit extract: Prospective, randomised, placebo controlled study. *Br Med J*, *322*, 134–137.

Shamberger, R. J. (2003). Calcium, magnesium, and other elements in the red blood cells and hair of normals and patients with premenstrual syndrome. *Biol Trace Elem Res*, *94*, 123–129.

Steege, J. F., & Blumenthal, J. A. (1993). The effects of aerobic exercise on premenstrual symptoms in middle-aged women: A preliminary study. *J Psychosom Res*, *37*, 127–133.

Sternfeld, B., Swindle, R., Chawla, A., Long, S., & Kennedy, S. (2002). Severity of premenstrual symptoms in a health maintenance organization population. *Obstet Gynecol*, *99*, 1014–1024.

Stevinson, C., & Ernst, E. (2000). A pilot study of *Hypericum perforatum* for the treatment of premenstrual syndrome. *BJOG*, *107*, 870–876.

Stevinson, C., & Ernst, E. (2001). Complementary/alternative therapies for premenstrual syndrome: A systematic review of randomized controlled trials. *Am J Obstet Gynecol*, *185*, 227–235.

Stoddard, J. L., Dent, C. W., Shames, L., & Bernstein, L. (2007). Exercise training effects on premenstrual distress and ovarian steroid hormones. *Eur J Appl Physiol*, *99*, 27–37.

Takeda, T., Tasaka, K., Sakata, M., & Murata, Y. (2006). Prevalence of premenstrual syndrome and premenstrual dysphoric disorder in Japanese women. *Arch Women's Ment Health*, *9*, 209–212.

Thys-Jacobs, S. (2000). Micronutrients and the premenstrual syndrome: The case for calcium. *J Am Coll Nutr*, *19*, 220–227.

Thys-Jacobs, S., Starkey, P., Bernstein, D., & Tian, J. (1998). Calcium carbonate and the premenstrual syndrome: Effects on premenstrual and menstrual symptoms. Premenstrual Syndrome Study Group. *Am J Obstet Gynecol*, *179*, 444–452.

Trock, B. J., Hilakivi-Clarke, L., & Clarke, R. (2006). Meta-analysis of soy intake and breast cancer risk. *J Natl Cancer Inst*, *98*, 459–471.

Van Die, M. D., Burger, H. G., Teede, H. J., & Bone, K. M. (2013). Vitex agnus-castus extracts for female reproductive disorders: A systematic review of clinical trials. *Planta Medica, 79,* 562–575. doi:10.1055/s-0032-1327831

Vaneslow, W., Dennerstein, L., Greenwood, K. M., & de Lignieres, B. (1996). Effect of progesterone and its 5 alpha and 5 beta metabolites on symptoms of premenstrual syndrome according to route of administration. *J Psychosom Obstetr Gynaecol, 17,* 29–38.

Van Zak, D. B. (1994). Biofeedback treatments for premenstrual and premenstrual affective syndromes. *Int J Psychosom, 41,* 53–60.

Walker, A. F., De Souza, M. C., Vickers, M. F., Abeyasekera, S., Collins, & M. L., Trinca, L. A. (1998). Magnesium supplementation alleviates premenstrual symptoms of fluid retention. *J Womens Health, 7,* 1157–1165.

Walsh, M. J., & Polus, B. I. (1999). The frequency of positive common spinal clinical examination findings in a sample of premenstrual syndrome sufferers. *J Manipulative Physiol Ther, 22,* 216–220.

Webster, D. E., Lu, J., Chen, S. N., Farnsworth, N. R., & Wang, J. Z. (2006). Activation of the mu-opiate receptor by Vitex agnus-castus methanol extracts: Implication for its use in PMS. *J Ethnopharmacol, 106,* 216–221.

Winter, J., & Bokkenheuser, V. D. (1987). Bacterial metabolism of natural and synthetic sex hormones undergoing enterohepatic circulation. *J Steroid Biochem, 27,* 1145–1149.

Wood, S. H., Mortola, J. F., Chan, Y. F., Moossazadeh, F., & Yen, S. S. (1992). Treatment of premenstrual syndrome with fluoxetine: A double-blind, placebo-controlled, crossover study. *Obstet Gynecol, 80*(3 Pt 1), 339–344.

Wurtman, J. J. (1990). Carbohydrate craving. Relationship between carbohydrate intake and disorders of mood. *Drugs, 39*(Suppl 3), 49–52.

Wyatt, K. M., Dimmock, P. W., Jones, P. W., & Shaughn O'Brien, P. M. (1999). Efficacy of vitamin B-6 in the treatment of premenstrual syndrome: Systematic review. *Br Med J, 318,* 1375–1381.

Yakir, M., Kreitler, S., Brzezinski, A., Vithoulkas, G., Oberbaum, M., & Bentwich, Z. (2001). Effects of homeopathic treatment in women with premenstrual syndrome: A pilot study. *Br Homeopath J, 90,* 148–153.

Yu, J. N., Liu, B. Y., Liu, Z. S., & Robinson, V. (2005). Evaluation of clinical therapeutic effects and safety of acupuncture treatment for premenstrual syndrome. *Zhongguo Zhen Jiu, 25,* 377–382.

Zhao, G., Wang, L., & Qu, C. (1998). Prevalence of premenstrual syndrome in reproductive women and its influential factors. *Zhonghua Fu Chan Ke Za Zhi, 33,* 222–224.

13

Vaginitis

PRISCILLA ABERCROMBIE

CASE STUDY

Tanisha is a 25-year-old African American woman who suffers from recurrent vaginal infections. She says, "I feel like I have an infection every month. Sometimes it's BV [bacterial vaginosis], and sometimes it's yeast." She is embarrassed by the vaginal odor and the amount of vaginal discharge. In addition, she experiences vaginal irritation and itching. She hopes that there is some kind of treatment that will stop this cycle of recurrent infection. She is particularly interested in using something other than antibiotics; she does not like taking them so frequently and she also feels like they have failed to produce "a cure."

Tanisha's story is not unusual. Vaginal symptoms are a common complaint accounting for approximately 10 million office visits per year (Kent, 1991). Bacterial vaginosis (BV) is the most common vaginal infection (22% to 50%) followed by vulvovaginal candidiasis (VVC) (17% to 39%) and the sexually transmitted infection trichomoniasis (4% to 35%) (Anderson, Klink, & Cohrssen, 2004). The primary focus of this chapter is on the integrative management of acute and recurrent VVC and BV.

Although conventional treatments have been studied extensively and are highly effective for acute infection, many women suffer from recurrent vaginitis and may choose not to use antibiotics on a long-term basis. Other women simply prefer a more "natural" treatment for vaginitis. In a study with 100 women (Nyirjesy, Weitz, Grody, & Lorber, 1997), 42% of women seen for chronic vaginal symptoms had used some type of alternative therapy: acidophilus pills orally (50%) or vaginally (11.4%), yogurt orally (20.5%) or vaginally (18.2%), vinegar douches (13.6%), or boric acid (13.6%). In another larger study of 480 women 65% of women with chronic vaginitis reported using complementary and alternative therapies, with acidophilus and yogurt the most common treatments cited (Nyirjesy, Robinson, Mathew, Lev-Sagie, Reyes, & Culhane, 2011). The evidence for alternative treatments in the management of acute vaginitis is not as strong as conventional medicine, yet the risk is also low. Accepting less compelling evidence may be reasonable for women who wish to avoid prescription medications and their side effects. Additionally, some of these treatments may play an important role in the prevention of recurrent vaginitis.

Vaginal Ecosystem

Lactobacilli play a particularly important role in the vaginal ecosystem. At menarche, the ovaries begin to produce estrogen, which causes the vaginal epithelium to become glycogenated. Glycogen promotes the growth of *Lactobacilli*, which play a number of roles. One is to assist in the breakdown of glucose-producing lactic acid, which helps maintain a normal vaginal pH of 4.0 (3.8 to 4.2). This acidic milieu is hostile to the proliferation of pathogenic organisms. *Lactobacilli* produce hydrogen peroxide that is damaging to anaerobic microflora, such as those found in BV. Finally, the *Lactobacilli* micropili adhere to vaginal epithelial cell receptors and prevent adherence of pathogens. Molecular-based techniques are providing new information about the vaginal microbiome, including the discovery of species of *Lactobacilli* that could not be studied by culture (Lamont et al., 2011). In addition, racial diversity has been found; in a study of 400 women, 80% of the Asian women and 90% of the Caucasian women had a vaginal microbiome dominated by *Lactobacilli*, while only about 60% of black and Hispanic women did. In addition, pH varied with ethnicity with higher average pH found in black and Hispanic women (between 4.7–5.0) (Ravel et al., 2011).

Psychosocial Impact

Women not only endure the physical symptoms of vaginal infections but also suffer psychosocial ramifications. Women with recurrent VVC have been found to have more depression, less satisfaction with life, poorer self-esteem, and increased perceived life stress, and they report feeling their symptoms seriously interfered with sexual and emotional relationships (Irving, Miller, Robinson, Reynolds, & Copas, 1998). A prospective study of 44 multiethnic women with vaginitis indicated that they were distressed by their vaginal symptoms, and two-thirds felt the symptoms were somewhat moderate to very serious (Karasz & Anderson, 2003). Misperceptions about the cause of vaginitis included infidelity, cancer, and past sexual behavior. In another study, women with recurrent BV were frustrated and distressed by vaginal odor and discharge, it impeded social, personal, and work relationships and led to hypervigilant hygiene routines (Payne, Cromer, Stanek, & Palmer, 2010). Although healthcare providers may view vaginitis as a bothersome condition with few troublesome consequences, women can be quite distressed.

Assessment

Many women with vaginal symptoms are incorrectly diagnosed. Specialists correctly diagnose vaginitis in about 80% to 90% of cases (Sobel, 1990), whereas primary care providers correctly make the diagnosis in only 50% to 60% of cases (Schaaf, Perez-Stable, & Borchardt, 1990). FDA-approved testing kits are available for VVC, BV, and trichomoniasis. These tests are both sensitive and specific and can help providers who do not have access to, or expertise in, microscopy (Bradshaw et al., 2006).

Vulvovaginal Candidiasis

Roughly 75% of women will experience acute VVC in their lifetime; 40% to 50% will have a recurrence (Hurley & De Louvois, 1979). Risk factors for VVC include antibiotics, systemic corticosteroids, allergic rhinitis, oral contraceptives, spermicides, and receptive oral sex (Watson & Calabretto, 2007). In addition, there may be a genetic basis for why some women are susceptible to recurrent VVC. They may possess different mutations and polymorphisms in their immune genes that alter their mucosal immune response to yeast (Watson & Calabretto, 2007). The vast majority of VVC infections are caused by *Candida albicans*. Efforts are underway to develop methods of molecular genotyping or DNA-fingerprinting to better detect different strains of *C. albicans* and the appropriate azoles for treatment (Bai, 2014).

The signs and symptoms of VVC include vaginal itching with thick white "curdy or cottage cheese" discharge, vulvitis, fissures or rash, and normal vaginal pH (<4.5). Microscopy shows the saline field with few white blood cells, rare or no clue cells, and the presence of *Lactobacilli*. The 10% potassium hydroxide (KOH) field will show pseudohyphae and absence of amine smell.

> ### Clinical Pearl
>
> I highly recommend using pH paper for the diagnosis of vaginitis. Women with candida vaginitis will have a normal pH of <4.5. If the pH is >5 then suspect BV or trichomoniasis.

TREATMENT

A Cochrane review found no difference in effectiveness between oral and intravaginal antifungals for the treatment of uncomplicated VVC (Nurbhai et al., 2007). Many women find oral fluconazole easier to use, and while it has excellent efficacy, it can take up to 48 hours before symptoms resolve. Therefore, women with vulvar irritation and/or inflammation may find that topical treatment with one of the azole creams has more immediate benefit. According to the Centers for Disease Control and Prevention (Workowski & Berman, 2006), azoles are effective in 80% to 90% of women who complete therapy. During pregnancy, topical intravaginal regimens should be prescribed for 7 days.

Diagnosis of VVC based on symptoms can be problematic. One study using telephone triage found that vaginal discharge was not predictive of a diagnosis of candidiasis, though patient-reported scores for vaginal burning of 6 or greater, and for vulvar itching of 5 or greater, were predictive of a positive yeast culture result (Hoffstetter, Barr, LeFevre, & Gavard, 2012). In another study by the same group there was no correlation between wet mount or self-reported symptoms with positive yeast cultures (Hoffstetter, Barr, LeFevre, Leong, & Leet, 2008). One study found that only 34% of 95 symptomatic women who purchased over-the-counter (OTC) antifungal products actually had yeast (Ferris et al., 2002). Self-medication should only be recommended for women who have been previously diagnosed with VVC and suffer from a recurrence of the same symptoms. Any woman whose symptoms persist after using an OTC preparation should be seen for an examination.

While VVC is not a sexually transmitted infection, partner treatment may be considered in women with recurrent VVC or in partners who are symptomatic (Workowski & Berman, 2006). Women should be informed that the azole creams are oil-based and can weaken latex condoms and diaphragms.

Clinical guidelines for the management of patients with sexually transmitted infections and vaginitis are available and updated regularly by the

CDC: http://www.cdc.gov/sTD/treatment/2010/default.htm. The guidelines can also be downloaded for free to your mobile device.

Clinical Pearl

Women with poorly controlled diabetes will require a 14-day therapy. A Cochrane review found no trials addressing treatment of VVC in HIV-positive women (Ray, Ray, George, & Swaminathan, 2011). In HIV-infected women, use of oral agents is associated with colonization of non-*albicans* species. Routine prophylaxis with fluconazole is not recommended (Workowski, & Berman, 2006). A consensus guideline for the treatment of candida in HIV infected patients recommends the use of topical therapy for VVC (Lortholary et al., 2012).

Recurrent Vulvovaginal Candidiasis

Recurrent VVC is defined as having four or more episodes in 1 year and affects approximately 5% to 8% of women (Foxman, Marsh, Gillespie, & Sobel, 1998). Vaginal culture can be used to confirm the diagnosis and identify unusual species of *Candida* (Hoffstetter et al., 2008), though colonization with non-*albicans* species is rare. One study found that 94% of women ($n = 427$) with recurrent VVC had *C. albicans* (Sobel et al., 2004). The recommended treatment for recurrent VVC is 7 to 14 days of topical or oral azole therapy followed by maintenance therapy one to two times weekly for 6 months with the goal of suppressing colonization. Unfortunately, relapse rates, after maintenance therapy, are as high as 30% to 50%. Typical dosing for oral fluconazole is 150 mg on days 1, 4, and 7 and then weekly for 6 months. This regimen produced a 91% cure at 6 months compared with 36% for placebo. The results at 1 year were 43% symptom-free in the treatment group versus 22% in the placebo arm ($p < .0001$). A systematic review and meta-analysis found that weekly fluconazole was effective for the treatment of recurrent VVC over 6 months (Rosa et al., 2013).

BORIC ACID

In a review of 14 studies, including two randomized controlled trials (RCTs), boric acid was compared with nystatin and numerous azoles (Iavazzo, Gkegkes, Zarkada, & Fandalagas, 2011). The mycologic cure rate was 40%–100% for boric acid compared with 50%–100% with azoles. The recurrence rates were

0–46% and there was no statistically significant difference between the therapies. Boric acid was well tolerated with reports of vaginal burning in <10%, watery discharge, and vaginal erythema. There is little systemic absorption of boric acid from the vagina.

Boric acid also shows promise in the treatment of *non-albicans* species. Cure rates of VVC with *Candida glabrata* were 64% in one study (Sobel, Chaim, Nagappan, & Leaman, 2003). In diabetic women with *C. glabrata*, 14 days of boric acid was shown to have a higher mycological cure rate than a single dose of fluconazole, although at 3 months the cure rates were similar (Ray, Goswami, Banerjee, et al., 2007; Ray, Goswami, Dadhwal, Goswami, Banerjee, & Kochupillai, 2007). Boric acid is both fungistatic and bacteriostatic (De Seta, Schmidt, Vu, Essmann, & Larsen, 2009), so it is also discussed as a treatment for bacterial vaginosis.

The usual dose of boric acid is 600 mg in a gelatin capsule inserted in the vagina daily for two weeks. A maintenance dose of twice weekly can be used to prevent recurrences. There is little systemic absorption with vaginal administration, but ingestion of large amounts of oral boric acid has been shown to be toxic. Another advantage is its inexpensive price. Boric acid should not be used during pregnancy.

OTHER TREATMENTS FOR VULVOVAGINAL CANDIDIASIS

Some small studies suggest that the hormonal contraceptive depot medroxy-progesterone acetate produces a less estrogenic environment in the vagina and leads to a reduction in the colonization of *Candida* (Dennerstein, 1986; Toppozada, Onsy, Fares, Amir, & Shaala, 1979). Numerous botanicals have been tested in vitro and found to be effective against *C. albicans* and non-*albicans* species, but clinical studies are lacking. See Table 13.1.

Clinical Pearl

Over-the-counter vaginal pH kits such as the Vagisil Screening Kit (Combe Incorporated) can assist women in determining their pH and help them decide whether they should try OTC treatment for VVC (pH < 4.5) or seek medical care (pH ≥ 5.0).

Table 13.1. Evidence for Botanicals Used for the Treatment of Vaginitis

Botanical	In Vitro C. albicans	In Vitro Non-Albicans species	In Vitro Other Vaginitis	Clinical studies
Tea tree oil (*Melaleuca alternifolia*)	Mondello et al. (2006) D'Auria et al. (2001) Ergin, A., & Arikan, S. (2002)	Ergin & Arikan (2002) Hammer et al. (1998)	For Trich: Mondello et al. (2006)	For BV: Hammer et al. (1999)
Propolis				For BV: Blackwell (1991) and Imhof et al., 2005
Garlic (*Allium sativum*)	(Moore & Atkins, 1977; Santana Perez et al. (1995)	Moore & Atkins, 1977		
Indian barberry (contains berberine) (*Berberis aristata*)			For Trich: Moore & Atkins (1977)	
Bergamot (*Citrus bergamia*)	Soffar et al. (2001)	Romano et al. (2005)		
Seaweed extract (*Ulva pertusa*)			For *Gardnerella vaginalis* in vitro: Ha et al. (2014)	
Clove oil	(Ahmad et al., 2005)			
Mentha suaveolens essential oil	In vitro/In vivo mice: Pietrella (2011)			
Geranium essential oil (*Pelargonium* spp)	In vivo mice: Maruyama (2008)			
Lavender oil (*Lavandula angustofolia*)	D'Auria et al. (2005)			

Bacterial Vaginosis

Bacterial vaginosis is the most common vaginal infection, with a prevalence of 29% among reproductive age women in the United States (Allsworth & Peipert, 2007). Bacterial vaginosis occurs when *Lactobacilli* in the vagina are replaced with high concentrations of anaerobic bacteria. It is not fully understood why there is a change in vaginal milieu, nor is it clear whether a sexually transmitted pathogen is involved. Risk factors for BV include multiple male or female sex partners, a new sex partner, douching, lack of condom use, and lack of vaginal *Lactobacilli* (Workowski & Berman, 2010). Women with BV are at increased risk for acquisition of some sexually transmitted diseases including HIV, complications after gynecologic surgery, complications of pregnancy, and recurrence of BV (Workowski & Berman, 2010). All symptomatic women should be treated. Symptomatic women who are pregnant should be treated with oral therapy. Bacterial vaginosis in pregnancy has been associated with adverse outcomes, but the only known benefit of therapy is reduction of symptoms. Studies investigating the treatment of asymptomatic high-risk pregnant women with BV have shown mixed results.

The diagnosis of BV is based on clinical exam and microscopic findings. The Amsel criteria for BV are three out of four of the following: pH $\geq$ 4.7, positive amine or whiff test, presence of >20% clue cells, or homogeneous gray discharge. The gold standard uses Nugent's criteria, but this is not practical in most clinical settings, as it requires a gram stain. A Nugent's score is obtained from evaluating three morphotypes in the vaginal fluid on a score of 1 to 10. A score of 7 or greater is considered diagnostic for BV.

Clinical Pearl

Fungal organisms noted on a Pap smear are not necessarily an indicator of a pathologic infection. A confirmatory wet mount and/or clinical symptoms are needed before treatment. "Predominance of *coccobacilli* consistent with shift in vaginal flora" noted on Pap smear is highly suggestive but not diagnostic of BV (Fitzhugh & Heller, 2008).

TREATMENT

Several conventional treatment protocols are available for BV. They include:

Metronidazole 500 mg orally twice daily for 7 days
Metronidazole gel 0.75%, 5 g intravaginally once daily for 5 days

Clindamycin cream 2%, 5 g intravaginally once daily for 7 days (Workowski & Berman, 2010).

Oral treatments are recommended in pregnancy and include:

Metronidazole 500 mg orally twice daily for 7 days
Metronidazole 250 mg orally three times daily for 7 days
Clindamycin 300 mg twice daily for 7 days

Consider a follow-up exam one month after treatment of high-risk pregnant women. In a Cochrane review of 24 clinical trials, clindamycin, oral metronidazole, and oral or intravaginal lactobacillus were found to be effective in the treatment of BV (Oduyebo, Anorlu, & Ogunsola, 2009). Metronidazole had more side effects than clindamycin. Hydrogen peroxide douche and triple sulphonamide cream were not effective.

Recurrent BV

In BV, recurrence rates are high; typical rates are 30% 3 months after treatment and 80% within 9 months (Sobel, 1999). Recurrence is associated with past history of BV, regular sex partner, and female sexual partners (Bradshaw et al., 2006). Recurrence is inversely associated with the use of hormonal contraception (Vodstrcil et al., 2013). The treatment strategies for recurrent BV include longer treatment period (2 weeks), change to a different antibiotic, or prophylactic maintenance therapy. Examples of maintenance therapies include vaginal metronidazole twice weekly or oral metronidazole three times a week. Pilot testing of a 750-mg vaginal metronidazole suppository twice weekly for 3 months showed very low recurrence rates (1 in 10) though once treatment was stopped remission rates were high (6 in 9) (Aguin, Akins, & Sobel, 2014). The use of combination therapies to prevent recurrence has not yielded impressive results. For example, in an RCT combining oral metronidazole with vaginal clindamycin or vaginal probiotic, the recurrence rates were the same (28%) at 6 months (Bradshaw et al., 2012). Triple therapy with 7 days of nitroimidazole, 21 days of vaginal boric acid 600 mg daily, and then metronidazole gel twice weekly for 16 weeks had a recurrence rate of 50% at 36 weeks (Reichman, Akins, & Sobel, 2009). It was hypothesized that the addition of boric acid would dissolve the vaginal biofilm that contains the bacterial pathogens adherent to epithelial cells in BV. Secondary VVC is common with maintenance therapy (Sobel et al., 2006).

ACIDIFYING AGENTS

A number of research trials have investigated the use of acidifying agents in the treatment and prevention of BV. The goal is to lower vaginal pH in order to support the growth of *Lactobacilli*. The results of these studies have been mixed. In a randomized double-blind placebo-controlled trial, a silicon-coated 250-mg vaginal tablet of ascorbic acid was twice as effective in preventing BV than placebo at 6 months (16% vs. 32%) but not at 3 months (Krasnopolsky et al., 2013). In a double-blinded RCT ($n = 29$), an acetic acid–based vaginal gel was not effective in treating BV (Holley, Richter, Varner, Pair, & Schwebke, 2004). Another RCT showed an acid-buffering gel to be less effective than high-dose metronidazole gel for the treatment of symptomatic BV (Simoes et al., 2006). However, when a lactic acid gel was added to metronidazole for the treatment of BV ($n = 90$), there was a significantly higher growth of *Lactobacilli*, suggesting that acidifying agents may play a role in the prevention of recurrent BV (Decena et al., 2006).

Treatments for Vulvovaginal Candidiasis and Bacterial Vaginosis

PROBIOTICS

The study of probiotics and their role in vaginal health has evolved over the years (MacPhee, Hummelen, Bisanz, Miller, & Reid, 2010). Originally, the focus was on probiotics that produce antimicrobial substances like hydrogen peroxide, adhere to epithelial cells, and exhibit in vitro inhibitory activity against BV pathogens. Researchers now focus on the probiotic's ability to survive intestinal transit, cope with hormonal changes, modulate host immune responses, and outcompete pathogenic organisms. Uropathogens are known to form dense biofilms. This disruption of biofilms may be one of the mechanisms by which probiotics reduce urinary tract infection (UTI) and prevent BV. For instance, the probiotics *Lactobacillus rhamnosus* GR-1 and *Lactobacillus reuteri* RC-14 have been shown to disrupt uropathogenic biofilms in vitro (McMillan et al., 2011). One of the challenges in the development of probiotics is the delivery method. When given orally they must survive transport through the gastrointestinal tract and then colonize in the vagina. Although administration of probiotics directly into the vagina would be preferable, they are more costly to develop and require FDA approval.

Probiotics containing *Lactobacilli* have been used as an alternative treatment for vaginitis for many years. In BV, there is a clear pathophysiologic relationship between the lack of *Lactobacilli* and the development of vaginitis; thus, promoting colonization in the vagina is logical. On the other hand, the role of *Lactobacilli* in the development of VVC is less clear. *Lactobacilli* can be quite plentiful in the acidic vaginal environment in which fungal organisms thrive. In vitro studies have shown that *Lactobacilli* can inhibit the growth of *C. albicans* and its adherence to vaginal epithelium, yet a review of the literature found limited evidence for the use of probiotics in the prevention of recurrent VVC (Falagas, Betsi, & Athanasiou, 2006). The strains showing the most promise are *Lactobacillus acidophilus, L. rhamnosus* GR-1, and *Lactobacillus fermentum* RC-14. It could be that certain species of *Lactobacilli* inhibit the growth of fungal organisms, however more research is needed.

A rigorous meta-analysis of 12 RCTs found that probiotics significantly improved the cure rate of BV when used alone or with an antibiotic whether administered orally or vaginally (Huang, Song, & Zhao, 2014). However, a previous review of clinical trials and a Cochrane review concluded that there was insufficient evidence for or against recommending probiotics for BV (Mastromarino, Vitali, & Mosca, 2013; Senok, Verstraelen, Temmerman, & Botta, 2009). The study of probiotics has also been plagued with methodological issues such as small sample size, lack of culture confirmation of *Candida* or documentation of the colonization of *Lactobacilli*, and lack of placebo or comparison group. Numerous strains of *Lactobacilli* have been studied using different doses and forms and for various durations. In some cases the species have not even been identified. These limitations, as well as the heterogeneity of the studies, has limited the ability to draw firm conclusions regarding effectiveness.

When combing through the data, however, certain probiotics may be more promising in combating BV than others. The probiotics cited most in rigorous trials were: *L. acidophilus, Lactobacillus casei rhamnosus, L. rhamnosus* GR-1, and *L. reuteri* RC-14 (Huang et al., 2014). Successful vaginal colonization with *L. crispatus* has been associated with a reduction in the growth of BV-associated bacteria (Ngugi et al., 2011). The addition of estrogen to the probiotic may foster the colonization of *Lactobacilli*. In a review of 16 studies, the use of a vaginal preparation containing *L. acidophilus* KS400 and 0.03 mg estriol (Gynoflor) improved the vaginal epithelium as well as the growth of *Lactobacilli* (Unlu & Donders, 2011). More rigorous studies are needed to demonstrate the effectiveness of these probiotics in the treatment and prevention of BV.

Conducting BV research poses many challenges (Lamont et al., 2011). Bacterial vaginosis is a syndrome comprising different bacterial compositions, symptoms, and responses to antimicrobials. Women with BV have different microbial profiles, and there is considerable biodiversity between women. For instance, 7%–33% of healthy women lack an appreciable number of *Lactobacilli* species in the vagina. The *Lactobacilli* are replaced by other lactic acid–producing bacteria, and the health of the vagina is maintained as long as production of lactic acid continues. This complexity explains why BV is so challenging to treat, especially in the setting on ongoing recurrence.

USE OF PROBIOTICS

Look for products that contain *Lactobacillus* found in vagina. One such probiotic is the OTC (Femdophilus): 5 billion *L. rhamnosus* GR-1 and *L. reuteri* RC-14; take 1–2 daily).

Take one capsule twice daily between meals for 7–14 days. In addition, it may be helpful to eat live-culture yogurt daily.

Botanicals

The most popular of the herbal therapies is tea tree oil (*Melaleuca alternifolia*) delivered as a vaginal suppository. It has been shown to have antifungal and antibacterial properties (Hammer, Carson, & Riley, 1999; Cox et al., 2000). It inhibited the growth of *C. albicans* in vitro (D'Auria et al., 2001) and in mice (Mondello, De Bernardis, Girolamo, Cassone, & Salvatore, 1998). It has been found to be effective against non-*albicans* species *C. glabrata* and *Candida parapsilosis* (Hammer, Carson, & Riley, 1998). There are no controlled trials for review; one case study describes successful treatment of BV with tea tree oil suppositories (Blackwell, 1991).

Most suppositories contain 10% tea tree oil or 200 mg per suppository. Directions are to insert intravaginally for 6 nights. Rarely, women may experience a hypersensitivity reaction to tea tree oil (Wolner-Hanssen & Sjoberg, 1998). Tea tree oil should not be used during pregnancy.

> Let us come back to Tanisha from our case study at the beginning of the chapter. She has had recurrent mixed vaginal infections, both VVC and BV. She prefers not to take antibiotics. I would start her on either tea tree oil or boric acid suppositories because they have both antibacterial and antifungal activity. Then, I would suggest a course of probiotics for 3 to 6 months to recolonize the vagina with *Lactobacilli* and prevent BV. In addition, I would discuss the risk factors for recurrent vaginal infections including sexual practices and family planning methods, as behavioral changes may decrease her risk of recurrence (see Box 13.1).

Box 13.1 Important Points for Patient Education

- If you have a history of frequent vaginal yeast infections, request an antifungal treatment when you are given a prescription for antibiotics.
- Abstain from vaginal or oral sex during treatment.
- Condoms are at increased risk for breakage when used with vaginal creams.
- Using condoms for 1 month after treatment may reduce the risk of recurrence.
- Do not insert penis, fingers, or sex toys into the vagina after insertion in the anus.
- Come in for an exam when you are symptomatic.
- Do not douche.

Conclusion

Vaginitis is a common women's health issue. Although conventional treatments have excellent efficacy for acute vaginitis, relapse rates are high. Both probiotics and boric acid show evidence for efficacy and play an important role in the prevention of recurrent vaginitis. There are few safety concerns from these two treatments.

REFERENCES

Aguin, T., Akins, R. A., & Sobel, J. D. (2014). High-dose vaginal maintenance metronidazole for recurrent bacterial vaginosis: A pilot study. *Sex Transm Dis, 41*, 290–291.

Ahmad, N., Alam, M. K., Shehbaz, A., et al. (2005). Antimicrobial activity of clove oil and its potential in the treatment of vaginal candidiasis. *J Drug Target, 13*(10), 555–561.

Allsworth, J. E., & Peipert, J. F. (2007). Prevalence of bacterial vaginosis: 2001–2004 national health and nutrition examination survey data. *Obstet Gynecol, 109*, 114–120.

Anderson, M. R., Klink, K., & Cohrssen, A. (2004). Evaluation of vaginal complaints. *JAMA, 291*, 1368–1379.

Bai, F. Y. (2014). Association of genotypes with infection types and antifungal susceptibilities in *Candida albicans* as revealed by recent molecular typing strategies. *Mycology, 5*, 1–9.

Blackwell, A. L. (1991). Tea tree oil and anaerobic (bacterial) vaginosis. *Lancet, 337*, 300.

Bradshaw, C. S., Morton, A. N., Hocking, J., et al. (2006). High recurrence rates of bacterial vaginosis over the course of 12 months after oral metronidazole therapy and factors associated with recurrence. *J Infect Dis, 193*, 1478–1486.

Bradshaw, C. S., Pirotta, M., De Guingand, D., et al. (2012). Efficacy of oral metronidazole with vaginal clindamycin or vaginal probiotic for bacterial vaginosis: Randomised placebo-controlled double-blind trial. *PLoS One, 7*, e34540.

Cox, S. D., Mann, C. M., Markham, J. L., et al. (2000). The mode of antimicrobial action of the essential oil of *Melaleuca alternifolia* (tea tree oil). *J Appl Microbiol, 88*, 170–175.

D'Auria, F. D., Laino, L., Strippoli, V., et al. (2001). In vitro activity of tea tree oil against *Candida albicans* mycelial conversion and other pathogenic fungi. *J Chemother, 13*, 377–383.

D'Auria, F. D., Tecca, M., Strippoli, V., Salvatore, G., Battinelli, L., & Mazzanti, G. (2005). Antifungal activity of lavandula angustifolia essential oil against candida albicans yeast and mycelial form. *Med Mycol: Off Publ Int Soc Human Ani Mycol, 43*(5), 391–396.

De Seta, F., Schmidt, M., Vu, B., Essmann, M., & Larsen, B. (2009). Antifungal mechanisms supporting boric acid therapy of candida vaginitis. *J Antimicrob Chemother, 63*, 325–336.

Decena, D. C., Co, J. T., Manalastas, R. M., Jr., et al. (2006). Metronidazole with lactacyd vaginal gel in bacterial vaginosis. *J Obstet Gynaecol Res, 32*, 243–251.

Dennerstein, G. J. (1986). Depo-provera in the treatment of recurrent vulvovaginal candidiasis. *J Reprod Med, 31*, 801–803.

Ergin, A., & Arikan, S. (2002). Comparison of microdilution and disc diffusion methods in assessing the in vitro activity of fluconazole and *Melaleuca alternifolia* (tea tree) oil against vaginal candida isolates. *J Chemother, 14*, 465–472.

Falagas, M. E., Betsi, G. I., & Athanasiou, S. (2006). Probiotics for prevention of recurrent vulvovaginal candidiasis: A review. *J Antimicrob Chemother, 58*, 266–272.

Ferris, D. G., Nyirjesy, P., Sobel, J. D., Soper, D., Pavletic, A., & Litaker, M. S. (2002). Over-the-counter antifungal drug misuse associated with patient-diagnosed vulvovaginal candidiasis. *Obstet Gynecol, 99*, 419–425.

Fitzhugh, V. A., & Heller, D. S. (2008). Significance of a diagnosis of microorganisms on pap smear. *J Low Genit Tract Dis, 12*, 40–51.

Foxman, B., Marsh, J. V., Gillespie, B., & Sobel, J. D. (1998). Frequency and response to vaginal symptoms among white and African American women: Results of a random digit dialing survey. *J Women's Health, 7*, 1167–1174.

Ha, Y. M., Choi, J. S., Lee, B. B., Moon, H. E., Cho, K. K., & Choi, I. S. (2014). Inhibitory effects of seaweed extracts on the growth of the vaginal bacterium gardnerella vaginalis. *J Environ Biol/Acad Environ Biol, India, 35*(3), 537–542.

Hammer, K. A., Carson, C. F., & Riley, T. V. (1998). In-vitro activity of essential oils, in particular melaleuca alternifolia (tea tree) oil and tea tree oil products, against Candida spp. *J Antimicrob Chemother, 42*, 591–595.

Hammer, K. A., Carson, C. F., & Riley, T. V. (1999). In vitro susceptibilities of lactobacilli and organisms associated with bacterial vaginosis to *Melaleuca alternifolia* (tea tree) oil. *Antimicrob Agents Chemother, 43*, 196.

Hoffstetter, S. E., Barr, S., LeFevre, C., Leong, F. C., & Leet, T. (2008). Self-reported yeast symptoms compared with clinical wet mount analysis and vaginal yeast culture in a specialty clinic setting. *J Reprod Med, 53*, 402–406.

Hoffstetter, S., Barr, S., LeFevre, C., & Gavard, J. A. (2012). Telephone triage: Diagnosis of candidiasis based upon self-reported vulvovaginal symptoms. *J Low Genit Tract Dis, 16*, 251–255.

Holley, R. L., Richter, H. E., Varner, R. E., Pair, L., & Schwebke, J. R. (2004). A random-ized, double-blind clinical trial of vaginal acidification versus placebo for the treat-ment of symptomatic bacterial vaginosis. *Sex Transm Dis*, *31*, 236–238.

Huang, H., Song, L., & Zhao, W. (2014). Effects of probiotics for the treatment of bacte-rial vaginosis in adult women: A meta-analysis of randomized clinical trials. *Arch Gynecol Obstet*, *289*, 1225–1234.

Hurley, R., & De Louvois, J. (1979). Candida vaginitis. *Postgrad Med J*, *55*, 645–647.

Iavazzo, C., Gkegkes, I. D., Zarkada, I. M., & Falagas, M. E. (2011). Boric acid for recur-rent vulvovaginal candidiasis: The clinical evidence. *J Women's Health (Larchmt)*, *20*, 1245–1255.

Imhof, M., Lipovac, M., Kurz, C., Barta, J., Verhoeven, H. C., & Huber, J. C. (2005). Propolis solution for the treatment of chronic vaginitis. *Int J Gynaecol Obstet: Off Org Int Feder Gynaecol Obstet*, *89*(2), 127–132.

Irving, G., Miller, D., Robinson, A., Reynolds, S., & Copas, A. J. (1998). Psychological factors associated with recurrent vaginal candidiasis: A preliminary study. *Sex Transm Infect*, *74*, 334–338.

Karasz, A., & Anderson, M. (2003). The vaginitis monologues: Women's experiences of vaginal complaints in a primary care setting. *Soc Sci Med*, *56*, 1013–1021.

Kent, H. L. (1991). Epidemiology of vaginitis. *Am J Obstet Gynecol*, *165*(4 Pt 2), 1168–1176.

Krasnopolsky, V. N., Prilepskaya, V. N., Polatti, F., et al. (2013). Efficacy of vitamin C vaginal tablets as prophylaxis for recurrent bacterial vaginosis: A randomised, double-blind, placebo-controlled clinical trial. *J Clin Med Res*, *5*, 309–315.

Lamont, R. F., Sobel, J. D., Akins, R. A., et al. (2011). The vaginal microbiome: New information about genital tract flora using molecular based techniques. *BJOG*, *118*, 533–549.

Lortholary, O., Petrikkos, G., Akova, M., et al. (2012). ESCMID guideline for the diag-nosis and management of Candida diseases 2012: Patients with HIV infection or AIDS. *Clin Microbiol Infect*, *18*(Suppl 7), 68–77.

MacPhee, R. A., Hummelen, R., Bisanz, J. E., Miller, W. L., & Reid, G. (2010). Probiotic strategies for the treatment and prevention of bacterial vaginosis. *Expert Opin Pharmacother*, *11*, 2985–2995.

Maruyama, N., Takizawa, T., Ishibashi, H., et al. (2008). Protective activity of geranium oil and its component, geraniol, in combination with vaginal washing against vagi-nal candidiasis in mice. *Biol Pharm Bull*, *31*(8), 1501–1506.

Mastromarino, P., Vitali, B., & Mosca, L. (2013). Bacterial vaginosis: A review on clini-cal trials with probiotics. *New Microbiol*, *36*, 229–238.

McMillan, A., Dell, M., Zellar, M. P., et al. (2011). Disruption of urogenital biofilms by lactobacilli. *Colloids Surf B Biointerfaces*, *86*, 58–64.

Mondello, F., De Bernardis, F., Girolamo, A., Cassone, A., & Salvatore, G. (1998). In vivo activity of terpinen-4-ol, the main bioactive component of *Melaleuca alterni-folia* cheel (tea tree) oil against azole-susceptible and -resistant human pathogenic candida species. *BMC Infect Dis*, *1998*, *6*, 158.

Moore, G. S., & Atkins, R. D. (1977). The fungicidal and fungistatic effects of an aqueous garlic extract on medically important yeast-like fungi. *Mycologia*, *69*(2), 341–348.

Ngugi, B. M., Hemmerling, A., Bukusi, E. A., et al. (2011). Effects of bacterial vaginosis-associated bacteria and sexual intercourse on vaginal colonization with the probiotic *Lactobacillus crispatus* CTV-05. *Sex Transm Dis, 38*, 1020–1027.

Nurbhai, M., Grimshaw, J., Watson, M., Bond, C., Mollison, J., & Ludbrook, A. (2007). Oral versus intra-vaginal imidazole and triazole anti-fungal treatment of uncomplicated vulvovaginal candidiasis (thrush). *Cochrane Database Syst Rev*, 4:CD002845.

Nyirjesy, P., Robinson, J., Mathew, L., Lev-Sagie, A., Reyes, I., & Culhane, J. F. (2011). Alternative therapies in women with chronic vaginitis. *Obstet Gynecol, 117*, 856–861.

Nyirjesy, P., Weitz, M. V., Grody, M. H., & Lorber, B. (1997). Over-the-counter and alternative medicines in the treatment of chronic vaginal symptoms. *Obstet Gynecol, 90*, 50–53.

Oduyebo, O. O., Anorlu, R. I., & Ogunsola, F. T. (2009). The effects of antimicrobial therapy on bacterial vaginosis in non-pregnant women. *Cochrane Database Syst Rev, 3*:CD006055.

Payne, S. C., Cromer, P. R., Stanek, M. K., & Palmer, A. A. (2010). Evidence of African-American women's frustrations with chronic recurrent bacterial vaginosis. *J Am Acad Nurse Pract, 22*, 101–108.

Pietrella, D., Angiolella, L., Vavala, E., et al. (2011). Beneficial effect of mentha suaveolens essential oil in the treatment of vaginal candidiasis assessed by real-time monitoring of infection. *BMC Compl Altern Med, 11*, 18-6882-11-18.

Ravel, J., Gajer, P., Abdo, Z., et al. (2011). Vaginal microbiome of reproductive-age women. *Proc Natl Acad Sci U S A, 108*(Suppl 1), 4680–4687.

Ray, A., Ray, S., George, A. T., & Swaminathan, N. (2011). Interventions for prevention and treatment of vulvovaginal candidiasis in women with HIV infection. *Cochrane Database Syst Rev, 8*:CD008739.

Ray, D., Goswami, R., Banerjee, U., et al. (2007). Prevalence of *Candida glabrata* and its response to boric acid vaginal suppositories in comparison with oral fluconazole in patients with diabetes and vulvovaginal candidiasis. *Diabetes Care, 30*, 312–317.

Ray, D., Goswami, R., Dadhwal, V., Goswami, D., Banerjee, U., & Kochupillai, N. (2007). Prolonged (3-month) mycological cure rate after boric acid suppositories in diabetic women with vulvovaginal candidiasis. *J Infect, 55*, 374–377.

Reichman, O., Akins, R., & Sobel, J. D. (2009). Boric acid addition to suppressive antimicrobial therapy for recurrent bacterial vaginosis. *Sex Transm Dis, 36*, 732–734.

Rosa, M. I., Silva, B. R., Pires, P. S., et al. (2013). Weekly fluconazole therapy for recurrent vulvovaginal candidiasis: A systematic review and meta-analysis. *Eur J Obstet Gynecol Reprod Biol, 167*, 132–136.

Santana Perez, E., Lugones Botell, M., Perez Stuart, O., & Castillo Brito, B. (1995). Vaginal parasites and acute cervicitis: Local treatment with propolis. preliminary report. [Parasitismo vaginal Y cervicitis agudoi tratamiento local an propoleo. Informe preliminar] *Revista Cubana De Enfermeria, 11*(1), 51–56.

Schaaf, V. M., Perez-Stable, E. J., & Borchardt, K. (1990). The limited value of symptoms and signs in the diagnosis of vaginal infections. *Arch Intern Med, 150*, 1929–1933.

Senok, A. C., Verstraelen, H., Temmerman, M., & Botta, G. A. (2009). Probiotics for the treatment of bacterial vaginosis. *Cochrane Database Syst Rev, 4*:CD006289.

Simoes, J. A., Bahamondes, L. G., Camargo, R. P., et al. (2006). A pilot clinical trial comparing an acid-buffering formulation (ACIDFORM gel) with metronidazole gel for the treatment of symptomatic bacterial vaginosis. *Br J Clin Pharmacol, 61,* 211–217.

Sobel, J. D. (1990). Vaginitis in adult women. *Obstet Gynecol Clin North Am, 17,* 851–879.

Sobel, J. D. (1999). Vulvovaginitis in healthy women. *Compr Ther, 25,* 335–346.

Sobel, J. D., Chaim, W., Nagappan, V., & Leaman, D. (2003). Treatment of vaginitis caused by candida glabrata: Use of topical boric acid and flucytosine. *Am J Obstet Gynecol, 189,* 1297–1300.

Sobel, J. D., Ferris, D., Schwebke, J., et al. (2006). Suppressive antibacterial therapy with 0.75% metronidazole vaginal gel to prevent recurrent bacterial vaginosis. *Am J Obstet Gynecol, 194,* 1283–1289.

Sobel, J. D., Wiesenfeld, H. C., Martens, M., et al. (2004). Maintenance fluconazole therapy for recurrent vulvovaginal candidiasis. *N Engl J Med, 351,* 876–883.

Soffar, S. A., Metwali, D. M., Abdel-Aziz, S. S., el-Wakil, H. S., & Saad, G. A. (2001). Evaluation of the effect of a plant alkaloid (berberine derived from berberis aristata) on trichomonas vaginalis in vitro. *J Egypt Soc Parasitol, 31*(3), 893–904 + 1p plate.

Toppozada, M., Onsy, F. A., Fares, E., Amir, S., & Shaala, S. (1979). The protective influence of progestogen only contraception against vaginal moniliasis. *Contraception, 20,* 99–103.

Unlu, C., & Donders, G. (2011). Use of lactobacilli and estriol combination in the treatment of disturbed vaginal ecosystem: A review. *J Turk Ger Gynecol Assoc, 12,* 239–246.

Vodstrcil, L. A., Hocking, J. S., Law, M., et al. (2013). Hormonal contraception is associated with a reduced risk of bacterial vaginosis: A systematic review and meta-analysis. *PLoS One, 8,* e73055.

Watson, C., & Calabretto, H. (2007). Comprehensive review of conventional and non-conventional methods of management of recurrent vulvovaginal candidiasis. *Aust N Z J Obstet Gynaecol, 47,* 262–272.

Wolner-Hanssen, P., & Sjoberg, I. (1998). Warning against a fashionable cure for vulvovaginitis: Tea tree oil may substitute candida itching with allergy itching. *Lakartidningen, 95,* 3309–3310.

Workowski, K. A., & Berman, S. M.; Centers for Disease Control and Prevention. (2006). Sexually transmitted diseases treatment guidelines, 2006. *MMWR Recomm Rep, 55*(RR-11), 1–94.

Workowski, K. A., & Berman, S.; Centers for Disease Control and Prevention (CDC). (2010). Sexually transmitted diseases treatment guidelines, 2010. *MMWR Recomm Rep, 59*(RR-12), 1–110.

14

Preconception Counseling and Fertility

VICTORIA MAIZES

CASE STUDY

Sally is a 30-year-old woman who is on track for tenure at a major university. She has been taking oral contraceptives since she was 18. Recently married, Sally is sure she wants children, but given her career aspirations, wants to wait until she is 34 or 35 years old. She worries about the impact waiting will have on her fertility. Her conventionally trained OB/GYN, who has seen many young women wrestle with infertility, advised that she freeze embryos as a safety net. What would you advise?

Introduction

From early childhood, many girls play with dolls and imagine becoming parents. The ability to bear children is often assumed, and when it does not occur with ease, or at all, it can be a source of great suffering. In most religions, bearing children is considered a blessing, and traditional societies commonly encourage elaborate preparation for conception. This chapter outlines preconception advice that enhances the likelihood both of conception and of giving birth to a healthy child.

In Western countries, the ability to control fertility with reliable contraception began in the 1960s, conferring new freedoms and increasing the average age of first childbirth from 21 to 26 years. Conventional medicine has made tremendous advances in assisted reproductive technologies (ART), thereby helping couples struggling to conceive. Sir Robert Edwards, PhD, was awarded the

Nobel Prize in 2010 for developing in vitro fertilization (IVF), which allowed couples that may never have conceived to become parents. However, the focus on high-tech solutions such as IVF, and the highly profitable industry it spawned, has reduced the emphasis on the simpler, more natural, less invasive, lower-cost and lower-risk strategies that are the strength of integrative medicine. While IVF can be miraculous, the cost and higher risks to mother and baby should make it a second-line choice except under unusual circumstances.

Nutrition

Substantial research supports the role of a healthy diet in conception (Chavarro, Rich-Edwards, Rosner, & Willett, 2007a). An optimal fertility diet is made up of freshly prepared, whole food and includes abundant vegetables and fruits, sufficient omega-3 fatty acids, and vegetable sources of protein. The diet is low in processed foods, meats, and rapidly digesting, high glycemic load carbohydrates. One such whole food diet, the Mediterranean diet, has been studied and is associated with a 44% lower risk of infertility in women attempting to conceive naturally, and a 40% greater likelihood of conception in couples using IVF to conceive (Estefania, et al., 2011; Vujkovic, et al., 2010).

The Nurse's Health Study II (NHS II), used food frequency questionnaires to determine the macro- and micronutrients that influence the risk of ovulatory infertility. (Ovulatory infertility is the most common cause of infertility in women and includes polycystic ovarian syndrome, luteal phase dysfunction, hypothalamic problems, and stress-induced infertility.)

The NHS II found increased ovulatory infertility in women who ate high glycemic index (GI) carbohydrates. Breakfast cereals stood out—they nearly doubled the risk of ovulatory infertility (Chavarro, Rich-Edwards, Rosner, & Willett, 2007b). Flour, the first ingredients in many breakfast cereals, is a high GI carbohydrate that is rapidly metabolized into blood sugar, followed by spikes in insulin with subsequent inflammation. Higher levels of insulin also reduce sex-hormone-binding globulin, which results in higher levels of circulating free testosterone. Another high GI carbohydrate, soda, has been linked to longer time to conception in two studies (Chavarro, Rich-Edwards, Rosner, & Willett, 2009; Hatch et al., 2012). And, previously undiagnosed celiac disease has been shown to be the underlying cause of infertility in about 4% of women.

The type of protein women ate was also related to the risk of ovulatory infertility (Chavarro, Rich-Edwards, Rosner, & Willett, 2008a). In women older than 32 years, each additional daily serving of red meat, chicken, or turkey increased the risk of ovulatory infertility by nearly one-third, fish and eggs had no effect, and vegetable protein reduced the risk by 50%.

In 2014, the Food and Drug Administration (FDA) and the Environmental Protection Agency changed their joint recommendation to pregnant women and women of childbearing age about consuming fish. Evidence had shown that 90% of women, in response to the 2004 warning, were consuming less than the FDA-recommended amount of fish, placing themselves and their baby at risk for having insufficient levels of omega-3 fatty acids. In June 2014, new draft guidelines were published that recommended a minimum intake of 8 to 12 ounces of a variety of fish each week from choices that are lower in mercury (Food and Drug Administration, 2014). The agencies continued to advise against eating shark, swordfish, king mackerel, and tilefish, and limiting albacore tuna to 6 ounces or less per week.

MICRONUTRIENTS

Vitamins

The American Academy of Pediatrics, the American College of Obstetrics and Gynecology, the American Academy of Family Physicians, and the US Preventive Services Task Force all recommend that women of childbearing age take a multivitamin with folic acid. When taken prior to conception and through the first trimester of pregnancy, these supplements reduce the risk of neural tube defects, heart defects, musculoskeletal defects, and orofacial defects (Goh, Bollano, Einarson, & Koren, 2006).

The NHS II found that multivitamins make it easier for women to conceive and less likely to miscarry (Chavarro, Rich-Edwards, Rosner, & Willett, 2008b). Three separate studies revealed an association between the use of folic acid prior to conception and a 40% lower prevalence of autism (Roth et al., 2011; Schmidt et al., 2011; Surén et al., 2013). Yet, the 2011 National Health and Nutrition Examination Survey (NHANES), revealed that only 34% of women between the ages of 20–39 get the recommended amount of supplemental folic acid.

Prenatal multivitamins are not tightly regulated and may contain very different ingredients. Iodine is only present in 51% of prenatal multivitamins (National Institutes of Health, 2011). Some women will need higher doses than the 400–800 mcg of folic acid found in most prenatal vitamins. This includes women with a personal or family history of bearing a child with a neural tube defect, those who have inflammatory bowel disease, obesity with BMI >35, or diabetes. Higher doses are also indicated for women who take anticonvulsant medications or folate antagonists (e.g., methotrexate, sulfonamides), smoke cigarettes, or belong to higher-risk ethnic groups (Sikh, Celtic, Northern Chinese; Kennedy & Koren, 2012). While some advocate use of 5 methyltetrahydrofolate to address polymorphisms, there are no trials to date (Czeizel et al., 2011; see Box 14.1).

SUPPLEMENTS

Women who are consuming less than the recommended 12 ounces of fish per week may benefit from supplementing with omega-3 fatty acids. A consensus statement from the World Association of Perinatal Medicine recommends a dose of at least 200 mg of docosahexaenoic acid (DHA) during pregnancy (Koletzko et al., 2008). No consensus was formed around the dose of eicosapentaenoic acid (EPA), but the group noted that intakes of up to 1 g/day DHA

Box 14.1 Preconception Multivitamin Ingredients

- Vitamin A: the current recommended dietary allowance (RDA) of preformed vitamin A is 700 retinol activity equivalents (RAEs) or 2,300 IU/day, with a tolerable upper intake level for pregnancy of 3,000 RAEs/day or 10,000 IU/day (Barker, 2004). Most experts say no more than 5,000 IU per day should be preformed because we also get vitamin A in our food and through food fortification. (The RDA during pregnancy is 2,567 IU/day preformed vitamin A and 4,300 IU/day for lactating women.)
- Iron: 18 mg (once pregnant, 27 mg, and 9 mg when lactating) (Barker, 2004)
- Iodine: 150 mcg (once pregnant, 220 mcg/day from all sources for pregnant women and 290 mcg/day for lactating women) (Barker, 2004)
- Folic acid: 400 mcg or more (once pregnant 600 mcg or more) (Barker, 2004)
- Vitamin D: 600 IU (Barker, 2004) (or more based on assessment of vitamin D level). Both vitamins D2 and D3 are effective.
- Vitamin B12: 2.4 mcg (once pregnant 2.6 mcg)
- Vitamin E: 22.4 IU/day for women over age 14, including while pregnant, and 28.4 while lactating (Barker, 2004)
- Calcium: the Food and Nutrition Board (FNB) at the Institute of Medicine recommends 1,000 mg to women over 19 and 1,300 mg a day for girls age 9–18 (Barker, 2004). This is from all sources—food and supplements—so it is useful to do a calculation of calcium in a woman's diet and then recommend a supplement dose if needed.
- Trace minerals: small amounts of copper, zinc, magnesium, and potassium

or 27 g/day omega 3 have been used in randomized clinical trials without significant adverse effects (Koletzko et al., 2007). Other supplements to consider include probiotics, n-acetyl cysteine, and Fertility Blend (a mixed antioxidant formula). All have some small studies that support their potential benefit in enhancing fertility.

Herbal Medicine

Herbal medicines have long been used to support fertility. *Vitex agnus-castus* is perhaps the best studied. Vitex has been shown to reduce levels of follicle-stimulating hormone and increase luteinizing hormone, thereby reducing estrogen and increasing progesterone. At higher doses, it can inhibit prolactin levels. Thus, it can be especially helpful in women who have luteal phase disorders (Gerhard, Patek, Monga, Blank, & Gorkow, 1998).

Herbs are also used to help women cleanse or detoxify before pregnancy. Schisandra (*Schisandra chinensis*) fruit is said to tonify and strengthen the hypothalamus, pituitary gland, ovaries, and adrenals (Upton, 1999). Milk thistle (*Silybum marianum*) is another very safe choice. It is thought to maximize the ability of the liver to detoxify chemical pollutants. Other commonly used herbs include the adaptogenic herbs shatavari root (discussed later) and damiana (*Turnera aphrodisiaca*), a traditional wedding gift in the southwest United States and Mexico.

Environmental Chemicals

Shockingly, testing of umbilical cord blood revealed that babies have an average of 232 environmental chemicals in their bodies at the time of birth (Fimrite, 2009). These chemicals can increase a child's risk of ADHD, autism, and leukemia, and later in life they increase the risk of diabetes and heart disease (Stillerman, Mattison, Giudice, & Woodruff, 2008). While terribly disturbing, lifestyle modification can reduce exposures to toxic chemicals in parents, thereby reducing the risk to the fetus (American College of Obstetricians and Gynecologists, 2013).

For most people, food and beverages are a significant source of environmental toxin absorption. Choosing organic meat, poultry, pork, and produce, whenever possible, is the best way to reduce pesticide exposure and genetically modified organisms (GMO). When the cost of organic is prohibitive, selectively purchasing the least contaminated conventionally grown vegetables and fruits is a wise alternative. The Environmental Working Group keeps an updated list (www.ewg.org) and has calculated that you can reduce your pesticide exposure by 92% when you eat from the "clean fifteen" rather than the "dirty dozen" (EWG, 2011).

Many resources currently exist to guide us to safer food, water, and cleaning and personal care products (see the chapter "Environmental Exposures and Women's Health"; Maizes, Chapter 35 of this book). Adopting new behaviors can significantly and rapidly reduce the body burden of many, but not all, environmental toxins. For example, a 2011 San Francisco study revealed that adults dropped their urinary bisphenol A levels by two-thirds in three days when they were provided with fresh, catered meals that avoided canned foods and the use of plastic containers (Gerona et al., 2013; Rudel et al., 2010; vom Saal et al., 2014).

Mind–Body

Human fertility is affected by stress. From an evolutionary biology perspective, this makes perfect sense. The meta-message is: Now is the time to focus on survival, not reproduction. The ovary and testes have cortisol receptors; too much cortisol signals the ovaries directly, as well as through feedback loops to the pituitary gland and hypothalamus, to tone down reproductive capacity.

Potentially furthering the downward fertility spiral, infertility can take a huge toll on well-being. In a survey of 121 couples with infertility, 19% of the women had moderate depression and 13% were severely depressed; in addition, 26% were at high risk for sexual dysfunction (Nelson et al., 2008).

Mind–body therapies have been studied as a way to normalize reproductive function and mitigate the stress of infertility diagnoses. A small study examined hypnosis in 12 women with functional hypothalamic amenorrhea; each had one hypnotherapy session and was followed for 12 weeks. The women were asked about their menstrual cycle and overall state of well-being and self-confidence. Nine of the 12 participants resumed menstruating, and all 12 described improvement in well-being and confidence. While a tiny sample, it is remarkable that one hypnotherapy session led three-quarters of the women to resume menstruating and had a broad salutogenic effect on all (Tschugguel, & Berga, 2003).

Another trial evaluated cognitive-behavioral therapy (CBT) for functional hypothalamic amenorrhea. Fifteen women were enrolled in the 20-week trial. Six of the eight women randomized to CBT resumed ovulating; the remaining two women had partial recovery of ovarian function. Only two of the women in the control group experienced renewed ovarian activity (Berga et al., 2003).

Mind–body groups are commonly designed as multiple-session, skill-building classes that teach a wide range of practices including yoga, guided imagery, breath work, mindfulness, journaling, body scanning, and cognitive restructuring (Domar et al., 2000). A meta-analysis of psychological interventions for infertility showed these skill-building groups to be more effective than either educational programs or individual therapy (Boivin, Griffiths, & Venetis, 2011). A second meta-analysis showed that mind–body groups lasting six or more sessions were more effective than those with fewer sessions (Hammerli, Znoj, & Barth, 2009).

Physical Activity

While we generally counsel people to be more physically active, in the preconception setting we sometimes need to ask women to cut back on their activity. Up to 44% of athletic women will experience intermittent or regular amenorrhea, an even higher percentage will have intermittent luteal phase dysfunction (De Souza, 2003). Vigorous exercise, more frequent exercise, or exercising to exhaustion significantly increased the time it took to conceive in one large population study (Gudmundsdottir, Flanders, & Augestad, 2009). The exception is women who are overweight or obese, in whom exercise reduces the time it takes to conceive (Wise et al., 2012). Walking and gentle forms of yoga can be encouraged in place of running, cycling, and vigorous forms of yoga for women who are having difficulty conceiving.

Acupuncture

Traditional Chinese medicine (TCM) includes acupuncture, herbs, tui na, moxibustion, dietary advice, and more. Acupuncture is the modality most commonly studied for its impact on fertility. However, most studies have only examined the impact of acupuncture on the success of embryo transfer during IVF. While many individual trials show benefit, three meta-analyses with contradictory findings have been published (Manheimer, van der Windt, et al., 2013; Manheimer, Zhang, et al., 2008; Zheng, Huang, Zhang, & Wang, 2012). The contradiction likely is due to the challenge of finding an appropriate sham for acupuncture. Some researchers have suggested that noninsertive needling at true acupoints is actually an active, not sham, treatment.

Ayurveda

Ayurveda is even less frequently studied than TCM for its impact on fertility. And yet, it has a rich set of traditional practices designed to prepare couples for pregnancy ranging from panchakarma (detoxification practices) to abstinence before attempting conception, select meditations, and consuming specific foods and herbs. The most commonly recommended herb for female fertility is shatavari (*Asparagus racemosus*). In Sanskrit, *Shatavari* means "she who possesses a hundred husbands," suggesting its ability to promote fertility and vitality.

Spirituality

The mystical perspective holds that there are three parties involved in creating a new life: a woman, a man, and God. Some adults come to conception with this spiritual perspective and may seek religious or secular ceremonies as they prepare to become the vessel that holds a newly forming life.

Struggling to conceive can lead to a crisis of spirit. Couples struggle with existential questions and the inherent unfairness. "Why is this happening to me?" lies just below the surface of many healthcare interactions. Religious traditions can be of help to some women and pose conflicts for others when religion prohibits certain reproductive treatment. Every religion has prayers that focus on fertility. Ceremonies can be designed to help women acknowledge their longing for a child, their frustration at not conceiving with ease, the loss of a child to miscarriage, or the loss of the dream of bearing children.

Conventional Medicine

Approximately 15% of couples will struggle to conceive. Infertility is somewhat arbitrarily defined as an inability to conceive despite 12 months of unprotected intercourse; however, of the 15% of couples deemed infertile, 43%–63% of women younger than 40 years will conceive naturally within the second year of trying (Dunson, Baird, & Colombo, 2004). For women who struggle with infertility, modern medicine can provide more options than ever before. Combine conventional treatment with the lifestyle recommendations for greatest effect.

Natural procreative technologies (NPT) are based on the Creighton Model FertilityCare System, which helps women identify ovulation through daily observations of cervical fluid. It was developed in response to the Catholic

Church's prohibition against IVF. Pre- and postovulatory estradiol and progesterone levels are sometimes assessed to diagnose hormonal deficiencies, and, when needed, medications are prescribed to enhance cervical mucus production (such as vitamin B6, guaifenesin, or antibiotics) or to increase luteal hormones (oral, vaginal, or transbuccal progesterone or human chorionic gonadotropin injections). Natural procreative technology has been studied in Ireland and Canada and has been shown to significantly increase birthrates over a 2-year period (Stanford, Parnell, & Boyle, 2008; Tham, Schliep, & Stanford, 2012).

The full range of ART for impaired fertility is beyond the scope of this chapter. While OB/GYNs and primary care physicians may offer some fertility services referral to a reproductive endocrinologist is appropriate for:

- Intrauterine insemination
- Clomid and other ovulation-inducing medications
- Recurrent miscarriage
- IVF

When to Begin Preparing for Conception

While living a healthy lifestyle is always of value, the evidence points most strongly to the 3- to 4-month window prior to conception when the oocyte matures. This period of time can used for physical, emotional, mental, and spiritual time for preparation. Changes in lifestyle, environmental chemical avoidance, and detoxification can be practiced. The fetal origins theory affirms the critical importance of the uterine environment and its influence on an individual's health over the course of their entire life (Barker, 2004). It is a compelling reason to follow a healthy lifestyle when trying to conceive as well as during pregnancy.

Susan's Case Revisited

Susan generally prefers a more natural approach and did not want to proceed with IVF and embryo freezing. I recommended to Susan that she stop her oral contraceptive to discover her natural menstrual cycle. When she did, she found it was a regular 31 days with 5–6 days of bleeding. Her temperature spike was consistent at day 17, and she had copious slippery cervical mucus. These signs suggest that she is currently fertile. We discussed keeping tabs on these fertility indicators and should a change occur, she might wish to alter her timing. She also is planning to negotiate with her department a job share that would allow her to begin attempting to conceive at age 32.

Summary: Preconception Counseling

1. Counsel all women about the impact of age on fertility. Explain that IVF success is also impacted by age.
2. Discuss the physical signs of fertility and set appropriate expectations for the time it will take to conceive.
3. Discuss discontinuation of dangerous behaviors (e.g., smoking, illicit drugs, and alcohol).
4. Discuss avoidance of environmental toxin exposures.
5. Assess immunizations. Recommended vaccines include MMR, varicella, DPT, and influenza.
6. Recommend an appropriate multivitamin.
7. Discuss a healthy fertility diet.
8. Review prescribed and over-the-counter medications and supplements carefully and make a plan to discontinue any that present risk or are not absolutely necessary.
9. Consider the need for genetic counseling and refer as needed.
10. Consider whether additional support is needed and consider supplements, herbal medicines, acupuncture, or referral to a reproductive endocrinologist.

REFERENCES

American College of Obstetricians and Gynecologists Committee on Health Care for Underserved Women, American Society for Reproductive Medicine Practice Committee, The University of California, San Francisco Program on Reproductive Health and the Environment. (2013). Committee Opinion Number 575, October 2013. *Obstet Gynecol, 122,* 931–935.

Barker, D. J. (2004). Developmental origins of adult health and disease. *J Epidemiol Community Health, 58,* 114–115. doi:10.1136/jech.58.2.114.

Berga, S. L., Marcus, M. D., Loucks, T. L., Hlastala, S., Ringham, R., & Krohn, M. A. (2003). Recovery of ovarian activity in women with functional hypothalamic amenorrhea who were treated with cognitive behavior therapy. *Fertil Steril, 80,* 976–981.

Boivin, J., Griffiths, E., & Venetis, C. A. (2011). Emotional distress in infertile women and failure of assisted reproductive technologies: Meta-analysis of prospective psychosocial studies. *BMJ, 342,* d223. doi: 10.1136/bmj.d223

Chavarro, J. E., Rich-Edwards, J. W., Rosner, B. A., & Willett, W. C. (2007a). Diet and lifestyle in the prevention of ovulatory disorder infertility. *Obstet Gynecol, 110*, 1050–1058.

Chavarro, J. E., Rich-Edwards, J. W., Rosner, B. A., & Willett, W. C. (2007b). A prospective study of dietary carbohydrate quantity and quality in relation to risk of ovulatory infertility. *Eur J Clin Nutr, 63*, 78–86. doi: 10.1038/sj.ejcn.1602904

Chavarro, J. E., Rich-Edwards, J. W., Rosner, B. A., & Willett, W. C. (2008a). Protein intake and ovulatory infertility. *Amer J Obstet Gynecol, 198*, 210, e1–e7. doi: http:// dx.doi.org/10.1016/j.ajog.2007.06.057

Chavarro, J. E., Rich-Edwards, J. W., Rosner, B. A., & Willett, W. C. (2008b). Use of multivitamins, intake of B vitamins, and risk of ovulatory infertility. *Fertil Steril, 89*, 668–676. doi: http://dx.doi.org/10.1016/j.fertnstert.2007.03.089

Chavarro, J. E., Rich-Edwards, J. W., Rosner, B. A., & Willett, W. C. (2009). Caffeinated and alcoholic beverage intake in relation to ovulatory disorder infertility. *Epidemiology, 20*, 374–381.

Czeizel, A. E., I Dudás, I., Paput, L., et al. (2011). Prevention of neural-tube defects with periconceptional folic acid, methylfolate, or multivitamins? *Ann Nutr Metab, 58*.

De Souza, M. J. (2003). Menstrual disturbances in athletes: A focus on luteal phase defects. *Med Sci Sports Exerc, 35*, 1553–1563.

Domar, A. D., Clapp, D., Slawsby, E. A., Dusek, J., Kessel, B., & Freizinger, M. (2000). Impact of group psychological interventions on pregnancy rates in infertile women. *Fertil Steril, 73*, 805–811.

Dunson, D., Baird, D., & Colombo, B. (2004). Increased infertility with age in men and women. *Obstet Gynecol, 103*, 51–56. doi: 10.1097/01.AOG.0000100153.24061.45

Environmental Working Group (EWG). (2011). *EWG'S 2011 shopper's guide helps cut consumer pesticide exposure*. Retrieved March 6, 2014, from http://www. ewg.org/news/news-releases/2011/06/13/ewgs-2011-shoppers-guide-helps-cu t-consumer-pesticide-exposure

Estefania, T., Lopez-del Burgo, C., Ruiz-Zambrana, A., et al. (2011). Dietary patterns and difficulty conceiving: A nested case–control study. *Fertil Steril, 96*, 1149–1153. doi: http://dx.doi.org/10.1016/j.fertnstert.2011.08.034

Fimrite, P. (2009). Chemicals, pollutants found in newborns. *San Francisco Chronicle*, December 3.

Food and Drug Administration. (2014). *Fish: What pregnant women and parents should know*. Draft updated advice by FDA and EPA. Retrieved June 23, 2014, from http:// www.fda.gov/Food/FoodborneIllnessContaminants/Metals/ucm393070.htm

Gerhard, I., Patek, A., Monga, B., Blank, A., & Gorkow, C. (1998). Matodynon® for female sterility [abstract in English]. *Forsch Komplementarmed, 5*, 272–278. doi:10.1159/000021154

Gerona, R. R., Woodruff, T. J., Dickenson, C. A., et al. (2013). BPA, BPA glucuronide, and BPA sulfate in mid-gestation umbilical cord serum in a northern California cohort. *Environ Sci Technol, 47*, 12477–12485. doi: 10.1021/es402764d

Goh, Y. I., Bollano, E., Einarson, T. R., & Koren, G. (2006). Prenatal multivitamin supplementation and rates of congenital anomalies: A meta-analysis. *J Obstetric Gynaecol Canada, 28*, 680–689.

Gudmundsdottir, S. L., Flanders, W. D., & Augestad, L. B. (2009). Physical activity and fertility in women: The North-Trøndelag Health Study. *Hum Reprod, 24,* 3196–3204. doi: 10.1093/humrep/dep337

Hammerli, K., Znoj, H., & Barth, J. (2009). The efficacy of psychological interventions for infertile patients: A meta-analysis examining mental health and pregnancy rate. *Hum Reprod, 15,* 279–295.

Hatch, E. E., Wise, L. A., Mikkelsen, E. M., et al. (2012). Caffeinated beverage and soda consumption and time to pregnancy. *Epidemiology, 23,* 393–401.

Kennedy, D., & Koren, G. (2012). Identifying women who might benefit from higher doses of folic acid in pregnancy. *Can Fam Physician, 58,* 394–397.

Koletzko, B., Cetin, I., & Brenna, J. T.; for the Perinatal Lipid Intake Working Group. (2007). Consensus statement: Dietary fat intakes for pregnant and lactating women. *Brit J Nutr, 98,* 873–877.

Koletzko, B., Lien, E., Agostoni, C., et al.; World Association of Perinatal Medicine Dietary Guidelines Working Group. (2008). The roles of long-chain polyunsaturated fatty acids in pregnancy, lactation and infancy: Review of current knowledge and consensus recommendations. *J Perinat Med, 36,* 5–14.

Maizes, V. (n.d.). *Reduce your environmental chemical exposure.* Retrieved March 6, 2014 from http://victoriamaizesmd.com/approaching-your-health/reduce-your-environmental-chemical-exposure

Manheimer, E., van der Windt, D., Cheng, K., et al. (2013). The effects of acupuncture on rates of clinical pregnancy among women undergoing in vitro fertilization: A systematic review and meta-analysis. *Human Reproduction Update, 19,* 696–713. doi:10.1093/humupd/dmt026

Manheimer, E., Zhang, G., Udoff, L., et al. (2008). Effects of acupuncture on rates of pregnancy and live birth among women undergoing in vitro fertilisation: systematic review and meta-analysis. *BMJ, 336,* 545–549. doi: 10.1136/bmj.39471.430451.BE

National Institutes of Health. (2011). *Iodine: Fact sheet for professionals.* Reviewed June 24, 2011. Retrieved January 2, 2015, from http://ods.od.nih.gov/factsheets/Iodine-HealthProfessional/

Nelson, C. J., Shindel, A. W., Naughton, C. K., et al. (2008). Prevalence and predictors of sexual problems, relationship stress, and depression in female partners of infertile couples. *J Sex Med, 5,* 1907–1914. doi: 10.1111/j.1743-6109.2008.00880.x

Roth, C, Magnus, P., Schjølberg, S., et al. (2011). Folic acid supplements in pregnancy and severe language delay in children. *JAMA, 306,* 1566–1573.

Royal College of Obstetricians and Gynaecologists. (2013, May). *Chemical exposures during pregnancy: Dealing with potential, but unproven, risks to child health.* Scientific Impact Statement No. 37.

Rudel, R. A., Gray, J. M., Engel, C. L., et al. (2010). Food packaging and bisphenol a and bis(2-ethyhexyl) phthalate exposure: Findings from a dietary intervention. *Environ Health Perspect, 119,* 914–920. doi: 10.1289/ehp.1003170.

Schmidt, R. J., Hansen, R. L., Hartiala, J., et al. (2011). Prenatal vitamins, one-carbon metabolism gene variants, and risk for autism. *Epidemiology, 22,* 476–485.

Stanford, J. B., Parnell, T. A., & Boyle, P. C. (2008). Outcomes from treatment of infertility with natural procreative technology in an Irish general practice. *J Am Board Fam Med, 21,* 375–384. doi: 10.3122/jabfm.2008.05.070239.

Stillerman, K. P., Mattison, D. R., Giudice, L. C., & Woodruff, T. J. (2008). Environmental exposures and adverse pregnancy outcomes: A review of the science. *Reproductive Sciences, 15,* 631–650. doi: 10.1177/1933719108322436

Surén, P., Roth, C., Bresnahan, M., et al. (2013). Association between maternal use of folic acid supplements and risk of autism spectrum disorders in children. *JAMA, 309,* 570–577.

Tham, E., Schliep, K., & Stanford, J. (2012). Natural procreative technology for infertility and recurrent miscarriage: Outcomes in Canadian family practice. *Can Fam Physician, 58,* e267–e274.

Tschugguel, W., & Berga, S. L. (2003). Treatment of functional hypothalamic amenorrhea with hypnotherapy. *Fertil Steril, 80,* 982–985.

Upton, R., ed. (1999). *Schisandra berry: Schisandra chinensis: Analytical, quality control, and therapeutic monograph.* Santa Cruz, CA: American Herbal Pharmacopoeia.

vom Saal, F. S., VandeVoort, C. A., Taylor, J. A., Welshons, W. V., Toutain, P. L., Hunt, P. A. (2014). Bisphenol A (BPA) pharmacokinetics with daily oral bolus or continuous exposure via silastic capsules in pregnant rhesus monkeys: Relevance for human exposures. *Reproductive Toxicology, 45,* 105–116. doi: 10.1016/j.reprotox.2014.01.007

Vujkovic, M., de Vries, J. H., Lindemans, J., et al. (2010). The preconception Mediterranean dietary pattern in couples undergoing in vitro fertilization/intracytoplasmic sperm injection treatment increases the chance of pregnancy. *Fertil Steril, 94,* 2096–2101. doi: http://dx.doi.org/10.1016/j.fertnstert.2009.12.079

Wise, L. A., Rothman, K. J., Mikkelsen, E. M., Sørensen, H. T., Riis, A. H., & Hatch, E. E. (2012). A prospective cohort study of physical activity and time to pregnancy. *Fertil Steril, 97,* 1136–1142, e4. doi: http://dx.doi.org/10.1016/j.fertnstert.2012.02.025

Zheng, C. H., Huang, G. Y., Zhang, M. M., & Wang, W. (2012). Effects of acupuncture on pregnancy rates in women undergoing in vitro fertilization: A systematic review and meta-analysis. *Fertil Steril, 97,* 599–611. doi: http://dx.doi.org/10.1016/j.fertnstert.2011.12.007

SUGGESTED RESOURCES

Domar, A. (2004). *Conquering infertility.* New York, NY: Penguin.

Indichova, J. (2001). *Inconceivable: A woman's triumph over despair and statistics.* New York, NY: Three Rivers Press.

Maizes, V. (2013). *Be fruitful: The essential guide to maximizing fertility and giving birth to a healthy child.* New York, NY: Scribner.

Wechsler, T. (2006). *Taking charge of your fertility, 10th anniversary edition.* New York, NY: Collins.

15

Pregnancy and Lactation

JACQUELYN M. PAYKEL

CASE STUDY

Teresa is a 24-year-old gravida 2, para 1 Hispanic female who presents for her first OB appointment at 8 weeks gestation. She is complaining of moderate nausea with occasional emesis, constipation, and headaches. Her first pregnancy was complicated by headaches, fetal macrosomia (normal diabetic screening), and induction at 39 weeks gestation for pregnancy-induced hypertension. Her son was born vaginally weighing 9 pounds 6 ounces and is 13 months old. Teresa's BMI is 32.5, BP 132/78, hematocrit 31%; she is, otherwise, healthy. She has a dedicated spouse and excellent familial support. She states that her most bothersome symptoms include nausea and "feeling tired all the time."

The journey of pregnancy is unique in medicine as it offers healthcare providers the opportunity to collaborate with women and assist them in maximizing preventive health measures that can last a lifetime. It is our opportunity as integrative clinicians to reinforce healthy lifestyle choices and encourage new self-care practices by engaging the whole person: mind, body, spirit, and community. Most women are motivated during pregnancy to improve their health because they sense that their actions will have a direct impact on the growing life within.

It is important to respect the impact of conventional medicine on the decline of perinatal and maternal morbidity and mortality over the last century. Maternal mortality in the United States has decreased from 850/100,000 in 1900 to 18.5/100,000 in 2013 (Kassenbaum et al., 2013). Engaging women in an *integrative* approach to their pregnancies—combining the best of conventional and the mind-body-spirit-community approach—can result in better maternal/neonatal health and a richer pregnancy experience.

Preconception

PRECONCEPTION COUNSELING

Preconception counseling is intended to open a dialogue about a woman's reproductive health and educate her about the importance of pregnancy planning so that she may optimize her health and take actions to optimize her baby's health (American College of Obstetricians and Gynecologists [ACOG], 2005). Collaboration with a trusted healthcare professional encourages the transition from knowledge acquisition to implementation of a healthy lifestyle. For example, in one study, though 80% of women knew the benefits of folic acid supplementation to prevent birth defects, only 27% regularly consumed multivitamins with at least 400 µg of folic acid prior to pregnancy (Lorenz et al., 2007). In another study, 89% of participants who were not currently taking a supplement indicated they would take a vitamin if recommended by their healthcare provider (March of Dimes, 2004). In general, women who participate in preconception counseling are more likely than their counterparts to change behaviors associated with adverse pregnancy outcomes (e.g., folic acid supplementation and eliminating alcohol consumption) (Elsinga, 2008).

Since approximately 50% of all pregnancies are unintended, it is important to offer preconception screening at routine annual exams to all women of reproductive age—not solely to the 15% of women who intentionally seek medical advice in preparation for pregnancy (Henshaw, 1998; Lorenz et al., 2007). Currently, only 16% of primary care physicians in the United States offer preconception counseling during routine annual exams (Henderson, Weisman, & Grason, 2002).

MATERNAL WEIGHT

The abundance of processed foods containing trans fats and refined carbohydrates, and the simultaneous lack of fresh fruits, vegetables, whole grains, and low-fat meats in the typical American diet contribute not only to the public's health but also specifically to pregnancy outcomes.

The negative effects are synergized by the sedentary nature of our society. Today, over 50% of women of childbearing age in the United States are either overweight or obese (Flegal, 2012). Obesity during pregnancy increases a woman's risk of miscarriage, fetal malformations (including neural tube defects [NTDs]), gestational diabetes, hypertensive disorders of pregnancy, thromboembolism, preterm labor, and intrauterine fetal demise. Delivery complications include an increased rate of labor induction, oxytocin augmentation, longer labors, and instrumental deliveries. Obese women are twice as likely as their normal-weight counterparts to have a cesarean delivery due to labor dystocia or fetal intolerance. If cesarean delivery occurs, they are more likely to experience intraoperative or postoperative complications such as hemorrhage, endometritis, and wound breakdown (ACOG, 2013b).

In addition, maternal obesity increases the risk of fetal macrosomia, and the subsequent risk of birth injury is twice as high. Children of obese mothers are three times more likely than their counterparts to be overweight by the age of 7 years and to suffer from a number of health problems including diabetes and its comorbidities.

On the other extreme of the weight spectrum, approximately 13.2% of childbearing aged women are underweight (CDC, 2007). Women with a BMI of less than 19.7 kg/m^2 at the time of conception are more likely to experience preterm labor and deliver low-birth-weight infants—both of which contribute to neonatal morbidity.

The preconception period, when a woman's focus turns to getting pregnant and optimizing her health for her child's welfare, is an opportune time to utilize motivational interviewing (MI) techniques, which foster a spirit of collaboration between provider and patient and encourage the mother-to-be to embrace a healthier lifestyle including dietary changes and increased physical activity (ACOG, 2009).

NUTRITION

Healthy nutrition during the preconception period can be thought of as the foundation for a lifetime of healthy choices. Two priorities should be emphasized regarding food choices: (1) improved nutritional value of caloric intake and (2) reduction of chemical load. One example of such a diet is the Mediterranean diet, which emphasizes whole grains; fruits and vegetables; iron- and calcium-rich foods; plant protein; animal protein from fish, poultry, and dairy; and monounsaturated fats while minimizing red meat, sweets, and processed foods. A recent study showed that women who were overweight or obese prior to pregnancy were less likely to deliver preterm if they followed the Mediterranean diet during pregnancy (Saunders et al., 2014). Another study demonstrated that children whose mothers consumed a high-quality Mediterranean diet throughout pregnancy experienced an 88% reduction in wheeze and a 45% reduction in allergy in their first 6 years of life (Chatzi et al., 2008).

The chemical load in our food supply is of concern for women anticipating pregnancy and the developing fetus. Decreasing one's exposure to pesticides, preservatives, additives, artificial sweeteners, and processed foods is advised.

> If a woman's budget does not allow for an all-organic diet, use the Environmental Working Group's list of "least contaminated" and "most contaminated" foods as a guide, available at www.ewg.org. Hormone-free foods such as milk, eggs, and meat are also readily available (Fischer-Rasmussen, Kjaer, Dahl, & Asping, 1991; Roscoe & Matteson, 2002).

ALCOHOL CONSUMPTION

Prenatal alcohol consumption, especially binge drinking, is a leading cause of preventable developmental disabilities and mental retardation in children. Well-woman visits are an optimal time to discuss the effects of alcohol on the developing embryo early in pregnancy—when most women do not know that they are pregnant. Alcohol consumption by women of reproductive age is common. A recent survey of 345,076 women aged 18–44 in the United States revealed that just over 50% of women consumed "any alcohol" and 15% had participated in binge drinking (four or more drinks on any occasion) within the past 30 days (CDC, 2012). Binge drinking has been found to be higher among women who smoked, those not planning a pregnancy, and those with low self-esteem (Tough, Tofflemire, Clarke, & Newburn-Cook, 2006). Most women, however, do change their behavior when they realize they are pregnant. One epidemiologic study in Canada consisted of 1,042 phone interviews with women who had recently delivered. Eighty percent of the respondents reported consuming alcohol preconceptually, 50% during early pregnancy before they were aware of pregnancy, and 18% after pregnancy awareness. Binge-drinking percentages were 32% during preconception, 11% during early conception, and 0% after pregnancy awareness. Women need to be educated about the risks of alcohol consumption during early pregnancy and encouraged to minimize alcohol intake during their reproductive years.

SUPPLEMENTS

Theoretically, our food supply should provide all the vitamins and minerals we need. In reality, most of us do not eat well enough to meet the recommended dietary allowances (RDA) published by the Institute of Medicine. In addition, the requirements for folic acid, calcium, iron, and vitamins D, C, and B increase during pregnancy. Supplements should be initiated in the preconception period and continued throughout pregnancy (Gardiner et al., 2008).

Prenatal Vitamins

While there is debate regarding the necessity of a daily prenatal vitamin during pregnancy, a number of reviews have found benefit. A large randomized controlled trial (RCT) demonstrated a decreased incidence of NTD, cardiovascular defects, limb defects, cleft palate, and other birth defects in the offspring of mothers who consumed a daily multivitamin (Czeizel, 2004). A systematic review of nine trials ($n = 15,378$) found a decrease in the number of low-birth-weight, small-for-gestational-age babies, and maternal anemia when low- or middle-income women took multivitamins most days during pregnancy (Rumbold, Middleton, & Crowther, 2005). While additional outcomes-based research is needed including a review of side effects and potential overdose (Haider & Bhutta, 2006), current recommendations suggest that, unless contraindicated, all women of reproductive age should take a daily multivitamin containing at least 400 µg of folic acid.

Folic Acid

Folate is a naturally occurring, water-soluble vitamin readily found in green leafy vegetables that is important for the health of DNA, production of red blood cells, metabolism of amino acids, and growth of the fetus and placenta. Folic acid is a synthetic compound that is used as a folate supplement. Folic acid consumption before conception and during the first trimester reduces the incidence of primary and secondary NTD such as spina bifida and anencephaly as well as certain congenital heart defects (De-Regil et al., 2010; Locksmith & Duff, 1998; Lumley, Watson, Watson, & Bower, 2001).

The RDA for folic acid, 400 μg, was first established as by the US Public Health Service in 1992 for all women of childbearing age (CDC, 1992). If a personal or family history of children born with NTD exists, this recommendation is increased to 4,000 μg of folic acid. It is estimated that at least 70% of NTD could be prevented if mothers consumed an adequate amount of folic acid (CDC, 1992).

Calcium

Most women in the United States do not consume the RDA of calcium prior to or during pregnancy (Harville, 2004; Thomas & Weisman, 2006). Calcium is important for adequate fetal bone development. Adequate calcium intake during pregnancy has been associated with decreased preterm delivery rates, higher birth weights, and decreased risk of maternal hypertensive illnesses. The current recommendation for calcium intake (diet plus supplement) during the preconception period and throughout pregnancy and lactation is 1,000–1,300 mg daily (Institute of Medicine, 2011). Depending on the woman, dietary intake of calcium could suffice. In general, one cup of green leafy vegetables contains 100 mg calcium, milk has 300 mg per 8 ounces, and cheese contains 400 mg per 2-ounce serving. When considering supplements, it is helpful to remember that calcium citrate is more easily absorbed than calcium carbonate (Reinwald, 2008).

Vitamin D

Vitamin D has many functions in the body, including maintenance of bone integrity and calcium homeostasis. Maternal vitamin D deficiency can contribute to bone diseases of the infant including rickets and osteomalacia (Pawley & Bishop, 2004). Research has suggested that vitamin D deficiency may also be associated with severe preeclampsia, gestational diabetes, increased risk of infection, cesarean delivery, and low offspring birth weight. However, a 2012 Cochrane review stated that the benefits of vitamin D supplementation to avert such complications during pregnancy are yet to be determined.

Populations at highest risk for vitamin D deficiency are African Americans, women not exposed to enough sunlight, women with inadequate dietary vitamin D intake, and women who wear head coverings (Wolpowitz & Gilchrest, 2006). The debate continues regarding the recommended daily dosage, safety of higher doses, and benefits that will be realized with vitamin D supplementation. Currently, the Food and Nutrition Board recommends 600 IU, the Endocrine Society 1,500–2,000 IU and the Vitamin D Council 4,000–6,000 IU of vitamin D3 daily (Vitamin D Council, 2014). More research is needed before definitive recommendations can be made.

Iron

Women experience a dilutional anemia during pregnancy. Normally, the maternal blood supply expands 40% during a singleton pregnancy, and over 50% with multiple gestations. Anemia during pregnancy is defined as hemoglobin and hematocrit of less than 11 g/dL and 33% in the first or third trimester and 10.5 g/dL and 32% in the second trimester. If supplementation is warranted, iron supplements should be taken with vitamin C to maximize absorption. Calcium-rich foods should not be consumed simultaneously, as calcium impairs iron absorption. A systematic review of forty trials (n = 12,706) revealed less postpartum anemia in women who routinely took iron supplementation during pregnancy. However, the effect on maternal and infant outcomes remains uncertain. It was concluded that more studies are needed before a recommendation can be made about routine iron supplementation during pregnancy (Peña-Rosas & Viteri, 2006).

Vitamin A

Vitamin A contributes to fetal vision, immunity, skin development, and overall growth. There are two forms of vitamin A. *Preformed vitamin A* comes from animal sources such as liver (e.g., cod liver oil, which is a source of highly concentrated vitamin A) and whole milk; this form of vitamin A is easily absorbed and is readily converted to retinol—the active form of vitamin A. *Provitamin A carotenoids* (e.g., beta-carotene), found in fruits and vegetables, are more difficult to absorb and less readily converted to retinol. The RDA for retinol in pregnancy is 2,500 IU per day and 4,300 IU per day during lactation. The tolerable upper intake level (UL) of retinol for pregnant and lactating women is 10,000 IU (Institute of Medicine, Food and Nutrition Board, 2001). Higher levels may result in adverse effects such as miscarriage, birth defects, osteoporosis, and central nervous system disorders (Bendich, 1989). Vitamin A toxicity generally arises from excessive supplementation rather than dietary intake.

ESSENTIAL FATTY ACIDS: FISH AND FISH OIL SUPPLEMENTS

The essential fatty acids (EFAs), such as omega-6 and omega-3 fatty acids, are essential for cellular function and structure. They are considered *essential* because they cannot be synthesized by the body and must be consumed in the food supply. There are three major types of omega-3 fatty acids ingested in the diet, alpha-linolenic acid (ALA), eicosapentaenoic acid (EPA), and docosahexaenoic acid (DHA). Several studies have shown an association between increased DHA and enhanced cognitive, motor, and visual development in infants (Jacobson et al., 2008). There is also evidence that fish oil taken during pregnancy may increase the length of gestation by two to three days, slightly increase birth weight, and decrease the number of babies born before 34 weeks gestation (Facchinetti, Fazzio, & Venturini, 2005; Makrides, Duley, & Olsen, 2006).

There is a public concern about mercury toxicity with the consumption of fish. Excessive mercury consumption can cause neurologic impairment in developing brains. For this reason, in 2004 the Environmental Protection Agency and other officials recommended that pregnant and nursing women should limit fish intake to "no more than two servings per week." The Environmental Protection Agency changed course in 2014, stating that women who are pregnant or nursing *should* eat 2–3 servings of a variety of low-mercury fish weekly (about 8–12 ounces) (Environmental Protection Agency, 2014). Officials state that health benefits of consuming most types of fish far outweigh any risk. Fish known to contain high levels of mercury (tilefish from the Gulf of Mexico, king mackerel, swordfish, and shark) should still be avoided by pregnant and nursing women. White (albacore) tuna should be limited to 6 ounces per week. Many regions in the United States also have additional local fish consumption advisories. See the US Environmental Protection Agency's website for more details: http://www.epa.gov/waterscience/fish/advice/index.html).

Although there are no current guidelines regarding optimal DHA intake during pregnancy (Greenberg, Bell, & Van Ausdal, 2008), many experts recommend 200 to 350 mg/day. Most fish oil supplements contain less than 1 to 2 ppb of mercury. Because the amount of fish oil used (1–2 g/day) is far less than the amount of seafood recommended (200 g twice a week) supplements have an inconsequential risk of mercury toxicity (Greenberg et al., 2008).

PROBIOTICS

Probiotic supplements contain live microorganisms that replenish beneficial gut flora. Improved gut biome results in a healthier gastrointestinal tract and improved bowel motility and potentially decreases absorption of allergens.

Atopy and other allergic conditions are on the rise around the world. It is well known that women with atopic skin disorders are more likely to have an offspring with the same; however, atopy is on the rise in all children, not just those whose mothers are affected. One double-blinded RCT found that when pregnant women were supplemented with *Lactobacillus rhamnosus* HN001 from 35 weeks gestation through 6 months if breastfeeding, and infants were supplemented from birth to 2 years of age, there was a significant reduction in the risk of developing atopic dermatitis and possibly also atopic sensitization in high-risk infants to age 6 years (Wickens et al., 2013).

Another study evaluated the use of probiotics, both orally and vaginally, on the rate of preterm delivery. The vaginal application of yogurt with live cultures resulted in an 81% reduction of recurrent bacterial vaginosis during pregnancy, but this was not powered adequately to assess the effect on preterm labor and delivery rates (Othman, Neilson, & Alfirevic, 2007). A study published in 2014 demonstrated that daily prenatal probiotic therapy has the potential to reduce group B strep colonization (Hanson et al., 2014). Larger randomized controlled trials are needed before formal recommendations can be made.

Probiotics do not appear to pose any safety concerns for pregnant and lactating women (Elias, Bozzo, & Einarson, 2011).

Early Pregnancy

NAUSEA AND VOMITING OF PREGNANCY

It is estimated that 90% of pregnant women experience nausea and vomiting of pregnancy (NVP), which usually starts between 4 and 6 weeks gestation, peaks around 9 weeks, and resolves by 16 weeks (ACOG, 2004; Ebrahimi, Maltepe, & Einarson, 2010). Up to 10% of women will experience NVP throughout their entire pregnancy, and 2% will experience hyperemesis gravidarum, which is characterized by protracted vomiting, electrolyte imbalance, an inability to take in adequate nutrition, and weight loss greater than 5% (ACOG, 2004). The etiology of NVP is elusive, but pregnancy-related hormonal fluctuations and delayed gastric emptying are thought to play a role. Reassurance, dietary changes, lifestyle changes, acupressure wrist bands, ginger (*Zingiber officinale*), vitamin B6, doxylamine, and prescription antiemetics are all useful while supporting a woman through NVP.

Dietary Changes

Simple changes in food selections and the manner of consumption may reduce NVP. Typical recommendations include eating small meals or sipping liquids every 2 hours, consuming bland foods and foods rich in vitamin B6 (e.g., chicken, avocados, bananas, whole grains, and corn) and avoiding spicy food, fatty food, and food with strong smells. Postprandial nausea can be ameliorated by sucking on peppermint candy, drinking peppermint tea, or brushing teeth. Eating simple, dry carbohydrates before getting out of bed, snacking on nuts between meals, and consuming very cold or frozen liquids to reduce the metallic taste in one's mouth are also helpful (Ebrahimi et al., 2010). There is little published evidence that dietary changes affect NVP, with the exception of a small study indicating that meals high in protein were more likely to eliminate NVP than fatty or carbohydrate-laden meals (ACOG, 2004; Latva-Pukkila, Isolauri, & Laitinen, 2010). Prenatal vitamins should be taken before bed or changed to a chewable vitamin containing 400 μg of folic acid until NVP resolves.

Acupressure of P6

Acupressure, acupuncture, or nerve stimulation of the pericardium 6 (P6) on the wrist (approximately three finger breadths above the crease on the volar aspect of the forearm) has been proposed to decrease nausea and vomiting in pregnancy (Belluomini, Litt, Lee, & Katz, 1994; Knight et al., 2001; O'Brien, Relyea, & Taerun, 1996). The Food and Drug Administration has approved Sea-Bands, which are commercially available for this purpose. A review of two large RCTs and another standardized review, however, found equivocal results (see Figure 15.1). Despite conflicting evidence of efficacy, acupressure is a safe, noninvasive, and inexpensive treatment that helps some women with NVP.

Botanicals

Ginger (*Zingiber officinale*), chamomile (*Matricaria recutita*), peppermint (*Mentha piperita*) leaf, and pickled umeboshi (a member of the apricot family) are botanicals traditionally used to decrease nausea during pregnancy. Only ginger has been adequately studied during pregnancy. Multiple studies support its efficacy for nausea during pregnancy (Borrelli et al., 2005; Fischer-Rasmussen, Kjaer, Dahl, & Asping, 1991; Vutyavanich, Kraisarin, & Ruangsri, 2001). A review of 12 studies concluded that daily dosages of

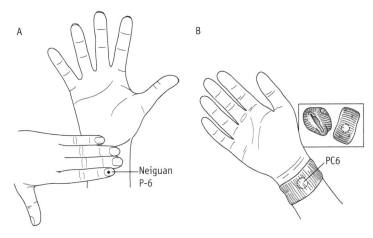

FIGURE 15.1. Demonstration of pericardium 6 acupressure point. *Source*: Adapted from Reikel D, *Integrative Medicine*. 2nd ed. Philadelphia, Pennsylvania: Saunders Elsevier; 2007.

less than 1,500 mg reduced nausea but did not have a significant impact on vomiting episodes. This review concluded that ginger did not pose a risk for adverse events during pregnancy (Viljoen, 2014). The German Commission E contraindicates ginger during pregnancy; however, no reason is provided. The US Food and Drug Administration lists it as generally regarded as safe as a food additive. Dried ginger is a stronger antiemetic than fresh. Standard dosing in RCTs is 250 to 1,000 mg of dried ginger per day taken in 3 to 4 divided doses (White, 2007). Doses over 4 g/day can theoretically act as an anticoagulant.

Vitamin B6 (Pyridoxine)

Vitamin B6 has also been shown to reduce NVP. The typical dose of pyridoxine for NVP is 40 to 60 mg/day. To prevent adverse neurological effects, the maximum dose should not exceed 100 mg/day. Combining vitamin B6 with doxylamine (Unisom) is safe and even more effective (ACOG, 2004; Thaver, Saeed, & Bhutta, 2006). In randomized trials, the combination of Vitamin B6 (10–25 mg every 8 hours) and doxylamine (25 mg before bed and in the morning and afternoon) yielded a 70% reduction in NVP. The American College of Obstetricians and Gynecologists recommends it as a first-line therapy (ACOG, 2004). The combination of pyridoxine and doxylamine is now available as a prescription drug. In 2013, the FDA approved Diclegis for NVP refractory to nonpharmacologic treatment.

Homeopathic Remedies

Homeopathic remedies include *Arsenicum, Colchicum, Ipecac, Nux vomica, Phosphorus, Pulsatilla,* and *Sepia.* There is no compelling evidence that any of these remedies significantly reduce NVP. A trained homeopath should be consulted if a woman desires this approach (DiGaetano, 2007).

THREATENED ABORTION

Twenty percent of all pregnancies are affected by bleeding prior to 20 weeks gestation (i.e., threatened abortion); 50% of these women will miscarry (Everett, 1997). When a woman calls with a complaint of first-trimester bleeding, she should be evaluated. Not only will she need emotional support during this anxiety-provoking time, but a thorough history, physical exam including cervical cultures, a wet prep, and pelvic ultrasound should be performed. A woman can be reassured that if fetal cardiac activity is present on ultrasound, the risk of miscarrying decreases from 50% to 3% (Scroggins, Smucker, & Krishen, 2000). Laboratory evaluation should include complete blood count, Rh typing, and serum hCG (Griebel, Halvorsen, Golemon, & Day, 2005).

Sensitive communication and reassurance for a woman who is experiencing a threatened abortion are vital: (1) Explain the potential concerns about early gestational bleeding, including spontaneous abortion (SAB), ectopic pregnancy, and the potential for heavy vaginal bleeding. (2) Address any feelings of guilt she might be experiencing regarding herself being the cause of the potential miscarriage. (3) Inform her that 50% of SABs are due to chromosomal abnormalities and that her actions, including recent sexual activity, have not been found to contribute to miscarriage rates.

Bed rest has not been adequately studied to recommend it to prevent miscarriage (Aleman, 2005). However, low-stress activities, a supportive network community, and reliance on one's spirituality during a potentially stressful time could be of emotional benefit.

ABDOMINAL CRAMPING

As the uterus grows, women may experience cramping and be concerned about a potential miscarriage. Round ligament pain is typically described as a "cramping" pain that is associated with prolonged standing or sudden twist-ing movements; the discomfort can usually be reproduced on exam. Inquiring about additional symptoms to rule out miscarriage, ectopic pregnancy, con-stipation, or urinary tract infection is important. Supportive interventions included rest, application of heat, chamomile tea, red raspberry leaf tea, and acetaminophen.

Herbal Teas

Chamomile (*Matricaria recutita)* and red raspberry (*Rubus* spp.) leaf tea have been traditionally used to decrease menstrual cramps. No formal studies have been completed to prove efficacy in alleviating uterine cramping during preg-nancy. The Natural Medicines Comprehensive Database lists these herbs as generally recognized as safe when used in amounts commonly found in foods. Two to four cups of tea per day is probably more than sufficient and carries a low risk of adverse events (Evans & Aronson, 2005).

CONSTIPATION, GAS, AND BLOATING

Increased progesterone throughout pregnancy slows transit in the gastrointes-tinal tract, which can result in constipation, gas, and bloating. Dietary recom-mendations include hydration, 30 minutes of exercise per day, consumption of frequent small meals throughout the day, and an increase in dietary fiber (i.e., vegetables and fruits like prunes, dates, and raisins). A tablespoon of ground flax seed or wheat germ added to cereal, cottage cheese, yogurt, or salads also serves as an excellent source of fiber. One meta-analysis compared fiber supplements and mild laxatives. The laxatives were more helpful than fiber supplements but were more likely to cause diarrhea and abdominal pain (Jewell & Young, 2001).

Probiotics may also prove helpful for functional constipation. One recent pilot study ($N = 20$) demonstrated that a multispecies probiotic mixture containing *Bifidobacterium bifidum* W23, *Bifidobacterium lactis* W52, *Bifidobacterium longum* W108, *Lactobacillus casei* W79, *Lactobacillus plantarum* W62, and *Lactobacillus rhamnosus* W71 resulted in a signifi-cant increase in the number of bowel movements per week, with decreased straining, and a reduction in abdominal pain and reflux (de Milliano et al., 2012).

Mid and Late Pregnancy

EXERCISE

Exercise transmits an improved sense of well-being and may improve maternal health during pregnancy. Very few high-quality studies have assessed either positive or detrimental effects on maternal or fetal well-being. One systematic review indicated there is insufficient data available to make a recommendation regarding the risks or benefits of aerobic exercise for either mother or baby (Kramer & Kakuma, 2006).

BACK PAIN

Two-thirds of women suffer from back pain during pregnancy. Recommended lifestyle changes include wearing comfortable shoes, correcting one's posture, sitting and standing with support, lifting from bent knees, sleeping with extra pillows, and taking warm baths (Evans & Aronson, 2005b). Interventions include maternity binders, massage, chiropractic, physical therapy, acupuncture, back exercises, application of hot and cold compresses, and rest. Valerian (*Valeriana officinalis*) has been recommended for back pain because of its muscle-relaxant qualities. Valerian is generally recognized as safe as a flavoring agent, but it has an unknown safety profile during pregnancy when consumed in medicinal amounts. There are no contraindications to valerian during pregnancy in the literature, including the German Commission E and the *American Herbal Products Botanical Safety Handbook, 2nd Edition* (Gardner & McGuffin, 2013).

Very little research has been conducted to prove the efficacy of treatments for back pain during pregnancy. In a systematic review of multiple modalities water exercises, pelvic-tilt exercises, physiotherapy, and acupuncture were shown to help relieve back pain more than usual prenatal care (Pennick & Young, 2007). A more recent prospective randomized trial of 66 women demonstrated a significant improvement of pain and quality of life after 4 to 8 weeks of progressive muscle relaxation accompanied by music. The authors acknowledged the need for larger RCTs to confirm their findings (Akmese & Oran, 2014).

HEARTBURN

Gastroesophageal reflux disease (GERD) affects 80% of women in late pregnancy. Current treatment recommendations include dietary changes (elimination of caffeine and spicy and tomato-based foods), other lifestyle changes, antacids, antihistamines, and proton-pump inhibitors. No studies have been done to assess dietary and lifestyle interventions. A systematic review of three RCTs (N = 286) using three medicinal protocols (IM prostigmine, antacid, and antacid plus ranitidine) found favorable results in the treatment groups. More data is needed to make recommendations about treatment of heartburn in pregnancy (Dowswell & Neilson, 2008).

STRETCH MARKS

Striae gravidarum (SG) generally start to appear after the 24th week of pregnancy. Stretch marks most commonly develop on the gravid abdomen, thighs, buttocks, and breasts. Over 50% of women will develop this cosmetic concern. Younger maternal age and higher maternal weight gain during pregnancy are associated with SG. Higher fetal birth weight, family history of SG, and increasing gestational age at delivery are associated with moderate-to-severe SG (Asman et al., 2007). Many products are available on the market purporting to improve the cosmetic appearance of SG; most are not helpful. Studies have demonstrated that neither cocoa butter nor olive oil reduced the formation or severity of stretch marks when compared with placebo (Buchanan, Fletcher, & Reid, 2010; Osman et al., 2008; Soltanipour et al., 2014). One study (n = 100) comparing Trofolastin (active ingredient *Centella asiatica* extract) with placebo found that women in the active arm developed fewer stretch marks (Young & Jewell, 1996).

VARICOSE VEINS

Increased blood volume, obstructed venous flow, and hormonally mediated relaxation of the vasculature during pregnancy all contribute to the development of varicose veins. Lower extremity elevation may decrease symptoms but does not alleviate varicosities (Jones & Carek, 2008). Compression stockings are frequently offered as a conservative therapy. No studies have proven efficacy (Bamigboye & Smyth, 2007), but compression stockings have been shown to improve leg symptoms caused by varicose veins (Thaler et al., 2001).

The botanicals butcher's broom (*Ruscus aculeatus*) and horse chestnut (*Aesculus hippocastanum*) seed extract have been used for treating chronic venous insufficiency. Although there are several studies addressing the use of a specific horse chestnut extract during pregnancy in the German literature, there is insufficient evidence of safety to recommend its use. The same is true for butcher's broom (Jones & Carek, 2008).

HEMORRHOIDS

Warm water soaks, application of ice, hygiene measures, and avoidance of prolonged sitting are practical interventions for the treatment of hemorrhoids during pregnancy. Dietary modifications such as increasing fiber and fluids, and topical application of witch hazel (*Hammamelis virginiana*), have not been adequately studied during pregnancy (Quijano & Abalos, 2005). Some practitioners recommend homeopathic arnica gel for external hemorrhoids though the safety profile is unknown. Nonhomeopathic arnica gels should not be used during pregnancy.

PREECLAMPSIA

Preeclampsia affects 2% to 8% of women, most frequently in women with chronic hypertension, obesity, those over the age of 34, or nulliparous. The definition of preeclampsia has recently changed. It is now defined by the ACOG as persistent elevation in blood pressure (moderate: 140–159/90–109 mm Hg or severe: greater than or equal to 160/100 mm Hg measured on two occasions at least 4 hours apart) that is associated with proteinuria (300 mg in 24 urine protein collection) *or* new onset of thrombocytopenia, impaired liver function, renal insufficiency, pulmonary edema, or visual or cerebral disturbances. Preeclampsia may result in uteroplacental insufficiency with decreased blood flow to the fetus. The precise etiology of this condition continues to elude science, which makes prevention difficult.

Low-Dose Aspirin

Women with a history of early-onset preeclampsia and preterm delivery before 34 weeks gestation may benefit from low-dose aspirin starting in the late first trimester (ACOG, 2013a).

Supplements

There is insufficient evidence to recommend Vitamin D, fish oil, or garlic supplementation to reduce the incidence of preeclampsia at this time (ACOG, 2013a). In a systematic review of 12 trials ($N = 15,206$), calcium supplementation has been found to decrease the risk of pregnancy induced hypertension and preeclampsia. The effect was greatest in high-risk groups (e.g., prior history of preeclampsia) and those with a low baseline calcium intake. Given this data, women should be encouraged to obtain the recommended daily intake for calcium (Hofmeyr, Atallah, & Duley, 2006).

Lifestyle Modification

Salt restriction and bed rest have not been shown to reduce the incidence of preeclampsia. Large RCTs are needed to assess exercise as a means to reverse endothelial dysfunction and decrease risk of developing preeclampsia (ACOG, 2013a).

FETAL MALPRESENTATION AT TERM

Breech presentation occurs in 3% to 4% of term pregnancies (Vetura, Martin, Curtin, & Mathews, 1999) The Term Breech Trial (an international, multicenter RCT) demonstrated significantly higher rates of perinatal mortality, neonatal mortality, and serious neonatal morbidity for planned vaginal breech deliveries compared with planned cesarean delivery (ACOG, 2006b; Hannah et al., 2000). If the fetus remains breech at 36 weeks gestation, the options in conventional medicine are (1) await spontaneous version; if this does not occur, proceed with cesarean delivery during the 39th week of pregnancy; (2) attempt an external cephalic version (ECV) after 36 weeks gestation. An ECV involves applying pressure to the maternal abdomen to cause the fetus to somersault to vertex presentation. This should be performed in a hospital setting and is successful approximately 58% of the time (ACOG, 2001).

Moxibustion to the Bladder 67 Point

Moxibustion entails burning a stick of mugwort to warm the Bladder 67 acupuncture point on the lateral aspect of the fifth toes. A systematic review of three trials ($N = 597$) found that moxibustion reduced the need for external cephalic version (RR 0.47, 95% CI 0.33–0.66), though the quality of the studies was not considered rigorous (Coyle, Smith, & Peat, 2012).

Knee–Chest Position to Modify Oxiput-Posterior or Oxiput-Transverse to Oxiput-Anterior

In one small trial, women who assumed the knee–chest (compared with sitting upright) position for 10 minutes were more successful in converting an occiput-posterior (OP) or occiput-transverse (OT) presentation to an occiput-anterior (OA) position (RR 0.26, 95% CI 0.18–0.38). However, the recommendation of this same practice for 10 minutes twice daily before the onset of labor was not helpful to correct a malpresentation. Assuming this position during labor also reduced backache (Hunter, Hofmeyr, & Kulier, 2007).

ANTEPARTUM PERINEAL MASSAGE

Studies show that 70% of women who deliver babies need some sort of perineal repair after vaginal delivery, which can cause pain, discomfort, and impaired sexual function. A systematic review of four trials ($N = 2,480$) evaluated antepartum perineal massage (APM) and the need for perineal repair after vaginal delivery. Practiced as little as two times/week starting at 35 weeks, APM decreased the risk of perineal trauma that required sutures in nulliparous women. One trial involving 376 multiparous women showed a statistical decrease in ongoing perineal pain 3 months after delivery. The reviewers recommended that women be informed about the likely benefits of APM and given instructions how to do it (Beckmann & Garrett, 2006). This, however, should not be confused with intrapartum perineal massage, which has been found to have little value (Stamp, Kruzins, & Crowther, 2001).

Post-Term Pregnancy and Cervical Ripening

The rate of post-term pregnancies is 10%. This figure is reduced by labor inductions and cesarean deliveries that occur before 40 complete weeks of gestation. The first trimester ultrasound, the most accurate means of dating a pregnancy, reduces the rate of post-term pregnancy (Neilson, 1998). Post-term pregnancies can impact maternal and fetal well-being. Maternal risks include increased risk for fetal macrosomia, prolonged labor, perineal injury, and double the risk of cesarean delivery. Fetal risks include perinatal mortality, shoulder dystocia, neurologic injury, meconium-stained amniotic fluid, and altered cord pH. There is evidence to support cervical ripening to decrease maternal and neonatal morbidity and mortality associated with post-term pregnancies (Poma, 1999).

ACUPUNCTURE

A 2008 Cochrane Review of 14 trials ($N = 2,220$) concluded that there is a need for well-designed RCT on acupuncture and labor induction before recommendations can be made (Smith & Crowther, 2013).

HERBAL SUPPLEMENTS

Commonly prescribed herbs for labor induction include evening primrose (*Oenothera biennis*), black cohosh (*Actaea racemosa*), blue cohosh (*Caulophylum thalictoides*), and red raspberry leaves. Evening primrose oil is generally massaged into the cervix, whereas the others are taken orally. The role of herbs in cervical ripening and labor is still uncertain (Belew, 1999). The safety of black and blue cohosh during pregnancy is questionable and probably best avoided.

CASTOR OIL, BATH, AND/OR ENEMA

Castor oil has been used as a labor inducer dating back to ancient Egypt. Only one trial ($N = 100$) assessed castor oil as a labor induction agent as compared with no treatment. The study was of poor quality and had too few participants to confirm efficacy, though 57.7% of women in the treatment arm went into labor within 24 hours versus 4.2% of the control arm. Ingestion of castor oil can cause watery stools and abdominal cramping (Adair, 2000; Kelly, Kavanagh, & Thomas, 2013).

HOMEOPATHY

A systematic review of two double-blind RCTs of moderate quality ($N = 133$) demonstrated no difference between the women who received homeopathic *Caulophyllum* to induce labor and the control groups. There is insufficient evidence to recommend homeopathy for labor induction at this time. However, the hallmark of homeopathy is individualized treatment, and therefore, standardization of the treatment of a particular herb violates classical homeopathic treatment. Rigorous evaluations of individualized homeopathic therapies for labor induction are needed (Smith, 2003).

BREAST STIMULATION

Nipple stimulation causes the release of oxytocin from the posterior pituitary gland, resulting in increased uterine contractions, the onset of labor, and a decreased risk of post-term pregnancy and postpartum hemorrhage. Historically, midwives have used nipple stimulation to stimulate labor. A meta-analysis including six trials ($N = 719$) demonstrated an increased probability of labor initiation within 72 hours of nipple stimulation and reduced postpartum hemorrhage rates. The safety of this intervention has not been fully evaluated especially in high-risk populations (Kavanagh, Kelly, & Thomas, 2005).

SEXUAL INTERCOURSE

Sexual relations are frequently recommended as a natural method of labor initiation because breast stimulation results in oxytocin secretion and uterine contractions; theoretically, intercourse may stimulate the lower uterine segment directly resulting in the localized release of prostaglandins. Semen also contains prostaglandins, which may induce cervical ripening. A randomized trial of 210 women demonstrated no difference in earlier onset of labor in women who had increased sexual activity versus the control group (Tan, Yow, & Omar, 2007). In general, studies evaluating the effect of coitus on labor are of questionable quality and show equivocal results. There *is* an association between intercourse and preterm labor (Kavanagh et al., 2001; Summers, 1997).

MEMBRANE SWEEPING

A systematic review of 22 trials ($N = 2,797$) compared membrane sweeping, starting at 38 weeks gestation with no intervention or with prostaglandin use. Membrane sweeping resulted in a decrease in the duration of pregnancy and the number of women reaching 41 weeks gestation; it did not result in an increased cesarean rate or an increase in maternal and neonatal infection. However, women in the treatment group experienced more bleeding, irregular contractions, and pain during cervical exam (Boulvain, Stan, & Irion, 2005). The number needed to treat to avoid labor induction was eight (Goldberg, 2007).

ISOLATED AMNIOTOMY FOR LABOR INDUCTION
OR LABOR AUGMENTATION

A systematic review of two trials (N = 310) found insufficient data supporting amniotomy alone for labor induction (Bricker & Luckas, 2000). Another review published in 2007 (14 studies, N = 4,893) found that amniotomy to augment spontaneous labor was of no value in shortening the first stage of labor and may actually increase the cesarean delivery rate. Therefore, amniotomy is not recommended for labor induction or labor augmentation in either normally progressing labors or in prolonged labors (Smyth, Alldred, & Markham, 2007).

Labor and Delivery

NUTRITION DURING LABOR

In 1999 the American Society of Anesthesiology Task Force on Obstetrical Anesthesia recommended only "sips and chips" during labor because of the fear of aspiration if a cesarean delivery under general anesthesia was eventually needed (which is a rare occurrence). This recommendation was based on expert opinion due to the lack of evidence available at that time. A recent Cochrane Review assessed five studies (N = 3,130) that collectively demonstrated no benefits or harms of restricting fluids and foods during labor in women at low risk of needing anesthesia (Singata, Tranmer, & Gyte, 2013). In many countries outside of the United States, women are allowed to eat and drink during labor (Berghella, Baster, & Chauhan, 2008).

PAIN CONTROL IN LABOR

Pain modulation during labor is multifaceted. A woman's expectations, preparation for delivery through childbirth classes, and perception of control throughout the delivery experience can all impact her sense of pain control during labor (McCrea & Wright, 1999). The physical environment and relationships that she maintains with people present at delivery, including the hospital personnel, can also significantly impact pain control during labor. All these affect her overall level of satisfaction with the birth experience. It is recommended that the physical environment be kept as calm as possible and that the laboring woman and her partner be included in the decision-making process.

Home-Like Versus Institutional Settings for Birth

A 2005 systematic review of six trials ($N = 8,677$) found that women who delivered in a home-like setting were more likely to have a spontaneous vaginal delivery, initiate breastfeeding, and have a higher satisfaction with their birth experience. They were less likely to need pain medication during labor or to have an episiotomy. However, there was a trend toward higher perinatal mortality in the home-like setting (five trials, $N = 8,529$; RR 1.83, 95% CI 0.99–3.38) (Hodnett, Downe, Edwards, & Walsh, 2005).

Doulas

In many traditions, birthing women are surrounded by a group of women whom they usually trust and personally select. As birthing moved into the hospital setting, less support was available for women, and many women deliver babies supported only by their partner and the hospital staff. A 2007 systematic review of 14 studies and over 13,000 women found that women who have a continuous labor support person (whether a doula, childbirth educator, friend, stranger, or family member, other than her partner) had a better birth experience, needed less analgesia, had faster labors, and were more likely to have a vaginal birth (Hodnett, Gates, Hofmeyr, & Sakala, 2007).

Midwife-Led Care

A systematic review of 12,276 women in 11 trials found several benefits and no adverse effects for mothers and their babies who experienced midwife-led care during pregnancy. There was a decreased pregnancy loss rate before 24 weeks gestation and less regional analgesia in labor; women were more likely to feel in control during the labor process, have a spontaneous vaginal delivery, and initiate breastfeeding after delivery (Hatem et al., 2008).

Complementary and Alternative Therapies

A systematic review of 14 trials ($N = 1,537$) evaluated different complementary and alternative modalities for pain control in labor. Although shown to personalize and improve the birth experience, there is insufficient evidence to support the benefits of aromatherapy, music, massage, relaxation techniques, or white noise. Additional research is needed before recommendations can be made regarding these modalities (Smith, Collins, Cyna, & Crowther, 2006). The use of TENS (transcutaneous electrical nerve stimulation) units during labor have also met with mixed results (Goldberg & Zasloff, 2007).

Acupuncture and Acupressure

Multiple systematic reviews have found acupuncture beneficial for pain control in labor (Lee & Ernst, 2004; Smith et al., 2006). One meta-analysis including two studies ($n = 496$) demonstrated a decreased use of epidural and conventional analgesia in those women receiving acupuncture (Goldberg & Zasloff, 2007). In one randomized, patient-blinded, placebo-controlled trial, women receiving acupuncture used fewer narcotics during labor and less epidural analgesia compared to controls (Skilnand, Fossen, & Heiberg, 2002). Authors of a more recent systematic review stated that, "Trials of acupuncture and acupressure show promise, but further studies are required" (Levett et al., 2014).

Self-Hypnosis Instruction

A total of 288 women in five separate trials experienced a decreased need for analgesia during labor when instructed in self-hypnosis during the antepartum period (Mantle, 2000; Smith et al., 2006).

Water Immersion

Water immersion during the *first stage* of labor significantly reduces a woman's perception of pain and use of epidural, spinal, or paracervical analgesia/anesthesia as reported in a systematic review of eight trials ($N = 2,939$). Furthermore, there was no increased risk of Apgar scores of less than 7 at five minutes, neonatal intensive care unit admissions, or instrumental or cesarean delivery. Only limited data is available for water immersion during the *second stage* of labor. The ACOG (2014) has recommended that due to the lack of evidence of maternal or fetal benefit and rare but potentially serious adverse effects, "the practice of immersion in the second stage of labor (underwater delivery) should be considered an experimental procedure that only should be performed within the context of an appropriately designed clinical trial with informed consent." No studies have looked at water immersion during the *third stage* of labor (Cluett, Nikodem, McCandlish, & Burns, 2002).

Botanicals and Homeopathic Remedies

Red raspberry leaf, motherwort (*Leonurus cardiaca*) and skullcap (*Scutellaria lateriflora*) are herbs commonly used for pain control during labor. Homeopathic remedies include *Arnica, Belladonna, Caulophyllum,* and *Cimicifuga.* There are insufficient data on the efficacy and safety of these substances to recommend them for use during labor (Goldberg & Zasloff, 2007).

Epidural for Pain Control in Labor

When compared with nonepidural pain management or no analgesia in labor, epidurals provide better pain relief. Epidurals are associated with a higher rate of operative vaginal delivery, a longer second stage, pitocin augmentation, maternal hypotension, a decrease in mobility after delivery, difficulty when urinating, and increase in the risk of fever. Use of an epidural did not impact the rate of cesarean delivery, long-term backache, or detrimental effects on the newborn (Anim-Somuah, Smyth, & Howell, 2005). Other pharmaceuticals used for pain control during labor such as antihistamines and narcotics will not be covered here; it is recommended that the reader refer to the ACOG Practice Bulletin No. 36 (ACOG, 2002).

Peripartum Perineal Care

PERINEAL SHAVING

Perineal shaving is a routine labor intervention in many countries. Three randomized trials ($N = 389$) found there is no evidence to suggest that routine perineal shaving in labor decreases the risk of infection, wound breakdown, or maternal satisfaction with the delivery. Overall, this is an unnecessary practice (Basevi & Lavender, 2000).

EPISIOTOMY

Routine episiotomy is no longer recommended. It can lead to third- and fourth-degree lacerations, a need for additional suturing, increased pain, and other long-term morbidities (ACOG, 2006a; Carroli & Belizan, 1999).

SUTURE CHOICE FOR PERINEAL REPAIR
AFTER VAGINAL DELIVERY

A recent systematic review of eight trials comparing catgut with synthetic absorbable suture showed that the absorbable suture material for perineal repair caused less short-term postpartum perineal pain and less suture dehiscence (Kettle & Johanson, 1999). There was no difference in long-term pain or dyspareunia between the two suture types.

COLD PACKS TO PERINEUM POST TRAUMA

A review of seven RCTs ($N = 859$) supports the use of localized treatment of the perineum with cold packs after vaginal delivery. When compared with no treatment, pain was reduced in the 24 to 72 hours period after delivery (East et al., 2007).

DELIVERY POSITIONING

Two meta-analyses, which reviewed 20 trials of variable quality and methodology ($N = 6,135$), found that the upright or lateral positioning during the second stage of labor is preferable to the supine or lithotomy position. Sitting, squatting, standing or side-lying were associated with shorter labors, fewer episiotomies and operative deliveries, less pain during and for 3 days after delivery, and less problems with the fetal heartbeat. However, there may be an increased risk of second-degree perineal lacerations and increased risk of postpartum hemorrhage (RR 1.63, 95% CI 1.29–2.05). More standardized studies are needed to make recommendations (Gupta & Hofmeyr, 2003; Gupta, Hofmeyr, & Smyth, 2004). Encouraging a woman to alter her positioning during labor seems to be of benefit. A recent Italian study of 225 women demonstrated that women who spent less than 50% of labor in the recumbent position had shorter labors, less need for analgesia, and lower episiotomy rate; experienced less persistence of fetal occiput posterior position; and had fewer operative deliveries (Gizzo et al., 2014).

Third Stage of Labor and Beyond

CORD CLAMPING

Delayed cord clamping of 30 to 120 seconds results in fewer transfusions and less intraventricular hemorrhage in *preterm* infants (Rabe, Reynolds, &

Diaz-Rossello, 2004). *Full-term* neonates also benefit from this practice. A recent study demonstrated that the position of the newborn before cord clamping does not seem to affect the volume of placental transfusion. Therefore, putting the baby to mother's chest immediately after delivery while waiting to clamp the cord not only enhances maternal-infant bonding, but also decreases the risk of neonatal anemia (Vain et al., 2014).

PLACENTAL CORD DRAINAGE

An RCT (n = 147) showed placental cord drainage in the management of the third stage of labor reduces the length of the third stage of labor an average of 5 minutes. Placental cord drainage has also been found to significantly reduce the risk of retained placenta for 30 minutes after birth in an RCT of 477 deliveries (RR 0.28, 95% CI 0.10–0.73) (Soltani, Dickinson, & Symonds, 2005).

UTERINE MASSAGE

In 2004, a joint statement by the International Federation of Gynecologists and Obstetricians and the International Confederation of Midwives indicated that uterine massage (UM) after the placenta delivers decreases the risk of postpartum hemorrhage. This statement was supported by an RCT (N = 200) that compared UM every 10 minutes for 60 minutes following delivery with no massage after the active management of the third stage of labor (i.e., use of oxytocin and cord traction to expeditiously deliver the placenta). Uterine massage decreased the risk of postpartum hemorrhage by 50% and the need for additional uterotonics by 80% (Hofmeyr, Abdel-Aleem, & Abdel-Aleem, 2008).

BREASTFEEDING

Breast milk is the most complete form of nutrition for infants. In 2003, the World Health Organization recommended that, when possible, children should be exclusively breastfed until 6 months of age. Breast milk digests easily, possesses the right amount of nutrients, protects infants from intestinal infections, increases IQ levels, and decreases the risks of adult obesity. Mothers who breastfeed experience less postpartum bleeding and more rapid weight loss and realize an immediate cost savings. Long-term benefits for women include lower risks of BRCA-1 (but not BRCA-2) related breast cancer (Kotsopolous et al., 2012), epithelial ovarian cancer (Luan et al., 2013), and type 2-diabetes (Jager et al., 2014). Increased caloric intake of 300 kcal is recommended while lactating.

Maternal Education

By engaging women early in the prenatal course, healthcare providers can significantly increase the number of women who choose to breastfeed (ACOG, 2007a). Postpartum support is also vital to success in breast-feeding. Identifying support personnel in the community and offering this list to women prior to delivery gives them sensitive resources to approach with questions and concerns while breastfeeding. A large meta-analysis of 30,000 women from 14 countries showed that women are much more likely to exclusively breastfeed for 6 months if supported either by lay or professional persons (Britton, McCormick, Renfrew, Wade, & King, 2007).

Early Skin-to-Skin Contact

A meta-analysis of ten studies (N = 552 mother–infant dyads) found that babies who experienced early skin-to-skin contact (babies placed prone on the mother's bare chest at birth and covered with a warm blanket) interacted more with their mothers, cried less, and stayed warmer. They were also more likely to continue breastfeeding for 1 to 4 months after discharge from the hospital (Moore, Anderson, & Bergman, 2007).

Methods of Breast Milk Expression

For those babies that cannot breastfeed within the first week of life, mothers often use either manual or mechanical methods for breast milk expression. A review of 12 studies (397 mothers) found that electric and foot-pedal breast pumps yielded more breast milk than manual expression. There was no difference in the contamination of the milk supply among the groups. Pumping both breasts simultaneously saved time and did not reduce yield (Fewtrell et al., 2001). Another study demonstrated that mothers who listened to relaxation tapes while pumping produced a higher volume of breast milk than those who did not (Becker, McCormick, & Renfrew, 2008).

Galactogogues

Galactogogues are foods, herbs, or medications used to stimulate milk production. Foods that are thought to increase milk production include apricots, asparagus, barley, beer, beet greens, carrots, dandelion greens, green beans, oatmeal, peas, pecans, sweet potatoes, and watercress (Mallory, 2008).

Herbs traditionally used to increase milk supply include fenugreek (*Trigonella foenum graecum*), goat's rue (*Galega officinalis*), blessed thistle (*Cnicus benedictus*), borage leaf (*Borago officinalis*), and alfalfa (*Medicago sativa*). Insufficient information is available to recommend most herbs as galactogogues. Fenugreek is an exception. Fenugreek is generally regarded as safe as a food additive (Natural Medicines Comprehensive Database, n.d.). The galactogogue dose is 3 to 6 g/day, and is generally effective within 1 to 3 days (Co, 2002; Mallory, 2008; Swafford & Berens, 2000). One RCT ($N = 66$) demonstrated that women who consumed a galactogogue tea (containing fenugreek) experienced increased breast milk production and the practice also facilitated neonatal weight gain (Turkyilmaz, et al., 2011).

MASTITIS

Lactational mastitis is caused by milk stasis and affects 2%–33% of the world's maternal population. It may or may not be associated with infection. Infectious mastitis affects 2% to 9.5% of breastfeeding women (ACOG, 2007b). The main etiological agents are *Staphylococci, Streptococci,* and/or *Corynebacterium*. Symptoms include breast tenderness, edema, erythema, and fever. If a breastfeeding woman calls with symptoms of mastitis, she should be examined to rule out abscess formation. Delayed diagnosis and treatment may result in abscess formation, breast tissue damage, and discontinuation of breastfeeding.

Prescription medications, including antibiotics, given for 10 to 14 days generally improve outcomes, however according to a recent Cochrane review, there is little evidence from the available RCT to adequately assess the efficacy of antibiotic therapy on mastitis (Jahanfar, Ng, & Teng, 2013). If an abscess has formed, surgical intervention may be needed. If possible, women suffering from mastitis should be encouraged to breastfeed or pump the affected breast.

Specific probiotics have been found as effective as antibiotics in the treatment of infectious mastitis. A recent randomized trial evaluated the efficacy of two strains of *Lactobacilli* naturally present in breast milk (*Lactobacillus fermentum* CECT5716 or *Lactobacillus salivarius* CECT5713) compared with traditional antibiotics. The use of either *Lactobacillus* species "appears to be an efficient alternative to the use of commonly prescribed antibiotics for the treatment of infectious mastitis during lactation (Arroyo, et al., 2010).

Breast engorgement is a condition of overfilled breasts when the tissues become swollen, hard, and painful. Cabbage leaves applied directly to the breast have been used for symptomatic relief of breast engorgement for centuries. One meta-analysis of eight studies ($N = 424$) demonstrated that cabbage leaves were as effective as gel packs for reduction in symptoms. However, the reviewers found no overall benefit in using cabbage leaves or cabbage leaf extracts to decrease the pain of engorgement (Mangesi & Muzonzini, 2008). Common homeopathic remedies for mastitis include *Belladonna*, *Bryonia*, *Silicea*, and *Phytolacca*. All except *Silicea* are considered unsafe for use during pregnancy and lactation (Natural Medicines Comprehensive Database, n.d.).

Summary

Pregnancy is a *natural* state that reinforces the importance of the mind-body-spirit-community connection in a woman's life. Whether in anticipation of pregnancy or during the journey, women generally seek knowledge desiring the best outcome for their baby and themselves. They frequently request "natural" and "safe" therapies for common physiological and psychological changes brought on by the pregnant state. Because of this, an integrative approach to pregnancy can result in a collaboration around wellness that could potentially have a lifelong impact on both mother and baby.

REFERENCES

Adair, C. D. (2000). Nonpharmacologic approaches to cervical priming and labor induction. *Clin Obstet Gynecol, 43*, 447–454.

Akmese, B. Z., & Oran, N. T. (2014, June 25). Effects of progressive muscle relaxation exercises accompanied by music on low back pain and quality of life during pregnancy. *J Midwifery Womens Health*. doi: 10.1111/jmwh.12176.

Aleman, A., Althabe, F., Belizán, J. M., & Bergel, E. (2005). Bed rest during pregnancy for preventing miscarriage. *Cochrane Database Syst Rev*, 2:CD003576.

American College of Obstetricians and Gynecologists (ACOG). (2001). External cephalic version. ACOG Practice Bulletin 2000 No. 13. *Obstet Gynecol*.

American College of Obstetricians and Gynecologists (ACOG). (2002). Obstetric analgesia and anesthesia. ACOG Practice Bulletin No. 36. *Obstet Gynecol, 100*, 177–191.

American College of Obstetricians and Gynecologists (ACOG). (2004). Nausea and vomiting of pregnancy. ACOG Practice Bulletin No. 52. *Obstet Gynecol, 103*, 803–815.

American College of Obstetricians and Gynecologists (ACOG). (2005). The importance of preconception care in the continuum of women's health care. ACOG Committee Opinion No. 313. *Obstet Gynecol, 106,* 665–666.

American College of Obstetricians and Gynecologists (ACOG). (2006a). Episiotomy. ACOG Practice Bulletin No. 71. *Obstet Gynecol, 107,* 957–962.

American College of Obstetricians and Gynecologists (ACOG). (2006b). Mode of term singleton breech delivery. ACOG Committee Opinion No. 340. *Obstet Gynecol, 108,* 235–237.

American College of Obstetricians and Gynecologists (ACOG). (2007a). Breastfeeding: Maternal and infant aspects. ACOG Committee Opinion No. 361. *Obstet Gynecol, 109,* 279–280.

American College of Obstetricians and Gynecologists (ACOG). (2007b). Breastfeeding: Maternal and infant aspects. Committee on Health Care for Underserved Women. Committee on Obstetric Practice. *ACOG Clin Rev, 12,* 5S.

American College of Obstetricians and Gynecologists (ACOG). (2009). Motivational interviewing: A tool for behavior change. ACOG Committee Opinion No. 423. *Obstet Gynecol, 113,* 243–246.

American College of Obstetricians and Gynecologists (ACOG). (2013a). Task force on hypertension in pregnancy. *ACOG, 2013,* 27–29.

American College of Obstetricians and Gynecologists (ACOG). (2013b). Obesity in pregnancy. Committee Opinion No. 549. *Obstet Gynecol, 121,* 213–217.

American College of Obstetricians and Gynecologists (ACOG). (2014). Immersion in water during labor and delivery. Committee Opinion No. 594. *Obstet Gynecol, 123,* 912–915.

American Society of Anesthesiologist Task Force on Obstetrical Anesthesia. (1999). Practice guidelines for obstetrical anesthesia: A report by the American Society of Anesthesiologist Task Force on Obstetrical Anesthesia. *Anesthesiology, 90,* 600–611.

Anim-Somuah, M., Smyth, R., & Howell, C. (2005). Epidural versus non-epidural or no analgesia in labour. *Cochrane Database Syst Rev, 4:*CD000331.

Arroyo R., et al. (2010). Treatments of infectious mastitis during lactation: Antibiotics versus oral administration of Lactobacilli isolated from breast milk. *Clin Infect Dis, 50*(12), 1551-1558.

Asman, H., et al. (2007). Risk factors for the development of striae gravidarum. *Am J Obstet Gynecol, 196,* e1–e5.

Bamigboye, A. A., & Smyth, R. (2007). Interventions for varicose veins and leg oedema in pregnancy. *Cochrane Database Syst Rev, 1:*CD001066.

Basevi, V., & Lavender, T. (2000). Routine perineal shaving on admission in labour. *Cochrane Database Syst Rev, 4:*CD001236.

Becker, G. E., McCormick, F. M., & Renfrew, M. J. (2008). Methods of milk expression for lactating women. *Cochrane Database Syst Rev, 4:*CD006170.

Beckmann, M. M., & Garrett, A. J. (2006). Antenatal perineal massage for reducing perineal trauma. *Cochrane Database Syst Rev, 1:*CD005123.

Belew, C. (1999). Herbs and the childbearing woman: Guidelines for nurse-midwives. *J Nurse Midwifery, 44,* 231–252.

Belluomini, J., Litt, R. C., Lee, K. A., & Katz, M. (1994). Acupressure for nausea and vomiting in pregnancy: A randomized, blinded study. *Obstet Gynecol, 84,* 245–248.

Bendich, A., & Langseth, L. (1989). Safety of vitamin A. *Am J Clin Nutr, 49,* 358–371.

Berghella, V., Baster, J. K., & Chauhan, S. P. (2008). Evidence-based labor and delivery management. *Am J Obstet Gynecol, 199,* 445–454.

Borrelli, F., Capasso, R., Aviello, G., et al. (2005). Effectiveness and safety of ginger in the treatment of pregnancy-induced nausea and vomiting. *Obstet Gynecol, 105,* 849.

Boulvain, M., Stan, C., & Irion, O. (2005). Membrane sweeping for induction of labour. *Cochrane Database Syst Rev,* 1:CD000451.

Bricker, L., & Luckas, M. (2000). Amniotomy alone for induction of labour. *Cochrane Database Syst Rev,* 4:CD002862.

Britton, C., McCormick, F. M., Renfrew, M. J., Wade, A., & King, S. E. (2007). Support for breastfeeding mothers. *Cochrane Database Syst Rev,* 1:CD001141.

Buchanan, K., Fletcher, H. M., & Reid, M. (2010). Prevention of striae gravidarum with cocoa butter cream. *Int J Gynaecol Obstet, 108,* 65–68.

Carroli, G., & Belizan, J. (1999). Episiotomy for vaginal birth. *Cochrane Database Syst Rev,* 3:CD000081.

CDC. (1992). Recommendations for the use of folic acid to reduce the number of cases of spina bifida and other neural tube defects. *MMWR, 41*(RR–14), 1–7.

CDC. (2007). Preconception and interconception health status of women who recently gave birth to a live-born infant: Pregnancy Risk Assessment Monitoring System (PRAMS), United States, 26 Reporting Areas, 2004. Surveillance Summaries, December 14, 2007. *MMWR, 56*(SS–10).

CDC. (2012). Alcohol use and binge drinking among women of childbearing age—United States, 2006–2010. *MMWR, 61,* 534–538.

Chatzi, L., Torrent, M., Romieu, I., et al. (2008). Mediterranean diet in pregnancy is protective for wheeze and atopy in childhood. *Thorax, 63,* 507–513.

Cluett, E. R., Nikodem, V. C., McCandlish, R. E., & Burns, E. E. (2002). Immersion in water in pregnancy, labour and birth. *Cochrane Database Syst Rev,* 2:CD000111.

Co, M. M., Hernandez, E. A., & Co, B. G. (2002). A comparative study on the efficacy of the different galactogogues among mothers with lactational insufficiency (Abstract). *AAP Section on Breastfeeding, 2002,* 125.

Coyle, M. E., Smith, C. A., & Peat, B. (2012). Cephalic version by moxibustion for breech presentation. *Cochrane Database Syst Rev,* 5:CD003928.

Czeizel, A. E. (2004). The primary prevention of birth defects: Multivitamins or folic acid? *Int J Med Sci, 1,* 50–61.

De Milliano, I., et al. (2012). Is a multispecies probiotic mixture effective in constipation during pregnancy? A pilot study. *Ntr J, 11,* 80.

De-Regil, L. M., et al. (2010). Effects and safety of periconceptional folate supplementation for preventing birth defects. *Cochrane Database Syst Rev,* 10.

De-Regil, L. M., Palacios, C., Ansary, A., Kulier, R. A., Peña-Rosas, J. P. (2012). Vitamin D supplementation for women during pregnancy. *Cochrane Database of Syst Rev,* 2.

DiGaetano, A. (2007). Nausea and vomiting in pregnancy. In D. Rakel (Ed.), *Integrative medicine* (2nd ed.). Philadelphia, PA: Saunders Elsevier.

Dowswell, T., & Neilson, J. P. (2008). Interventions for heartburn in pregnancy. *Cochrane Database Syst Rev*, 4:CD007065.

East, C. E., Begg, L., Henshall, N. E., et al. (2007). Local cooling for relieving pain from perineal trauma sustained during childbirth. *Cochrane Database Syst Rev*, 4:CD006304.

Ebrahimi, N., Maltepe, C., & Einarson, A. (2010). Optimal management of nausea and vomiting of pregnancy. *Int J Womens Health*, *2*, 241–248.

Elias, J., Bozzo, P., & Einarson, A. (2011). Are probiotics safe during pregnancy and lactation? *Can Fam Physician*, *57*, 299–301.

Elsinga, J. (2008). The effect of preconception counseling on lifestyle and other behavior before and during pregnancy. *Womens Health Issues*, *18*, S117–S125.

Environmental Protection Agency and US Food and Drug Administration. (2014). Advice encourages pregnant women and breastfeeding mothers to eat more fish that are lower in mercury. http://yosemite.epa.gov/opa/admpress.nsf/docf6618525a9efb85257359003f b69d/b8edc48od8cfe29b85257cf20065f826!opendocument Accessed 8/1/2014.

Evans, J. M., & Aronson, R. (2005a). The emotional and physical world of early pregnancy: Cramps. In J. M. Evans (Ed.), *The whole pregnancy handbook: An obstetrician's guide to integrating conventional and alternative medicine before, during and after pregnancy*. New York, NY: Penguin Group.

Evans, J. M., & Aronson, R. (2005b). Pregnancy's effects: back pain. In J. M. Evans (Ed.), *The whole pregnancy handbook: An obstetrician's guide to integrating conventional and alternative medicine before, during and after pregnancy*. New York, NY: Penguin Group.

Everett, C. (1997). Incidence and outcome of bleeding before the 20th week of pregnancy: Prospective study from general practice. *Br Med J*, *315*, 32–34.

Facchinetti, F., Fazzio, M., & Venturini, P. (2005). Polyunsaturated fatty acids and risk of preterm delivery. *Eur Rev Med Pharmacol Sci*, *9*, 41–48.

FDA. (2013). *Announcement: FDA approves diclegis for pregnant women experiencing nausea and vomiting*. Retrieved July 21, 2014, from www.fda.gov/NewsEvents/ Newsroom/PressAnnouncements/ucm347087.htm

Fewtrell, M. S., et al. (2001). Randomized trial comparing the efficacy of a novel manual breast pump with a standard electric breast pump in mothers who delivered preterm infants. *Pediatrics*, *107*, 1291–1297.

Fischer-Rasmussen, W., Kjaer, S. K., Dahl, C., & Asping, U. (1991). Ginger treatment of hyperemesis gravidarum. *Eur J Obstet Gynecol Reprod Biol*, *38*, 19–24.

Flegal, K. M., et al. (2012). Prevalence of obesity and trends in the distribution of body mass index among U.S. adults, 1999–2010. *JAMA*, *307*, 491–497.

Gardiner, P. M., Nelson, L., Shellhaas, C. S., et al. (2008). The clinical content of preconception care: Nutrition and dietary supplements. *Am J Obstet Gynecol*, *199*(6 Suppl 2), S296–S309.

Gardner, Z., & McGuffin, M. (2013). *American herbal products association's botanical safety handbook* (2nd ed.). Boca Raton, FL: CRC Press.

Gizzo, S., et al. (2014). Women's choice of position during labour: Return to the past or a modern way to give birth? A cohort study in Italy. *Biomed Res Int*, *2014*, 638093. doi: 10.1155/2014/638093

Goldberg, D. (2007). Post-term pregnancy. In D. Rakel (Ed.), *Integrative medicine* (2nd ed.). Philadelphia, PA: Saunders Elsevier.

Goldberg, D., & Zasloff, E. (2007). Labor pain management. In D. Rakel (Ed.), *Integrative medicine* (2nd ed.). Philadelphia, PA: Saunders Elsevier.

Greenberg, J. A., Bell, S. J., & Van Ausdal, W. (2008). Omega-3 fatty acid consumption during pregnancy. *Rev Obstet Gynecol, 1,* 162–169.

Griebel, C. P., Halvorsen, J., Golemon, T. B., & Day, A. A. (2005). Management of spontaneous abortion. *Am Fam Physician, 72,* 1243–1250.

Gupta, J. K., & Hofmeyr, G. J. (2003). Position for women during second stage of labour. *Cochrane Database Syst Rev,* 3:CD002006.

Gupta, J. K., Hofmeyr, G. J., & Smyth, R. (2004). Position in the second stage of labour for women without epidural anaesthesia. *Cochrane Database Syst Rev,* 1:CD002006.

Haider, B. A., & Bhutta, Z. A. (2006). Multiple-micronutrient supplementation for women during pregnancy. *Cochrane Database Syst Rev,* 4:CD004905.

Hannah, M. E., Hannah, W. J., Hewson, S. A., et al. (2000). Planned cesarean section versus planned vaginal birth for breech presentation at term: A randomized multicenter trial. Term Breech Trial Collaborative Group. *Lancet, 356,* 1375–1383.

Hanson, L., et al. (2014). Feasibility of oral prenatal probiotics against maternal group B strep vaginal and rectal colonization. *J Obstet Gynecol Neonatal Nurs, 43,* 294–304.

Harville, E. W. (2004). Calcium intake during pregnancy among white and African-American pregnant women in the United States. *J Am Coll Nutr, 23,* 43–50.

Hatem, M., Sandall, J., Devane, D., et al. (2008). Midwife-led versus other models of care for childbearing women. *Cochrane Database of Syst Rev,* 4:CD004667.

Henderson, J. T., Weisman, C. S., & Grason, H. (2002). Are two doctors better than one? Women's physician use and appropriate care. *Womens Health Issues, 12,* 139–149.

Henshaw, S. D. (1998). Unintended pregnancy in the United States. *Fam Plann Perspect, 30,* 24–29, 46.

Hodnett, E. D., Downe, S., Edwards, N., & Walsh, D. (2005). Home-like versus conventional institutional settings for birth. *Cochrane Database Syst Rev,* 1:CD000012.

Hodnett, E. D., Gates, S., Hofmeyr, G. J., & Sakala, C. (2007). Continuous support for women during childbirth. *Cochrane Database Syst Rev,* 3:CD003766.

Hofmeyr, G. J., Abdel-Aleem, H., & Abdel-Aleem, M. A. (2008). Uterine massage for preventing postpartum haemorrhage. *Cochrane Database Syst Rev,* 3:CD006431.

Hofmeyr, G. J., Atallah, A. N., & Duley, L. (2006). Calcium supplementation during pregnancy for preventing hypertensive disorders and related problems. *Cochrane Database Syst Rev,* 3:CD001059.

Hunter, S., Hofmeyr, G. J., & Kulier, R. (2007). Hands and knees posture in late pregnancy or labour for fetal malposition (lateral or posterior). *Cochrane Database Syst Rev,* 4:CD001063.

Institute of Medicine, Food and Nutrition Board. (2001). *Dietary reference intakes for vitamin A, vitamin K, arsenic, boron, chromium, copper, iodine, iron, manganese, molybdenum, nickel, silicon, vanadium, and zinc.* Washington, DC: National Academy Press.

Institute of Medicine, Food and Nutrition Board, National Academy of Sciences. (2011). *Recommended dietary allowance and adequate intake values, vitamins and elements*. Institute of Medicine. Updated September 12, 2011. www.iom.edu/Activities/Nutrition/SummaryDRIs/DRI-Tables.aspx

Jacobson, J. L., Jacobson, S. W., Muckle, G., et al. (2008). Beneficial effects of a poly-unsaturated fatty acid on infant development: Evidence from the Inuit of arctic Quebec. *J Pediatr, 152*, 356–364.

Jager, S., et al. (2014). Breast-feeding and maternal risk of type 2 diabetes: A prospective study and meta-analysis. *Diabetologia, 57*, 1355–1365. doi: 10.1007/s00125-014-3247-3

Jahanfar, S., Ng, C. J., & Teng, C. L. (2013). Antibiotics for mastitis in breastfeeding women. *Cochrane Database System Rev, 2*: CD005458.

Jewell, D. J., & Young, G. (2001). Interventions for treating constipation in pregnancy. *Cochrane Database Syst Rev, 2*:CD001142.

Jewell, D., & Young, G. (2003). Interventions for nausea and vomiting in early pregnancy. *Cochrane Database Syst Rev, 4*:CD000145.

Jones, R. H., & Carek, P. J. (2008). Management of varicose veins. *Am Fam Physician, 78*, 1289–1294.

Kassenbaum, N. J., et al. (2014, May 2). Global, regional and national levels and causes of maternal mortality during 1990–2013: A systematic analysis for the Global Burden of Disease Study 2013. *Lancet*. Early online publication. doi:10.1016/S0140-6736(14)60696-6

Kavanagh, J., Kelly, A. J., & Thomas, J. (2001). Sexual intercourse for cervical ripening and induction of labour. *Cochrane Database Syst Rev, 2*:CD003093.

Kavanagh, J., Kelly, A. J., & Thomas, J. (2005). Breast stimulation for cervical ripening and induction of labour. *Cochrane Database Syst Rev, 3*:CD003392.

Kelly, A. J., Kavanagh, J., & Thomas, J. (2013). Castor oil, bath and/or enema for cervical priming and induction of labour. *Cochrane Database Syst Rev, 7*:CD003099.

Kettle, C., & Johanson, R. (1999). Absorbable synthetic versus catgut suture material for perineal repair. *Cochrane Database Syst Rev, 4*:CD000006.

Knight, B., Mudge, C., Openshaw, S., et al. (2001). Effect of acupuncture on nausea and pregnancy: A randomized, controlled trial. *Obstet Gynecol, 97*, 184–188.

Kotsopoulos, J., et al. (2012). Breastfeeding and the risk of breast cancer in BRCA1 and BRCA2 mutation carriers. *Breast Cancer Res, 14*, R42.

Kramer, M. S., & Kakuma, R. (2002). Optimal duration of exclusive breastfeeding. *Cochrane Database Syst Rev, 1*:CD003517.

Kramer, M. S., & McDonald, S. W. (2006). Aerobic exercise for women during pregnancy. *Cochrane Database Syst Rev, 3*:CD000180.

Latva-Pukkila, U., Isolauri, E., & Laitinen, K. (2010). Dietary and clinical impacts of nausea and vomiting during pregnancy. *J Hum Nutr Diet, 23*, 69–77.

Lee, H., & Ernst, E. (2004). Acupuncture for labor pain management: A systematic review. *Am J Obstet Gynecol, 191*, 1573.

Levett, K. M., et al. (2014). Acupuncture and acupressure for pain management in labour and birth: A critical narrative review of current systematic review evidence. *Complement Ther Med, 22*, 523–540.

Locksmith, G. J., & Duff, P. (1998). Preventing neural tube defects: The importance of periconceptional folic acid supplements. *Obstet Gynecol, 91*, 1027–1034.

Lorenz, D., Lincoln, A., Dooley, S., et al. (2007). Surveillance of preconception health indicators among women delivering live-born infants, Oklahoma, 2000–2003. *MMWR, 56*, 631–634.

Luan, N. N., et al. (2013). Breastfeeding and ovarian cancer risk: A meta-analysis of epidemiologic studies. *Am J Clin Nutr, 98*, 1020–1031.

Lumley, J., Watson, L., Watson, M., & Bower, C. (2001). Periconceptional supplementation with folate and/or multivitamins for preventing neural tube defects. *Cochrane Database Syst Rev, 3*:CD001056.

Makrides, M., Duley, L., & Olsen, S. F. (2006). Marine oil, and other prostaglandin precursor, supplementation for pregnancy uncomplicated by pre-eclampsia or intrauterine growth restriction. *Cochrane Database Syst Rev, 3*:CD003402.

Mallory, J. (2008). *Supplement sampler: Natural galactogogues.* University of Wisconsin Integrative Medicine Department of Family Medicine. http://www.fammed.wisc.edu/files/webfm-uploads/documents/outreach/im/ss_galactogogues.pdf

Mangesi, L., & Muzonzini, G. (2008). Treatments for breast engorgement during lactation (Protocol). *Cochrane Database Syst Rev, 1*:CD006946.

Mantle, F. (2000). The role of hypnosis in pregnancy and childbirth. In D. Tiran & S. Mack (Eds.), *Complementary therapies for pregnancy and childbirth* (2nd ed.). New York, NY: Balliere Tindall.

March of Dimes Birth Defects Foundation. (2004). *Folic acid and the prevention of birth defects: A national survey of pre-pregnancy awareness and behavior among women of childbearing age, 1995–2004.* White Plains, NY: March of Dimes.

McCrea, B. H., & Wright, M. E. (1999). Satisfaction in childbirth and perceptions of pain control in pain relief during labour. *J Adv Nurs, 29*, 877.

Moore, E. R., Anderson, G. C., & Bergman, N. (2007). Early skin-to-skin contact for mothers and their healthy newborn infants. *Cochrane Database Syst Rev, 3*:CD003519.

National Women's Health Information Center. US Department of Health and Human Services. Office on Women's Health. (n.d.). *Breastfeeding.* http://www.womenshealth.gov/breastfeeding/index.cfm?page=227

Natural Medicines Comprehensive Database. (n.d.). *Mastitis.* Retrieved February 14, 2009, from http://www.naturaltherapypages.com.au/article/mastitis

Neilson, J. P. (1998). Ultrasound for fetal assessment in early pregnancy. *Cochrane Database Syst Rev, 4*:CD000182.

O'Brien, B., Relyea, M. J., & Taerun, T. (1996). Efficacy of P6 acupressure in the treatment of nausea and vomiting during pregnancy. *Am J Obstet Gynecol, 174*, 708–715.

Osman, H., Usta, I. M., Rubeiz, N., Abu Rustum, R., Charara, I., & Nassar, A. H. (2008). Cocoa butter lotion for prevention of striae gravidarum: A double-blind, randomized and placebo-controlled trial. *BJOG, 115*, 1138–1142.

Othman, M., Neilson, J. P., & Alfirevic, Z. (2007). Probiotics for preventing preterm labour. *Cochrane Database Syst Rev*, 1:CD005941.

Pawley, N., & Bishop, N. J. (2004). Prenatal and infant predictors of bone health: The influence of vitamin D. *Am J Clin Nutr, 80*, 1748S–1751S.

Peña-Rosas, J. P., & Viteri, F. E. (2006). Effects of routine oral iron supplementation with or without folic acid for women during pregnancy. *Cochrane Database Syst Rev*, 3:CD004736.

Pennick, V., & Young, G. (2007). Interventions for preventing and treating pelvic and back pain in pregnancy. *Cochrane Database Syst Rev*, 2:CD001139.

Poma, P. A. (1999). Cervical ripening: A review and recommendations for clinical practice. *J Reprod Med, 44*, 657–668.

Quijano, C. E., & Abalos, E. (2005). Conservative management of symptomatic and/or complicated haemorrhoids in pregnancy and the puerperium. *Cochrane Database Syst Rev*, 3:CD004077.

Rabe, H., Reynolds, G., & Diaz-Rossello, J. (2004). Early versus delayed umbilical cord clamping in preterm infants. *Cochrane Database Syst Rev*, 4:CD003248.

Rakel, D. (2007). *Integrative medicine* (2nd ed.). Philadelphia, PA: Saunders Elsevier.

Reinwald, S. (2008). The health benefits of calcium citrate malate: A review of the supporting science. *Adv Food Nutr Res, 54*, 219–346.

Roscoe, J. A., & Matteson, S. E. (2002). Acupressure and acustimulation bands for control of nausea: A brief review. *Am J Obstet Gynecol, 186*, S244–S247.

Rumbold, A., Middleton, P., & Crowther, C. A. (2005). Vitamin supplementation for preventing miscarriage. *Cochrane Database Syst Rev*, 2:CD004073.

Saunders, L., et al. (2014). Effect of a Mediterranean diet during pregnancy on fetal growth and preterm delivery: Results from a French Caribbean Mother-Child Cohort Study (TIMOUN). *Paediatr Perinat Epidemiol, 28*, 235–244.

Scroggins, K. M., Smucker, W. D., & Krishen, A. E. (2000). Spontaneous pregnancy loss: Evaluation, management and follow-up counseling. *Prim Care, 27*, 153–167.

Singata, M., Tranmer, J., & Gyte, G. M. L. (2013). Restricting oral fluid and food intake during labour. *Cochrane Database Syst Rev*, 8:CD003930.

Skilnand, E., Fossen, D., & Heiberg, E. (2002). Acupuncture in the management of pain in labor. *Acta Obstet Gynecol Scand, 81*, 943.

Smith, C. A. (2003). Homoeopathy for induction of labour. *Cochrane Database Syst Rev*, 4:CD003399.

Smith, C. A., Collins, C. T., Cyna, A. M., & Crowther, C. A. (2006). Complementary and alternative therapies for pain management in labour. *Cochrane Database Syst Rev*, 4:CD003521.

Smith, C. A., & Crowther, C. A. (2013). Acupuncture for induction of labour. *Cochrane Database Syst Rev*, 8:CD002962..

Smyth, R. M. D., Alldred, S. K., & Markham, C. (2007). Amniotomy for shortening spontaneous labour. *Cochrane Database Syst Rev*, 4:CD006167.

Soltani, H., Dickinson, F., & Symonds, I. (2005). Placental cord drainage after spontaneous vaginal delivery as part of the management of the third stage of labour. *Cochrane Database Syst Rev*, 4:CD004665.

Soltanipore, F., et al. (2014). The effect of olive oil and Saj cream in prevention of striae gravidarum: A randomized clinical controlled trial. *Complement Ther Med*, 22, 220–225.

Stamp, G., Kruzins, G., & Crowther, C. (2001). Perineal massage in labour and prevention of perineal trauma: Randomized controlled trial. *Br Med J*, 322, 1277–1280.

Summers, L. (1997). Methods of cervical ripening and labor induction. *J Nurse Midwifery*, 42, 71–85.

Swafford, S., & Berens, P. (2000, September 11–13). *Effect of fenugreek on breast milk volume*. Abstract. 5th International Meeting of the Academy of Breastfeeding Medicine, Tucson, AZ.

Tan, P. C., Yow, C. M., & Omar, S. Z. (2007). Effect of coital activity on onset of labor in women scheduled for labor induction: A randomized controlled trial. *Obstet Gynecol*, 110, 820–826.

Thaler, E., et al. (2001). Compression stockings prophylaxis of emergent varicose veins in pregnancy: A prospective randomised controlled trial. *Swiss Med Wkly*, 131(45–46), 659–62.

Thaver, D., Saeed, M. A., & Bhutta, Z. A. (2006). Pyridoxine (vitamin B6) supplementation in pregnancy. *Cochrane Database Syst Rev*, 2:CD000179.

Thomas, M., & Weisman, S. M. (2006). Calcium supplementation during pregnancy and lactation: Effects on the mother and the fetus. *Am J Obstet Gynec*, 194.

Tough, S., Tofflemire, K., Clarke, M., & Newburn-Cook, C. (2006). Do women change their drinking behaviors while trying to conceive? An opportunity for preconception counseling. *Clin Med Res*, 4, 97–105.

Turkyilmaz C., et al. (2011). The effect of galactagogue herbal tea on breast milk production and short-term catch-up of birth weight in the first week of life. *J Altern Complement med*, 17(2), 139-142.

Vain, N. E., et al. (2014, April 16). Effect of gravity on volume of placental transfusion: A multicenter, randomised, non-inferiority trial. *Lancet*. pii: S0140-6736(14)60197–60195

Vetura, S. J., Martin, J. A., Curtin, S. C., & Mathews, T. J. (1999). Births: Final data for 1997. *Natl Vital Stat Rep*, 47, 1–96.

Viljoen, E., Visser, J., Koen, N., & Musekiwa, A. (2014). A systematic review and meta-analysis of the effect of ginger in the treatment of pregnancy-associated nausea and vomiting. *Nutr J*, 13, 20.

Vitamin D Council. (2013). *Vitamin D during pregnancy and breastfeeding*. Vitamin D Council. January 30, 2013. Retrieved June 15, 2014, from https://www.vitamind-council.org/further-topics/vitamin-d-during-pregnancy-and-breastfeeding/

Vutyavanich, T., Kraisarin, T., & Ruangsri, R. (2001). Ginger for nausea and vomiting in pregnancy: Randomized, double-masked, placebo-controlled trial. *Obstet Gynecol, 97*, 577–582.

White, B. (2007). Ginger: An overview. *Am Fam Physician, 75*, 1689–1691.

Wickens, K., Stanley, T. V., Mitchell, E. A., et al. (2013). Early supplementation with *Lactobacillus rhamnosus* HN001 reduces eczema prevalence to 6 years: Does it also reduce atopic sensitization? *Clin Exp Allergy, 43*, 1048–1057.

Wolpowitz, D., & Gilchrest, B. A. (2006). The vitamin D questions: How much do you need and how should you get it? *J Am Acad Dermatol, 54*, 301–317.

Young, G. L., & Jewell, D. (1996). Crams for preventing stretch marks in pregnancy. *Cochrane Database Syst Rev,* 1:CD000066.

16

Polycystic Ovary Syndrome

BRIDGET S. BONGAARD

CASE STUDY

Denise came into my office despondent and desperate. She was 19 years old and increasingly concerned about her erratic menstrual cycles, sometimes going months without having a period. Embarrassed by the increasing amount of dark hair that was growing on her chin, upper lip, and now around her nipples, Denise admitted also feeling somewhat depressed about her weight, as she had gained roughly 40 pounds in the last 3 years. After taking a personal and family history and ordering pertinent laboratory tests, I explained that she had a condition known as polycystic ovary syndrome and that together we would create a plan that would help her lose weight, regulate her menstrual cycle, and slow the growth of unwanted hair.

Introduction

Polycystic ovary syndrome (PCOS) is the most common premenopausal endocrine disorder in women, affecting 5% to 10% percent of all women of reproductive age. It generally starts at puberty with an increased incidence of menstrual abnormalities, hirsutism, acne, and infertility. If left unmanaged it can lead to miscarriage, cardiovascular complications, endometrial cancer, and a sevenfold greater risk of type II diabetes (Avery & Braunack-Mayer, 2007). The presentation at the time of diagnosis varies with the symptom complex and the age of the patient. Some women may seek evaluation for obesity, acne, or hirsutism, while others might have a relatively lean body mass and present with menstrual irregularities or difficulty conceiving. While it was once considered a "benign nuisance," PCOS should be regarded as a real threat to a woman's health because of the increased risk of cancer, diabetes, and coronary artery disease (Sheehan, 2004).

Pathophysiology

There is no single cause of PCOS; it is an intertwined dysregulation of elevated androgens, estrogen, and hyperinsulinemia. Ovarian insulin receptors stimulate thecal cell production of excessive androgens (Kodaman & Duleba, 2008). Androstenedione, the immediate precursor to testosterone, is normally converted to estrone and estradiol by aromatase in the ovaries. However in PCOS, aromatase is impaired, leading to high levels of androstenedione entering the circulation. Intra-abdominal adipose tissue, which has a higher expression of 17-beta hydroxysteroid dehydrogenase than aromatase, preferentially converts androstenedione to testosterone. High levels of insulin decrease sex hormone binding globulin (SHBG) levels, which further increase free testosterone, and increase cardiovascular risk by lowering high-density lipoprotein (HDL) and increasing low-density lipoprotein (LDL), triglycerides, and very low density lipoprotein (VLDL) (Kodaman & Duleba, 2008). The increase in androgen production may be enough to cause male pattern hair production (i.e., chin, chest, back), male pattern hair loss, and/or acne.

Approximately 80% of women with PCOS suffer from anovulation, which results in oligomenorrhea, amenorrhea, dysfunctional uterine bleeding, and/or infertility (Sheehan, 2004). Menstrual irregularity is the result of high and sustained production of estrogens. Without the normal rise and fall in estrogen that occurs in cycling women, anovulation occurs. Fertility is impaired in many PCOS patients. If and when pregnancies do occur, the first trimester rate of miscarriage is as high as 30% to 50% (Sheehan, 2004). Prolonged anovulation can also predispose women to the development of uterine fibroids (Wise, Palmer, Stewart, & Rosenberg, 2007). The prolonged exposure to unopposed estrogen with progesterone deficiency and androgen excess increases the risk of gynecologic cancers later in life (Karadeniz et al., 2007).

Insulin resistance is independent of obesity, although obesity plays an amplifying role (Corbould & Dunaif, 2007). Simply said, women with PCOS may have insulin resistance whether or not they are obese.

Comorbid Diseases

Increased cardiovascular mortality in women with PCOS has not been conclusively demonstrated. Some studies suggest increased cardiac events, while other studies reveal no increase when compared with normal cycling women (Cho, Randeva, & Atkin, 2007). Hypertension may develop due to hyperinsulinemia, which stimulates the release of insulin-like growth factor-1 (IGF-1). The IGF-1 causes vascular smooth muscle hypertrophy and the release of angiotensin II, which in turn increases sodium retention and stimulates vascular endothelial dysfunction. Elevated angiotensin II levels further aggravate insulin resistance. Hyperinsulinemia enhances clotting by elevating plasminogen activator inhibitor (PAI-1) and reducing fibrinolysis.

Patients with PCOS are also predisposed to an increased state of inflammation. Fat cells are metabolically active and secrete inflammatory agents such as tumor necrosis factor (TNF), interleukin 6 (IL-6), PAI-1, leptin, resistin, adiponectin, and angiotensinogen (Cho et al., 2007). The TNF stimulates the production of C-reactive protein and IL-6. These inflammatory compounds produce increased oxidative stress even in lean women with PCOS (Cho et al., 2007).

Diabetes is a well-known risk factor for cardiovascular disease. One study found that 31% of patients newly diagnosed with PCOS had impaired glucose tolerance, while 7.5% met the criterion for type II diabetes mellitus regardless of overall body mass (Sheehan, 2004). By the age of 40, up to 40% of women with PCOS will have type II diabetes, or impaired glucose tolerance (Lord, Flight, & Norman, 2003). The risk of gestational diabetes is increased 10-fold, compared with the general population (Sheehan, 2004).

Screening and Diagnosis of Polycystic Ovary Syndrome

The clinical features of PCOS include oligo- or amenorrhea, infertility or first-trimester miscarriage, truncal or central obesity, hirsutism, acne, acanthosis nigricans, and male pattern balding. Excluding diagnoses that can mimic PCOS is the first priority. Congenital adrenal hyperplasia, Cushing's disease, and androgen-secreting tumors of the ovary or adrenal gland must be ruled out (Cho et al., 2007).

Even in the early stages of PCOS, 30% to 40% of women are unable to regulate their glucose levels. It is recommended that women be screened with a 2-hour glucose tolerance test (Lau, 2007). Other recommended laboratory evaluation includes a cholesterol panel and free and total testosterone levels (should be less than 200 ng/dL). The LH/FSH ratio is also measured. A ratio of ≥2.0 is suggestive of PCOS, but is not highly sensitive or specific and can be affected by the use of oral contraceptives (Sheehan, 2004).

Ovarian ultrasound can be helpful in identifying women with PCOS, but is not completely reliable. Ultrasound criteria for PCOS are increased ovarian area (>5.5 cm²) or volume (11 mL), and/or presence of ≥12 follicles measuring 2 to 9 mm in diameter (mean of both ovaries); when present, the diagnosis of PCOS can be made with 99% specificity and a 75% sensitivity (Sheehan, 2004).

Integrative Treatment Options

Due to the complex endocrine and metabolic nature of PCOS, the treatment plan requires a multipronged approach. Pharmacologic agents, dietary supplements, acupuncture, and mind–body therapies can all play a role in reversing the disease process and improving quality of life.

Pharmaceuticals

METFORMIN

Metformin is an effective first-line treatment of metabolic syndrome and decreases hirsutism by improving insulin resistance and hyperandrogenism (Cho et al., 2007). In one study, normalization of menstrual cycles and ovulation occurred in 40% of women taking metformin, with 79% of these women becoming pregnant within 3 months of starting the medication (Sheehan, 2004). The addition of clomiphene to induce ovulation increased the pregnancy rate to 89%. Metformin also reduced the rate of first-trimester miscarriages. Since metformin may stimulate ovulation in women with PCOS, a discussion on contraceptive therapy may be warranted with those who are not planning a pregnancy.

Metformin does not change waist-to-hip ratio or reduce BMI, yet has a significant impact on lipids by lowering total cholesterol and LDL, but not triglycerides, HDL, or blood pressure (Wulffele et al., 2004). The clinically effective dose is generally 1,500 mg/day, however, it is important to start with 500 mg daily and increase the dose in 500-mg increments after 1 to 2 weeks to minimize the commonly seen GI side effects (nausea, diarrhea, abdominal cramping). There is also data that show long-term metformin can deplete vitamin B12. Metformin should not be used in women with a creatinine clearance below 30 mL/min.

THIAZOLIDINEDIONE DRUGS

Thiazolidinediones (TZDs) such as pioglidizone (Actos) and roziglidazone (Avandia) are a class of insulin-sensitizing drugs; TZDs decrease hyperandrogenism and hirsutism and improve menstrual cycle regulation in patients with PCOS. However, in October 2013 the Endocrine Society Guidelines for the Diagnosis and Management of PCOS concluded that "thiazolidinediones have an unfavorable risk-benefit ratio." These drugs therefore should no longer be used.

ORAL CONTRACEPTIVES

For decades, the mainstay of PCOS treatment has been oral contraceptive pills (OCPs) because of their ability to regulate unpredictable menstrual periods. Oral contraceptive pills also increase SHBG, thereby increasing the binding of free testosterone and decreasing circulating androgens.

Low-dose combined contraceptives are effective and considered a first-line therapy in reestablishing menstrual function and treating hyperandrogenic symptoms in women under the age of 35 who are not attempting conception (Tan, Yap, & Tan, 2001). One effective combination is ethinyl estradiol and the low androgen progesterone agent drospirenone (EE/DRSP). When combined with 100 mg of spironolactone, a synergistic improvement in hirsutism and drop in androgen levels was found. However, there were no improvements in glucose tolerance, BMI, cholesterol, or triglycerides, and an elevation of high-sensitivity C-reactive protein and homocysteine were found (Harmanci et al., 2013).

Oral contraceptives inhibit 5-alpha-reductase and androgen receptor binding and suppress luteinizing hormone (LH), which stimulates increased production of SHBG. Careful monitoring of glucose tolerance is recommended as oral contraceptives can increase insulin resistance. Oral contraceptive pills should not be used in women with a hypercoagulable state, a history of deep venous thrombosis, or those older than 35 years who smoke (Sheehan, 2004).

Medroxyprogesterone can be used to regulate cycles in women who have increased cardiovascular risk (Kelly, 2000). Cyclic progestin/progesterone therapy is used to treat abnormal uterine bleeding and to prevent endometrial hyperplasia (Hunter & Sterrett, 2000; Slowey, 2001).

Spironolactone confers a mild antiandrogen effect; however, it can take months to work and may increase serum potassium levels. Creams such as eflornithine hydrochloride 13.9% (Vaniqa) can act as a mild depilatory agent. Plucking or shaving and electrolysis can further diminish unsightly hair.

Lifestyle Modification

DIET AND EXERCISE

Although obesity is not the cause of PCOS, it may aggravate the associated insulin resistance and metabolic abnormalities. Significant weight loss reduces hyperinsulinemia and subsequently hyperandrogenemia (Sheehan, 2004) by increasing SHBG and reducing basal levels of insulin (Cho et al., 2007). A 2013 meta-analysis found weight loss is most effectively achieved by limiting caloric intake to a maximum of 1,200–1,500 kcal per day (Ravn, Haugen, & Glintborg, 2013). When a low calorie diet is combined with metformin increased weight loss and lower androgen levels are found when compared with diet alone (Ravn et al., 2013). An exercise program consisting of a brisk daily 20-minute walk resulted in a 7% weight loss (Sheehan, 2004). In addition to weight loss, exercise improves insulin sensitivity; both aerobic exercise and resistance training are beneficial.

A meta-analysis of lifestyle modification (LSM) of nine trials including 583 women found a significant reduction in BMI, fasting blood sugar, and fasting insulin levels (Domecq et al., 2013). Interestingly, the addition of metformin did not significantly improve blood sugar or insulin levels. No significant improvement of pregnancy rates or hirsutism was noted with LSM. Not surprisingly, collectively there was an attrition rate of ~24%, limiting findings. Given the vast amount of evidence that supports the use of LSM (i.e., healthy diet, physical activity, weight management) in diabetes and cardiovascular health, clinicians should encourage these behaviors at every opportunity.

ALCOHOL

The effect of alcohol consumption on the development of type II diabetes is variable, depending on the amount ingested. Mild to moderate alcohol consumption, defined as between 6 and 48 g/day lowers insulin resistance and decreases the risk of the development of diabetes by 30% (Kopper et al., 2005).

Alcohol-containing beverages have different alcohol content, which may vary according to the country. Box 16.1 gives a tool for defining a "standard

---

Box 16.1 Defining a "Standard Drink"

Equivalent beverages would be:

1 shot of 80 proof liquor
1 glass of wine/ 5 fluid oz
1 12-oz can of beer

Source: Wikipedia.com.

---

drink" in the United States. Each drink proportion is measured as 0.6 fluid ounce or 18 mL, and contains 14 g of pure alcohol.

Excessive alcohol consumption increases the risk of diabetes and reverses the positive effects on lipids and blood pressure. Moderate chronic intake also leads to menstrual abnormalities and decreases ovarian volume and follicle numbers (Na et al., 2013) and therefore should be discouraged in PCOS patients seeking fertility.

TEA AND COFFEE

Tea and coffee consumption can effect the inflammatory milieu in PCOS patients. Moderate intake of caffeine results in increased insulin sensitivity. Both coffee and tea possess antioxidants that afford protection against diabetes, cardiovascular disease, and cancer (Isu et al., 2006). Intake of 3 to 4 cups of tea per day or up to 6 cups of coffee per day decreases the risk of diabetes by 20% (Huxley et al., 2009) without impairment of fecundity (Taylor et al., 2011).

Dietary Supplements

CHROMIUM

Chromium is an essential trace element that is required for carbohydrate and lipid metabolism. Chromium enhances glucose metabolism, decreases cardiovascular risk, and may benefit atypical depression (Pattar, Tackett, Liu, & Elmendorf, 2006). Despite many studies, the evidence for chromium in patients with insulin resistance or type II diabetes is mixed; it appears to have the greatest benefit in obese, insulin-resistant individuals. The typical dose is 200–1,000 mcg daily of chromium picolinate.

CINNAMON (*CINNAMOMUM VERUM, C. ZEYLANICUM, C. CASSIA*)

Cinnamon is another insulin-sensitizing agent that can be added to the diet. It stimulates glucose uptake and synthesis by fat cells (lowering glucose and insulin levels), lowers blood pressure, and improves abnormal lipid profiles. Use of cinnamon extract in one study increased lean body mass even after controlling for smoking, physical activity, dietary habits, blood pressure, glucose, and lipid levels (Zeigenfuss, Hofheins, Mendel, Landis, & Anderson, 2006). A small study of 15 women with PCOS with an average BMI of 28.8 found that 1 gram of cinnamon extract was superior to placebo in reducing fasting glucose and insulin resistance (Wang et al., 2007). Other studies have used doses ranging from 1 to 6 grams of cinnamon and shown dose-dependent decreases in fasting blood glucose and lipid levels (Zeigenfuss et al., 2006). This inexpensive spice can be added to the diet.

GINSENG (*PANAX GINSENG, PANAX QUINQUEFOLIUS*)

Ginseng demonstrates antidiabetic effects as well. Three grams of ginseng extract administered prior to an oral glucose tolerance test resulted in a decrease of blood sugar in both diabetic and nondiabetic patients (Vuksan et al., 2000). However, it is difficult to offer specific recommendations, as a meta-analysis of ginseng studies reveals variability depending on the species (Seivenpiper et al., 2003; Seivenpiper et al., 2004) and plant parts (root, leaf, stem, berry) used (Dey et al., 2003).

VITAMIN D

There is limited evidence that vitamin D may benefit women with PCOS. A small open study of 13 women with PCOS found that vitamin D supplementation improved their symptoms. Five of the women had serum 25(OH) D levels less than 9 ng/mL and three had borderline low vitamin D. All of the women were treated with a daily dose of 1,500 mg calcium and a weekly dose of 50,000 IU vitamin D2 to maintain a serum level of 30–40 ng/mL. Of the nine women who had oligomenorrhea at baseline, seven normalized their cycles within 2 months, and the other two became pregnant (Thys-Jacobs, Donovan, Papadopoulos, Sarrel, & Bilezikian, 1999).

N-ACETYLCYSTEINE

N-acetylcysteine (NAC) is derived from the sulfur-containing amino acid cysteine. It is used as a pharmaceutical agent for the management of acetaminophen overdose and as a mucolytic. N-acetylcysteine may reduce insulin resistance and improve fertility. A double-blind placebo-controlled trial of 150 overweight or obese women with PCOS who had failed to ovulate with clomiphene citrate were randomized to receive 1,000 mg/day clomiphene and either 600 mg NAC twice daily or placebo for 5 days starting on day 3 of their menstrual cycles. The ovulation rate for the active group was 49.3% versus 1.3% for placebo ($p < .0001$) and the pregnancy rate was 21.3% versus 0% ($p = .00006$). No cases of ovarian hyperstimulation occurred, and there were two miscarriages in NAC group (Rizk, Bedaiwy, & Al-Inany, 2005).

WHITE PEONY ROOT (*PAEONIA LACTIFLORA*)

Paeonia lactiflora has been used for gynecological conditions for centuries in traditional Chinese medicine, and Western herbalists commonly employ it for similar purposes. White peony increases progesterone and reduces testosterone levels. In vitro, the active constituent paeoniflorin has been shown to effect the ovarian follicle by enhancing the activity of aromatase. The daily dose for white peony root is 3–5 grams. White peony is contraindicated during pregnancy, as it has abortifacient properties.

SHAKUYAKU-KANZO-TO

Shakuyaku-kanzo-to, a combination of equal parts of licorice root and white peony root, has been studied in PCOS. Several small studies have shown that it reduces testosterone levels and increases pregnancy rates in women with PCOS. Glycyrrhetinic acid, a metabolite of glycyrrhizin from licorice, blocks the enzymes that convert 17-hydroxyprogesterone to androstenedione in vitro, lowering testosterone levels. Licorice can elevate blood pressure and induce hypokalemia. Prolonged use of licorice at doses of 1,000 mg, or higher, should include monitoring of potassium and blood pressure.

SAW PALMETTO (*SERENOA REPENS*)

While saw palmetto is primarily considered for men with mild symptoms of benign prostatic hyperplasia (BPH), it is also used for women with PCOS and/ or hirsutism. Saw palmetto inhibits 5-alpha-reductase, an enzyme that appears to play a role in the pathogenesis of PCOS. The dose and preparation of saw palmetto in PCOS is similar to that used in men with BPH: 320 mg/day of an extract standardized to contain 80%–95% fatty acids.

CHASTE TREE (*VITEX AGNUS CASTUS*)

Chaste tree berry is commonly used for irregular menstruation, particularly for normalizing menstruation in women with hyperprolactinemia, an under-lying cause of corpus luteal insufficiency. Constituents within chaste tree bind to dopamine receptors, resulting in the inhibition of prolactin. Some women with PCOS have elevated prolactin levels, thus chaste tree might be considered as a useful addition to the treatment protocol.

> Safety in pregnancy has not been established for Shakuyaku-kanzo-to, saw palmetto, or higher doses of chromium.

ACUPUNCTURE

Acupuncture lowers sympathetic nervous system tone, leading to increased blood flow to the ovaries, potentially improving ovulation. In a small study of 24 patients with PCOS (Stener-Victorin et al., 2000), low frequency electro-acupuncture induced ovulation in one-third of the subjects. Those with the lowest androgen levels before treatment responded most favorably.

Acupuncture has been also been found to decrease circulating testosterone and improve menstrual irregularity in women diagnosed with PCOS. In a randomized controlled trial from Sweden (Johansson et al., 2013) acupuncture was performed twice a week for 10 to 13 weeks on lean and overweight PCOS patients. Ovulation frequency during treatment increased while circulating levels of estrogen, androgens (DHEA, DHEAS, and free and total testosterone), inhibin B, anti-mullerian hormone, and serum cortisol decreased.

Acupuncture can also improve symptoms of anxiety, depression, and impaired health-related quality of life (HRQoL) that sometimes accompany the experience of infertility. A 16-week study of 72 women with PCOS

(Stener-Victorin et al., 2013) compared acupuncture, exercise, and a control group (who received oral information about the benefits of exercise). The acupuncture group showed an improvement in depression and anxiety; acupuncture and exercise both led to an improvement in HRQoL; while exercise improved infertility. Positive effects were still present 16 weeks post trial.

MIND–BODY MEDICINE

While there are studies on mind–body approaches for cardiovascular risk reduction and diabetes, there are none that specifically address PCOS. It is reasonable to include mind–body approaches in the treatment of PCOS, as they can reduce inflammation and anxiety and help balance the autonomic nervous system. The resulting reduction in stress hormones may decrease blood pressure and blood sugar levels. Mind–body therapies such as yoga, guided visualization, hypnosis, biofeedback, and aromatherapy can be used.

RECOMMENDATIONS

For women presenting primarily with ovarian dysfunction (irregular menses or anovulation) and insulin resistance without central obesity; oral contraceptives may be a good choice if not contraindicated. A low-glycemic diet and routine exercise program should be highly recommended. Acupuncture may help restore ovulation, and referral to a traditional Chinese medicine provider who specializes in women's health can be considered.

In women with more advanced symptoms, including infertility or amenorrhea, hyperandrogenemia, and increasing insulin resistance in the form of metabolic syndrome, it is imperative that a more extensive treatment plan be initiated. These women are at high risk for developing diabetes, cardiovascular disease, nonalcoholic steatohepatitis, and estrogen-driven cancers. In addition to the measures mentioned above, women can be advised to use insulin sensitizers (cinnamon and chromium) and start metformin.

When treating PCOS comorbidities, one should follow the patient with biannual lipid panels to assess cardiovascular risk and fasting blood sugars to screen for the development of hyperglycemia while recommending diet and exercise lifestyle modifications to decrease the development of type II diabetes. Treatments should be individualized and the mind–body component not forgotten.

SUMMARY

Women affected by PCOS may have a broad range of symptoms that are challenging physically and emotionally. There is not one simple treatment strategy to recommend, as each woman presents with her own unique combination of symptoms and disease manifestations. It is best to try and understand the underlying pathophysiology and craft a comprehensive treatment plan that includes integrative strategies. Women should be taught about their pathophysiology so that they can be champions for their own healing. Sharing treatment options can empower a woman to participate more fully in her care and improve her overall outcome.

REFERENCES

Avery, J. C., & Braunack-Mayer, A. J. (2007). The information needs of women diagnosed with polycystic ovarian syndrome: Implications for treatment and health outcomes. *BMC Women's Health, 7*, 1–10.

Cho, L. W., Randeva, H. S., & Atkin, S. L. (2007). Cardiometabolic aspects of polycystic ovarian syndrome. *Vascular Health Risk Manag, 3*, 55–63.

Corbould, A., & Dunaif A. (2007). The adipose cell lineage is not intrinsically insulin resistant in polycystic ovary syndrome. *Metabolism, 56*, 716–722.

Dey, L., Xie, J. T., Wang, A., et al. (2003). Antihyperglycemic effects of ginseng: Comparison between root and berry. *Phytomedicine, 10*, 600–605.

Domecq, J. P., Prutsky, G., Mullan, R. J., et al. (2013). Adverse effects of the common treatments for polycystic ovary syndrome: a systematic review and meta-analysis. *J Clin Endocrinol Metab, 98*, 4646–4654.

Harmanci, A., Cinar, N., Bayraktar, M., et al. (2013). Oral contraceptive plus antiandrogen therapy and cardiometabolic risk in polycystic ovary syndrome. *Clin Endocrinol, 78*, 120–125.

Hunter, M. H., & Sterrett, J. J. (2000). Polycystic ovary syndrome: it's not just infertility. *Am Fam Physician, 62*,1079–1088, 1090.

Huxley, R., Ying Lee, C. M., Barzi, F., et al. (2009). Coffee, decaffeinated coffee, and tea consumption in relation to incident type 2 diabetes. *Arch Intern Med, 169*, 2053–2063.

Isu, H., Date, C., Wakai, K., Fukui, M., Tamakoshi, A., & the JACC Study Group. (2006). The relationship between green tea and total caffeine intake and risk among Japanese adults. *Ann Intern Med, 144*, 554–562.

Johansson, J., Redman, L., Veldhuis, P. P., Sazonova, A., Labrie, F., Holm, G., ... Stener-Victorin, E. (2013). Acupuncture for ovulation induction in polycystic ovary syndrome: A randomized controlled trial. *Am J Physiol Endocrinol Metab, 304*, E934–E943.

Karadeniz, M., Erdongan, M., Gerdeli, A., et al. (2007). The progesterone receptor PROGINS polymorphism is not related to oxidative stress factors in women with polycystic ovary syndrome. *Cardiovasc Diabetol, 6*, 29.

Kelly, G. S. (2000). Insulin resistance: lifestyle and nutritional interventions. *Altern Med Rev: J Clin Therapeut, 5*,109–132.

Kodaman, P. H., & Duleba, A. J. (2008). Statins in the treatment of polycystic ovary syndrome. *Semin Reprod Med, 26*, 127–138.

Kopper, L. L., Dekker, J. M., Hendriks, H. F., et al. (2005). Moderate alcohol consumption lowers risk of type 2 diabetes care. *Diabetes Care, 28*, 719–725.

Lau, D. C. W. (2007). Screening for diabetes in women with polycystic ovary syndrome. *CMAJ, 176*, 951.

Lord, J. M., Flight, I. H. K., & Norman, R. J. (2003). Metformin in polycystic ovary syndrome: Systematic review and meta-analysis. *Br Med J, 327*, 1–6.

Na, L., Fu, S., Zhu, F., et al. (2013). Alcohol intake diminishes ovarian reserve in childbearing age women. *J Obst Gyn Res, 39*, 516–521.

Pattar, G. R., Tackett, L., Liu, P., & Elmendorf, J. S. (2006). Chromium picolinate positively influences the glucose transporter system via affecting cholesterol homeostasis in adipocytes cultured under hyperglycemic conditions. *Mutat Res, 610*, 93–100.

Ravn, P., Haugen, A. G., & Glintborg, D. (2013). Overweight in polycystic ovary syndrome: An update on evidence based advice on diet, exercise and metformin use for weight loss. *Minerva Endocrinol, 38*, 59–76.

Rizk, A. Y., Bedaiwy, M. A., & Al-Inany, H. G. (2005). N-acetyl-cysteine is a novel adjuvant to clomiphene citrate in clomiphene citrate-resistant patients with polycystic ovary syndrome. *Fertil Steril, 83*, 367–370.

Seivenpiper, J. L., Amason, J. T., Leiter, L. A., et al. (2003). Variable effects of American Ginseng: a batch of American Ginseng (*Panax quinquefolius* L.) with a depressed ginsenoside profile does not affect post prandial glycemia. *Eur J Clin Nutr, 57*, 243–248.

Seivenpiper, J. L., Arnason, J. T., Leiter, L. A., et al. (2004). Decreasing, null and increasing effects of eight popular types of ginseng on acute postprandial glycemic indices in healthy humans: The role of ginsenosides. *J Am Coll Nutr, 23*, 248–258.

Sheehan, M. T. (2004). Polycystic ovarian syndrome: diagnosis and management. *Clin Med Res, 2*, 13–27.

Slowey, M. J. (2001). Polycystic ovary syndrome: new perspective on an old problem. *South Med J, 94*, 190–196.

Stener-Victorin, E., Holm, G., Janson, P. O., Gustafson, D., & Waern, M. (2013). Acupuncture and physical exercise for affective symptoms and health-related quality of life in polycystic ovary syndrome: Secondary analysis from a randomized controlled trial. *BMC Complement Altern Med, 13*, 131.

Stener-Victorin, E., Waldenstrom, U., Tagnfors, U., et al. (2000). Effects of electro-acupuncture on anovulation in women with polycystic ovary syndrome. *Acta Obstet Gynecol Scand, 79*, 180–188.

Tan, W. C., Yap, C., & Tan, A. S. (2001). Clinical management of PCOS. *Acta Obstet Gynecol Scand, 80*, 689–696.

Taylor, K. C., Small, C. M., Dominguez, C. E., et al. (2011). Alcohol, smoking and caffeine in relationship to fecundibility, with effect modification by NAT 2. *Ann Epidemiol, 21,* 864–872.

Thys-Jacobs, S., Donovan, D., Papadopoulos, A., Sarrel, P., & Bilezikian, J. P. (1999). Vitamin D and calcium dysregulation in the polycystic ovarian syndrome. *Steroids, 64,* 430–435.

Vuksan, V., Sievenpiper, J. L., Koo, V. Y. Y., Francis, T., Beljan-Zdravkovic, U., Xu, Z., & Vigden, E. (2000). American ginseng (*Panax quinquefolius* l) reduces postprandial glycemia in nondiabetic subjects and subjects with type 2 diabetes mellitus. *Arch Intern Med, 160,* 1009–1013.

Wang, J. G., Anderson, R. A., Graham, G. M., Chu, M. C., Sauer, M. V., Guarnaccia, M. M., & Lobo, R. A. (2007). The effect of cinnamon extract on insulin resistance parameters in polycystic ovary syndrome: a pilot study. *Fertil Steril, 88,* 240–243.

Wikipedia.com. (2014). *Alcoholic beverages: Standard drink section.* Retrieved December 12, 2014.

Wise, L. A., Palmer, J. R., Stewart, E. A., & Rosenberg, L. (2007). Polycystic ovary syndrome and risk of uterine leiomyomata. *Fertil Steril, 87,* 1108–1115.

Wulffele, M. G., Kooy, A., deZeeuw, D., et al. (2004). The effect of metformin on blood pressure, plasma cholesterol and triglycerides in type 2 diabetes mellitus: a systematic review. *J Intern Med, 256,* 1–14.

Zeigenfuss, T. N., Hofheins, J. E., Mendel, R. W., Landis, J., & Anderson, R. A. (2006). Effects of water soluble cinnamon extract on body composition and features of the metabolic syndrome in prediabetic men and women. *J Int Soc Sports Nutr, 3,* 45–53.

17

Endometriosis

MARGEVA MORRIS COLE

CASE STUDY

Ellen is a 28-year-old magazine editor who is eager to conceive. She and her husband have tried for more than 1 year without success. She has predictable monthly menses and her testing for ovulation has been normal. Her husband, Tom, just received results documenting a normal semen analysis. Ellen has no history of sexually transmitted diseases, and her hysterosalpingogram showed a normal uterine cavity and patent tubes.

Further discussion with Ellen reveals that she has had severe cramping with her menses since she was a teen. She requires large doses of ibuprofen for control. Her cramping has been better during the years she was on oral contraceptives (OCs). Ellen is active physically but admits to eating whatever is available because of her busy schedule. Her stress at work and the concern over possible infertility has caused her great anxiety. Her tension and irritability is starting to put a strain on her emotional and sexual relationship with her husband, Tom.

After discussion with the couple, Ellen opts to undergo a diagnostic laparoscopy at which multiple endometriosis implants are noted throughout the pelvis. The visible implants are excised or ablated using laser and cautery. She recovers well. When the surgical findings are reviewed with the couple, Ellen's physician explains the impact of endometriosis on fertility. Ellen has several choices: to suppress the endometriosis with a gonadotropin-releasing hormone (GnRH) agonist for several months, to proceed with infertility therapy such as in vitro fertilization with a specialist, or to continue to try on their own for several more months.

Ellen is eager to continue to try on her own for 6 more months. She does not want the delay that Lupron would require and is not ready yet to move on to assisted reproductive interventions. Her physician discusses with her an approach to suppression of inflammation in her body through a healthy diet with fresh fruits and vegetables, whole grains, and healthy oils. Preconception nutrition with supplementation of folic acid, vitamin D, and omega-3 fatty acids is also reviewed. Herbal therapies are not encouraged at this time because of lack of data on efficacy and safety in early pregnancy. The physical and psychological benefits of stress reduction through yoga and mindfulness-based stress reduction techniques are emphasized. Options for couples counseling and group forums to explore the stresses of and responses to infertility are also offered. Ellen's physician makes her confident that whenever she is ready to return to discuss other avenues, the door will be open.

Introduction

Endometriosis is a common but enigmatic condition, affecting up to 50% of asymptomatic reproductive age women (Fauconnier & Chapron, 2005; Box 17.1).

Box 17.1 How Many Women Have Endometriosis?

1% of women undergoing major surgery for all gynecologic indications
1%–7% of women undergoing tubal sterilization
12%–32% of women of reproductive age undergoing laparoscopy for pelvic pain
9%–50% of women undergoing laparoscopy for infertility
50% of teenagers undergoing laparoscopy for evaluation of chronic pelvic pain or dysmenorrhea

Sources: Chatman and Ward (1982); Sangi-Haghpeykar and Poindexter (1995); Missmer et al. (2004).

Its diagnosis and management are hampered by poor correlation between the degree of symptoms and the extent of disease (Fedele, Parazzini, Bianchi, Arcaini, & Candiani, 1990; Vercellini et al., 1996).

Pathogenesis

Endometriosis can be defined as the presence of ectopic implants of endometrial glands and stroma outside the uterus. Several theories of pathogenesis attempt to explain its variable presentations (Schenken, 1989; Table 17.1).

Endometriosis most commonly affects the pelvic peritoneal surfaces and the external surfaces of the ovary, fallopian tubes, and uterus (Jenkins, Olive, & Haney, 1986; Figure 17.1). More severe disease can involve invasion into the bowel and bladder or distant metastases to other organs such as the lungs (Fauconnier et al., 2002). Endometriosis can also develop in the abdominal wall, most often in the incision following Cesarean section (Minaglia, Mishell, & Ballard, 2007).

The cause of endometriosis is still unclear, but many factors may influence its development in a given individual (Hadfield, Mardon, Barlow, & Kennedy, 1997; Hediger, Hartnett, & Louis, 2005; Houston, 1984; Olive & Henderson, 1987; Sangi-Haghpeykar & Poindexter, 1995; Simpson, Elias, Malinak, & Buttram, 1980; Box 17.2).

Table 17.1. Theories of Pathogenesis

Name	Theory	Supporting Evidence
Retrograde menstruation	Implantation of endometrial cells onto peritoneum due to retrograde flow of menses through the fallopian tube	Increased incidence of endometriosis in women with congenital obstruction of the reproductive tract
Coelomic metaplasia	Transformation of multipotential peritoneal cells into endometrial glands	Development of endometriosis in women with uterine agenesis
Hematologic or lymphatic spread	Transport of endometrial glands through the vascular and lymphatic systems	Presence of endometriosis in sites outside the abdominal cavity
Direct transplantation	Iatrogenic displacement of cells into the body wall at the time of surgery	Endometriosis implants in scars from Cesarean sections and episiotomies

Source: Schenken (1989).

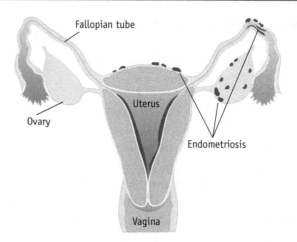

FIGURE 17.1. Common locations for endometriosis implants in the pelvis.

One study has suggested a higher prevalence of endometriosis in women with other autoimmune inflammatory diseases such as hypothyroidism, asthma, allergies, chronic fatigue syndrome, and fibromyalgia (Sinaii, Cleary, Ballweg, Nieman, & Stratton, 2002). Another study suggests the possible role of environmental factors such as exposure to dioxins and PCBs (Foster & Agarwal, 2002).

Symptoms/Diagnosis

Symptoms of endometriosis vary in intensity, confounding attempts at diagnosis. Cyclic severe dysmenorrhea may be the most common presenting

---

Box 17.2 Risk Factors for Endometriosis

Nulliparity (Simpson, Elias, Malinak, & Buttram, 1980)

Delayed childbearing (Simpson et al., 1980)

Family history/genetic factors (Simpson et al., 1980; Hadfield, Mardon, Barlow, & Kennedy, 1997)

Decreased BMI (Hediger, Hartnett, & Louis, 2005)

Increased height (Hediger et al., 2005)

Caucasian race (Sangi-Haghpeykar & Poindexter, 2995; Houston, 1984)

Congenital anatomic variations that obstruct menstrual flow — (blind uterine horn, cervical agenesis, transverse vaginal septum) (Olive & Henderson, 1987)

symptom, but chronic pelvic pain, dyspareunia, delayed fertility, and abnormal bleeding can also be associated with endometriosis (Kennedy et al., 2005; Sinaii et al., 2008). Overlapping symptoms such as cyclic bowel and bladder symptoms and sharp pelvic pain can complicate the differentiation of endometriosis from irritable bowel syndrome, inflammatory bowel disease, interstitial cystitis, and pelvic inflammatory disease (Husby, Haugen, & Moen, 2003).

Pain from endometriosis appears to arise from release of proinflammatory substances such as cytokines and prostaglandins as well as direct infiltration of local nerves (Harada, Momoeda, Taketani, Hoshiai, & Terakawa, 2001; Lebovic, Mueller, & Taylor, 2001; Ryan et al., 1995; Van Langendonckt, Casanas-Roux, & Donnez, 2002).

Though certain physical examination findings can be suggestive of endometriosis, the physical examination is often entirely unremarkable (Vercellini et al., 1996; Box 17.3). Radiologic imaging is generally not sensitive enough to detect endometriosis unless an endometrioma is present on one or both ovaries (Abrao et al., 2007; Guerriero et al., 1996; Kinkel, Frei, Balleyguier, & Chapron, 2006; Moore et al., 2002).

Definitive diagnosis is made by biopsy at laparoscopy (Stratton et al., 2002; Walter, Hentz, Magtibay, Cornella, & Magrina, 2001). Sensitivity and accuracy of diagnosis at the time of laparoscopy depends on the experience and diligence of the surgeon. Implants can be subtle and variable in appearance. They can hide behind ovaries and other structures or under the peritoneal surface, or involve less obvious locations such as the surface of the appendix (Gustofson, Kim, Liu, & Stratton, 2006). Careful surveillance and multiple biopsies increase the rate of detection (Wykes, Clark, & Khan, 2004). If extensive implants are visible, diagnosis by photography and biopsy can be straightforward and conclusive (Marchino et al., 2005). Despite careful evaluation, the extent of findings at laparoscopy does not always correlate well with the magnitude of the patient's symptoms or chances for fertility (Fedele et al., 1990).

Box 17.3 Physical Examination Findings in Endometriosis

Adnexal mass
Fixed, retroverted uterus
Nodularity of uterosacral ligaments, rectovaginal septum, or posterior cul-de-sac
Shortening of cardinal ligament
Pain with palpation of uterus, cul-de-sac, or uterosacral ligaments

Psychological Effects

Endometriosis can have a dramatic effect on a woman's well-being. Aside from the impact of cyclic or chronic pelvic pain, sexual relationships and enjoyment can also be affected by deep dyspareunia. In addition, approximately 30%–50% of patients with endometriosis may have difficulty conceiving (Winkel, 2003). These difficulties can affect a woman's sense of wholeness and her ability to cope with stress, resulting in increased rates of depression (Lorencatto, Petta, Navarro, Bahamondes, & Matos, 2006).

Management

Management of endometriosis focuses on both the reduction of symptoms and improvement in the quality of life. These approaches may also minimize the extent of disease.

MEDICAL INTERVENTION

Medical management of endometriosis offers a variety of options for treatment. Nonsteroidal anti-inflammatory drugs (NSAIDs) are often the first-line therapy for dysmenorrhea (Allen, Hopewell, Prentice, & Gregory, 2005). Hormonal treatments can be offered to those not currently seeking pregnancy. Most commonly, oral contraceptives are used in either a cyclic or continuous fashion. They induce a progestin-dominant hormonal state that causes decidualization and atrophy of endometrial tissue. Oral contraceptives are more effective in reducing dysmenorrhea than dyspareunia (Harada et al., 2008; Winkel, 2003).

Other sources of progestins can have a similar effect with varying side-effect profiles. Oral progestins such as medroxyprogesterone and norethindrone have been used continuously for suppression of endometriosis with good success (Prentice, Deary, & Bland, 2000). Injectable depot medroxyprogesterone acetate (DMPA or DepoProvera) reduced dysmenorrhea and pelvic pain significantly in one study (Crosignani, Luciano, Ray, & Bergqvist, 2006). Several studies now also point to the successful use of the levonorgestrel IUD for reduction of pelvic pain and dysmenorrhea (Lockhat, Emembolu, & Konje, 2005; Petta et al., 2005; Vercellini et al., 1999; Vercellini et al., 2003).

Danazol is another oral agent used with great success for suppression of symptoms associated with endometriosis. Its use in recent years has decreased because of its extensive side-effect profile, including hirsutism, acne, weight gain, and depression (Selak, Farquhar, Prentice, & Singla, 2007).

> I have found that the Mirena levonorgestrel IUD is invaluable in women looking for long-term relief from dysmenorrhea who are not interested in hysterectomy. It is equally effective in cases of primary dysmenorrhea, endometriosis, and adenomyosis, thus avoiding the need for laparoscopy if the IUD gives relief. The Mirena can simply be replaced every 5 years until the woman is menopausal.

Gonadotropin-releasing hormone agonists have become the mainstay of medical therapy for patients with moderate to severe pain. The medication induces a hypoestrogenic state, mimicking menopause. The removal of estrogenic stimulation then induces atrophy of active endometriosis lesions (Ling, 1999; Prentice, Deary, Goldbeck-Wood, Farquhar, & Smith, 2000). A 6-month course of intramuscular or intranasal therapy can lead to 85%–100% improvement in symptoms (Winkel & Scialli, 2001). The side effects of the medication also mimic menopause (hot flashes, vaginal dryness, bone loss) and are eliminated by hormonal "add-back" therapy without loss in GnRH efficacy (Surrey, 1999).

Newer medications used in endometriosis therapy include progesterone antagonists, selective progesterone receptor modulators, and aromatase inhibitors (Prentice, Deary, & Bland, 2000). All are being used effectively in early pilot studies (Attar & Bulun, 2006; Chwalisz et al., 2005; Patwardhan et al., 2008). Ovarian suppression with GnRH agonists should be considered when using aromatase inhibitors due to their potential for causing development of painful ovarian cysts in ovulatory women (Remorgida, Abbamonte, Ragni, Fulcheri, & Ferrero, 2007).

SURGICAL MANAGEMENT

Surgical management allows definitive diagnosis but also incurs surgical risk. It is often the preferred path of therapy for those wishing to conceive as soon as possible, since the medical therapies either preclude or are contraindicated in pregnancy. Surgery can be definitive or conservative. Definitive surgery involves hysterectomy with or without removal of the ovaries. This route is often pursued by women with severe unrelenting disease who do not wish future childbearing. In most instances, hysterectomy should be discouraged in young women who may later choose to have children (MacDonald,

Klock, & Milad, 1999). Recurrence of endometriosis is rare after hysterectomy (Namnoum, Hickman, Goodman, Gehlbach, & Rock, 1995).

Conservative surgery usually involves laparoscopy to investigate the pelvis and treat as much of the endometriosis as possible while leaving the pelvic organs in place (Crosignani et al., 1996). Endometriosis lesions can be excised sharply or ablated with laser or electrosurgery. The extent of treatment can be limited by the proximity of implants to important pelvic structures such as ureters and pelvic vessels and nerves.

When present, endometriomas may require only excision of the cyst or partial/total oophorectomy. Interruption of the presacral or uterosacral nerve pathways at the time of laparoscopy has not been found to increase the success rate after surgery (Proctor, Latthe, Farquhar, Khan, & Johnson, 2005). Follow-up after conservative surgery suggests good short-term relief at 6 months but significant recurrence of symptoms at 1 to 2 years (Jacobson, Barlow, Garry, & Koninckx, 2001; Sutton, Ewen, Whitelaw, & Haines, 1994). A significant number of women will require repeat surgery over time (Shakiba, Bena, McGill, Minger, & Falcone, 2008). Postoperative therapy with GnRH agonists or levonorgestrel IUD appears to delay recurrence of symptoms (Hornstein, Hemmings, Yuzpe, & Heinrichs, 1997; Vercellini et al., 2003).

Integrative Approaches

Integrative approaches to endometriosis often focus on reducing the inflammatory response that fosters the pain experienced by the patient as well as moderating the psychological and emotional stress engendered by chronic pain.

As in other areas of medicine, one of the primary areas of emphasis should be education about the role of the anti-inflammatory diet. Simple interventions such as reducing intake of processed foods and red meat and increasing intake of fresh fruits, green vegetables, and omega-3 fatty acids can help ameliorate a patient's symptoms (Fjerbaek & Knudsen, 2007; Fugh-Berman & Kronenberg, 2003; Parazzini et al., 2004). For more information on the anti-inflammatory diet, see the chapter "Nutrition."

The experience of pain and dysmenorrhea has a significant effect on a woman's psychological and emotional well-being. Similarly, significant social stressors and weak social networks can aggravate the intensity of dysmenorrhea (Alonso & Coe, 2001). Mind–body techniques such as mindfulness-based stress reduction, cognitive-behavioral therapy, hypnosis, guided imagery, and biofeedback have been used for decades to reduce stress and increase coping skills. Symptoms of dysmenorrhea and pelvic pain may be reduced with these behavioral interventions, which can reduce the body's responsiveness to the stress of pain (Proctor, Murphy, Pattison, Suckling, & Farquhar, 2007). In the setting of endometriosis, these techniques offer the woman a measure of self-control as she learns to cope with her symptoms. The ability to relax, to alleviate accumulated stress, and to allay anxiety can be powerful tools while other interventions begin to take effect. The woman may feel more whole when she gains more control over her body's response to stress.

> Patients with chronic pain often develop a panicky response to each episode of pain or to new stimuli such a pelvic examination. Teaching them coping skills such as breathing exercises or imagery can help them weather each experience with less fear and tension.

Chronic tension in the muscles of the abdomen, legs, and pelvic floor may result from years of conditioned response to pelvic pain. Regular exercise can decrease the amount of pain experienced (Fugh-Berman & Kronenberg, 2003). Stretching and yoga may increase the patient's day-to-day functioning and sense of well-being. Targeted pelvic floor physical therapy with a specially trained therapist can reduce pain scores, especially in chronic pelvic pain and dyspareunia. Massage can also be a relaxing adjunctive therapy. There are no clinical trials of the use of these modalities with endometriosis. Research on frequently used spinal manipulation techniques has not been shown to be effective in cases of primary or secondary dysmenorrhea (Proctor, Hing, Johnson, & Murphy, 2006).

> In patients who have years of pelvic pain due to endometriosis, pain may persist after effective treatment due to "trigger points" or "knots" in the muscles of the abdominal wall due to years of guarding against the pain. I have found that these patients are often best served with a referral to a skilled physical therapist with specialized training in techniques focused on the pelvis. Other excellent referral options include experienced acupuncturists or practitioners skilled in manual interventions such as the counterstrain technique.

Acupuncture has been posited as a possible effective treatment for endometriosis-related pelvic pain and dysmenorrhea due to its descending pain inhibition and possible reduction in cytokine release (Lundeberg & Lund, 2008; Wayne et al., 2008). At this time, no large studies have been completed to examine this treatment approach. Two small pilot studies suggest that acupuncture may be a safe, well-accepted and possibly effective treatment

Table 17.2. Medicinal Herbs and Natural Compounds Used in the Treatment of Endometriosis and Their Anti-inflammatory Effects

Herbs	Antiproliferative	Antinociceptive, Sedative	Anti-inflammatory Action			
			Antioxidant	Suppression		
				COX-2	Cytokines	NF-KappaB
Bupleurum	+				+	+
Chinese angelica	+	+	+		+	
Dahurian angelica root	+	+		+	+	+
Cattail pollen					+	
Cinnamon twigs		+		+		
Cnidium fruit	+	+				
Corydalis		+			+	
Curcuma (turmeric)	+	+	+	+	+	+
Cyperus	+		+			
Frankincense	+	+			+	+
Licorice root	+	+		+	+	+
Myrrh		+	+		+	
Persica					+	
Poria	+	+		+	+	
Red peony root			+			
Rhubarb	+	+			+	+
Salvia root		+	+			+
Scutellaria	+			+	+	
Sparganium		+			+	
Tortoise shell						+
White peony root				+	+	

Source: Wieser et al. (2007), by permission of Oxford University Press.

for endometriosis in adolescents (Highfield et al., 2006; Wayne et al., 2008). Several other smaller studies have focused on the relief of dysmenorrhea not specific to endometriosis. These have found that acupuncture reduces the intensity of both dysmenorrhea up to 6 months after treatment, although secondary dysmenorrhea may be less responsive than primary (Helms, 1987; Iorno et al., 2008; Witt et al., 2008).

Botanical therapies have been used for centuries to reduce pain in the pelvis as well as elsewhere in the body. Studies suggest that these herbs and their multiple constituent bioactive compounds may work through COX-2 inhibition, suppression of cytokines, antioxidant effects, and direct sedative and antinociceptive properties (Wieser et al., 2007; Table 17.2).

At this time, there are few high-quality evidence-based studies that examine the efficacy, side effects, and interactions of these medicinal herbal compounds in women, although protocols are currently underway (Flower, Lewith, & Little, 2007; Zhu, Proctor, Bensoussan, Smith, & Wu, 2008). Commonly used herbs with a benign safety profile include chaste tree berry, black cohosh, black haw, cramp bark, dong quai, and ginger. No studies exist to assess their efficacy in endometriosis and dysmenorrhea (Low Dog & Micozzi, 2005; Table 17.3).

Small studies have evaluated pycnogenol and the traditional Japanese herbal formula Toki-shakuyaku-san and found them to be helpful in reducing dysmenorrhea (Kohama, Herai, & Inoue, 2007; Suzuki et al., 2008; Tanaka, 2003). Traditional Chinese medicine has used many herbal compounds alone and in combination to battle dysmenorrhea through a reduction of qi stasis in the liver (Table 17.4). Early research data on these compounds exists in a few Chinese language studies (Jia et al., 2006). The primary side effects of these compounds seem to be interaction with anticoagulant medications (Wieser et al., 2007).

My Approach With a Woman With Severe Dysmenorrhea

Thorough history including:

- Menstrual and sexual history including age of onset of menses, age of onset of dysmenorrhea, frequency of menses, age of first coitus, pain throughout menstrual cycle, and dyspareunia
- General medical history of other inflammatory conditions, depression, and pain syndromes
- Surgical history of prior abdominal procedures
- Family history of endometriosis, fibroids, early hysterectomy

- Social history (diet, stressors)
- Current medications and supplements

Careful physical examination to evaluate for abnormalities as noted in Box 17.3.If abnormalities of uterus or ovaries are noted on physical examination, then I will order imaging by ultrasound. Significant evidence of scarring and nodularity will prompt me to consider laparoscopy earlier in the evaluation.

Initial therapy usually involves prescription-strength NSAIDs such as Naproxen and oral contraceptives unless there is a medical contraindication to estrogen. I usually start with cyclic OCs and then move to continuous OCs after 3 months if the cyclic therapy has not been sufficient. Some patients will do well with Depo-Provera or oral norethindrone.

We also discuss the anti-inflammatory diet, stress reduction, stretching, exercise, and application of heat. Referrals for physical therapy, acupuncture, or other complementary modalities are offered to the patient according to her needs and interests.

If continuous OCs do not control the patient's dysmenorrhea or if the patient declines OC therapy, we discuss laparoscopy or empiric GnRH agonist therapy.

At the time of laparoscopy, all evident lesions are ablated or excised. Postoperative suppression of endometriosis follows with continuous OCs, oral or injectable progestin, GnRH agonist injections, or levonorgestrel IUD. The GnRH agonist therapy usually lasts 6 months. I use add-back with either norethindrone acetate 5 mg/day or low-dose ethinyl estradiol 1 mg/norethindrone acetate 5 mg/day (Femhrt, Warner Chilcott). If this is started at the time of the first GnRH agonist injection, patients rarely experience the classic hot flashes associated with GnRH therapy.

After the 6-month course, the patient then chooses suppression with OCs, progestins, or levonorgestrel IUD long-term unless she wishes to try for pregnancy.

Most patients will have several years of relief before recurrence of symptoms.

Summary

Endometriosis is a medical condition with unclear etiology and aggravating factors. Currently, the most well studied approaches involve surgery, nonsteroidal use, and hormonal therapies. Alternative therapies offer a less-invasive approach focused on reducing the pain associated with endometriosis implants, but, as yet, there is minimal scientific evidence to support its efficacy.

Table 17.3. Commonly Used Herbs

Common Name	Scientific Name	Effect	Side Effects	Contraindications
Chaste tree berry	*Vitex agnus castus*	Enhances progesterone activity/binding		
Black cohosh	*Cimicifuga racemosa*	Antispasmodic, Anti-inflammatory		Pregnancy, lactation
Black haw	*Viburnum prunifolium*	Uterine relaxant		Active oxalate-containing kidney stones
Cramp bark	*Viburnum opulus*	Uterine relaxant		
Dong quai	*Angelica sinensis*	Uterine relaxation and stimulation, anti-inflammatory, analgesic	Prolongation of prothrombin time	Pregnancy, warfarin use
Ginger	*Zingiber officinale*	antispasmodic		Active gallstone disease
Kava	*Piper methysticum*	Muscle relaxant, sedative	CNS depression, possible hepatotoxicity	Pregnancy, lactation, depression
Pulsatilla	*Anemone pulsatilla*	Antispasmodic, sedative, analgesic		Pregnancy, lactation
Cotton root bark	*Gossypium* spp.	Atrophy of endometrial tissue (possibly antiprogestational)	Hypokalemia	Pregnancy, lactation
Yellow vine	*Tripterygium wilfordii*	Anti-inflammatory, immunosuppressive	Menstrual irregularities	Pregnancy, lactation

Source: Low and Micozzi (2005).

Table 17.4. TCM Herbs Commonly Used for Dysmenorrhea

Pharmacopia Name	Binomial
Caulis Sargentodoxae	Sargentodoxa cuneata
Cortex Cinnamomi Cassiae	Cinnamomum cassia
Cortex Moutan	Paeonia suffruticosa
Faeces Trogopterorum	Trogopterus xanthipes or Pteromys volans
Flos Carthami	Carthamus tinctorius
Flos Rosae Chinensis	Rosa chinensis
Fructus Akebiae	Akebia quinata
Fructus Foeniculi	Foeniculum vulgare
Fructus Jujubae	Ziziphus jujuba
Herba Leonuri and Fructus Leonuri	Leonurus heterophyllus
Herba Selaginellae	Selaginella tamariscina
Herba Lycopi	Lycopus lucidus
Herba Verbenae	Verbena officinalis
Lignum Sappan	Lignum sappan
Pollen Typhae	Typha angustifolia
Radix Angelicae Sinensis	Angelicae sinensis
Radix Astragali	Astragalus membranaceus
Radix Curcumae	Aromaticae Curcuma aromatica
Radix Linderae	Lindera strychnifolia
Radix Paeoniae Alba and Radix Paeoniae Rubra	Paeonia veitchii and Paeoni lactiflora
Radix Rehmanniae	Rehmannia glutinosa
Radix Salviae Miltiorrhizae	Salvia miltiorrhiza
Rhizoma Chuanxiong	Ligusticum chuanxiong
Rhizoma Corydalis	Corydalis yanhusuo
Rhizoma Curcumae Longae	Curcuma longa
Rhizoma Cyperi	Cyperus rotundus
Semen Persicae	Prunus persica
Semen Vaccariae	Vaccaria segetalis

Source: Jia et al. (2006).

REFERENCES

Abrao, M. S., Gonçalves, M. O., Dias, J. A., Jr., Podgaec, S., Chamie, L. P., & Blasbalg, R. (2007). Comparison between clinical examination, transvaginal sonography and magnetic resonance imaging for the diagnosis of deep endometriosis. *Hum Reprod*, 22, 3092–3097.

Allen, C., Hopewell, S., Prentice, A., & Gregory, D. (2005). Non-steroidal anti-inflammatory drugs for pain in women with endometriosis. *Cochrane Database Syst Rev*, 4:CD004753.

Alonso, C., & Coe, C. L. (2001). Disruptions of social relationships accentuate the association between emotional distress and menstrual pain in young women. *Health Psychol*, 20, 411–416.

Attar, E., & Bulun, S. E. (2006). Aromatase inhibitors: The next generation of therapeutics for endometriosis? *Fertil Steril*, 85, 1307–1318.

Chatman, D. L., & Ward, A. B. (1982). Endometriosis in adolescents. *J Reprod Med*, 27, 156–160.

Chwalisz, K., Perez, M. C., Demanno, D., Winkel, C., Schubert, G., & Elger, W. (2005). Selective progesterone receptor modulator development and use in the treatment of leiomyomata and endometriosis. *Endocr Rev*, 26, 423–438.

Crosignani, P. G., Luciano, A., Ray, A., & Bergqvist, A. (2006). Subcutaneous depot medroxyprogesterone acetate versus leuprolide acetate in the treatment of endometriosis-associated pain. *Hum Reprod*, 21, 248–256.

Crosignani, P. G., Vercellini, P., Biffignandi, F., Costantini, W., Cortesi, I., & Imparato, E. (1996). Laparoscopy versus laparotomy in conservative surgical treatment for severe endometriosis. *Fertil Steril*, 66, 706–711.

Fauconnier, A., & Chapron, C. (2005). Endometriosis and pelvic pain: Epidemiological evidence of the relationship and implications. *Hum Reprod Update*, 11, 595–606.

Fauconnier, A., Chapron, C., Dubuisson, J. B., Vieira, M., Dousset, B., & Bréart, G. (2002). Relation between pain symptoms and the anatomic location of deep infiltrating endometriosis. *Fertil Steril*, 78, 719–726.

Fedele, L., Parazzini, F., Bianchi, S., Arcaini, L., & Candiani, G. B. (1990). Stage and localization of pelvic endometriosis and pain. *Fertil Steril*, 53, 155–158.

Fjerbaek, A., & Knudsen, U. B. (2007). Endometriosis, dysmenorrhea and diet: What is the evidence? *Eur J Obstet Gynecol Reprod Biol*, 132, 140–147.

Flower, A., Lewith, G. T., & Little, P. (2007). Seeking an oracle: Using the Delphi process to develop practice guidelines for the treatment of endometriosis with Chinese herbal medicine. *J Altern Complement Med*, 13, 969–976.

Foster, W. G., & Agarwal, S. K. (2002). Environmental contaminants and dietary factors in endometriosis. *Ann N Y Acad Sci*, 955, 213–229; discussion 230–232, 396–406.

Fugh-Berman, A., & Kronenberg, F. (2003). Complementary and alternative medicine (CAM) in reproductive-age women: A review of randomized controlled trials. *Reprod Toxicol*, 17, 137–152.

Guerriero, S., Mais, V., Ajossa, S., Paoletti, A. M., Angiolucci, M., & Melis, G. B. (1996). Transvaginal ultrasonography combined with CA-125 plasma levels in the diagnosis of endometrioma. *Fertil Steril, 65*, 293–298.

Gustofson, R. L., Kim, N., Liu, S., & Stratton, P. (2006). Endometriosis and the appendix: A case series and comprehensive review of the literature. *Fertil Steril, 86*, 298–303.

Hadfield, R. M., Mardon, H. J., Barlow, D. H., & Kennedy, S. H. (1997). Endometriosis in monozygotic twins. *Fertil Steril, 68*, 941–942.

Harada, T., Iwabe, T., & Terakawa, N. (2001). Role of cytokines in endometriosis. *Fertil Steril, 76*, 1–10.

Harada, T., Momoeda, M., Taketani, H., Hoshiai, H., & Terakawa, N. (2008). Low-dose oral contraceptive pill for dysmenorrhea associated with endometriosis: A placebo-controlled, double-blind, randomized trial. *Fertil Steril, 90*, 1583–1588.

Hediger, M. L., Hartnett, H. J., & Louis, G. M. (2005). Association of endometriosis with body size and figure. *Fertil Steril, 84*, 1366–1374.

Helms, J. M. (1987). Acupuncture for the management of primary dysmenorrhea. *Obstet Gynecol, 69*, 51–56.

Highfield, E. S., Laufer, M. R., Schnyer, R. N., Kerr, C. E., Thomas, P., & Wayne, P. M. (2006). Adolescent endometriosis-related pelvic pain treated with acupuncture: Two case reports. *J Altern Complement Med, 12*, 317–322.

Hornstein, M. D., Hemmings, R., Yuzpe, A. A., & Heinrichs, W. L. (1997). Use of nafarelin versus placebo after reductive laparoscopic surgery for endometriosis. *Fertil Steril, 68*, 860–864.

Houston, D. E. (1984). Evidence for the risk of pelvic endometriosis by age, race and socioeconomic status. *Epidemiol Rev, 6*, 167–191.

Husby, G. K., Haugen, R. S., & Moen, M. H. (2003). Diagnostic delay in women with pain and endometriosis. *Acta Obstet Gynecol Scand, 82*, 649–653.

Iorno, V., Burani, R., Bianchini, B., Minelli, E., Martinelli, F., & Ciatto, S. (2008). Acupuncture treatment of dysmenorrhea resistant to conventional medical treatment. *Evid Based Complement Alternat Med, 5*, 227–230.

Jacobson, T. Z., Barlow, D. H., Garry, R., & Koninckx, P. (2001). Laparoscopic surgery for pelvic pain associated with endometriosis. *Cochrane Database Syst Rev*, 4:CD001300.

Jenkins, S., Olive, D. L., & Haney, A. F. (1986). Endometriosis: Pathogenetic implications of the anatomic distribution. *Obstet Gynecol, 67*, 335–338.

Jia, W., Wang, X., Xu, D., Zhao, A., & Zhang, Y. (2006). Common traditional Chinese medicinal herbs for dysmenorrhea. *Phytother Res, 20*, 819–824.

Kennedy, S., Bergqvist, A., Chapron, C., et al. (2005). ESHRE guideline for the diagnosis and treatment of endometriosis. *Hum Reprod, 20*, 2698–2704.

Kinkel, K., Frei, K. A., Balleyguier, C., & Chapron, C. (2006). Diagnosis of endometriosis with imaging: A review. *Eur Radiol, 16*, 285–298.

Kohama, T., Herai, K., & Inoue, M. (2007). Effect of French maritime pine bark extract on endometriosis as compared with leuprorelin acetate. *J Reprod Med, 52*, 703–708.

Lebovic, D. I., Mueller, M. D., & Taylor, R. N. (2001). Immunobiology of endometriosis. *Fertil Steril, 75*, 1–10.

Ling, F. W. (1999). Randomized controlled trial of depot leuprolide in patients with chronic pelvic pain and clinically suspected endometriosis. Pelvic Pain Study Group. *Obstet Gynecol, 93*, 51–58.

Lockhat, F. B., Emembolu, J. O., & Konje, J. C. (2005). The efficacy, side-effects and continuation rates in women with symptomatic endometriosis undergoing treatment with an intra-uterine administered progestogen (levonorgestrel): A 3 year follow-up. *Hum Reprod, 20*, 789–793.

Lorencatto, C., Petta, C. A., Navarro, M. J., Bahamondes, L., & Matos, A. (2006). Depression in women with endometriosis with and without chronic pelvic pain. *Acta Obstet Gynecol Scand, 85*, 88–92.

Low Dog, T., & Micozzi, M. S. (2005). *Women's health in complementary and integrative medicine: A clinical guide*. St. Louis, MO: Elsevier Churchill Livingstone.

Lundeberg, T., & Lund I. (2008). Is there a role for acupuncture in endometriosis pain, or "endometrialgia"? *Acupunct Med, 26*, 94–110.

MacDonald, S. R., Klock, S. C., & Milad, M. P. (1999). Long-term outcome of non-conservative surgery (hysterectomy) for endometriosis-associated pain in women <30 years old. *Am J Obstet Gynecol, 180*(6 Pt 1), 1360–1363.

Marchino, G. L., Gennarelli, G., Enria, R., Bongioanni, F., Lipari, G., Massobrio, M. (2005). Diagnosis of pelvic endometriosis with use of macroscopic versus histologic findings. *Fertil Steril, 84*, 12–15.

Minaglia, S., Mishell, D. R., Jr., & Ballard, C. A. (2007). Incisional endometriomas after Cesarean section: A case series. *J Reprod Med, 52*, 630–634.

Missmer, S. A., Hankinson, S. E., Spiegelman, D., Barbieri, R. L., Marshall, L. M., & Hunter, D. J. (2004). Incidence of laparoscopically confirmed endometriosis by demographic, anthropometric, and lifestyle factors. *Am J Epidemiol, 160*, 784–796.

Moore, J., Copley, S., Morris, J., Lindsell, D., Golding, S., & Kennedy, S. (2002). A systematic review of the accuracy of ultrasound in the diagnosis of endometriosis. *Ultrasound Obstet Gynecol, 20*, 630–634.

Namnoum, A. B., Hickman, T. N., Goodman, S. B., Gehlbach, D. L., & Rock, J. A. (1995). Incidence of symptom recurrence after hysterectomy for endometriosis. *Fertil Steril, 64*, 898–902.

Olive, D. L., & Henderson, D. Y. (1987). Endometriosis and mullerian anomalies. *Obstet Gynecol, 69*, 412–415.

Parazzini, F., Chiaffarino, F., Surace, M., et al. (2004). Selected food intake and risk of endometriosis. *Hum Reprod, 19*, 1755–1759.

Patwardhan, S., & Nawathe, A., Yates, D., et al. (2008). Systematic review of the effects of aromatase inhibitors on pain associated with endometriosis. *BJOG, 115*, 818–822.

Petta, C. A., Ferriani, R. A., Abrao, M. S., et al. (2005). Randomized clinical trial of a levonorgestrel-releasing intrauterine system and a depot GnRH analogue for the treatment of chronic pelvic pain in women with endometriosis. *Hum Reprod, 20,* 1993–1998.

Prentice, A., Deary, A. J., & Bland, E. (2000). Progestagens and anti-progestagens for pain associated with endometriosis. *Cochrane Database Syst Rev,* 2:CD002122.

Prentice, A., Deary, A. J., Goldbeck-Wood, S., Farquhar, C., & Smith, S. K. (2000). Gonadotrophin-releasing hormone analogues for pain associated with endometriosis. *Cochrane Database Syst Rev,* 2:CD000346.

Proctor, M. L., Hing, W., Johnson, T. C., & Murphy, P. A. (2006). Spinal manipulation for primary and secondary dysmenorrhoea. *Cochrane Database Syst Rev,* 3:CD002119.

Proctor, M. L., Latthe, P. M., Farquhar, C. M., Khan, K. S., & Johnson, N. P. (2005). Surgical interruption of pelvic nerve pathways for primary and secondary dysmenorrhoea. *Cochrane Database Syst Rev,* 4:CD001896.

Proctor, M. L., Murphy, P. A., Pattison, H. M., Suckling, J., & Farquhar, C. M. (2007). Behavioural interventions for primary and secondary dysmenorrhoea. *Cochrane Database Syst Rev,* 3:CD002248.

Remorgida, V., Abbamonte, L. H., Ragni, N., Fulcheri, E., & Ferrero, S. (2007). Letrozole and desogestrel-only contraceptive pill for the treatment of stage IV endometriosis. *Aust N Z J Obstet Gynaecol, 47,* 222–225.

Ryan, I. P., Tseng, J. F., Schriock, E. D., Khorram, O., Landers, D. V., & Taylor, R. N. (1995). Interleukin-8 concentrations are elevated in peritoneal fluid of women with endometriosis. *Fertil Steril, 63,* 929–932.

Sangi-Haghpeykar, H., & Poindexter, A. N., III. (1995). Epidemiology of endometriosis among parous women. *Obstet Gynecol, 85,* 983–992.

Schenken, R. S. (1989). *Endometriosis: Contemporary concepts in clinical management.* Philadelphia, PA: Lippincott.

Selak, V., Farquhar, C., Prentice, A., & Singla, A. (2007). Danazol for pelvic pain associated with endometriosis. *Cochrane Database Syst Rev,* 4:CD000068.

Shakiba, K., Bena, J. F., McGill, K. M., Minger, J., & Falcone, T. (2008). Surgical treatment of endometriosis: a 7-year follow-up on the requirement for further surgery. *Obstet Gynecol, 111,* 1285–1292.

Simpson, J. L., Elias, S., Malinak, L. R., & Buttram, V. C., Jr. (1980). Heritable aspects of endometriosis: I. Genetic studies. *Am J Obstet Gynecol, 137,* 327–331.

Sinaii, N., Cleary, S. D., Ballweg, M. L., Nieman, L. K., & Stratton, P. (2002). High rates of autoimmune and endocrine disorders, fibromyalgia, chronic fatigue syndrome and atopic diseases among women with endometriosis: A survey analysis. *Hum Reprod, 17,* 2715–2724.

Sinaii, N., Plumb, K., Cotton, L., et al. (2008). Differences in characteristics among 1,000 women with endometriosis based on extent of disease. *Fertil Steril, 89,* 538–545.

Stratton, P., Winkel, C. A., Sinaii, N., Merino, M. J., Zimmer, C., & Nieman, L. K. (2002). Location, color, size, depth, and volume may predict endometriosis in lesions resected at surgery. *Fertil Steril, 78,* 743–749.

Surrey, E. S. (1999). Add-back therapy and gonadotropin-releasing hormone agonists in the treatment of patients with endometriosis: Can a consensus be reached? Add-Back Consensus Working Group. *Fertil Steril, 71*, 420–424.

Sutton, C. J., Ewen, S. P., Whitelaw, N., & Haines, P. (1994). Prospective, randomized, double-blind, controlled trial of laser laparoscopy in the treatment of pelvic pain associated with minimal, mild, and moderate endometriosis. *Fertil Steril, 62*, 696–700.

Suzuki, N. K., Uebaba, K., Kohama, T., Moniwa, N., Kanayama, N., & Koike, K. (2008). French maritime pine bark extract significantly lowers the requirement for analgesic medication in dysmenorrhea: A multicenter, randomized, double-blind, placebo-controlled study. *J Reprod Med, 53*, 338–346.

Tanaka, T. (2003). A novel anti-dysmenorrhea therapy with cyclic administration of two Japanese herbal medicines. *Clin Exp Obstet Gynecol, 30*, 95–98.

Van Langendonckt, A., Casanas-Roux, F., & Donnez, J. (2002). Oxidative stress and peritoneal endometriosis. *Fertil Steril, 77*, 861–870.

Vercellini, P., Aimi, G., Panazza, S., De Giorgi, O., Pesole, A., & Crosignani, P. G. (1999). A levonorgestrel-releasing intrauterine system for the treatment of dysmenorrhea associated with endometriosis: A pilot study. *Fertil Steril, 72*, 505–508.

Vercellini, P., Frontino, G., De Giorgi, O., Aimi, G., Zaina, B., & Crosignani, P. G. (2003). Comparison of a levonorgestrel-releasing intrauterine device versus expectant management after conservative surgery for symptomatic endometriosis: a pilot study. *Fertil Steril, 80*, 305–309.

Vercellini, P., Trespidi, L., De Giorgi, O., Cortesi, I., Parazzini, F., & Crosignani, P. G. (1996). Endometriosis and pelvic pain: Relation to disease stage and localization. *Fertil Steril, 65*, 299–304.

Walter, A. J., Hentz, J. G., Magtibay, P. M., Cornella, J. L., & Magrina, J. F. (2001). Endometriosis: Correlation between histologic and visual findings at laparoscopy. *Am J Obstet Gynecol, 184*, 1407–1411; discussion 1411–1413.

Wayne, P. M., Kerr, C. E., Schnyer, R. N., et al. (2008). Japanese-style acupuncture for endometriosis-related pelvic pain in adolescents and young women: Results of a randomized sham-controlled trial. *J Pediatr Adolesc Gynecol, 21*, 247–257.

Wieser, F., Cohen, M., Gaeddert, A., et al. (2007). Evolution of medical treatment for endometriosis: Back to the roots? *Hum Reprod Update, 13*, 487–499.

Winkel, C. A. (2003). Evaluation and management of women with endometriosis. *Obstet Gynecol, 102*, 397–408.

Winkel, C. A., & Scialli, A. R. (2001). Medical and surgical therapies for pain associated with endometriosis. *J Womens Health Gend Based Med, 10*, 137–162.

Witt, C. M., Reinhold, T., Brinkhaus, B., Roll, S., Jena, S., & Willich, S. N. (2008). Acupuncture in patients with dysmenorrhea: A randomized study on clinical effectiveness and cost-effectiveness in usual care. *Am J Obstet Gynecol, 198*, 166, e1–e8.

Wykes, C. B., Clark, T. J., & Khan, K. S. (2004). Accuracy of laparoscopy in the diagnosis of endometriosis: A systematic quantitative review. *BJOG, 111*, 1204–1212.

Zhu, X., Proctor, M., Bensoussan, A., Smith, C. A., & Wu, E. (2008). Chinese herbal medicine for primary dysmenorrhoea. *Cochrane Database Syst Rev, 2*:CD005288.

18

Chronic Pelvic Pain

BETTINA HERBERT

Chronic pelvic pain (CPP), the subject of whispered complaints and misplaced shame, diminishes the quality of life and overall well-being for almost one in four women (Zondervan et al., 2001). It is the second most common gynecological complaint and accounts for 13% to 20% of gynecological consultations and up to 52% of diagnostic laparoscopy (Ghaly & Chien, 2000).

The "disease with 20 names" has many often overlapping physical, functional, and psychological etiologies (Hahn, 2001). It can be challenging to elucidate the pain generators (Anderson, 2006). For many women, despite enduring multiple interrogations and procedures, there will be no definitive diagnosis (Mathias, Kuppermann, Liberman, Lipschutz, & Steege, 1996).

Often symptom relief, rather than resolution, is the treatment goal. After a brief respite, pain may return, treatment side effects may become intolerable, and the woman is forced either back into the medical maze or to resign herself to living her life in pain (McGowan, Luker, Creed, & Chew-Graham, 2007).

This is not a comprehensive overview of CPP. Rather it is a look at the difficult journeys of three women that illustrate, in part, the oft-overlooked role of nonphysiologic changes in body mechanics impacting somatic structures (muscle, fascia, ligament, tendon). Such imbalances can, over time, be the cause of considerable pain and discomfort; the effects can multiply as the body accumulates layers of compensation. The result may be hard to identify and treat unless malalignment or somatic dysfunction is included in the differential diagnosis. Of the many different etiologies, 22% of women have musculoskeletal causes of CPP (Gyang, Hartman, & Lamvu, 2013).

Another often underdeduced contributor to chronic pain is past or present abuse: physical, sexual, and emotional, including neglect. This is by far the most delicate part of a patient's history to explore, and yet, it may be as important to address as the physiologic changes. In fact, abuse can impact physiology and anatomy through the effects of a chronically overactive, hypervigilant sympathetic nervous system (Van der Kolk, 1994).

Biochemical imbalances and endogenous or exogenous toxins may be perpetuating factors as well, contributing to an inflammatory milieu that may impede healing. Sufficient assimilation of nutrients is foundational to optimal healing and function. If pelvic pain is not isolated but is part of a systemic response, investigation of other triggers is warranted. These include not only malabsorption and poor nutrition but also toxic exposures (heavy metals, persistent organic pollutants), mold, yeast, or multiple chemical sensitivity disorder. These additional approaches can expand our diagnostic and therapeutic options and help diminish both patient and provider's feelings of disappointment and inadequacy.

CASE STUDY 18.1

DYSMENORRHEA: SOMETIMES MORE THAN HORMONES

Pamela's gynecologist referred her for recent-onset dysmenorrhea. Up until 8 months prior, she had been free of premenstrual and menstrual morbidities. At age 38, her cramps became so severe that she started to miss work. Lab results and imaging studies failed to reveal any abnormalities. A detailed history that included questions about trauma and injury uncovered a traumatic sprained ankle about 18 months prior. It had taken weeks to heal, and the only therapy had been ice and rest.

Physical examination revealed tenderness at both sacroiliac joints. The ankle had normal range of motion and no residual talofibular ligamentous laxity. A twitch response in the inferior rectus abdominus identified a trigger point. Osteopathic palpatory diagnosis revealed tenderness at the superior aspect of the pubic symphysis and a "listening" (restriction) of the right broad and round ligaments.

Using osteopathic manipulative treatment (OMT) and viscerofascial techniques, Pamela was treated three times over 6 weeks for alignment of the pelvic bowl and sacrum, rebalancing the pelvic floor muscles and pelvic organs using external maneuvers. A short course of physical therapy corrected a lack of proprioception at the ankle (common after sprains and a source of chronic reinjury), and Pamela's dysmenorrhea resolved.

Discussion

Malalignment of anatomical structures can have a dramatic effect on physiology (Korr, 1997; Schamberger, 2002). Once there is a disruption in the biomechanical relationships within the body, all surrounding and supporting structures work to compensate (Alexander, 2005). Changes include asymmetries in muscle length, power, and weight-bearing and can affect circulation and neurophysiology as well as entire organ systems (Prendergast & Weiss, 2003)

In Pamela's case, the ankle was abruptly inverted past its physiologic limit, transmitting a traumatic force through the femur to the pelvic floor muscles, pelvis, and fascia (Brous, 1997; Schiowitz, 1997). The resulting malalignment affected not only the connective tissue and organs but also the circulatory and neural elements within the connective tissue (Smutney & Hitchcock, 1997).

The "ligaments" of the pelvis, unlike most in the body, contain blood vessels and nerves, therefore acting more like mesenteries. Over time, and amplified by many movements, somatic dysfunction can develop. Untreated, this positive feedback cycle could, over time, impact autonomic innervation and induce vasoconstriction and visceral spasm with a concomitant slowing of venolymphatic flow (Barral, 1993). The "ripple effect" can transmit even further and often leads to a reorganization of structures that results in pain far removed in time and location from the initial injury.

Musculoskeletal dysfunction can affect internal organs that are innervated at the same spinal cord segment (Holtzman, Petrocco-Napuli, & Burke, 2008). Similarly, visceral afferents can create somatic dysfunction (Kuchera & Kuchera, 1994) that may also include active trigger points that are often present in women with CPP, irrespective of the presence or type of the underlying pathology (Ling & Slocumb, 1993). In a study of 177 patients with CPP, 74% had abdominal wall trigger points (Gyang et al., 2013). They may be of autonomic reflexive origin or the result of muscles being either too long or too short. While treatment with injection (Slocumb, 1984), dry needling, or OMT such as positional release and muscle energy is very useful (Holtzman et al., 2008; Kuchera & Kuchera, 1994; Travell & Simons, 1983, 1992), sometimes it does not result in permanent relief. Both structural and visceral elements need to be evaluated. Other therapies to consider include physical therapy, pelvic floor therapy (Montenegro et al., 2010), visceral manipulation, biofeedback or quantitative EEGs (neurobiofeedback), low allergenic diet, and mindful meditation (Fox, Flynn, & Allen, 2011; Boxes 18.1 and 18.2).

Box 18.1 Fascia

More than just fibroelastic connective tissue, fascia is a mobius strip in the body.

The fibers of supportive structures, such as ligaments and tendons, peritonea and pleura, and periosteum and dura, and interdigitate with each other, forming a continuous web throughout the body. Thus a disruption in one area can affect not only the immediately surrounding structures but also those distal in increasing layers of compensatory movements (Prendergast & Weiss, 2003)

Box 18.2 Somatic Dysfunction

Impaired or altered function of related components of the somatic (body framework) system: skeletal, arthrodial, and myofascial structures as well as related vascular, lymphatic, and neural elements. Three elements define somatic dysfunction: tissue texture abnormality (effusions, laxity, stability, tone of soft tissue); asymmetry (misalignment, defects, masses, crepitation); and restriction of motion. Often there is a fourth criterion: tenderness. The mnemonic is TART.

These are diagnosed using observation, for example, shoulder height discrepancy (Brous, 1997), and skilled palpation—a tension in muscles, ligaments, fascia, and other connective tissue. The abnormal feel of tissue is often due to muscle hypertonicity, second to increased alpha motor neuron stimulation. The altered activity of skin may be due to altered pilomotor, vasomotor, and sudomotor functions under the control of the sympathetic nervous system.

ICD-10 codes for somatic dysfunction are separated into 10 anatomic regions including abdomen, pelvis, cervical spine, and so forth.

CASE STUDY 18.2

POSTPARTUM PAIN AND STRESS INCONTINENCE—EXAMINING
THE PELVIC BOWL

Since the birth of her son 6 months prior, Susie continued to have low back and pelvic pain. She had experienced an uneventful pregnancy and delivery with some mild low back pain after the 32nd week. Now raising a leg to get her son strapped into his car seat, getting dressed, and climbing stairs hurt the most. Her pain was 5/10, and much worse ("just about unbearable") when climbing stairs. Clearly upset, Susie also reported ongo-ing stress incontinence and a mood that grew darker daily. She was increasingly distraught about the future and the idea that she would not be able to keep up with her son when he started crawling and walking.

Imaging: Lumbar spine and pelvic X-rays were unremark-able; bone scan, normal.

Physical examination revealed tenderness to palpation at the right quadratus lumborum, anterior inferior iliac spine, poste-rior superior iliac spine, and ischial tuberosity with decreased one-legged balance. Osteopathic palpation revealed tenderness at the symphysis pubis and asymmetry of the pubic tubercles (left tubercle cephalad). Sacral sulci were asymmetric. The left medial umbilical ligament was shortened and a restric-tion noted over the right pubovesicular (PV) ligament. After reassurance and explaining what had happened and the treat-ment approach, OMT, including myofascial techniques (muscle energy), utilized adductor activation while realigning the pubic tubercles; then the inguinal ligament was gently released; and sacral torsion (asymmetry) was treated using a balanced liga-mentous tension approach.

To address the stress incontinence, the left medial umbili-cal ligament was restored to normal length using external vis-cerofascial manipulation. Tension of the right PV ligament had already resolved. Finally, a short course of acupuncture helped release remaining muscle tension as well as help restore Susie's normally sunny disposition. In short order she was back to cel-ebrating and giving a mother's special love.

Discussion

Somatic dysfunction frequently occurs in the context of normal imaging. While there was no disruption of the symphysis pubis and despite the absence of radiological evidence of oseitis pubis, Susie had both connective tissue and myofascial pain generators (Costello, 1998).

The body may not regain its previous physiologic relationship after the pro-found changes of pregnancy (Tettambel, 2005). In this case, nonphysiologic alignment affected the symphysis pubis—and therefore the pelvic bowl—as well as the suspensory structures of the bladder. The slight change in the fibro-cartilaginous symphysis pubis altered the muscle length and power of certain hip flexors that, in turn, exacerbated the already irritated symphysis. This relatively small deviation also affected the alignment of the sacrum between the ilia (Lee, 2004). Each step over the past 6 months had increased the discomfort and inflammation and reinforced the altered, painful alignment of structures.

Stress incontinence may affect up to 10% of women at 3 months postpartum (Torrisi et al., 2007).

In this case, the shortened medial umbilical ligament plus the pelvic floor disruption lessened the acute angle of the bladder neck, leading to decreased inhibition of urine flow during valsalva maneuvers. Realigning both specific cystic fascia and the supporting structures of the pelvis resolved the stress incontinence (Barral, 1993). Visceral dysfunction from many etiologies—childbirth, surgery, infection, and trauma (both physical and emotional)—can affect the soma (Nelson, 2006a, 2006b, 2006c; Nelson & Rottman, 2006). Adding this approach to a treatment plan has helped relieve many CPP syndromes (Barral, 1989).

CASE STUDY 18.3

THE INVISIBLE PANDEMIC—ABUSE: CAN I TRUST YOU?

Katherine had suffered for 30 years with debilitating back and right leg pain and ulcerative colitis. She had broken several vertebrae in two severe automobile crashes and often lost her balance and fell, sometimes from spinal "lightning strikes." Despite this, Katherine had excelled in an international career, combating the pain until finally, at 52, she could no longer work.

Imaging (CT): old anterior-posterior compression fracture of pelvis; complex fracture posterior pelvis; flexion/ distraction fractures T5-T8; transverse process fractures L2-L5.

Physical examination revealed a thin woman with kyphosis, missing spinous processes of T5-T8 with numerous well-healed scars over her entire body. The right anterior superior iliac spine was painful to palpation, and her right iliopsoas muscle was in spasm. She demonstrated decreased one-legged balance, no right great toe or ankle proprioception, and right-sided myoclonic jerks.

Despite the CT findings and somatic guarding of her pelvis, Katherine complained only of leg and spine pain. Although it was clear that she had pelvic pain, her wishes were respected, and her pelvis was treated only indirectly (from surrounding areas) until the time she might say more.

After 6 months of weekly treatment yielding steady but slow progress, one day Katherine was unable to lie on the treatment table, arching her pelvis into the air. Looking away, she hesitatingly confessed to previously unspoken pain "shooting from the right hip across to my left," that today was "louder than the beast in my spine."

Several months earlier, well into the therapy, answers to questions about trauma (physical, emotional, sexual and spiritual), other than the vehicle crashes, had been negative on all counts. On this day she described the childhood beatings, acts of cruelty and vertebrae broken long before the car accidents.

With Katherine's consent and her psychologist's active involvement, monthly four-handed sessions were added using somatoemotional release (SER) (a body-centered therapy for uncovering residual effect of trauma) to address the pelvic pain. In that "understanding, safe room" she was able to slowly allow images and associations to develop in response to gentle palpation, positional support, and a few open-ended questions at appropriate times.

The sessions allowed a controlled, safe return to key traumatic events. Skilled palpation revealed parts of her body that were "holding"—the expression of the sentient overload of her tissue. With the subtle support of "listening" hands, Katherine began to revisit certain traumas, the effects of which were stored in her body. Unfortunately it came as no surprise that she had been a victim of severe emotional and sexual abuse as well as the relentless beatings. Based on her physical expression and dramatic body movements, the nonverbal periods took her to a hell where only brutality and danger had existed. Often her body was just silently supported as it moved seemingly of its own volition into various postures.

During the third SER session, a child's tremulous voice emerged during Katherine's semitrance state asking, "Can I trust you?" She was greeted and told, "I can't answer that. You will have to decide for yourself." She grew quiet. Although the patient did not have any recall of this, we informed her psychologist of the event.

One month later that child's voice returned, identifying herself as Katherine's inner healer who had decided she could trust us and proceeded to guide both the therapy and her healing. That dialogue blossomed over the ensuing sessions into the purest expression of the patient's aspect of inner healer, the patient and physicians working in partnership.

At first, Katherine could access this innate healing knowledge only during the sessions. As her inner healer and psyche grew stronger and matured, Katherine started being able to "hear" her without going into a trance-like state. In this way, she learned self-care that had not been demonstrated in her childhood. Gradually she made significant life changes: terminated an abusive relationship; started an anti-inflammatory diet; added supplements, botanicals, and key nutrients; and started to meditate, though at first she was afraid to close her eyes and opted for walking meditation instead.

Her analgesic regimen of Kadian 1,800 mg/day and Valium 10 mg three times daily changed to buprenorphine 28 mg/day in divided doses with devils claw (*Harpagophytum procumbens*) (Low Dog, 2008) as well as hops (*Humulus lupulus*) and wild yam (*Dioscorea villosa*) for the cramping of her ulcerative colitis. Valerian (*Valeriana officinalis*), passion flower (*Passiflora incarnata*), kava kava (*Piper methysticum*) (Pittler & Ernst, 2003), and ashwagandha (*Withania somniferum*) were also added. As her pain subsided, so did her myoclonic jerks. Other providers added to her team included an endocrinologist for the hormonal changes caused by long-term opioid use and the effects of chronic trauma (Heim, Newport, Bonsall, Miller, & Nemeroff, 2001), a specialist in post-traumatic stress disorder (PTSD) who used eye movement desensitization therapy (EMDR), and a physical therapist for balance training.

Nine months into this intensive multidisciplinary approach, Katherine started being able to access memories while wide awake and identify and lessen the effects of triggers in the environment. Over time, this ability became integrated into her conscious awareness and behavior. The "beast" in her spine and pelvis, miraculously, became an ally, a harbinger of dangerous emotions, to be heeded, not battled.

Discussion

CHRONIC PAIN AND ABUSE

The Centers for Disease Control's 2005 report on Adverse Childhood Events reveals that in the general population women suffer childhood physical, sexual, and emotional abuse at rates of 27%, 24.7%, and 13.1% respectively.

In the chronic pain population, those percentages range as high as 50% (Davis, Luecken, & Zautra, 2005; Goldberg & Goldstein, 2000; Goldberg, Pachas, & Keith, 1999), and in CPP, up to 64% (Collett, Cordle, Stewart, & Jagger, 1998; Fry, Crisp, & Beard, 1997).While abuse may or may not be causal, it can affect coping with pain and recovery (Jarrell et al., 2005). Invisible trauma such as sexual and emotional abuse may often have a direct effect on the body (Drossman et al., 1990; Leserman, 2005; Lovy, 2006). Concomitant depression (Fillingim, Wilkinson, & Powell, 1999; Goldberg, 1994; Lampe et al., 2003) and anxiety along with hypervigilance (Gunter, 2008), a facilitated sympathetic nervous system, and alterations in the hypothalamic-pituitary-adrenal axis may contribute to the distress (Heim, Ehlert, Hanker, & Hellhammer, 1998).

Eliciting and treating this level of trauma calls for a primary therapeutic relationship of trust with a healthcare professional. For people who have been abused, trusting is difficult; betrayal always looms. Often emotional distress and not being taken seriously may lead patients to keep silent, especially during the initial visits (Price et al., 2006). It takes time, patience, and a consistently nonjudgmental demeanor to gain a patient's trust (Rubin, 2005).

Studies encourage practitioners to inquire about abuse and that is often the case in clinical practice (Hurst, MacDonald, Say, & Read, 2003; Read, McGregor, Coggan, & Thomas, 2006; Walker et al., 1992). However, some women would rather not be asked (Pikarinen, Saisto, Schei, Swahnberg, & Halmesmaki, 2007). If they are in states of denial, fear, or repression (Thomas, Moss-Morris, & Faquhar, 2006), one hopes to create a bond of trust and non-judgment (shame is frequently the overarching emotion) while remaining patient.

Another option for asking about abuse uses normalization (Leserman, 2005) to help remove the stigma, sense of isolation, and shame so many women feel (Kolko, 2000). A segue to asking about abuse, therefore, might be "in about half of women with pain similar to yours, we have found that people treated them badly, sometimes years earlier, even in childhood."

Chronic pelvic pain as a pain syndrome responds to a multidisciplinary team (Gunter, 2003; Peters et al., 1991). That ideally includes a mental health specialist who is willing to work openly and collaboratively (Sharp & Keefe, 2005). Over 30% of women referred to a CPP clinic had a positive screen for PTSD (Meltzer-Brody et al., 2007). The clinician may consider some of the mind–body therapies that are useful in other pain syndromes, such as progressive relaxation, mindfulness-based stress reduction (Grossman, Tiefenthaler-Gilmer, Raysc, & Kesper, 2007), hypnosis (Axelrad, Brown, & Wain, 2009), biofeedback, EEG biofeedback (neurofeedback), and guided imagery or approaches such as cognitive behavioral therapy (Robertson,

Humphreys, & Ray, 2004) and EMDR (Bisson et al., 2007) that may be useful in PTSD as well.

Body-centered therapies such as OMT, massage, gentle chiropractic, Feldenkrais, Alexander, myofascial release (Madore & Kahn, 2008), or trigger point therapy may be appropriate, as long as the practitioner is experienced and vigilant for signs of remembered or reexperienced trauma. Because no one wants to risk retraumatizing the patient, these cases should include the active involvement of a mental health professional for addressing emotions and memories that may arise.

Nutritional changes including, at times, an elimination diet, play a key role in ameliorating both gastrointestinal as well as inflammatory contributors to CPP (Parcell, 2008; Sulindro-Ma, Ivy, & Isenhart, 2008).

Educating the patient in ways of self-nourishment that contribute to healing can have positive effects in both physical and emotional arenas. Often a little improvement from implementing small changes, such as adding one vegetable portion daily, sipping chamomile tea, or eliminating refined sugar, can be a catalyst for embracing the long-term attitudinal changes about self-care.

Because of the intricate interweaving of abuse into every aspect of a woman's life and the lack of high-quality evidence for targeted treatments for specific patient subgroups, the clinician needs to use great delicacy, intuition, and understanding to be able to engage the woman and embark on a healing journey (Selfe, Matthews, & Stones, 1998). The wisdom gained from experience is extremely valuable. In presenting the possibility of a psychological component, the physical reality must still be validated or the woman who is already bathed in shame and fear may misinterpret and blame herself. Our challenge is to gently explain how psychophysiology may affect CPP (Elliott, 2002). Mind and body are a unity, despite our medical model of separate specialties (Greenman, 2003; Steege, 1998).

What You Can Do

1. Watch how your patient walks, in the waiting room, in the hallway, paying special attention to antalgic gait, asymmetry of pelvic movement, side-to-side pelvic movement, if one hip flares more than the other, or if the time spent on one leg is shorter than on the other. Any of these may indicate somatic dysfunction or "guarding" of an injured or painful area. Ask yourself "What isn't moving?"

2. In addition to a regular history, take a full history of trauma, physical, emotional, and sexual, including neglect. Be vigilant for subtle and

not-so-subtle changes in posture, eye contact, and vocal inflection, or for redirecting the question.

3. Take an additional history regarding diet and any gastrointestinal symptoms. Sometimes food intolerances and pro-inflammatory foods (e.g., sugar, highly refined carbohydrates, and processed foods) may aggravate an existing condition. Restoring gut function and trying an elimination diet are inexpensive, if labor-intensive, ways to test. Add anti-inflammatory and anxiolytic teas, herbs, and supplements as needed. You may also want to consider exposures to toxins, heavy metals, or mold.

4. Evaluate the pelvic bowl—check for asymmetry and/or tenderness (often both) at the superior aspect of the pubic symphysis or at the posterior part of the bowl, at the sacral sulci. Sometimes there can be symmetry but tenderness on both sides of the sacrum, common after childbirth.

5. Check the posterior superior iliac spines (PSIS) using the Gillet (stork) test. A thumb on the ipsilateral PSIS should move caudad while the knee is being raised to marching position (thigh parallel to the floor). If one PSIS does not move, there is dysfunction.

6. Forge partnerships with skilled providers in mental health, mind–body, integrative nutrition, and other medical paradigms such as acupuncture and osteopathy. If you are not one yourself, make referrals to physicians who are well versed in integrative, botanical, and/or functional medicine. You will create a referral network as well as a virtual "team approach" for each patient.

7. Consider referral to a physiatrist well trained in neuromusculoskel-etal medicine to help create and coordinate a treatment plan.

8. Offer a mind–body therapy such as mindfulness-based stress reduction, meditation, qigong, gentle yoga, or hypnosis as part of a treatment plan.

9. Manage expectations. This approach to correct underlying causes may take weeks or months before significant changes are noticed. Patient education about time frames and pointing out incremental improvement can reduce frustration and increase self-observation skills.

Summary

Though there are myriad etiologies of CPP, common therapeutic targets include inflammation, somatic dysfunction, and psychological disturbances.

Inflammation may be addressed not only with dietary changes including thoughtfully selected nutritional and botanical supplements, but also with mind–body therapies. Somatic dysfunction may respond to manipulative therapies provided by osteopaths (Greenman, 2003), naturopaths, chiropractors, and some physical therapists. Therapists may also offer visceral, craniosacral, myofascial, and other whole-body therapies. There are many women's clinics with therapists who specialize in pelvic floor alignment along with physical therapy. Mental health care may be key in many cases.

Integrative medicine offers evidence-informed therapies to support the human being's intrinsic capacity for healing, incorporating the wisdom of many therapies' origins (e.g., traditional Chinese medicine, indigenous medicine, Ayurveda, osteopathy, chiropractic, etc.) combined with the advances made by modern biomedicine.

Given the complexity and wide variation of etiologies and symptoms of CPP, using an integrative approach may offer an expanded selection of therapeutic approaches (Bailey & Stein, 2008). To serve our patients, we must expand our capacity to listen to each patient—with ears, eyes, mind, hands, and heart (Milne, 1995). Each treatment plan may then be tailored to the unique history and perspective that lie within the individual. Doing so requires the essential elements of time, skill and love.

Resources

While the best sources for referrals are in your own network and community and from patients and colleagues, the following websites can be used to find practitioners of the work described above. This is only a partial list of therapeutic approaches that may be useful for CPP.

- American Academy of Medical Acupuncture, www.medicalacupuncture.org
- American Academy of Osteopathy, www.academyofosteopathy.org
- American Academy of Physical Medicine and Rehabilitation (physiatrists), www.aapmr.org
- American Association of Acupuncture and Oriental Medicine, www.aaaomonline.org
- American Association of Naturopathic Physicians, www.naturopathic.org
- American Botanical Council (membership required), abc.herbalgram.org/site/PageServer

- American Physical Therapy Association, www.apta.org (Select "women's health" under expertise.)
- American Society of Clinical Hypnosis, www.asch.net
- Association for Applied Psychophysiology and Biofeedback, www.aapb.org/
- Biodynamics of Osteopathy (physicians trained in biodynamic cranial osteopathy), http://jamesjealous.com/
- Center for Mindfulness in Medicine, Health Care and Society, www.umassmed.edu/cfm/mbsr
- EMDR International Association, www.emdria.org
- Institute for Functional Medicine, http://functionalmedicine.org/
- International Society for Neurofeedback and Research, www.isnr.org
- Milne Institute (craniosacral therapists), www.milneinstitute.com
- National Association of Myofascial Trigger Point Therapists, www.namtpt.shuttlepod.org (Note: Many physicians, especially physiatrists, work with trigger points as well.)
- Natural Standard: The Authority on Integrative Medicine (membership required), www.naturalstandard.com
- The Alexander Technique, www.alexandertechnique.com
- The Barral Institute (for visceral manipulation), www.barralinstitute.com
- The Chikly Health Institute (for lymphatic drainage), www.chiklyinstitute.org
- The Feldenkrais Method of Somatic Education, www.feldenkrais.com
- The Osteopathic Cranial Academy (physicians trained in cranial osteopathy), www.cranialacademy.com
- The Upledger Institute, www.iahp.com/pages/search/index.php (Note: Search for therapists with many classes and experience in visceral, craniosacral, lymphatic, and/or somatoemotional release techniques.)

REFERENCES

Alexander, J. (2005). Trauma. In D. S. Jones (Ed.), *Textbook of functional medicine* (pp. 140–147). Gig Harbor, WA: Institute for Functional Medicine.

Anderson, R. U. (2006). Traditional therapy for chronic pelvic pain does not work: What do we do now? *Nat Clin Pract Urol, 3*, 145–156.

Axelrad, D. A., Brown, D., & Wain, H. (2009). Hypnosis. In B. J. Sadock, V. A. Sadock, & P. Ruiz (Eds.), *Kaplan and Sadock's comprehensive textbook of psychiatry* (9th ed., pp. 2804–2831). Philadelphia, PA: Lippincott Williams & Wilkins.

Bailey, A., & Stein, M. (2008). Integrative pain medicine models: Women's health programs. In J. F. Audette & B. Bailey (Eds.), *Integrative pain management: The science and practice of complementary and alternative medicine in pain management* (pp. 497–545). Totowa, NJ: Humana Press.

Barral, J. P. (1989). *Visceral manipulation II.* Seattle, WA: Eastland Press.

Barral, J. P. (1993). *Urogenital manipulation.* Seattle, WA: Eastland Press.

Bisson, J. I., Ehlers, A., Matthews, R., Pilling, S., Richards, D., & Turner, S. (2007). Psychological treatments for chronic post-traumatic stress disorder: Systematic review and meta-analysis. *Br J Psychiatry, 190,* 97–104.

Brous, N. (1997). Fascia. In E. L. DiGiovanna & S. Schiowitz (Eds.), *An osteopathic approach to diagnosis and treatment* (2nd ed., pp. 19–20). Philadelphia, PA: Lippincott-Raven.

Collett, B. J., Cordle, C. J., Stewart, C. R., & Jagger, C. (1998). A comparative study of women with chronic pelvic pain, chronic nonpelvic pain and those with no history of pain attending general practitioners. *Br J Obstet Gynaecol, 105,* 87–92.

Costello, K. (1998). Myofascial syndromes. In J. F. Steege, D. A. Metztger, & B. S. Levy (Eds.), *Chronic pelvic pain: An integrated approach* (pp. 251–266). Philadelphia, PA: Saunders.

Davis, D. A., Luecken, L. J., & Zautra, A. J. (2005). Are reports of childhood abuse related to the experience of chronic pain in adulthood? A meta-analytic review of the literature. *Clin Pain, 21,* 398–405.

Drossman, D. A., Leserman, Nachman, G., et al. (1990). Sexual and physical abuse in women with functional or organic gastrointestinal disorders. *Ann Intern Med, 113,* 828–833.

Elliott, M. L. (2002). Treating the patient with pelvic pain. In D. C. Turk & R. J. Gatchel (Eds.), *Psychological approaches to pain management: A practitioner's handbook* (2nd ed., pp. 455–469). New York, NY: Guilford Press.

Fillingim, R. B., Wilkinson, C. S., & Powell, T. (1999). Self-reported abuse history and pain complaints among young adults. *Clin J Pain, 15,* 85–91.

Fox, S. D., Flynn, E., & Allen, R. H. (2011). Mindfulness meditation for women with chronic pelvic pain: a pilot study. *J Reprod Med, 56,* 158–162.

Fry, R. P., Crisp, A. H., & Beard, R. W. (1997). Sociopsychological factors in chronic pelvic pain: A review. *Psychosom Res, 42,* 1–15.

Ghaly, A. F., & Chien, P. W. (2000). Chronic pelvic pain: Clinical dilemma or clinician's nightmare. *Sex Tranms Infect, 76,* 419–425.

Goldberg, R. T. (1994). Childhood abuse, depression, and chronic pain. *Clin J Pain, 10,* 277–281.

Goldberg, R. T., & Goldstein, R. (2000). A comparison of chronic pain patients and controls on traumatic events in childhood. *Disabil Rehabil, 22,* 756–763.

Goldberg, R. T., Pachas, W. N., & Keith, D. (1999). Relationship between traumatic events in childhood and chronic pain. *Disabil Rehabil, 21,* 23–30.

Grace, V. M. (1998). Mind/body dualism in medicine: The case of chronic pelvic pain without organic pathology: A critical review of the literature. *Int J Health Ser, 28,* 127–151.

Greenman, P. E. (2003). The manipulative prescription. In P. E. Greenman, *Principles of manual medicine* (3rd ed. pp. 45–52). Philadelphia. PA: Lippincott Williams & Wilkins.

Grossman, P., Tiefenthaler-Gilmer, U., Raysc, A., & Kesper, U. (2007). Mindfulness training as an intervention for fibromyalgia: Evidence of postintervention and 3-year follow-up benefits in well-being. *Psychother Psychosom, 76,* 226–233.

Gunter, J. (2003). Chronic pelvic pain: An integrated approach to diagnosis and treatment, *Obstet Gynecolog Surv, 58,* 615–623.

Gunter, J. (2008). The neurobiology of chronic pelvic pain. In J. M. Potts (Ed.), *Genitourinary pain and inflammation: Diagnosis and management* (pp. 3–17). Totowa, NJ: Humana Press.

Gyang, A., Hartman, M., & Lamvu, G. (2013). Musculoskeletal causes of chronic pelvic pain. *Obstet Gynecol, 121,* 645–650.

Hahn, L. (2001). Chronic pelvic pain in women: A condition difficult to diagnose—more than 70 different diagnoses can be considered [article in Swedish]. *Lakartidningen, 98,* 1780–1785.

Heim, C., Ehlert, U., Hanker, J. P., & Hellhammer, D. H. (1998). Abuse-related post-traumatic stress disorder and alterations of the hypothalamic-pituitary-adrenal axis in women with chronic pelvic pain. *Psychosom Med, 60,* 309–318.

Heim, C., Newport, D. J., Bonsall, R., Miller, A. H., & Nemeroff, C. B. (2001). Altered pituitary-adrenal axis responses to provocative challenge tests in adult survivors of childhood abuse. *Am J Psychiatry, 158,* 575–581.

Holtzman, D. A., Petrocco-Napuli, K. L., & Burke, J. R. (2008). Prospective case series on the effects of lumbosacral manipulation on dysmenorrhea. *Manipulative Physiol Ther, 31,* 237–246.

Hurst, C., MacDonald, J., Say, J., & Read, J. (2003). Routine questioning about non-consenting sex: A survey of practice in Australasian sexual health clinics. *Int J STD AIDS, 14,* 329–333.

Jarrell, J. F., Vilos, G. A., Allaire, L. C., et al; Chronic Pelvic Pain Working Group, SOGC. (2005). Consensus guidelines for the management of chronic pelvic pain [article in English and French]. *J Obstet Gynaecol Can, 27,* 869–910.

Kolko, D. J. (2000). How do I interview a child about alleged physical abuse? In H. Dubowitz & D. DePanfilis (Eds.), *Handbook for child protection practice* (pp. 75–79). Thousand Oaks, CA: Sage.

Korr, I. M. (1997). Hyperactivity of sympathetic innervation: A common factor in disease. In H. H. King (Ed.), *The collected papers of Irvin M. Korr* (Vol. 2, pp. 70–76). Ann Arbor, MI: American Academy of Osteopathy.

Kuchera, M. L., & Kuchera, W. A. (1994). *Osteopathic principles in practice.* (2nd ed.). Columbus, OH: Greyden Press.

Lampe, A., Doering, S., Rumpold, G., et al. (2003). Chronic pain syndromes and their relation to childhood abuse and stressful life events. *Psychosom Res, 54,* 361–367.

Lee, D. (2004). *The pelvic girdle: An approach to the examination and treatment of the lumbopelvic-hip region.* Philadelphia, PA: Churchill Livingstone.

Leserman, J. (2005). Sexual abuse history: Prevalence, health effects, mediators, and psychological treatment. *Psychosom Med, 67,* 906–915.

Ling, F. W., & Slocumb, J. C. (1993). Use of trigger point injections in chronic pelvic pain. *Obstet Gynecol Clin North Am, 20,* 809–815.

Lovy, A. (2006). The psychiatric patient. In K. E. Nelson & T. Glonek (Eds.), *Somatic dysfunction in osteopathic family medicine* (pp. 73–86). Philadelphia, PA: Lippincott, Williams and Wilkins.

Low Dog, T. (2008). Botanicals in the management of pain. In J. F. Audette & A. Bailey (Eds.), *Integrative pain management: The science and practice of complementary and alternative medicine in pain management* (pp. 447–470). Totowa, NJ: Humana Press.

Madore, A., & Kahn, J. R. (2008). Therapeutic massage and bodywork in integrative pain management. In J. F. Audette & B. Bailey (Eds.), *Integrative pain management: The science and practice of complementary and alternative medicine in pain management* (pp. 353–378). Totowa, NJ: Humana Press.

Mathias, S. D., Kuppermann, M., Liberman, R. F., Lipschutz, R. C., & Steege, J. F. (1996). Chronic pelvic pain: Prevalence, health-related quality of life, and economic correlates. *Obstet Gynecol, 87,* 321–327.

McGowan, L., Luker, K., Creed, F., & Chew-Graham, C. A. (2007). How do you explain a pain that can't be seen? The narratives of women with chronic pelvic pain and their disengagement with the diagnostic cycle. *Br Health Psychol, 12,* 261–274.

Meltzer-Brody, S., Leserman, J., Zolnoun, D., Steege, J., Green, E., & Teich, A. (2007). Trauma and posttraumatic stress disorder in women with chronic pelvic pain. *Obstet Gynecol, 109,* 902–908.

Milne, H. (1995). *The heart of listening: A visionary approach to craniosacral work.* Berkeley, CA: North Atlantic Books.

Montenegro, M. I., Mateus-Vasoconceles, E. C., Candido dos Reis, F. J., et al. (2010). Thiele massage as a therapeutic option for women with chronic pelvic pain caused by tenderness of pelvic floor muscles. *J Eval Clin Pract, 16,* 981–982.

Nelson, K. E. (2006a). Diagnosing somatic dysfunction. In K. E. Nelson & T. Glonek (Eds.), *Somatic dysfunction in osteopathic family medicine* (pp. 12–26). Philadelphia, PA: Lippincott, Williams and Wilkins.

Nelson, K. E. (2006b). The manipulative prescription. In K. E. Nelson & T. Glonek (Eds.), *Somatic dysfunction in osteopathic family medicine* (pp. 27–32). Philadelphia, PA: Lippincott, Williams and Wilkins.

Nelson, K. E. (2006c). Viscerosomatic and somatovisceral reflexes. In K. E. Nelson & T. Glonek (Eds.), *Somatic dysfunction in osteopathic family medicine* (pp. 33–55). Philadelphia, PA: Lippincott, Williams and Wilkins.

Nelson, K. E., & Rottman, J. (2006). The female patient. In K. E. Nelson & T. Glonek (Eds.), *Somatic dysfunction in osteopathic family medicine* (pp. 105–126). Philadelphia, PA: Lippincott, Williams and Wilkins.

Parcell, S. (2008). Biochemical and nutritional influences on pain. In J. F. Audette & B. Bailey (Eds.), *Integrative pain management: The science and practice of complementary and alternative medicine in pain management* (pp. 133–172). Totowa, NJ: Humana Press.

Peters, A. A., van Dorst, E., Jellis, B., van Zuuren, E., Hermans, J., & Trimbos, J. B. (1991). A randomized clinical trial to compare two different approaches in women with chronic pelvic pain. *Obstet Gynecol, 77*, 740–744.

Pikarinen, U., Saisto, T., Schei, B., Swahnberg, K., & Halmesmaki, E. (2007). Experiences of physical and sexual abuse and their implications for current health. *Obstet Gynecol, 109*, 1116–1122.

Pittler, M. H., & Ernst, E. (2003). Kava extract for treating anxiety. *Cochrane Database Syst Rev*, 2:CD003383.

Prendergast, S. A., & Weiss, J. M. (2003). Screening for musculoskeletal causes of pelvic pain. *Clin Obstet Gynecol, 46*, 773–782.

Price, J., Farmer, G., Harris, J., Hope, T., Kennedy, S., & Mayou, R. (2006). Attitudes of women with chronic pelvic pain to the gynaecological consultation: A qualitative study. *BJOG, 113*, 446–452.

Read, J., McGregor, K., Coggan, C., & Thomas, D. R. (2006). Mental health services and sexual abuse: The need for staff training. *Trauma Dissociation, 7*, 33–50.

Robertson, M., Humphreys, L., & Ray, R. (2004). Psychological treatments for posttraumatic stress disorders: Recommendations for the clinician based on a review of literature. *J Psychiatr Pract, 10*, 106–118.

Rubin, J. J. (2005). Psychosomatic pain: New insights and management strategies. *South Med J, 98*, 1099–1110; quiz 1111–1112, 1138.

Schamberger, W. (2002). *The malalignment syndrome: Implications for medicine and sport* (pp. 231–240). London, England: Churchill Livingstone.

Schiowitz, S. (1997). Static symmetry. In E. L. DiGiovanna & S. Schiowitz (Eds.), *An osteopathic approach to diagnosis and treatment* (2nd ed., pp. 37–47). Philadelphia, PA: Lippincott-Raven.

Selfe, S. A., Matthews, Z., & Stones, R. W. (1998). Factors influencing outcome in consultations for chronic pelvic pain. *J Womens Health, 7*, 1041–1048.

Sharp, J., & Keefe, B. (2005). Psychiatry in chronic pain: a review and update. *Curr Psychiatr Rep, 7*, 213–219.

Slocumb, J. C. (1984). Neurological factors in chronic pelvic pain: Trigger points and the abdominal pelvic pain syndrome. *Am J Obstet Gynecol, 149*, 536–543.

Smutney, C. J., & Hitchcock, M. E. (1997). Dysmenorrhea and premenstrual syndrome. In E. L. DiGiovanna & S. Schiowitz (Eds.), *An osteopathic approach to diagnosis and treatment* (2nd ed., pp. 455–459). Philadelphia, PA: Lippincott-Raven.

Steege, J. F. (1998). Philosophy of the integrated approach: Overcoming the mind-body split. In J. F. Steege, D. A. Metztger, & B. S. Levy (Eds.), *Chronic pelvic pain: An integrated approach* (pp. 5–12). Philadelphia, PA: Saunders.

Sulindro-Ma, M., Ivy, C. L., & Isenhart, A. C. (2008). Nutrition and supplements for pain management. In J. F. Audette & B. Bailey (Eds.), *Integrative pain management: The science and practice of complementary and alternative medicine in pain management* (pp. 417–446). Totowa, NJ: Humana Press.

Tettambel, M. A. (2005). An osteopathic approach to treating women with chronic pelvic pain. *Am Osteopath Assoc, 105*(9 Suppl 4), S20–S22.

Thomas, E., Moss-Morris, R., & Faquhar, C. (2006). Coping with emotions and abuse history in women with chronic pelvic pain. *Psychosom Res, 60,* 109–112.

Torrisi, G., Sampugnaro, E. G., Pappalardo, E. M., D'Urso, E., Vecchio, M., & Mazza, A. (2007). Postpartum urinary stress incontinence: Analysis of the associated risk factors and neurophysiological tests. *Minerva Ginecol, 59,* 491–498.

Travell, J. G., & Simons, D. G. (1983). *Myofascial pain and dysfunction: The trigger point manual.* Baltimore, MD: Lippincott Williams & Wilkins.

Travell, J. G., & Simons, D. G. (1992). *Myofascial pain and dysfunction: The trigger point manual* (Vol. 2). Baltimore, MD: Lippincott Williams & Wilkins.

Van der Kolk, B. A. (1994). The body keeps the score: Memory and the evolving psychobiology of posttraumatic stress. *Harv Rev Psychiatry, 1,* 253–265.

Walker, E. A., Katon, W. J., Hansom, J., et al. (1992). Medical and psychiatric symptoms in women with childhood sexual abuse. *Psychosom Med, 54,* 658–664.

Zondervan, K. T., Yudkin, P. L., Vessey, M. P., et al. (2001). The community prevalence of chronic pelvic pain in women and associated illness behaviour. *Br J Gen Pract, 51,* 541–547.

19

Menopause

TORI HUDSON

CASE STUDY

Martha is a 49-year-old woman who is seeking information about treatment options to relieve her menopausal symptoms. She has been experiencing less regular menses, vaginal dryness, hot flashes and night sweats that are moderate in frequency and intensity, and problems with sleep. She has been otherwise healthy, with normal lipids, glucose, thyroid, pap smears, and mammograms, although she has gained 10 pounds in the last year. She is very interested in a "natural approach" to addressing her menopausal symptoms. She is also interested in knowing if she is at risk for osteoporosis, and if so, what options might be available to her outside of taking hormonal therapy (HT).

The goals of an integrative medicine approach to perimenopause and menopause are to provide relief from common perimenopausal/menopausal symptoms and to prevent and/or treat osteoporosis, heart disease, and other conditions of aging while minimizing the risk of breast cancer, uterine cancer, blood clots, strokes, or gallbladder disease. The evaluation reveals a woman's symptoms, health habits, mental/emotional stressors, and risks for future diseases. The integrative provider then uses a spectrum of interventions including diet, exercise, stress management, nutritional supplements, herbal therapies, hormones, prescription and/or over-the-counter (OTC) medications.

The changes associated with perimenopause/menopause can be mild, moderate, or severe. Some women have very few symptoms, while others have progressive and problematic symptoms for many years. The most common symptoms are vasomotor (hot flashes and night sweats), sleep disturbances, and vaginal dryness. This chapter focuses primarily on menopausal symptom relief.

Menopause Evaluation

LESS TESTING, MORE LISTENING AND LEARNING

The onset of perimenopause/menopause is an important time for a comprehensive health and lifestyle evaluation. A thorough medical history and complete physical exam are essential prior to initiating menopausal HT of any kind, and preferably prior to any treatment plan, hormonal or not. Assessment of risk factors for stroke, coronary heart disease, venous thrombotic embolism, osteoporosis, diabetes, and breast/ovarian/uterine cancer is vital.

In addition to the history and physical exam, selective use of bone density (DEXA) testing, testing lipid profiles (including subfractions, lipoprotein a, homocysteine, apo B, and others), fasting glucose, hemoglobin A1c, and screening mammography should be performed according to national guidelines, age, medical judgment, and a conversation between practitioner and patient. Other selected tests depend on a woman's age, symptoms, and comorbidities.

There is no single test for perimenopause/menopause. Tests to determine ovarian function are not routinely conducted because the diagnosis of perimenopause or menopause is made primarily on the medical history. Practitioners can use hormone testing on an individual basis, mostly to differentiate menopause from thyroid problems, abnormal causes of a lack of menses such as elevated prolactin levels, or premature ovarian failure (premature menopause). The follicle stimulating hormone (FSH) test is not that helpful in the perimenopausal woman, as FSH levels fluctuate immensely during this time. In a woman who is still having menses, especially irregular/random cycles, her FSH fluctuates unpredictably and can easily be within normal range on one day and elevated on another.

Clinical Pearl

There are two common scenarios when one might order an FSH:

1. If a woman is suspected to be perimenopausal or possibly menopausal and is using contraception, the FSH can be useful in determining if she still needs contraception. When an FSH is above 30 mIU/mL, and remains greater than 30 mIU/mL one month later, then a diagnosis of menopause can be established and she will no longer need contraception. It is important to continue the contraception during that 1-month period until this is determined.

2. If a woman is reporting irregular menses, irritability, fatigue, and insomnia, ordering an FSH and thyroid stimulating hormone (TSH) test can help sort out whether her problems are perimenopause and/or hypothyroid.

Hormone Testing

There is a popular notion that salivary, serum, or urinary hormone testing can determine the optimal dosing of hormone management during menopause. There is questionable value for these tests in a perimenopausal woman, in whom estrogen/progesterone levels fluctuate greatly from day to day. Nor is there is adequate scientific evidence to support claims of increased efficacy, enhanced safety, or the need for testing in order to determine the optimal dosing of hormone prescriptions.

Even in postmenopausal women who are not on hormones, there are numerous problems with salivary testing of estrogen and progesterone (Du, et al., 2013; Gavrilova & Lindau, 2009): (1) Only a very small amount of these hormones is present in the saliva, (2) high false positive elevations are seen in those already taking sublingual hormones, (3) contamination of the saliva collection tube may occur if using topical hormone creams/gels, (4) there is insufficient proficiency testing, (5) variable technologies yield broad differences in results, (6) technical challenges are not adequately addressed by all laboratories conducting these tests, (7) there is insufficient scientifically proven accuracy, and (8) there are interfering components such as food, beverages, medications, and chewing gums. Not all practitioners are deterred by these challenges in salivary hormone testing, and there are clearly different approaches to menopause management that clinicians have taken. If they are an experienced and knowledgeable menopause practitioner, and they use these tests, then it is likely that they have an approach that they feel confident in, and helps them to achieve success with their patients.

Salivary testing of cortisol and dehydroepiandrosterone (DHEA) levels holds more promise, as these do not fluctuate so much from day to day, there is a known daily rhythm of cortisol production, and these hormones are naturally present in higher amounts in the saliva. Salivary cortisol testing can be useful in assessing disorders of the hypothalamic-pituitary axis (Raff, 2009) and possibly for selecting therapies for anxiety and/or insomnia in particular.

Serum testing of estrogen, progesterone, and testosterone is more accurate, however, is not generally necessary in perimenopausal/menopausal women. The reference ranges are wide, and a normal reference range for testosterone during the perimenopause/menopause has not been established. Again, in a perimenopausal woman, estrogen levels are fluctuating within a day and from day to day and therefore are not valuable in diagnosis or management. There are so many peaks and valleys and such erratic hormone activity that testing offers little value in most situations. In a postmenopausal woman, her estrogen and progesterone levels are predictably low, she is in a menopausal state and they are supposed to be low, making the purpose of testing unclear.

For women taking HT, it is tempting to think serum or salivary testing can guide the clinician in dosing. Hormone testing is a popular recommendation in some consumer menopause books and can be a practice style of some clinicians. However, there is no mathematical grid or equation comparing values of estrogen, progesterone, or testosterone levels in the blood or saliva and how these values equate with a specific dose of the comparable hormone. While there are reference ranges for these hormones, we do not know exactly what dose to give in order to keep the woman within the reference range. Women absorb, utilize and metabolize hormones differently, and the form of hormone and delivery method contributes to the variation.

In selective cases serum hormone testing may be helpful. These are generally when a woman is on HT and not doing well—despite our best efforts with a good medical history and adjusting the dose, she is still symptomatic. However, even if testing is done, it basically comes down to good clinical judgment and the willingness of the woman and her practitioner to try another dose, delivery, or option. There also may be a theoretical value in testing an estradiol level in a patient for whom you are concerned the dose is much higher than what she needs.

Urinary testing of estrogen metabolites can be considered when evaluating a woman's risk of conditions that may be associated with higher or lower levels of certain estrogen metabolites. While the data are limited, using estrogen metabolism testing to gain some insight for her risk of cervical or breast cancer or reduce her risk of cancer recurrence is a practice that is still unfolding. However, recent research has cast some doubt on the association of 2-hydroxyestrone/16-hydroxyestrone and breast cancer risk, though

4-hydroxyestrogen may still be fruitful territory (Arslan et al., 2014; Mackey et al., 2012; Obi, Vrieling, Heinz, & Chang-Claude, 2011).

Clinical Pearl

It is important to recognize and respect that clinicians think through patient management issues differently. However, the healthcare dollar has become more and more precious. Often in situations where we are feel we have less expertise, clinicians are vulnerable to three shortcomings—ordering unnecessary tests, too few tests, or the wrong tests. The more expertise one has in perimenopause/menopause, it is likely there is a lesser need for any hormone testing for patient management. We recognize that some patients want hormone testing for their menopause issues. It is important to respectfully listen to their needs, share your thoughts and provide pertinent education, make recommendations, and order the tests if they really want them, even if you do not appear to need them.

It might serve everyone if we could increase our vigilance in evaluation and testing with midlife women for metabolic syndrome, diabetes, and cardiovascular disease. We can make a dramatic difference in quality of life, morbidity, and mortality with comprehensive evaluation including laboratory testing and then optimize our prevention strategies and interventions based on these results with ongoing monitoring of progress.

The Integrative Medicine Approach

Once symptoms have been pinpointed and disease risks have been identified, the following treatment categories can be considered:

1. Diet, exercise, lifestyle, stress management
2. Nutritional supplementation
3. Botanical supplementation
4. Compounded bioidentical hormone preparations
5. Bioidentical conventionally available HT
6. Nonbioidentical conventional HT
7. Nonhormonal OTC and prescription medications
8. Traditional Chinese medicine including acupuncture and herbs
9. Mind–body approaches
10. Massage

Diet, exercise, lifestyle, and/or nutritional supplements and botanical therapies will be effective for the management of perimenopause/menopause symptoms in the majority of women. When these are not adequate, HT or other medications can be recommended.

Diet, Exercise, and Stress Management

NUTRITION

Nutrition is a cornerstone of integrative medicine. While dietary advice should be individualized, common themes include a diet rich in whole, organic, and unprocessed foods, with an emphasis on vegetables, whole grains, beans, seeds, nuts, fruits, lean proteins, healthy fats, and low in fried foods, simple carbohydrates, alcohol, sugar, and salt. Some foods, such as soy and flax, have been studied for their beneficial effects on menopause-related symptoms.

Soy

Soy foods are a rich source of phytoestrogens and may be useful in menopause for hot flashes, bone, cholesterol, blood pressure, and coronary artery disease. (See the chapters "Nutrition" and Cardiovascular Diseases in Women" for more details). With regard to hot flashes, studies have been contradictory; assessments complicated by varying dose, variation in isoflavone profile, and duration of trials. However, when sufficient doses of the isoflavone genistein are consumed, beneficial effects on hot flash frequency and severity are seen.

A 2012 meta-analysis concluded that ingestion of soy isoflavones (median, 54 mg; aglycone equivalents) for 6 weeks to 12 months significantly reduced the frequency of hot flashes by 20.6% (95% CI, -28.38 to -12.86; $p < .00001$) compared with placebo (heterogeneity $p = .0003$, I = 67%; random effects model). This analysis also found that isoflavones significantly reduced hot flash severity by 26.2% (95% CI: -42.23 to -10.15, $p = .001$) compared with placebo. Isoflavone supplements providing more than 18.8 mg of genistein (the median for all studies) were more than twice as potent at reducing hot flash frequency as supplements containing lower levels of the isoflavone (Taku, Melby, Kronenberg, Kurzer, & Messina, 2012).

Concerns have been raised about long-term soy consumption, particularly isolated isoflavones, as they may exert adverse estrogenic effects on breast and/ or endometrial tissue. These fears appear to be unfounded. An analysis of 9,514 breast cancer survivors who were followed for 7.4 years found that higher post-diagnosis soy intake was associated with a significant 25% reduction in tumor recurrence (Messina, 2014). Additionally, a 3-year study on two doses of soy isoflavones; 80 mg and 120 mg/day failed to find any adverse effect on endometrial thickness (Alekel et al., 2015).

Flaxseeds

Research is emerging that flaxseed (*Linum usitatissimum*) may offer potential health benefits in heart disease, diabetes, and even certain cancers (Goyal, Sharma, Upadhyay, Gill, & Sihag, 2014). The seeds are a rich source of the omega-3 fatty acid alpha-linolenic acid (ALA), fiber, and phytoestrogen lignans. Flaxseeds contain high levels of secoisolariciresinol diglucoside (SDG), a lignan metabolized by gut bacteria to enterodiol and enterolactone, both of which exert weak estrogenic and antiestrogenic effects (Adolphe et al., 2010). There have been fewer studies looking at the role of flax in menopause-related symptoms, and while small studies have shown benefit, a systematic review concluded that available evidence from controlled studies indicates no benefit (beyond placebo) of flax consumption on vasomotor symptoms in postmenopausal women (Dew & Williamson, 2013).

EXERCISE

The benefits of exercise for peri- and postmenopausal women are wide and deep. Regular exercise has many beneficial effects on health, including increased longevity, decreased risk of cardiorespiratory and metabolic diseases and some cancers (most notably colon and breast), maintenance of energy balance, and improved musculoskeletal, functional, and mental health (US Department of Health and Human Services, 2008). The data are mixed as to whether exercise can relieve vasomotor symptoms during the menopause transition. A review of more than 30 studies found that half showed no effect on hot flashes, with the majority of the balance showing an inverse relationship between exercise and hot flashes, and three studies reporting increased vasomotor symptoms with high levels of exercise (Sternfeld & Dugan, 2011). Given the overwhelming beneficial effects of exercise to human health, all clinicians should prescribe regular physical activity to their patients.

STRESS MANAGEMENT

The menopausal years can be a vulnerable time for many women. However, studies of women in midlife suggest that depression, as defined by the current

Diagnostic and Statistical Manual of Mental Disorders (DSM-5), is no more common in menopause than any other time of life (Freeman et al., 2004; Schmidt, Haw, & Rubinow, 2004). Clinicians should be aware of risk factors that may increase a woman's risk for depression during the menopausal transition including a personal history of depression (especially depression related to pregnancy or menstruation), vasomotor symptoms, surgical menopause, and adverse life events (Vivian-Taylor & Hickey, 2014). With this in mind, practitioners should screen for depression where indicated and help support women with appropriate strategies for managing stress such as meditation, yoga, breathing exercises, going for walks, and even taking long baths.

DIETARY SUPPLEMENTS

There are a number of dietary supplements that may be beneficial during the menopausal transition. In general, most women should probably take a good multivitamin that provides 70%–100% of the recommended daily intake of vitamins and minerals. The following dietary supplements are also sometimes recommended.

Bioflavonoids

Bioflavonoids, such as rutin, hesperidin, and quercetin, are known for their antioxidant and anti-inflammatory properties and their ability to strengthen capillaries. Some clinicians recommend it for menorrhagia, which can sometimes occur during the perimenopause. Some older and less-than-optimal studies show that bioflavonoids, taken in combination with vitamin C, helps relieve menopausal hot flashes (Smith, 1964). Ninety-four women with hot flashes were given a combination of 900 mg hesperidin, 300 mg hesperidin methylchalcone, and 1,200 mg of vitamin C every day for 4 weeks. Hot flashes were relieved in 53% of women and reduced in an additional 34% by the end of 1 month. There are no more recent studies for review.

Gamma-Oryzanol

Gamma-oryzanol, a mixture of substances such as sterols and ferulic acid generally derived from rice bran oil, is used in Japan for relieving anxiety and menopausal symptoms. Research did show beneficial effects on menopausal hot flashes in the early 1960s (Murase & Iishima, 1963), with at least one additional study confirming that finding (Ishihara, 1984). The dose used in the study was 300 mg/day. There are no more recent studies for review.

Fish Oil

When it comes to helping perimenopausal and menopausal women with hormone-related issues, there are three broad areas to be mindful of: symptom relief, disease prevention, and disease treatment. While it is common knowledge that fish oils can help prevent heart disease and strokes, it may not be such common knowledge that fish oils can help with hot flashes, dry skin, and dry eye syndrome, all issues that can plague menopausal women. One double-blind, placebo-controlled randomized trial reported a 55% decrease in hot flash frequency with approximately 60% of the women responding to one 500 mg capsules containing 350 mg eicosapentaenoic acid (EPA) and 50 mg docosahexaenoic acid (DHA) given three times per day. After 8 weeks, the hot flash frequency decreased in the fish oil group by a mean of 1.58 per day and only 0.50 per day in the placebo group. However, there were no differences in hot flash severity, and no differences were noted in the quality of life scores between the two groups (Lucas et al., 2009).

An open study of peri- or postmenopausal women given 2 g/day of fish oil (each gram contained 840 mg of EPA and 375 mg of DHA) reported a 50% reduction in the number of hot flashes as well as a high response rate with 8 weeks treatment. Dry eye syndrome can be influenced by age and the hormonal changes of menopause. Diets low in omega-3 fatty acids have been associated with a greater incidence of dry eye syndrome. Fish oils, as well as flax oil and sea buckthorn oil, are demonstrating positive results in this challenging area of women's health. Omega-3 deficiency may also be associated with dryness of the skin.

BOTANICALS

Herbalists commonly use combinations of herbs to treat menopause. There has been limited research in this area, and what follows are primarily studies of individual herbs. However, many of the OTC products that women use are in fact combinations.

Black Cohosh (Actaea racemosa, Cimicifuga racemosa)

Since the early 1980s, black cohosh has emerged as the most studied of the herbal alternatives to HT for menopause symptoms. Numerous randomized clinical trials have studied black cohosh extract with encouraging but mixed results. A 2012 Cochrane review of 16 randomized controlled trials (RCTs) of perimenopausal or postmenopausal women ($n = 2,027$) using oral mono preparations of black cohosh extract at a median daily dose of 40 mg for a mean duration of 23 weeks were reviewed (Leach, 2012). Comparator interventions included placebo, hormone therapy, red clover, and fluoxetine. The authors concluded that there is "currently insufficient evidence to support the use of black cohosh for menopausal symptoms. However, there is adequate justification for conducting further studies in this area." The review also found many methodological flaws in the trials, which limited any definite conclusions.

Perhaps combination therapies are better. In one placebo-controlled RCT using the combination of black cohosh and St. John's Wort (*Hypericum perforatum*), a popular treatment in Germany, the mean Menopause Rating Scale (MRS) score decreased 50% in the treatment group compared with 19.6% in the placebo group. The Hamilton Depression Rating Scale score decreased 41.8% in the treatment group and 12.7% in the placebo group. Both measures revealed the St. John's Wort plus black cohosh combination performed significantly better than placebo (Uebelhack et al., 2006).

Questions have been raised about the safety of black cohosh in women with breast cancer. A review of 14 RCTs, 7 uncontrolled trials, and 5 observational studies did not find an association between black cohosh and increased risk of breast cancer (Fritz et al., 2014). A prospective observational study was carried out in 50 menopausal breast cancer patients who were on tamoxifen, an anti-estrogen therapy that can induce or worsen menopausal symptoms (Rostock et al., 2011). All 50 women were post surgery, 87% were post radiation treatment, and approximately half had also received chemotherapy. All the women were treated with an isopropanolic extract of black cohosh (one to four tablets, 2.5 mg) for 6 months. Symptoms were recorded before therapy and after 1, 3, and 6 months using the Menopause Rating Scale (MRS II). The total MRS II score for women on black cohosh treatment reduced from 17.6 to 13.6, a statistically significant reduction. Symptoms of hot flashes, sweating, sleep problems, and anxiety improved, but there were no changes in vaginal dryness and body aches/pains. Ninety percent of the women reported the tolerability of the black cohosh extract as very good or good. No significant adverse effects were noted.

It should be noted that historically black cohosh was considered a useful herb for melancholy. A systematic review found that black cohosh significantly reduced depression and anxiety in all studies reviewed (Geller & Studee, 2007). The average recommended dose of standardized black cohosh extract is 40–80 mg/day, though clinical studies performed prior to 1996 used doses of up to 160 mg of standardized extract. There have been a small number of published case reports suggesting a rare, but possible, relationship between black cohosh consumption and liver damage. The US Pharmacopeia Dietary

Supplements Expert Information Council has published a thorough review of adverse events; they recommend that women with liver disease discontinue the use of black cohosh, as should any woman who develops nausea, vomiting, dark urine, or jaundice (Mahady et al., 2008).

Clinical Pearl

Despite the conflicting data, the collective research on black cohosh and our own clinical experience lead us to conclude that it can be effective for hot flashes, mood swings, sleep disorders, and body aches.

Chasteberry (Vitex agnus castus)

One of the most common changes to occur in the menopause transition is irregular menstruation. Some women will experience significant bleeding problems because of menses that are either too frequent or too heavy. This set of symptoms is often an indication for chaste tree berry. Chaste tree increases secretion of luteinizing hormone (LH), an effect that favors progesterone (Haller, 1961; Loch, 1989). This shifts the ratio of estrogen to progesterone and creates a "progesterone-like" effect. In perimenopausal women, this may be useful for managing dysfunctional uterine bleeding (DUB) associated with episodic anovulatory cycles. The dose is generally 500 mg/day of the crude fruit taken continuously throughout the month. If using an extract (generally a strength of 12–16:1), the dose is generally 20–40 mg/day.

Dong Quai (Angelica sinensis)

A 12-week study using dong quai, which traditionally has been used in combination with many other herbs, as a solo agent for the relief of menopausal symptoms such as hot flashes and sweats did not prove effective (Hirata et al., 1997). A randomized, double-blinded, placebo-controlled 6-month trial of the combination of dong quai and astragalus (*Astragalus membranaceus*) found a significant reduction in mild hot flashes, but the combination was no better than placebo for relief of moderate to severe hot flashes or night sweats (Haines, Lam, Chung, Cheng, & Leung, 2008). More research is necessary before any definite conclusions can be made regarding the use of dong quai in menopause.

Clinical Pearl

Dong quai may increase menstrual flow or bring on menstruation. In a perimenopausal woman with menorrhagia or who has not menstruated for several months, dong quai should be avoided.

Ginseng (Panax ginseng)

Panax ginseng, also known as Korean or Chinese ginseng root, is the most widely used of the ginseng species. Historically, ginseng has been used as a tonic. The German health authorities recognize its use as a "tonic for invigoration and fortification in times of fatigue and debility and for declining capacity for work and concentration." Ginseng can help in reducing mental or physical fatigue (D'Angelo et al., 1986; Hallstrom, Fulder, & Carruthers, 1982; Hikino, 1991; Shibata, Tanaka, Shoji, & Saito, 1985), enhancing the ability to adapt to various physical and mental stressors by supporting the adrenal glands (Bombardelli, Cirstoni, & Lietti, 1980).

A randomized, placebo-controlled study evaluated 200 mg per day of standardized ginseng extract in 384 postmenopausal women (Wiklund, Mattsson, Lindgren, & Limoni, 1999). While there was no improvement in hot flashes or night sweats, depression and well-being were significantly improved with ginseng. Another RCT found that 1 month of Korean red ginseng increased energy, and decreased insomnia and depression in menopausal women (Tode et al., 1999). Finally, a randomized, placebo-controlled, double-blinded clinical trial in 72 postmenopausal women randomly assigned them to either 3 g/day Korean red ginseng, containing 60 mg ginsenosides, or placebo for 3 months. The MRS score dropped significantly from 12.45 to 8.32 in the ginseng group compared with 10.23 to 9.26 in the placebo group. The hot flash score also reduced significantly in the red ginseng group. Importantly, dose and type of ginseng differed between the negative and positive studies.

The dose is generally 100–300 mg ginseng extract standardized to 4%–6% ginsenosides. Higher doses may be necessary to achieve desired effects. The use of ginseng in women with breast cancer is controversial and safety at this time is not known.

Hops (Humulus lupulus)

The dried female flowers of hops have been used to brew beer for centuries, however their use as medicine far surpasses this use. The German Commission

E approved hops strobiles for anxiety, restlessness, and sleep disruptions. One randomized, double-blinded, placebo-controlled study of 67 menopausal women that were given placebo, 100 mg, or 250 mg standardized hops extract for 12 weeks (Heyerick et al., 2006) found that at 6 weeks, the 100- and 250-mg doses were significantly superior to placebo, but not after 12 weeks. Even so, there was a more rapid decrease in menopause symptoms, especially hot flashes, for both doses of hops extract.

A 2010 randomized, double-blinded, placebo-controlled, crossover pilot study was done to examine the efficacy of a hops extract (standardized at 100 mcg 8-prenylnaringenin per day) for relief of menopausal symptoms (Erkkola et al., 2010). Thirty-six menopausal women were randomized to take either a placebo or hops extract for a period of 8 weeks and then were switched to the opposite group for another 8 weeks. Menopause-reporting forms including the Kummperman Index (KI), MRS, and a multifactorial visual analog scale (VAS) were used prior to starting the study, after 8 weeks, and after 16 weeks. After 8 weeks, both the hops and placebo groups had significant improvement in outcome measures compared with baseline (higher average reductions occurred in the placebo group.) After 16 weeks however, only the women who had received hops extract in the second 8-week period had a reduction in all outcome measures, whereas women in the placebo group in the second 8 weeks had an increase for all outcome measures. Although the overall treatment efficacy of hops compared with the placebo did not show a significant effect, the time-specific uses did indicate significant reductions in the kupperman index (KI) and the visual analog scale (VAS) for the hops group, and a marginal reduction in symptoms for the MRS after 16 weeks.

Hops may prove to be a useful herb for women suffering from common menopause symptoms such as hot flashes, night sweats, and insomnia. Hops contains phytoestrogens, which may account for its activity.

Kava (Piper methysticum)

Kava is a member of the pepper family native to the South Pacific islands, where the root has been and continues to be used both medicinally and ceremonially. It is predominantly used to relieve tension and anxiety. Research has shown that kava has analgesic, sedative, anxiolytic, muscle relaxant, and anticonvulsant effects. And while kava is not typically thought of as an herb for menopause, anxiety, irritability, tension, nervousness, and sleep disruption are common symptoms for many menopausal women. Four RCTs have investigated the value of kava for menopausal symptoms (Cagnacci et al., 2003;

De Leo et al., 2000; Warnecke, 1991; Warnecke, Pfaender, Gerster, & Gracza, 1990). Two studies showed significant reduction in anxiety and menopausal symptoms, while another showed the greatest improvement with kava plus HT. In the fourth, the study evaluated the effects of kava on anxiety, depression, and menopause symptoms in perimenopausal women for 3 months. Depression and anxiety were reduced in women receiving kava compared with the control group, but there was no improvement in hot flashes.

The dose is typically 100–400 mg/day of kava extract standardized to provide up to, but not more than, 240 mg per day of kavalactones. Women who have a liver disorder or who are taking medications that have the potential to induce liver toxicity should avoid the use of kava.

Maca (Lepidium peruvianum, L. meyenii)

Maca is a traditional plant common to the Andes used for centuries to enhance fertility, improve sexual function and energy and more. Maca belongs to the mustard family and is considered an adaptogen—an herb that is thought to help the body adapt to a variety of stressors.

A growing number of women and clinicians are using maca to relieve the symptoms of menopause, and its popularity continues to grow as more research confirms its effectiveness. A systematic review of four RCTs that tested the effects of maca on menopausal symptoms in healthy perimenopausal, early postmenopausal, and late postmenopausal women using the KI and the Greene Climacteric Score, found that all four RCTs demonstrated favorable effects of maca (Lee, Shin, Yang, Lim, & Ernst, 2011), however, three of these studies were conducted by the same research group.

Maca is also purported to improve sexual function in men and women, an issue that many women struggle with, particularly with aging. A systematic review that included two trials in women found a positive effect on sexual dysfunction or libido in menopausal women (Shin, 2010). While the evidence is limited, there does appear to be some benefit.

The commonly recommended dose of maca extract is 2,000–3,000 mg per day. There does not appear to be any significant adverse effects associated with maca.

Pine Bark (Pinus pinaster)

Pycnogenol is a proprietary extract from the bark of the French maritime pine tree (*Pinus pinaster*). Pycnogenol contains procyanidins and related compounds, and flavonoids similar to those found in green tea. A double-blinded study of 230 Taiwanese perimenopausal women aged 45–55 years, gave either placebo or 100 mg of pycnogenol twice daily for 6 months (Yang, Liao, Zhu, Liao, & Rohdewald, 2007). The Women's Health Questionnaire (WHQ) was used to evaluate the climacteric symptoms at baseline, and at 1, 3, and 6 months (Yang et al., 2007). Symptoms of depression, vasomotor symptoms, memory, anxiety, sexual function, and sleep all improved significantly in both severity and frequency ($p < .001$) as soon as 1 month after starting pycnogenol. Most symptoms also improved with placebo, but not significantly.

Another double-blinded, placebo-controlled study evaluated 30 mg of pycnogenol twice daily or placebo for 3 months in 170 perimenopausal women (Kohama & Negami, 2013). Symptoms were evaluated using the WHQ and KI. Pycnogenol was significantly more effective than placebo for improving hot flashes and night sweats and insomnia/sleep problems. The total KI severity score of perimenopausal symptoms was significantly better after 4 weeks of pycnogenol treatment and decreased overall by 56% in the pycnogenol group and 39% in the placebo group after 12 weeks.

The mechanism by which pycnogenol improves menopause-related symptoms is unknown. Research has shown that pine bark helps dilate the peripheral vascular system due to its effects on the vascular endothelium. Thermodysregulation is related to fluctuating estrogen levels at menopause, both in the blood and in the temperature-regulating center of the hypothalamus. Perhaps the vasodilating effect of pycnogenol helps the body emit excess heat. In any case, pycnogenol may be considered a reasonable option for hot flashes and night sweats, with potential cardiovascular benefits.

Pomegranate (Punica granatum)

The luscious fruit of the pomegranate tree has been cherished as a food and medicine for at least 4,000 years in Egypt, Greece, and China. Scientific studies confirm that it is rich in antioxidant and anti-inflammatory compounds (Zarfeshany, Asgary, & Javanmard, 2014). Traditional use suggested that this fruit might have some impact on hormones in both men and women. A 12-week RCT in 81 postmenopausal women tested the effectiveness of two daily doses of either 30 mg of pomegranate seed oil (PGS) containing 127 mcg of steroidal phytoestrogens per dose or a placebo (sunflower seed oil) to relieve hot flashes and other menopause-related symptoms. After the 12 weeks of treatment, PGS reduced the number of hot flashes by 4.3 per day versus by 2.5 per day in the placebo group, but the difference did not reach statistical significance (Auerbach et al., 2012). However, when reviewing clusters of symptoms within the MRS, there was a significant improvement in sleep disorders and joint/muscular discomfort ($p < 0.03$). Interestingly, after the trial ended, hot flashes more rapidly escalated in the placebo group versus those taking PGS. More research is needed.

Red Clover (Trifolium pratense)

Red clover blossom has long been used in folk medicine as a mild expectorant and nourishing herb for people of all ages. Red clover leaves were found to contain isoflavones, similar but not identical to soy, leading researchers to investigate their potential use in relieving menopausal symptoms. A 2007 meta-analysis of five red clover trials found a reduction in hot flash frequency in the active treatment group (40–82 mg isoflavones daily) compared with the placebo group (weighted mean difference -1.5 hot flashes daily; 95% CI −2.94 to 0.03; $p = 0.05$). The reviewers concluded that there is evidence of a marginally significant effect of red clover isoflavones for treating hot flashes in menopausal women (Coon, Pittler, & Ernst, 2007).

A more recent study using red clover in menopausal women, focused on the effect of a red clover extract in 109 postmenopausal women with depression and anxiety symptoms (Lipovac et al., 2010). The participants were randomly assigned to take either two capsules daily of a red clover extract totaling 80 mg of isoflavones or a placebo for 3 months. At the end of the 90 days, there was a 1-week break, and the two groups switched to take the opposite treatment for an additional 3 months. After taking the red clover extract, women had 75% reduction for anxiety and 78.3% reduction for depression scores on validated testing instruments. After taking the placebo pills, there was an average reduction of 21.7% for both depression and anxiety scores.

Long-term safety data for red clover extracts have not been established.

St. John's Wort (Hypericum perforatum)

St. John's Wort has been used for a wide range of medical conditions, the most common being depressive disorders. It is also the most thoroughly researched botanical used to alleviate depression (see the chapter "Depression" for more information), There has also been tremendous interest in evaluating St. John's Wort, alone or in combination with other herbs such as black cohosh, passionflower, and chasteberry, for the relief of menopause-related symptoms.

A 2014 systematic review and meta-analysis concluded that St. John's Wort and its combination with herbs were significantly superior to placebo (standard mean difference = –1.08; 95% confidence interval –1.38 to –0.77) and St. John's Wort extract alone was more effective than placebo in the treatment of menopause (Liu et al., 2014). Adverse events occurred in 53 (17.4%) patients on St. John's Wort preparations and 45 (15.4%) patients on placebo (relative risk = 1.16; 95% confidence interval 0.81–1.66).

St. John's Wort can be considered an option, alone or in combination with other herbs, such as black cohosh, for the relief of hot flashes and/or depression and/or mood swings. It has an excellent safety profile when used at the standard doses of 900–1,800 mg per day of extracts standardized to 0.3% hypericin and/or hyperforin, however, it is known to interact with a wide range of medications metabolized via CYP3A4. Caution should be used when combining St. John's Wort with prescription medications.

Siberian Rhubarb (Rheum rhaponticum)

Siberian rhubarb, or false rhubarb, belongs to the smartweed family and is not the same species as the garden rhubarb used for food. A special extract, known in the scientific literature as ERr 731, is made from the roots of Siberian rhubarb and has been in wide use in Germany since 1993, specifically for the treatment of menopause symptoms. ERr 731 does not contain any of the anthraquinone glycosides, or laxative compounds, found in many rhubarb species.

A 12-week double-blinded RCT evaluated the effects of one 250-mg tablet (ERr731 containing 4 mg of *R. rhaponticum* dry extract) or placebo in 109 perimenopausal women. The primary outcome was the change in MRS II. After 12 weeks, the MRS II total score and each MRS II symptom significantly decreased in the rhubarb extract group compared with the placebo group ($p < .0001$). The overall menopause quality of life score was also significantly better in the treatment group compared with placebo. No adverse events were observed (Hewger et al., 2006).

Another double-blinded RCT evaluated the same dose of the same extract in 109 perimenopausal women with menopause symptoms, including anxiety. After only 4 weeks of treatment the HAM-A (Hamilton Anxiety Scale) score for ERr 731 group decreased significantly. This was maintained after the 4 weeks and was even more significant after 12 weeks of treatment. Anxiety decreased from moderate or severe to slight, in 33 of 39 women treated with ERr 731. Quality of life issues also increased in the ERr 731 group far more significantly than in the placebo group (22.4 points vs. 7.6 points) (Kaszkin-Bettag et al., 2007).

In an observational study, 363 menopausal women with menopausal symptoms were given one tablet of ERr 731 for 6 months. A change in MRS was the primary outcome. After 6 months of treatment, 252 women completed the study. There was a significant decrease of the total MRS score from an average of 14.7 points at baseline to 6.9 points at the end of the 6 months (p < .0001). The most pronounced improvement was within the first 3 months of treatment, and in women who were the most symptomatic at baseline with MRS scores $= \geq 18$ points. The most significant improvement was for symptoms of hot flashes, irritability, sleep problems, depressive mood, and physical/mental exhaustion (Kaszkin-Bettag et al., 2008).

While promising, it is important to acknowledge that the aforementioned research has been conducted by one research team in one large cohort of women. Recommendations for use would be strengthened by independent research by outside investigators in a more diverse group of study participants.

Valerian (Valeriana officinalis)

Valerian has been used for centuries to aid with sleep and as a calmative, two uses that remain in modern times. Researchers are beginning to evaluate its use to improve sleep during the menopausal transition, as well as testing to see whether it can help reduce vasomotor symptoms. A double-blinded study randomized 68 perimenopausal women to receive 255-mg valerian capsules three times a day for 8 weeks or an identical-appearing placebo. The severity of hot flashes revealed a meaningful statistical reduction pre- and post-valerian treatment ($p < .001$) compared with placebo (Mirabi, 2013).

A randomized, blinded, placebo-controlled study evaluated the effectiveness of 530 mg of concentrated valerian extract or a placebo twice a day for 4 weeks in 100 postmenopausal women using the Pittsburgh Sleep Quality Index (PSQI) tool (Taavoni, Ekbatani, Kashaniyan, & Haghani, 2011). A statistically significant change was reported in the quality of sleep of the intervention group in comparison with the placebo group ($p < 0.001$); 30% of the participants in the intervention group and 4% in the placebo group showed an improvement in the quality of sleep ($p < 0.001$).

While additional studies are needed, valerian may prove to be beneficial for women moving through the menopausal transition experiencing hot flashes and/or insomnia. The safety profile for valerian is quite good. Dose is generally 2–3 grams of crude valerian root or equivalent extract.

ADDITIONAL COMBINATION HERBAL PRODUCTS FOR MENOPAUSE

Multiple combination products are available for use in menopausal women. Most combination products have not been researched, even though individual ingredients might have been. In one study of a five-herb combination formula for menopause symptoms, 13 peri- and postmenopausal women were randomly assigned to a treatment group or a placebo group. The treatment group received capsules of burdock root, licorice root, motherwort, dong quai, and wild yam root and took two capsules three times per day (Hudson & Standish, 1997). After 3 months, women receiving the herbal product showed a greater response rate than women in the placebo group. One hundred percent of women taking the botanical formula had a reduction in their symptom severity according to a symptom diary, while only 67% of women receiving placebo showed a decrease. Seventy-one percent of women taking the herbal formula reported a reduction in the total number of symptoms, while only 17% of the women taking placebo reported a decrease in the total number of their symptoms. The botanical formula was most effective in treating hot flashes, mood changes, and insomnia.

HORMONE THERAPY

Choosing to use hormones requires considerable understanding of the benefits and risks and ability to individualize the benefits and risks for each patient. Hormonal therapies should be used in the lowest dose, for the shortest duration, and in the safest manner possible. Each type of estrogen and progestogen, route of administration, timing of initiation, and duration of use have distinct benefits and adverse effects. For a current comprehensive review of the benefits and risks of hormone therapy for menopausal women, consider the 2012 position statement from the North American Menopause Society (NAMS, 2012). Research since the publication of that position statement continues to review the literature in the areas of the potential benefits (vasomotor symptoms, mood, quality of life, sleep, osteoporosis, fractures, type 2 diabetes, and more) and potential risks (breast cancer, cardiovascular disease, strokes, deep vein thrombosis, dementia, gall bladder disease, ovarian cancer, and lung cancer). Clinicians should regularly update their knowledge of the state of the science, as the data continues to shift and build.

BIOIDENTICAL OR NATURAL HORMONES

One of the greatest areas of confusion in menopause management today is the subject of bioidentical, or "natural" hormones. The bioidentical hormones most commonly used in menopause include estradiol, estrone, estriol, progesterone, and to a lesser extent, testosterone and DHEA. Bioidentical hormones are made from either beta-sitosterol extracted from soybeans or from diosgenin extracted from Mexican wild yam (*Dioscorea villosa*). These compounds are then processed to create hormones that are biochemically identical to those the human female produces.

Pharmaceutical estrogens can be bioidentical or not, synthetic, or derived from a natural substance (such as those found in the urine of pregnant mares). Nonbioidentical hormones include conjugated plant estrogens; conjugated equine estrogens (CEEs); synthetic estrogens; synthetic progestogens, called progestins; and synthetic testosterone. It is the *chemical structure* of a hormone, not its *source*, that determines whether a hormone is bioidentical or not.

Bioidentical estrogens require a prescription and are available from regular pharmacies or as nonpatented forms prepared by compounding pharmacies. Advantages of conventional pharmaceutical HT include years of scientific study and the assurance of standardization. Insurance coverage generally pays for pharmaceutical hormone prescriptions but often does not always pay for compounded hormones. Pharmaceutical preparations are limited in dosage forms and combinations; they also contain additives, binders, adhesives, and/ or preservatives. Occasionally these substances can cause side effects including skin reactions, headaches, and digestive problems.

A popular practice for prescribing compounded natural estrogens is to combine estriol with small doses of estradiol and estrone. Triple estrogen, "Tri-Est," is typically prescribed in a formula composed of 80% estriol, 10% estradiol, and 10% estrone. More commonly, a Bi-Est formulation eliminates the estrone and is prescribed 80% estriol, 20% estradiol.

The advantages for using compounded forms include customized combination and dosing regimens and a greater array of delivery options. Capsules, sublingual lozenges or pellets, creams, gels, vaginal creams/gels or tablets, nasal sprays, and even pellets that are implanted under the skin are available. Any combination of estradiol, estriol, estrone, progesterone, testosterone, and DHEA can be formulated in a compounded hormone prescription (Table 19.1).

Table 19.1. Examples of Commercially Available Bioidentical Hormone Replacement Therapy

Generic Name	Brand Names
17 Beta estradiol (E2)	Estrace
Delivered as:	
Estradiol tablet	Estrace
Transdermal estradiol patches	Climara, Vivelle, Alora, Esclim, Menostar, Estraderm
Transdermal estradiol gels/creams	Estrogel, Divigel, Elestrin, Estrasorb
Vaginal estradiol cream	Estrace
Vaginal estradiol tablet	Vagifem
Vaginal estradiol ring	Estring (dosed for local treatment) Femring (dosed for systemic treatment)
Oral micronized progesterone	Prometrium
Vaginal Progesterone	Procheive

There is currently no scientific evidence that bioidentical estradiol is safer than the nonbioidentical estrogen, except possibly in the area of strokes.

There is some evidence that oral micronized bioidentical progesterone has less adverse breast cancer risk than the synthetic medroxyprogesterone acetate.

Naturopathic physicians often use estriol to treat menopausal symptoms as it is thought to have a better safety profile than estradiol and estrone. Estriol is about one-fourth as potent as estradiol (Head, 1998). Estriol can be taken orally in capsules or tablets, and intravaginally as a cream. Vaginal estriol creams, gels, and suppositories have been shown to restore normal vaginal cytology (Cano et al., 2012) and, combined with pelvic floor exercises, to decrease the incidence of bladder infections (Capobianco et al., 2012). These creams most likely work by restoring the vaginal flora and increasing lubrication, elasticity, and thickness of vaginal cells. A common prescription is 1 mg of estriol per gram of cream; insert 1 gram cream vaginally daily for 2 weeks and then twice a week for maintenance.

Currently available conventional hormone prescriptions for women include

- Oral estrogens
- Oral estrogen/progestins
- Oral progestogens
- Oral estrogens/testosterone
- Transdermal estrogens
- Transdermal estrogens/progestogens

- Vaginal estrogens-systemic; local
- Vaginal progestogens

A list of all the current conventional hormone prescriptions can be obtained from the North American Menopause Society (www.northamericanmeno-pausesociety.org).

Ideal Prescribing Route

Estradiol has the least side effect on lipids and renin when delivered transdermally, as it avoids the first pass effect on the liver. This also permits much lower doses to be used with equal efficacy. Micronized progesterone is available in both oral and vaginal forms. When symptoms are primarily urogenital, vaginal forms of estrogen (CEE, estradiol, and estriol) can be used with minimal systemic absorption.

Progesterone

For women who have not had a hysterectomy, a progestogen must be added to any estrogen preparation to prevent endometrial hyperplasia and uterine cancer. *Progesterone* is a natural hormone made by the ovaries, and its main function is to support pregnancy *Progestin* is the term applied to the synthetic derivatives, which differ in biochemical structure from progesterone. Progestins used in conventional HT and birth control pills are what often account for the side effects that women experience, such as irritability, depression, bloating, and mood swings. Progestins tend to cause water retention, can interact with brain chemistry, and can alter other steroid pathways. *Progestogen* is the term applied to any substance possessing progesterone qualities. It can refer to progesterone or progestin.

The advantages of bioidentical progesterone over progestins are better validated than those for estrogens. Bioidentical progesterone minimizes the side effects associated with progestogens and has a more favorable effect on lipid profiles (Writing Group for the PEPI Trial, 1996) and cardiovascular function (Hermsmeyer, Thompson, Pohost, & Kaski, 2008). In some women, insomnia, fatigue, and mood swings may be more responsive to progesterone than estrogen.

The most compelling area for choosing bioidentical progesterone over progestins may be for breast cancer. While adding progestin to an estrogen will lead to a slight increase risk of breast cancer after approximately 4 years of use, there are now three observational French studies and one US study that demonstrate the potential mitigation of that slight risk by using progesterone rather than the progestin. This is in contrast to synthetic progestogens and particularly medroxyprogesterone acetate, which appears to have mitogenic effects on breast cells, in synergism with estrogen (L'Hermite, 2013). Estrogens alone appear to have a more breast-friendly impact than an estrogen with a progestin.

Progesterone is available with a prescription as oral capsules, sublingual drops, sublingual pellets, lozenges, transvaginal or rectal suppositories, and by injection. Progesterone is also available OTC as a cream. Progesterone is added to compounded biestrogen or triestrogen formulas at a minimum of 100 mg/day to protect the uterus (Table 19.2).

Testosterone

The majority of women treated with estrogen replacement have resolution of their menopausal symptoms. For those who do not, and especially for those women complaining of a loss of libido, estrogen with testosterone may be beneficial. There is no level of testosterone that defines a woman as being deficient in testosterone. However, there is a growing body of evidence to support the use of testosterone for the treatment of hypoactive sexual desire disorder (HSDD), or low sexual desire, in postmenopausal women (Davis & Worsley, 2014).

One study of early postmenopausal women (both natural and surgical) who were switched from estrogen alone to estrogen/testosterone therapy found overall symptom relief was superior to estrogen-only therapy. Sexual drive and satisfaction both increased (Dobay, Balos, & Willard, 1996). A double-blind study of women dissatisfied with their HT regimen showed that sexual desire, satisfaction, and frequency of sexual activity were

Table 19.2. Recommended Dose Ratios for Tri-estrogen and Bi-estrogen Formulations With Progesterone; and Vaginal Estriol

Tri-estrogen formulation considered comparable to:
0.625 mg Premarin/2.5 mg Provera =
Estriol 1 mg/estradiol 0.125 mg/estrone 0.125 mg/Progesterone 50 mg, 1 cap twice daily
Or
Estriol 2 mg/Estradiol 0.25 mg/ Estrone 0.25 mg/Progesterone 100 mg, 1 cap daily

Bi-estrogen formulation is considered comparable to:
0.625 mg Premarin/2.5 mg Provera =
Estriol 1 mg/Estradiol 0.250 mg/Progesterone 50 mg, 1 cap twice daily
OR
Estriol 2 mg/ Estradiol 0.50 mg/Progesterone 100 mg, 1 cap daily

Vaginal estriol: Estriol cream 1 mg/g—insert 1 gram nightly for 2 weeks then a maintenance dose of 1 gram twice weekly

increased when they used the estrogen/testosterone combination (Sarrel et al., 1998). Other studies have shown that the combination of 1.25 mg of esterified estrogen and 2.5 mg of methyltestosterone given daily for 2 years after surgical menopause significantly reduced the intensity of hot flashes and vaginal dryness in 81% and 73% of women, respectively (Watts et al., 1995). A 2008 RCT of 814 women with hypoactive sexual desire revealed that a 300-µg testosterone patch improved the frequency of satisfying sexual episodes and decreased distress in postmenopausal women (Davis et al., 2008). In this study, the women were not treated with estrogen or progesterone. Three excess cases of breast cancer were detected, but this increase was not statistically significant in the study.

A 2012 Australian review concluded that "randomized, double-blind, placebo-controlled studies have established the efficacy of the transdermal testosterone patch for relieving symptoms of HSDD in surgically and naturally menopausal women with and without concomitant estrogen or estrogen/progestin therapy. The main side effects reported in clinical trials were increased hair growth and acne. Available safety data for testosterone, although not conclusive, were reassuring with respect to cardiovascular, breast, and endometrial outcomes (Davis & Braunstein, 2012)." However, in the United States, the FDA has not approved testosterone to treat any sexual problems in women.

Currently, formulations of conventional prescriptions of estrogen and testosterone include either 1.25 or 0.625 mg esterified estrogens, combined with 2.5 or 1.25 mg of methyltestosterone, respectively. At present, bioidentical testosterone can only be obtained from a compounding pharmacy. Two or 3 milligrams of bioidentical testosterone are generally formulated alone or together with the biestrogen or triestrogen formulation. Testosterone cream applied to the genital region can be used as an alternate delivery method. Common prescriptions are anywhere from 1 to 10 mg/g of cream. The cream is applied to the external genitalia right before sexual activity to enhance sensation to touch and orgasm. This should not exceed twice per week to avert local testosterone side effects, such as clitoral enlargement.

The North American Menopause Society (NAMS, 2005) concluded, "Postmenopausal women with decreased sexual desire who have no cause other than being postmenopausal, may be candidates for testosterone treatment." Other causes of low libido should be ruled out, and laboratory testing of testosterone levels should be used to monitor for supraphysiologic levels before and during therapy.

Testosterone therapy is contraindicated in women with breast or uterine cancer and in women with cardiovascular or liver disease. Testosterone should be given at the lowest dose for the shortest time that meets treatment objectives (NAMS, 2005).

Additional Medications

Nonhormonal options for hot flashes include clonidine, usually 0.1 to 0.2 mg/day at bedtime. The neuroleptic neurontin is administered at 300 mg three times a day. Venlafaxine and paroxetine have shown a reduction in hot flashes in studies using 37.5–75 mg and 10–20 mg/day, respectively. However, selective serotonin reuptake inhibitors and selective norepinephrine reuptake inhibitors (SSRIs and SNRIs) have also been shown to actually cause vasomotor symptoms in men and women. Bellergal, an ergot and belladonna combination, was used for many years for vasomotor symptoms but is now only available from compounding pharmacies. There are no studies, and empirical reports show mixed results.

Traditional Chinese Medicine and Acupuncture

Acupuncture has a long historical tradition in women's medicine. Research on the use of acupuncture has shown some benefit in treating women with hot flashes. A modern multicenter, randomized, controlled trial, called the Acupuncture on Hot Flushes Among Menopausal Women (ACUFLASH) found that hot flash frequency decreased by 5.8 per 24 hours in the acupuncture group (n = 134) compared with 3.7 per 24 hours in the control group (n = 133). Hot flash intensity also decreased by 3.2 units in the acupuncture group and 1.8 units in the control group. The women in the acupuncture group also experienced significant improvements in sleep issues compared with the control group (Borud et al., 2009).

Chinese herbal medicines have not been the subject of robust research but one RCT in postmenopausal women compared traditional Chinese medicine (TCM) acupuncture, sham acupuncture, Chinese herbal medicine, and placebo. The TCM acupuncture group experienced a significant decline in hot flash severity and hot flash frequency and the MRS compared with sham acupuncture, however, there was no significant difference between the Chinese herbal medicine and placebo group. (Nedeljkovic et al., 2013).

Mind–Body Approaches

Mind–body medicine tends to include a wide range of therapies such as hypnosis; dance, music, and art therapy; prayer; relaxation and visual imagery; meditation; and yoga. Even though these therapies have been used all over the world for generations, modern clinical research now supports their effectiveness in improving quality of life and reducing anxiety and pain. There is also a growing amount of research to support their use in reducing menopausal symptoms. (For more detailed information, please refer to the chapter "Mind–Body Therapies").

HYPNOSIS

Hypnosis has been studied in a 12-week randomized, single blind, controlled, clinical trial in which 187 postmenopausal women with a minimum of seven hot flashes per day received five weekly sessions of either clinical hypnosis or structured attention control. The women in the clinical hypnosis group showed a mean reduction in hot flash score of 80% compared with 15% in the control group (Elkins, Fisher, & Johnson, 2011).

Hypnosis has also been shown to reduce self-reported hot flashes among breast cancer survivors. A randomized trial of sixty female breast cancer survivors with hot flashes received five hypnosis sessions per week or no treatment (Elkins et al., 2008). Hot flash scores decreased 68% from baseline to end point in the hypnosis arm. There were also significant improvements in self-reported anxiety, depression, interference of hot flashes on daily activities, and sleep in the hypnosis group.

Massage

Research data on therapeutic massage supports its use for relieving stress, and there have also been studies evaluating the role of massage in menopause. In one study, women with hot flashes were divided into three groups: therapeutic massage (TM), passive movement (PM), and control (CTL). Twice a week, women received either massage sessions or passive movement. The Beck Depression Inventory was decreased in the TM group and the Menopause Quality of Life improved in the TM group as compared with the other groups (Oliveira, Hachul, Goto, Tufik, & Bittencourt, 2012).

In a randomized placebo-controlled clinical trial of 90 women attending a menopause clinic, women were assigned to an aromatherapy massage group, a placebo massage group, or a control group. Each participant in the aromatherapy massage group received 30-minute aromatherapy treatment sessions twice a week for 4 weeks with aroma oil. Women in the placebo massage group received the same treatment with plain oil. Women in the control group received no treatment. After eight sessions of intervention, women in both the aromatherapy massage group and the plain oil massage group had a lower menopausal score than the control group; and when the aromatherapy massage and the placebo massage groups were compared, the menopausal score for the aromatherapy massage group was significantly lower (Darsareh, Taavoni, Joolaee, & Haghani, 2012).

Summary

Menopause is a normal and natural part of aging, and each woman experiences it in her own way. Using nutritional and botanical therapies, hormone therapy, other pharmaceuticals, or some combination of each, is a personal decision. The studious menopause practitioner is well versed in the research on lifestyle, nutrition, nutraceuticals, botanicals, hormones, and nonhormonal medications for the vast array of symptoms associated with menopause. However, the big picture of evaluating, preventing and treating conditions associated with post-menopausal aging is equally important. For conditions such as osteoporosis, Alzheimer's dementia, breast cancer, type 2 diabetes, and cardiovascular disease, it is the responsibility of the menopause practitioner to be up to date in testing, prevention, and treatment with a broad range of integrative medicine options. Menopause, aging, and our concerns about long-term health problems evolve over time. Balance is necessary, and overmedicalization of menopause is inappropriate. The integrative provider can remind women that menopause can be a time of positive, life-changing insights, empowerment, and personal growth.

REFERENCES

Abdali, K., Khajehei, M., & Tabatabaee, R. (2010). Effect of St. John's wort on severity, frequency, and duration of hot flashes in premenopausal, perimenopausal and postmenopausal women: A randomized, double-blind, placebo-controlled study. *Menopause, 17*, 326–331.

Adolphe, J. L., Whiting, S. J., Juurlink, B. H., Thorpe, L. U., & Alcorn J. (2010). Health effects with consumption of the flax lignan secoisolariciresinol diglucoside. *Br J Nutr, 103*, 929–938.

Auerbach, L., Rakus, J., Bauer, C., et al. (2012). Pomegranate seed oil in women with menopausal symptoms: A prospective randomized, placebo-controlled, double-blinded trial. *Menopause, 19*, 426–432.

Alekel, D. L., Genschel, U., Koehler, K. J., et al. (2015). Soy Isoflavones for Reducing Bone Loss Study: Effects of a 3-year trial on hormones, adverse events, and endometrial thickness in postmenopausal women. *Menopause, 22*(2), 185–197.

Arslan, A. A., Koenig, K. L., Lenner, P., et al. (2014). Circulating estrogen metabolites and risk of breast cancer in postmenopausal women. *Cancer Epidemiol Biomarkers Prev, 23*, 1290–1297.

Baber, R. J., Templeman, C., Morton, T., et al. (1999). Randomized placebo-controlled trial of an isoflavone supplement and menopausal symptoms in women. *Climacteric*, 2, 85–92.

Bai, W., Henneicke-von Zepelin, H., Wang, S., et al. (2007). Efficacy and tolerability of a medicinal product containing an isopropanolic black cohosh extract in Chinese women with menopausal symptoms: A randomized, double blind, parallel-controlled study versus tibolone. *Maturitas, 58*, 31–41.

Balderer, G., & Borbely, A. (1985). Effect of valerian on human sleep. *Psychopharmacology (Berl), 87*, 406.

Bombardelli, E., Cirstoni, A., & Lietti, A. (1980). The effect of acute and chronic (*Panax ginseng saponins*) treatment on adrenal function; biochemical and pharmacological. *Proceedings 3rd International Ginseng Symposium (September 8–10, 1980)* (pp. 9–16). Seoul, Korea: Korean Ginseng Research Institute.

Borrelli, F., & Ernst E. (2002). *Cimicifuga racemosa*: A systematic review of its clinical efficacy. *Eur J Clin Pharmacol, 58*, 235–241.

Borud, E. K., Alraek, T., White, A., et al. (2009). The Acupuncture on Hot Flushes Among Menopausal Women (ACUFLASH) study, a randomized controlled trial. *Menopause, 16*, 484–493.

Brown, W. J., Williams, L., Ford, J. H., et al. (2005). Identifying the energy gap: Magnitude and determinants of 5-year weight gain in midage women. *Obes Res, 13*, 1431–1441.

Cagnacci, A., Arangino, S., Rensi, A., et al. (2003). Kava-Kava administration reduces anxiety in perimenopausal women. *Maturitas, 44*, 103–109.

Cano, A., Estévez, J., Usandizaga, R., et al. (2012). The therapeutic effect of a new ultra low concentration estriol gel formulation (0.005% estriol vaginal gel) on symptoms and signs of postmenopausal vaginal atrophy: Results from a pivotal phase III study. *Menopause, 19*, 1130–1139.

Capobianco, G., Donolo, E., Borghero, G., et al. (2012). Effects of intravaginal estriol and pelvic floor rehabilitation on urogenital aging in postmenopausal women. *Arch Gynecol Obstet, 285*, 397–403.

Coon, J. T., Pittler, M. H., & Ernst, E. (2007). *Trifolium pratense* isoflavones in the treatment of menopausal hot flushes: A systematic review and meta-analysis. *Phytomedicine, 14*, 153–159.

D'Angelo, L., Grimaldi, R., Caravaggi, M., et al. (1986). A double-blind, placebo-controlled clinical study on the effect of a standardized ginseng extract on psychomotor performance in healthy volunteers. *J Ethnopharmacol, 16*, 15–22.

Darsareh, F., Taavoni, S., Joolaee, S., & Haghani, H. (2012). Effect of aromatherapy massage on menopausal symptoms: A randomized placebo-controlled clinical trial. *Menopause, 19*, 995–999.

Davis, S. R., & Braunstein, G. D. (2012). Efficacy and safety of testosterone in the management of hypoactive sexual desire disorder in postmenopausal women. *J Sex Med, 9*, 1134–1148.

Davis, S. R., Moreau, M., Kroll, R., et al.; APHRODITE Study Team. (2008). Testosterone for low libido in postmenopausal women not taking estrogen. *New Engl J Med, 359*, 2005–2017.

Davis, S. R., & Worsley, R. (2014). Androgen treatment of postmenopausal women. *J Steroid Biochem Mol Biol, 142*, 107–114.

De Leo, V., Marca, A., Lanzetta, D., et al. (2000). Valutazione dell'associazione di estratto di Kava-Kava e terapia ormonale sostitutiva nel trattamento d'ansia in post-menopausa. *Minerva Ginecol, 52*, 263–267.

Dew, T. P., & Williamson, G. (2013). Controlled flax interventions for the improvement of menopausal symptoms and postmenopausal bone health: A systematic review. *Menopause , 20*, 1207–1215.

Dobay, B., Balos, R., & Willard, N. (1996). *Improved menopausal symptom relief with estrogen-androgen therapy.* Presented at the Annual Conference of the North American Menopause Society, Chicago, IL, September.

Du, J. Y., Sanchez, P., Kim, L., Azen, C. G., Zava, D. T., & Stanczyk, F. Z. (2013). Percutaneous progesterone delivery via cream or gel application in postmenopausal women: A randomized cross-over study of progesterone levels in serum, whole blood, saliva, and capillary blood. *Menopause, 20*, 1169–1175.

Elkins, G. R., Fisher, W. I., & Johnson, A. K. (2011). Hypnosis for hot flashes among postmenopausal women study: A study protocol of an ongoing randomized clinical trial. *BMC Complement Altern Med, 11*, 92.

Elkins, G., Marcus, J., Stearns, V., et al. (2008). Randomized trial of a hypnosis intervention for treatment of hot flashes among breast cancer survivors. *J Clin Oncol, 26*, 5022–5026.

Erkkola, R., Vervarcke, S., Vansteelandt, S., et al. (2010). A randomized, double-blind, placebo-controlled, cross-over pilot study on the use of a standardized hop extract to alleviate menopausal discomforts. *Phytomedicine, 17*, 389–396.

Fitzpatrick, L., & Santen, R. (2002). Hot flashes: The old and the new, what is really true? *Mayo Clinic Proc, 77*, 1155–1158.

Freeman, E., Sammel, M., Liu, L., et al. (2004). Hormones and menopausal status as predictors of depression in women in transition to menopause. *Arch Gen Psych, 61*, 62–70.

Freeman, M., Hibbeln, J., Silver, M., et al. (2011). Omega-3 fatty acids for major depressive disorder associated with the menopausal transition: A preliminary open trial. *Menopause, 18*, 279.

Fritz, H., Seely, D., McGowan, J., et al. (2014). Black cohosh and breast cancer: A systematic review. *Integr Cancer Ther, 13*, 12–29.

Geller, S. E., & Studee, L. (2007). Botanical and dietary supplements for mood and anxiety in menopausal women. *Menopause, 14*(3 Pt 1), 541–549.

Goyal, A., Sharma, V., Upadhyay, N., Gill, S., & Sihag, M. (2014). Flax and flaxseed oil: An ancient medicine and modern functional food. *J Food Sci Technol, 51*, 1633–1653.

Gavrilova, N., & Lindau, S. T. (2009). Salivary sex hormone measurement in a national, population-based study of older adults. *Journal of Gerontology, 64*, 94–105.

Grube, B., Walper, A., & Whatley, D. (1999). St. John's wort extract: Efficacy for menopausal symptoms of psychological origin. *Adv Ther, 16*, 177.

Haines, C. J., Lam, P. M., Chung, T. K., Cheng, K. F., & Leung, P. C. (2008). A randomized, double-blind, placebo-controlled study of the effect of a Chinese herbal medicine preparation (Dang Gui Buxue Tang) on menopausal symptoms in Hong Kong Chinese women. *Climacteric, 11,* 244–251.

Haller, J. (1961). The influence of plant extracts in the hormonal exchange between hypophysis and ovary: An experimental endocrinological animal study. *A Geburtsh Gynakol, 156,* 274–302.

Hallstrom, C., Fulder, S., & Carruthers, M. (1982). Effect of ginseng on the performance of nurses on night duty. *Comp Med East West, 6,* 277–282.

Head, K. (1998). Estriol: Safety and efficacy. *Alt Med Rev, 3,* 101–113.

Hermsmeyer, K., Thompson, T., Pohost, G., & Kaski, J. (2008). Cardiovascular effects of medroxyprogesterone acetate and progesterone: A case of mistaken identity? *Nat Clin Pract Cardiovas Med, 5,* 387–395.

Hewger, M., Ventskiovskiy, B., Borzenko, I., et al. (2006). Efficacy and safety of a special extract of *Rheum rhaponticum* (ERr 731) in perimenopausal women with climacteric complaints: A 12 week randomized, double-blind, placebo-controlled trial. *Menopause,13,* 744–759.

Heyerick, A., Vervarcke, S., Depypere, H., et al. (2006). A first prospective, randomized, double-blind, placebo-controlled study on the use of a standardized hop extract to alleviate menopausal discomforts. *Maturitas, 54,* 164–175.

Hikino, H. (1991). Traditional remedies and modern assessment: The case of ginseng. In: R. Wijeskera (Ed.), *The medicinal plant industry* (pp. 149–166). Boca Raton, FL: CRC Press.

Hirata, J., Swiersz, L. M., Zell, B., et al. (1997). Does dong quai have estrogenic effects in postmenopausal women? A double-blind, placebo-controlled trial. *Fertil Steril, 68,* 981–986.

Hudson, T., & Standish, L. (1997). Clinical and endocrinological effects of a menopausal botanical formula. *J Naturo Med, 7,* 73–77.

Huntley, A., & Ernst, E. (2003). A systematic review of herbal medicinal products for the treatment of menopausal symptoms. *Menopause, 10,* 465–476.

Hustin, J., & Van den Eynde, J. (1977). Cytological evaluation of the effect of various estrogens given in postmenopause. *Acta Cytol, 21,* 225–228.

Ishihara, M. (1984). Effect of gamma-oryzanol on serum lipid peroxide levels and climacteric disturbances. *Asia Oceania J Obstet Gynecol, 10,* 317.

Jeri, A., & deRomana, C. (2000). The effect of isoflavone phytoestrogens in relieving hot flushes in Peruvian post-menopausal women. In *Proceedings of the 9th International Menopause Society World Congress on Menopause, Yokohama, Japan, October 17–21, 1999.* New York, NY: Parthenon.

Kaszkin-Bettag, M., Beck, S., Richardson, A., et al. (2008). Efficacy of the special extract ERr731 from Rhapontic rhubarb for menopausal complaints: A 6-month open observational study. *Alternative Therapies, 14,* 32–38.

Kaszkin-Bettag, M., Ventskovskiy, B., Kravchenko, A., et al. (2007). The special extract ERr 731 of the roots of Rheum rhaponticum decreases anxiety and improves health state and general well-being in perimenopausal women. *Menopause, 14,* 270–283.

Knight, D., Howes, J., & Eden, J. (1999). The effect of Promensil, an isoflavone extract, on menopausal symptoms. *Climacteric, 2,* 79–84.

Kohama, T., & Negami, M. (2013). Effects of low-dose French maritime pine bark extract on climacteric syndrome in 170 perimenopausal women. *J Reprod Med, 58,* 39–46.

Leathwood, P., & Chauffard, F. (1985). Aqueous extract of valerian reduces latency to fall asleep in man. *Planta Med, 51,* 144–148.

Leathwood, P., Chauffard, F., Heck, E., & Munoz-Box R. (1982). Aqueous extract of valerian root (*Valeriana officinalis* L.) improves sleep quality in man. *Pharmacol Biochem Behav, 17,* 65.

Lee, M. S., Shin, B. C., Yang, E. J., Lim, H. J., & Ernst, E. (2011). Maca (*Lepidium meyenii*) for treatment of menopausal symptoms: A systematic review. *Maturitas, 70,* 227–233.

L'Hermite, M. (2013). HRT optimization, using transdermal estradiol plus micronized progesterone, a safer HRT. *Climacteric, 16*(Suppl 1), 44–53.

Lipovac, M., Chedraui, P., Gruenhut, C., et al. (2010). Improvement of postmenopausal depressive and anxiety symptoms after treatment with isoflavones derived from red clover extracts. *Maturitas, 65,* 258–261.

Liu, Y. R., Jiang, Y. L., Huang, R. Q., Yang, J. Y., Xiao, B. K., & Dong, J. X. (2014). *Hypericum perforatum* L. preparations for menopause: A meta-analysis of efficacy and safety. *Climacteric, 17,* 325–335.

Loch, E. (1989). Diagnosis and therapy of hormonal bleeding disturbances. *TW Gynakol, 2,* 379–385.

Lucas, M., Asselin, G., Merette, C., et al. (2009). Effects of ethyl-eicosapentaenoic acid omega-3 fatty acid supplementation on hot flashes and quality of life among middle-aged women: A double-blind, placebo-controlled, randomized clinical trial. *Menopause, 16,* 357–366.

Mackey, R. H., Fanelli, T. J., Modugno, F., et al. (2012). Hormone therapy, estrogen metabolism, and risk of breast cancer in the Women's Health Initiative Hormone Therapy Trial. *Cancer Epidemiol Biomarkers Prev, 21,* 2022–2032.

Mahady, G. B., Low Dog, T., Sarma, D., et al. (2008). Review of case reports concerning hepatotoxicity and black cohosh (*Cimicifuga racemosa*). *Menopause, 15,* 628–638.

Matthews, K., Wing, R., Kuller, L., et al. (1990). Influences of natural menopause on psychological characteristics and symptoms of middle-aged healthy women. *J Consult Clin Psychol, 5,* 345–351.

Meissner, H., et al. (2006). Hormone-balancing effect of pre-gelatinized organic Maca (*Lepidium peruvianum* Chacon): III. Clinical responses of early-postmenopausal women to Maca in double blind, randomized, placebo-controlled, crossover configuration, outpatient study. *Int J Biomed Sci, 2,* 375–394.

Meissner H., Kapczynski W., Mscisz, A., et al. (2005). Use of a gelatinised maca (*Lepidium peruvianum*) in early-postmenopausal women—a pilot study. *Int J Biomed Sci, 1,* 33–45.

Messina, M. (2014). Soy foods, isoflavones, and the health of postmenopausal women. *Am J Clin Nutr, 100*(Suppl 1), 423S–430S.

Mirabi, P., & Mojab, F. (2013). The effects of valerian root on hot flashes in menopausal women. *Iran J Pharm Res, 12,* 217–222.

Murase, Y., & Iishima, H. (1963). Clinical studies of oral administration of gamma-oryzanol on climacteric complaints and its syndrome. *Obstet Gynecol Prac*, *12*, 147–149.

Nachtigall, L., La Grega, L., Lee, W., & Fenichel, R. (1999). The effects of isoflavones derived from red clover on vasomotor symptoms and endometrial thickness. In *Proceedings of the 9th International Menopause Society World Congress on Menopause, Yokohama, Japan, October 17–21, 1999*. New York, NY: Parthenon.

Nedeljkovic, M., Tian, L., Ji, P., et al. (2013). Effects of acupuncture and Chinese herbal medicine on hot flushes and quality of life in postmenopausal women: Results of a four-arm randomized controlled pilot trial. *Menopause*. [Epub ahead of print]

North American Menopause Society (NAMS). (2000). The role of isoflavones in menopausal health: Consensus opinion of the North American Menopause Society. *Menopause*, *7*, 215–229.

North American Menopause Society (NAMS). (2005). The role of testosterone therapy in postmenopausal women: Position statement of the North American Menopause Society. *Menopause*, *12*, 497–511.

North American Menopause Society (NAMS). (2012). The 2012 Hormone Therapy Position Statement of the North American Menopause Society. *Menopause*, *19*, 257–271).

Obi, N., Vrieling, A., Heinz, J., & Chang-Claude, J. (2011). Estrogen metabolite ratio: Is the 2-hydroxyestrone to 16α-hydroxyestrone ratio predictive for breast cancer? *Int J Womens Health*, *3*, 37–51.

Oliveira, D. S., Hachul, H., Goto, V., Tufik, S., & Bittencourt, L. R. (2012). Effect of therapeutic massage on insomnia and climacteric symptoms in postmenopausal women. *Climacteric*, *15*, 21–29.

Raff, H. (2009). Utility of salivary cortisol measurements in Cushing's syndrome and adrenal insufficiency. *J Clin Endocrinol Metab*, *94*, 3647–3655.

Raz, R., et al. (1993). A controlled trial of intravaginal estriol in postmenopausal women with urinary tract infections. *N Engl J Med*, *329*, 753–756.

Rostock, M., Fischer, J., Mumm, A., et al. (2011). Black cohosh (*Cimicifuga racemosa*) in tamoxifen-treated breast cancer patients with climacteric complaints—a prospective observational study. *Gynecol Endocrinol*, *27*, 844–848.

Sarrel, P., Dobay, B., & Wiita, B. (1998). Sexual behavior and neuroendocrine responses to estrogen and estrogen-androgen in postmenopausal women dissatisfied with estrogen-only therapy. *J Reprod Med*, *43*, 847–856.

Schmidt, P., Haw, N., & Rubinow, D. (2004). A longitudinal evaluation of the relationship between reproductive status and mood in perimenopausal women. *Am J Psychiatry*, *161*, 2238–2244.

Shibata, S., Tanaka, O., Shoji, J., & Saito, H. (1985). Chemistry and pharmacology of Panax. *Econ Med Plant Res*, *1*, 217–284.

Smith, C. (1964). Non-hormonal control of vaso-motor flushing in menopausal patients. *Chic Med*, *67*, 193–195.

Sternfeld, B., & Dugan, S. (2011). Physical activity and health during the menopausal transition. *Obstet Gynecol Clin North Am*, *38*, 537–566.

Stolze, H. (1985). An alternative to treat menopausal symptoms with a phytotherapeutic agent. *Med Welt, 36*, 871–874.

Taavoni, S., Ekbatani, N., Kashaniyan, M., & Haghani, H. (2011). Effect of valerian on sleep quality in postmenopausal women: A randomized placebo-controlled clinical trial. *Menopause, 18*, 951–955.

Taku, K., Melby, M. K., Kronenberg, F., Kurzer, M. S., & Messina, M. (2012). Extracted or synthesized soybean isoflavones reduce menopausal hot flash frequency and severity: Systematic review and meta-analysis of randomized controlled trials. *Menopause, 19*, 776–790.

Thompson, L., Robb, P., Serraino, M., & Cheung, F. (1991). Mammalian lignan production from various foods. *Nutr and Canc, 16*, 43–52.

Tice, J., Ettinger, B., Ensrud, K., et al. (2003). Phytoestrogen supplements for the treatment of hot flashes: The isoflavone clover extract (ICE) study. *JAMA, 290*, 207–214.

Tode, T., Kikuchi, Y., Hirata, J., et al. (1999). Effect of Korean red ginseng on psychological functions in patients with severe climacteric syndromes. *Int J Gynaecol Obstet, 67*, 169.

Uebelhack, R., Blohmer, J. U., Graubaum, H. J., et al. (2006). Black cohosh and St. John's wort for climacteric complaints. *Obstet Gynecol, 107*, 247–255.

US Department of Health and Human Services, Office of Disease Prevention and Health Promotion. (2008). *Physical activity guidelines advisory committee report.* Washington, DC: Author.

van de Weijer, P., & Barentsen, R. (2002). Isoflavones from red clover Promensil significantly reduce menopausal hot flush symptoms compared with placebo. *Maturitas, 42*, 187–193.

Vivian-Taylor, J., & Hickey, M. (2014). Menopause and depression: Is there a link? *Maturitas, 79*, 142–146.

Yang, H.-M., Liao, M.-F., Zhu, S.-Y., Liao, M.-N., & Rohdewald, P. (2007). A randomised, double-blind, placebo-controlled trial on the effect of Pycnogenol on the climacteric syndrome in perimenopausal women. *Acta Obstetricia et Gynecologica, 86*, 978–985.

Young Kim, S., Kyo Seo, S., Mi Choi, Y., et al. (2012). Effects of red ginseng supplementation on menopausal symptoms and cardiovascular risk factors in postmenopausal women: A double-blind randomized controlled trial. *Menopause, 19*, 461–466.

Warnecke, G. (1991). Psychosomatic dysfunction in the female climacteric: Clinical effectiveness and tolerance of kava extract WS 1490 (in German). *Fortschr Med, 109*, 119–122.

Warnecke, G., Pfaender, H., Gerster, G., & Gracza, E. (1990). Wirksamkeit von Kawa-Kawa-Extrakt beim klimakterischen Syndrom. *Zeitschrift Phytotherapie, 11*, 81–86.

Watts, N., Notelovitz, M., Timmons, M., et al. (1995). Comparison of oral estrogens and estrogens plus androgen on bone mineral density, menopausal symptoms, and lipid-lipoprotein profiles in surgical menopause. *Obstet Gynecol, 85*, 529–537.

Wiklund, I., Mattsson, L., Lindgren, R., & Limoni, C. (1999). Effects of a standardized ginseng on the quality of life and physiological parameters in symptomatic post-menopausal women: A double-blind, placebo-controlled trial. *Int J Clin Pharm Res*, *19*, 89–99.

Writing Group for the PEPI Trial. (1996). Effects of hormone replacement therapy on endometrial histology in postmenopausal women. The Postmenopausal Estrogen/ Progestin Interventions (PEPI) Trial. *JAMA*, *275*, 370–375.

Zarfeshany, A., Asgary, S., & Javanmard, S. H. (2014). Potent health benefits of pomegranate *Adv Biomed Res*, *3*, 100.

20

Prevention of Cervical Dysplasia and Cancer

LISE ALSCHULER

CASE STUDY

Sylvia was a healthy 35-year-old mother of two who had been happily and monogamously married for 10 years. Sylvia did not smoke or drink alcohol, she maintainted a healthy weight, and her only health issue was long-standing psoriasis. At Sylvia's routine gynecological examination, she was told that her cervix looked a little suspicious. The results of her subsequent Pap smear revealed cervical atypia. She was shocked. She was also panicked, as she was supporting her father who was dying from lung cancer and was worried about this being a precancerous condition. Her gynecologist told her not to worry and that any necessary treatment would be determined after a repeat Pap in three months. Sylvia could not sleep and realized that she could not simply wait for three more months. She sought my consultation. I recommended a comprehensive supplement, dietary, and stress management program. Sylvia adhered to the program with enthusiasm, experiencing a sense of wellness she had not realized that she was missing. In three months, her repeat Pap came back normal. Sylvia breathed a sigh of relief and vowed to continue to promote her health and wellness.

Introduction

Cervical cancer is the third most common cancer, after breast and colorectal cancers, in women worldwide, and is the leading cause of cancer-related death in many developing countries (Arbyn et al., 2011). Just a century ago, cervical cancer was the leading cause of death among women in the United States (Trimble et al., 2008). Over the past 30 years, widespread adoption of screening with Pap smears along with effective treatments for precancerous cervical conditions has cut the death rate from cervical cancer in half. The recent development of vaccines against the causative human papillomavirus (HPV) may reduce the prevalence of cervical cancer even further. Of significance too is the growing awareness of the role that lifestyle behaviors, diet, and selected nutrients and botanicals play in the prevention and treatment of cervical cancer.

Epidemiology

The worldwide incidence of cervical cancer is about 440,000 cases annually. In the United States, the overall rate of cervical cancer is 18.6 cases per 100,000 women and the incidence rises steadily with age, peaking at ages 65 to 69. Compared with white women, black women have double the incidence of cervical cancer, particularly in the 65 to 69 years age group. This recently confirmed age-related incidence suggests that women over the age of 65 are at the greatest risk for cervical cancer, however this is the age current guidelines suggest screenings may cease (Rositch, Nowak, & Gravitt, 2014). Of note, cervical cancer is rarely diagnosed in women over age 65 years who have participated in regular Pap test screening throughout adulthood. Additionally, these numbers represent a fraction of the total number of cervical abnormalities, which are considered risk factors for cervical cancer (Table 20.1).

Overall, the American Cancer Society estimates that there will be about 12,360 new diagnoses of invasive cervical cancer and 4,020 deaths in 2014 (American Cancer Society, 2014). The mortality rate for cervical cancer among non-Hispanic white women in the United States is 2.6 per 100,000 and 4.9 per 100,000 for African American women (Trimble et al., 2008). In the United States, cervical cancer is most prevalent and more deadly in socioeconomically disadvantaged black and Hispanic women.

Table 20.1. Prevalence of Cervical Atypia

Cervical Atypia	Number of Cases per Year
Atypical squamous cells of uncertain significance (ASCUS)	2,000,000
Low-grade squamous intraepithelial lesions (LGSIL)	1,250,000
High-grade squamous intraepithelial lesions (HGSIL)	300,000

Source: Rock et al. (2000).

Significant to the epidemiology of cervical cancer is the rate of HPV infection among women, some strains of which are considered causal agents. The incidence of HPV in women is alarmingly high. It is estimated that roughly 25 million women, between the ages of 14 and 59 years, are infected with HPV in the United States (Huh & Roden, 2008). Furthermore, it is predicted that 80% of all women will acquire genital HPV infection by 50 years of age (Huh & Roden, 2008). Genital HPVs, particularly HPV 16 and 18, and to a lesser extent HPV 6 and 11, are thought to cause two-thirds of all cervical cancers. Fortunately, the road from viral infection to cancer is not a one-way trajectory. Other factors including dietary habits, smoking, sexual partners, and nutrient status play a role in viral virulence, thus creating a window for a multifaceted integrative approach to prevention and treatment.

Declaring that cervical cancer should be eradicated is now a rational statement. Effective and low-cost screening, prevention vaccines, and targeted lifestyle practices can make cervical cancer a disease of the past. I hope that in my lifetime as a physician, the day will come when I will no longer witness anyone dying from cervical cancer.

PATHOPHYSIOLOGY AND DIAGNOSIS

There are three major histological types of cervical cancer. Squamous cell carcinoma is the most common type, followed by adenocarcinoma and then small cell carcinoma. Small cell carcinoma of the cervix is a very rare form and is associated with a worse prognosis and increased tendency for distant metastases (Chen, Macdonald, & Gaffney, 2008). Cervical cancer is often asymptomatic in early stages. When symptoms do occur, it is generally when the cancer is more advanced. These symptoms may include abnormal vaginal bleeding, heavy discharge, dyspareunia, dysuria, and pelvic pain. Advanced cervical cancer is characterized by metastases primarily to the abdomen and lung. Cervical cancer is diagnosed with cervical cytology (Pap smear) followed by biopsy and staged according to the International Federation of Gynecology and Obstetrics (FIGO) classification system (Box 20.1).

As mentioned earlier, cervical cancer is considered to be the result of infection with HPV, particularly types 16 and 18 (Munoz et al., 2003). The virus is introduced through sexual contact and proliferates in the basal cells of squamous epithelium. Host infection with HPV involves HPV early genes, namely E1, E2, E5, E6, and E7, the expression of which contributes to viral replication and abnormal proliferation. The HPV-infected cells do not fully differentiate and thus do not express many viral proteins on their surfaces. This allows for immune evasion. In addition, the infected cell matures in the deeper epithelial layers, which are located further away from the highest concentration of T-cells. Thus, the more mature (still not fully differentiated) cervical cells avoid contact with the cellular arm of our immune system. Individuals with defects in T-cell-mediated immunity, such as women with HIV, are especially vulnerable to HPV-associated cancer, as there is little chance at mounting a cytotoxic attack. Despite the adeptness of immune evasion, HPV infection does not necessarily lead to the development of cervical cancer. In fact, the majority of women infected with HPV are able to eradicate this infection or prevent the pathogenicity of the virus. This is the primary opportunity for disease prevention and control in HPV-infected women and is influenced by several behavioral and nutritional factors.

Box 20.1 Abbreviated FIGO Staging of Cervical Cancer

Stage I is carcinoma strictly confined to the cervix. The diagnosis of both Stages IA1 and IA2 should be based on microscopic examination of removed tissue, preferably a cone, which must include the entire lesion.

Stage II is carcinoma that extends beyond the cervix, but does not extend into the pelvic wall. The carcinoma involves the vagina, but not as far as the lower third.

Stage III is carcinoma that has extended into the pelvic sidewall. The tumor involves the lower third of the vagina.

Stage IV is carcinoma that has extended beyond the true pelvis or has clinically involved the mucosa of the bladder and/or rectum and includes spread to distant organs.

Source: TNM Classification of Malignant Tumours (2002).

In 2014, the cobas was approved by the FDA for use as a stand-alone test to detect all high-risk HPV genotypes, after being approved in 2011 as a follow-up or adjunctive test to cell cytology. In a comparative study, the sensitivity and specificity of cobas for detecting cervical high-grade intraepithelial lesions (CIN-2) was found to be 91.4% and 31.2% respectively. When considering only positive HPV-16 and/or HPV-18 genotype results, the cobas test showed a sensitivity and specificity of 51.9% and 86.6%, respectively (Binnicker et al., 2014). A positive result should be followed with a Pap test in order to determine the need for colposcopy.

Influencing the Pathogenicity of Human Papillomavirus Infection

There are well-established behavioral influences on HPV pathogenicity. Women with later sexual experiences, fewer sexual partners, female sexual partners, male sexual partners who use condoms, and who are nonsmokers are all at decreased risk of developing cervical cancer if infected with HPV (Rock, Michael, Reynolds, & Ruffin, 2000). As HPV is transmitted sexually, increased sexual activity increases exposure. Tobacco smoking is a direct carcinogen and cervical cells seem particularly vulnerable to its genotoxic effects. A high viral load combined with regular alcohol consumption has also been shown to increase the risk of persistent HPV infection in a prospective study (Oh et al., 2014). Specifically, among regular alcohol drinkers of greater than 15 g alcohol per day and also among women with a history of drinking for at least five years, high HPV load was associated with 1-year and 2-year persistence compared with nondrinkers, in whom HPV load was not associated with persistence risk (p for trend < .001). This suggests a synergistic effect of viral load and alcohol behaviors in the risk of HPV persistence. Counseling women about these factors should be the basis of a comprehensive integrative approach.

Dietary intake and serum concentrations of carotenoids, vitamin C, vitamin E, and folate are inversely correlated with persistence of cervical HPV infection and development of cervical cancer (Rock et al., 2000). A unifying theory for the protective role these nutrients play in preventing the development of cervical cancer in HPV-infected women centers around the role of peroxidation and DNA mutations. Reactive oxygen species (ROS) are considered to be involved in the initiation and progression of carcinogenesis via damage to oncogenes, the fragile genes in the DNA particularly susceptible to viral and oxidative damage. Low antioxidant activity has been observed in women with cervical cancer along with increased lipid peroxidation and suppressed cellular immunity compared with healthy controls ($n = 94$) (Kazbariene et al., 2004). Women with cervical cancer have lower levels of endogenous antioxidants, such as glutathione, vitamin E, vitamin C, and coenzyme Q10 (Palan et al., 2003). It has been postulated that this low antioxidative status results from depletion due to lipid peroxide scavenging (Manju, Sailaja, & Nalini, 2002). Over time, impaired antioxidation may allow virally and oxidatively induced carcinogenesis to persist.

In addition to providing general antioxidation, carotenoids, vitamin C, vitamin E, and folate possess antineoplastic activity against cervical cancer cells. Carotenes induce cell cycle arrest and apoptosis of dysplastic cells via a variety of intracellular actions (Donaldson, 2011). Vitamins C and E stimulate phagocytosis, protect cellular proteins and DNA against ROS damage, and may inhibit oncogene formation (Myung, Ju, Kim, & Kim, 2011). Folate supports DNA methylation, particularly of HPV-16 oncogenes, thus silencing neoplastic formation (Hublarova, Hrstka, & Vojtesek, 2008).

Some women may have even higher dietary requirements for antioxidants depending on where they live. Exposure to high levels of more than one air pollutant such as benzene, diesel particulate matter, and/or polycyclic aromatic hydrocarbons is positively associated with cervical dysplasia prevalence (p for trend = .004). Specifically, women living in census tracts with high levels of these hazardous air pollutants were approximately two to three times more likely to be diagnosed with cervical dysplasia than women living in areas with relatively low pollutant levels. Of note, 73% of both cases and controls were positive for HPV infection, underscoring the independent correlation with air pollution (Scheurer, Danysh, Follen, & Lupo, 2014).

Integrative Prevention Strategies

The role of individual nutrients in the pathogenesis of cervical cancer has been well elucidated and has given rise to specific lifestyle-based prevention strategies. A number of well-designed studies have demonstrated the protective link between certain nutrients and the development of cervical cancer. High intakes of vegetables, fruits, fiber, beta-carotenes, folic acid, retinols, vitamin E, and vitamin C are associated with up to 60% risk reduction for development of cervical cancer in HPV-positive women (Table 20.2).

It is important to note that the inverse relationship between these nutrients and cervical cancer has been specifically observed from food intake. This data does not directly support the use of individual dietary supplements for prevention.

Table 20.2. Protective Effects of Dietary Components Against Development of Cervical Cancer

Dietary Nutrients Studied	Study Design	Outcome	Citation
Fruits, vegetables	Prospective, $n = 299,649$ (253 cases invasive squamous cervical cancer)	17% lower risk of invasive squamous cervical cancer	Gonzalez et al. (2011)
Vegetables and fruits	Matched cohort study, $n = 328$	Lower intake of vegetables and fruit and higher viral load (≥ 15.5) associated with increased risk of CINII and CINIII (OR = 2.84) compared with low intake and lower viral load	Hwang, Lee, Kim, & Kim (2010)
Vegetables, fruits, beta-carotene, vitamins C, E, fiber	Matched case control, $n = 170$	22%–44% lower risk of developing cervical cancer	Atalah et al. (2001)
Vitamin A, retinol	Meta-analysis	Pooled odds ratios of cervical cancer 0.59 (95% CI, 0.49–0.72) for total vitamin A intake and 0.60 (95% CI, 0.41–0.89) for blood vitamin A levels	Zhang, Dai, Zhang, & Wang (2012)
Fiber, vitamins C, E, A, alpha-carotene, beta-carotene, lutein, folate, total fruit and vegetable intake	Hospital-based, case–control study, $n = 239$	Risk reduction of 40%–60% was observed for women in the highest versus lowest tertiles of dietary intake of each nutrient	Ghosh et al. (2008)

Any discussion of cervical cancer prevention would be incomplete without mention of HPV vaccination, as HPV 16 and 18 are responsible for causing 70% of all cases of cervical cancer (Hoops & Twiggs, 2008). The development of a vaccine that can protect a majority of women against pathogenic HPV infection, and thus cervical cancer, has led to widespread efforts to make this vaccine universally available. In addition to the positive impact on human suffering, cost-benefit analysis demonstrates significant cost savings (Prasad & Hill, 2008).

Two vaccines are available that contain virus-like particles: Cervarix contains particles derived from HPV 16 and 18 and Gardasil from HPV 6, 11, 16, and 18. In a Phase 3 study, Cervarix showed 84% (97.9% CI, 73.5%–91.1%) efficacy against 6-month persistent infections with HPV type 16 and 74% (97.9% CI, 49.1%–87.8%) efficacy against HPV type 18. Gardasil has been shown to be 98% effective in preventing CIN 2+ lesions associated with HPV types 16 and 18 (Huh & Roden, 2008). Clinical efficacy has been measured up to 5.5 years and the vaccine is predicted to provide lifelong protection in the majority of people. In the United States, the Advisory Committee on Immunization Practices recommends HPV vaccination for females aged 11–12 years—ideally before they become sexually active. "Catch-up" vaccination in females, aged 13–26, is also recommended as this group has the highest prevalence of HPV infection (Wright et al., 2008). In spite of the vaccine's effectiveness, only 33% of girls aged 13–17 years received the recommended 3-dose HPV vaccine series in 2012. By Centers for Disease Control and Prevention (CDC) estimates, increasing HPV vaccination to 80% in this age group would prevent an estimated 53,000 cases of cancer over the lifetimes of these girls (CDC, 2013). Even with the cervical cancer vaccine, women should be counseled to come in for their annual gynecological examination.

While the vaccine shows great promise, some authorities question whether universal HPV vaccination was recommended too quickly. The evidence shows that the vaccines can prevent infection with two out of 15 oncogenic HPV strains (HPV 16 and HPV 18) and the precancerous cervical intraepithelial neoplasia (CIN) 1–3 lesions. (Markowitz et al., 2007). These HPV strains were used as surrogate end points to cervical cancer as studies lasted only 5 years. In addition, Gardasil has been linked to a particularly large number of adverse drug reactions (ADRs). As of September 2012, 21,265 ADRs have been reported in the United States for Gardasil, including 78 deaths, 363 life-threatening ADRs, and 609 events that resulted in permanent disability. Compared with all other vaccines in women younger than 30, Gardasil alone was associated with >60% of all serious ADRs (including 61.9% of all deaths, 64.9% of all life-threatening reactions and 81.8% cases of permanent disability) (Tomljenovic & Shaw, 2012).

While these statistics are concerning, it is important to look at the totality of the data. According to the CDC, from June 2006 to March 2014, approximately 67 million doses of HPV vaccines were distributed and the Vaccine Adverse Event Reporting System (VAERs) received approximately 25,000 adverse event reports occurring in girls and women who received HPV vaccines; 92% were classified as nonserious. Adverse events in the HPV-vaccinated population were then compared with those in another appropriate population (such as adolescents vaccinated with vaccines other than HPV), including Guillain-Barré syndrome, stroke, venous thromboembolism (VTE), appendicitis, seizures, syncope (fainting), and allergic reactions. After a careful review it was shown that none of these adverse events were any more common after HPV vaccination than among comparison groups (CDC, 2014).

It is important that clinicians be aware of the controversy and the legitimate concerns many parents and women have when it comes to the HPV vaccine and be willing to have a frank and open conversation about both the risks and benefits.

Integrative Treatment

It is beyond the scope of this chapter to delve extensively into the conventional treatment for cervical cancer; please refer to appropriate texts and articles. For this chapter, I want to stress that the bulk of integrative therapies in the management of cervical carcinoma lies within the realm of preventing HPV-induced dysplasia from becoming carcinoma. The impact of several nutrients as chemopreventive agents has already been discussed.

A woman with cervical dysplasia is a prime candidate for lifestyle modification, dietary modification, and supplementation. We can assume that women with cervical dysplasia have some degree of immunosuppression given the presence of a viral pathology. It is well established that stress and chronic negative emotions (anger, anxiety, depression) can disrupt immunity. Conversely, positive emotional states (happiness, joy, optimism) support immunity. In many ways, cervical dysplasia can be viewed as an opportunity for women to assess their emotional well-being.

I am a strong proponent of giving women explicit permission to be happy and joyful (it astounds me how many women do not feel that they deserve to be happy) and will use the diagnosis of this precancerous condition to initiate this dialogue. A natural sequel to this conversation is a conversation about specific stress-management practices. Helping a woman discover effective stress-management techniques such as exercise, meditation, yoga, cooking, artwork, and so on will improve her immune function and incorporate wellness into her life. In addition to these important benefits, a lifestyle-based wellness program may also encourage her interest in, and compliance with, a nutritional supplement program.

It is common naturopathic practice to provide an aggressive dietary and supplement recommendations in order to reverse the dysplasia. Dietary recommendations constellate around a whole-foods diet replete with colorful (antioxidant rich) fruits and vegetables. Excessive consumption of refined sugar and alcohol should be avoided due to their immunosuppressant effects.

I have personally observed the benefits of additional supplementation. I routinely recommend several supplements. Low serum folate is associated with having high-grade (greater than 2) CIN (Piyathilake et al., 2007). Supplementation with folic acid to create sufficiency is indicated and dosages ranging from 400 mcg to 10 mg have been studied. The higher doses have not necessarily yielded clinically superior results (Marshall, 2003), thus dosing to achieve normal serum levels is most appropriate. While there is limited association between polymorphisms of key methylation genes, such as methylenetetrahydrofolate reductase (MTHFR) and methionine synthase (Zhu et al., 2013) and CIN, women with MTHFR polymorphisms are at increased risk of CIN if they also have low serum folate and vitamin B12 (Tong et al., 2011). In these women, using a methylated form of folate may provide additional benefit, particularly in supporting DNA methylation and in so doing downregulating HPV transcription. In addition, given the association between vitamins C and E and cervical cancer protection, combined with the fact that many Americans are functionally deficient in these antioxidants, their supplementation is often indicated. I typically recommend vitamin C at 500 mg at least three times daily and vitamin E (as mixed tocopherols) at 400 IU twice daily.

Several botanicals may be beneficial for women with cervical dysplasia. Green tea (*Camellia sinensis*) polyphenols, particularly polyphenon E (a decaffeinated, enriched green tea catechin extract), induce apoptosis, arrest the cell cycle, and decrease the production of epidermal growth factor receptor (EGFR), all of which are necessary for cervical cancer progression (Ahn et al., 2003). Green tea also supports hepatic detoxification (all phases) and provides antioxidation effects. However, a phase II randomized, double-blind, placebo-controlled trial of 98 women with persistent HPV infection and low grade CIN (CIN1) compared 800 mg per day of polyphenon E with placebo for 4 months (Garcia et al., 2014). There was no difference in the clearance of HPV or CIN between the intervention and placebo group. One can conclude that short-term use of polyphenon E extract is unlikely to be effective. Accepted clinical practice is to recommend green tea as a long-term prevention strategy in people at risk, not as a short-term treatment strategy. I recommend daily consumption of at least eight cups of good quality green tea or consumption of 600–1,200 mg standardized extract of green tea (standardized to 80% polyphenols, of which at least 50% is EGCG) taken in divided doses and always taken with food. If a woman is willing, I will also recommend a retention vaginal douche with cooled green tea. Topical treatment with green tea has demonstrated benefit for cervical dysplasia (Ahn et al., 2003).

For those women who refuse loop electrosurgical excision procedure (LEEP) conization or cryotherapy for precancerous cervical lesions, and in whom there is a satisfactory colposcopy, herbal escharotics treatment may be an option. This involves repeated application of enzyme and botanical agents in a sequential manner to the cervical tissue. I have used this treatment and found that, while it is more labor- and time-intensive, it is effective and offers the patient weekly opportunities for focused healing sessions in a supportive and safe environment. Naturopathic escharotic treatments involve twice-weekly applications of ablative agents to the cervix. Agents used in naturopathic escharotics treatments are sequentially painted on the cervix and consist of bromelain, compounded zinc chloride, blood root (*Sanguinaria canadensis*) tincture, and calendula (*Calendula officinalis*) succus tincture, followed by vaginal depletion packs, which are essentially tampons coated with a mixture of thuja (*Thuja occidentalis*) oil, goldenseal root (*Hydrastis canadensis*) tincture, tea tree (*Melaleuca alternifolia*) essential oil, bitter orange (*Citrus aurantium*) essential oil, vitamin A, and ferrous sulfate. The agents used in escharotics treatments debride the cervical tissue, reduce inflammation, support local immunity, and induce apoptosis of virally infected cells. A full course of naturopathic escharotics treatments requires at least one-and-a-half months. There are currently no clinical studies to validate the effectiveness of this treatment.

Indole-3-carbinol (I3C) and its gastric breakdown product, diindolylmethane (DIM), also available as a supplement, are useful natural agents for cervical dysplasia. Both I3C and DIM induce apoptosis of human cervical cancer cells and HPV-16 infected cervical cells (Chen et al., 2001). Both I3C and DIM induce 2-hydroxylation of estrogen over 16-hydroxylation via induction of cyp1A1 and inhibit 4-hydroxylation of estrogens via the inhibition of cyp1B1 (Bradlow, Sepkovic, Telang, & Osborne, 1999). Women with CIN 2 and 3 have a higher 16-hydroxylation to 2-hydroxylation ratio, which is problematic in that 16-hyroxylated estrogen metabolites are strongly estrogenic and carcinogenic. In contrast, 2-hydroxylated estrogen metabolites are weakly estrogenic and not carcinogenic. Of note, 4-hydroxylated estrogen metabolites are strongly estrogenic and carcinogenic. Administration of 200–400 mg of I3C can reverse CIN as demonstrated in a randomized control trial (n = 30) of women with CIN 2 or 3 (Bell et al., 2000). Unfortunately, there are no additional clinical trials available for review.

Curcuma longa, or turmeric, is an Indian culinary herb. The past decade has seen an outpouring of preclinical and some clinical studies regarding turmeric and one of its main constituents, curcumin (diferuloylmethane), as an antineoplastic agent. One such in vitro study demonstrated that curcumin induces apoptosis of cervical cancer cells in a concentration-dependent manner. Curcumin also selectively inhibits expression of viral oncogenes E6 and E7. Finally, curcumin downregulates NFkappaB, thus decreasing inflammation, a known potentiator of carcinogenesis (Divya & Pillai, 2006). A phase I clinical trial of curcumin included four patients with CIN. These patients, along with the other 21 patients in the study, tolerated doses of up to 8 g/day of curcumin without adverse effect. One of the four CIN patients demonstrated histological improvement and one of the four CIN patients proceeded to develop frank malignancy (Cheng et al., 2001). Of note, this study was not powered or designed to assess clinical effect. A phase II randomized controlled study of 287 HPV-positive women without high-grade cervical neoplasia were randomized to four intervention arms to be treated with topical polyherbal vaginal cream (extracts of *Curcuma longa*, *Aloe vera*, *Emblica officinalis*, and *n-docosanol*) vaginal cream (Basant cream), vaginal placebo cream, curcumin vaginal capsules, or vaginal placebo capsules for 30 days (Basu et al., 2013). The HPV clearance rate in the Basant arm (87.7%) was significantly higher than in the combined placebo arms (73.3%). The curcumin vaginal capsules were associated with a higher rate of clearance (81.3%) than placebo, though the difference did not reach statistical significance. Mild to moderate vaginal irritation and pruritis were reported after Basant application.

Turmeric may also be beneficial for those patients undergoing chemoradiation. In one in vitro study, curcuminoids were found to decrease MDR-1 gene expression in multi-drug-resistant human cervical carcinoma cells (Limtrakul, Anuchapreeda, & Buddhasukh, 2004). This suggests that curcuminoids may reduce MDR-1 production of P-glycoprotein, a major cell membrane protein involved in cellular efflux of, and therefore resistance to, chemotherapy agents. Another in vitro study demonstrated cervical cancer cell sensitization to the cytotoxic effects of Taxol when these cells were simultaneously exposed to curcumin. This sensitization effect was not observed in normal cervical cells (Bava et al., 2005). Finally, pretreatment of cervical cancer cells with curcumin resulted in significant dose-dependent radiosensitization of these cells, while normal cells were not affected (Javvadi et al., 2008). Preclinical data indicates that curcumin may have potential as a synergistic agent with chemoradiation treatment for cervical carcinoma. When recommending turmeric, I encourage women to use turmeric generously in their cooking and will also recommend supplementation with concentrated colloidal curcumin, turmeric extracts standardized to 95% curcuminoids, turmeric extract with piperine, or other optimized curcumin matrix products. Each curcumin product has different bioavailability claims that need to be considered when targeting a daily dose equivalent to 4–8 g of curcumin root powder.

Other potentially useful natural agents include ascorbic acid, *Agaricus blazei* (Brazilian sun mushroom), and acupuncture. One of the mechanisms of HPV carcinogenesis involves the viral degradation of p53 in cervical cancer cells, thereby interfering with the cell's apoptotic ability. An in vitro study demonstrated that ascorbic acid stabilized p53, restoring apoptosis. Intact apoptosis is necessary for successful chemotherapeutic response (Reddy, Khanna, & Singh, 2001). Thus, ascorbic acid may contribute to decreased tumor burden, particularly in conjunction with some chemotherapeutic agents. Of note, ascorbic acid has no known or theoretical interference with cisplatin, the standard first-line chemotherapy agent, and, in effect, may be synergistic with platin chemotherapy.

A small randomized placebo-controlled trial of 100 gynecologic patients, which included 61 cervical cancer patients, stages Ia–IIIb, received either carboplatin and etoposide or carboplatin and Taxol every 3 weeks with or without oral *Agaricus blazei* (as *Agaricus blazei* Murill Kyowa [ABMK], a patented extract) taken at a daily dosage of three liquid packs (30 mL) daily. Parameters of immune function and tolerance to treatment were observed. Those patients who received *A. blazei* had improved natural killer cell activity and appetite, less alopecia, better emotional stability, and less general weakness (Ahn et al., 2004). Of note, this study did not assess whether the *A. blazei* might have interacted with the chemotherapy in such a way as to decrease its efficacy.

One of the adverse effects of radiation therapy for cervical cancer can be radiation rectitis. In an open trial of 44 patients with cervical cancer, receiving radiation therapy and with radiation rectitis, acupuncture was administered once daily for up to 1 week. Of the patients, 73% of them experienced complete resolution of their radiation rectitis symptoms, 9% experienced marked improvement of symptoms, 18% experienced somewhat improved symptoms, and there were no patients that failed to report any benefit from acupuncture (Zaohua, 1987).

Acupuncture is also helpful in reducing radiation-induced fatigue and malaise. Acupuncture is a complementary therapy that should always be considered, given its low risk and high potential benefit.

Some natural agents have preliminary data that suggest direct antineoplastic action against cervical cancer cells. A mixture containing lysine, proline, arginine, ascorbic acid, and green tea demonstrated significant antiproliferative effects on human cervical cancer cells via inhibition of matrix metalloproteinases (Roomi et al., 2006). Whether this antimetastatic action occurs in vivo remains to be determined. Finally, another natural substance, coenzyme Q10, has been shown to inhibit the cell growth and induce apoptosis of human cervical cancer cells (Gorelick et al., 2004). Although this effect has not yet been studied in humans, the preliminary data, combined with the minimal toxicity profile of coenzyme Q10, should be given consideration in an integrative treatment plan.

Conclusions

The key to successful integrative management of cervical cancer is prevention and early diagnosis. Lifestyle adjustments, which rely heavily on dietary modifications and avoidance of tobacco use, form the cornerstone of an integrative approach. Supplementation of selected nutrients and herbs also has a place in prevention and quite possibly in the management of established cervical carcinoma. Ultimately, with the adoption of prevention-oriented lifestyles, the advent of preventive vaccinations and continued screening practices, cervical cancer will be a disease of the past and this chapter will become obsolete.

REFERENCES

Ahn, W. S., Huh, S. W., Bae, S. M., et al. (2003). A major constituent of green tea, EGCG, inhibits the growth of a human cervical cancer cell line, CaSki Cells, through apoptosis, G(1) arrest, and regulation of expression. *DNA Cell Biol, 22,* 217–224.

Ahn, W. S., Kim, D. J., Chae, G. T., et al. (2004). Natural killer cell activity and quality of life were improved by consumption of a mushroom extract, *Agaricus blazei* Murill Kyowa, in gynecological cancer patients undergoing chemotherapy. *Int J Gynecol Cancer, 14,* 589–594.

American Cancer Society. (2014). What are the key statistics about cervical cancer? Retrieved August 25, 2014, from http://www.cancer.org/cancer/cervicalcancer/detailedguide/cervical-cancer-key-statistics

Arbyn, M., Castellsague, X., de Sanjose, S., et al. (2011). Worldwide burden of cervical cancer in 2008. *Ann Oncol, 22*, 2675–2686.

Atalah, E., Urteaga, C., Rebolledo, A., et al. (2001). [Diet, smoking and reproductive history as risk factor for cervical cancer] (in Spanish). *Rev Med Child, 129*, 597–603.

Basu, P., Dutta, S., Begum, R., et al. (2013). Clearance of cervical human papillomavirus infection by topical application of curcumin and curcumin containing polyherbal cream: A phase II randomized controlled study. *Asian Pac J Cancer Prev, 14*, 5753–5759.

Bava, S., Puliappadamba, V., Deepti, A., et al. (2005). Sensitization of taxol-induced apoptosis by curcumin involves down-regulation of nuclear factor-kappaB and the serine/threonine kinase Akt and is independent of tubulin polymerization. *J Biol Chem, 280*, 6301–6308.

Binnicker, M. J., Pritt, B. S., Duresko, B. J., et al. (2014). Comparative evaluation of three commercial systems for the detection of high-risk human papillomavirus in cervical and vaginal ThinPrep PreservCyt samples with biopsy correlation. *J Clin Microbiol*. [Epub ahead of print]

Bell, M. C., Crowley-Nowick, P., Bradlow, H. L., et al. (2000). Placebo-controlled trial of indole- 3-carbinol in the treatment of CIN. *Gynecol Oncol, 78*, 123–129.

Bradlow, H. L., Sepkovic, D. W., Telang, N. T., & Osborne, M. P. (1999). Multifunctional aspects of the action of indole-3-carbinol as an antitumor agent. *Ann N Y Acad Sci, 889*, 204–213.

Centers for Disease Control and Prevention (CDC). (2013). National and state vaccination coverage among adolescents aged 13–17 years —United States, 2012. *Morbidity and Mortality Weekly Report (MMWR), 62*, 685–693.

Centers for Disease Control and Prevention (CDC). (2014). *Human papillomavirus (HPV) vaccine.* Retrieved September 1, 2014, from http://www.cdc.gov/vaccine-safety/vaccines/HPV/index.html

Chen, D., Qi, M., Auborn, K. J., et al. (2001). Indole-3-carbinol and diindolylmethane induce apoptosis of human cervical cancer cells and in murine HPV 16-transgenic preneoplastic cervical epithelium. *J Nutr, 131*, 3294–3302.

Chen, J., Macdonald, O., & Gaffney, D. (2008). Incidence, mortality, and prognostic factors of small cell carcinoma of the cervix. *Obstet Gynecol, 111*, 1394–1402.

Cheng, A., Hsu, C., Lin, J., et al. (2001). Phase I clinical trial of curcumin, a chemopreventive agent, in patients with high-risk or pre-malignant lesions. *Anticancer Res, 21*, 2895–2900.

Divya, C., & Pillai, M. (2006). Antitumor action of curcumin in human papillomavirus associated cells involves downregulation of viral oncogenes, prevention of NFkB and AP-1 translocation, and modulation of apoptosis. *Mol Carcinog, 45*, 320–332.

Donaldson, M. (2011). A carotenoid health index based on plasma carotenoids and health outcomes. *Nutrients, 3*, 1002–1022.

Garcia, F. A., Cornelison, T., Nuño, T., et al. (2014). Results of a phase II randomized, double-blind, placebo-controlled trial of Polyphenon E in women with persistent high-risk HPV infection and low-grade cervical intraepithelial neoplasia. *Gynecol Oncol, 132*, 377–382.

Ghosh, C., Baker, J., Moysich, K., et al. (2008). Dietary intakes of selected nutrients and food groups and risk of cervical cancer. *Nutrition Cancer, 60*, 331–341.

González, C. A., Travier, N., Luján-Barroso, L., et al. (2011). Dietary factors and in situ and invasive cervical cancer risk in the European Prospective Investigation Into Cancer and Nutrition Study. *Int J Cancer, 129*, 449–459.

Gorelick, C., Lopez-Jones, M., Goldberg, G., et al. (2004). Coenzyme Q10 and lipid-related gene induction in HeLa cells. *Am J Obstet Gynecol, 190*, 1432–1434.

Hoops, K., & Twiggs, L. (2008). Human papillomavirus vaccination: The policy debate over the prevention of cervical cancer—A commentary. *J Low Genit Tract Dis, 12*, 181–S184.

Hublarova, P., Hrstka, R., & Vojtesek, B. (2008). [The significance of methylation in HPV16 genome to cervix carcinogenesis] (in Czech). *Ceska Gynekol, 73*, 87–92.

Huh, W., & Roden, R. (2008). The future of vaccines for cervical cancer. *Gyn Oncol, 109*, S48–SS56.

Hwang, J. H., Lee, J. K., Kim, T. J., & Kim, M. K. (2010). The association between fruit and vegetable consumption and HPV viral load in high-risk HPV-positive women with cervical intraepithelial neoplasia. *Cancer Causes Control, 21*, 51–59.

Javvadi, P., Segan, A., Tuttle, S., et al. (2008). The chemopreventive agent curcumin is a potent radiosensitizer of human cervical tumor cells via increased reactive oxygen species production and overactivation of the mitogen-activated protein kinase pathway. *Mol Pharmacol, 73*, 1491–S14501.

Kazbariene, B., Prasmickiene, G., Krikstaponiene, A., et al. (2004). [Changes in the parameters of immune and antioxidant systems in patients with cervical cancer] (in Lithuanian). *Medicina (Kaunas), 40*, 1158–1164.

Limtrakul, P., Anuchapreeda, S., & Buddhasukh, D. (2004). Modulation of human multidrug-resistance MDR-1 gene by natural curcuminoids. *BMC Cancer, 17*, 4–13.

Manju, V., Sailaja, K., & Nalini, N. (2002). Circulating lipid peroxidation and antioxidant status in cervical cancer patients: A case-control study. *Clin Biochem, 35*, 621–625.

Markowitz, L. E., Dunne, E. F., Saraiya, M., Lawson, H. W., Chesson, H., & Unger, E. (2007). Quadrivalent human papillomavirus vaccine: Recommendations of the Advisory Committee on Immunization Practices (ACIP). *Recommendations and Reports, 56*(RR02), 1–24.

Marshall, K. (2003). Cervical dysplasia: Early intervention. *Altern Med Rev, 8*, 156–170.

Munoz, N., Bosch, X., Sanjose, S., et al. (2003). Epidemiologic classification of human papillomavirus types associated with cervical cancer. *NEJM, 348*, 518–527.

Myung, S.-K., Ju, W., Kim, S., & Kim, H. (2011). Vitamin or antioxidant intake (or serum level) and risk of cervical neoplasm: A meta-analysis. *BJOG: An International Journal of Obstetrics and Gynaecology, 118*, 1285–1291.

Oh, H. Y., Seo S.-S., Kim, M. K., et al. (2014). Synergistic effect of viral load and alcohol consumption on the risk of persistent high-risk human papillomavirus infection. *PLoS ONE, 9*, e104374.

Palan, P., Mikhail, M., Shaban, D., et al. (2003). Plasma concentrations of coenzyme Q10 and tocopherols in cervical intraepithelial neoplasia and cervical cancer. *Eur J Cancer Prev, 12*, 321–326.

Piyathilake, C. J., Macaluso, M., Brill, I., et al. (2007). Lower red blood cell folate enhances the HPV-16-associated risk of cervical intraepithelial neoplasia. *Nutrition, 23*, 203–210.

Prasad, S., & Hill, R. (2008). A cost-benefit analysis on the HPV vaccine in Medicaid-enrolled females of the Appalachian region of Kentucky. *J Ky Med Assoc, 106*, 271–276.

Reddy, V., Khanna, N., & Singh, N. (2001). Vitamin C augments chemotherapeutic response of cervical carcinoma HeLa cells by stabilizing p53. *Biochem Biophys Res Commun, 282*, 409–415.

Rock, C., Michael, C., Reynolds, R., & Ruffin, M. (2000). Prevention of cervix cancer. *Crit Rev Oncol/Hematol, 33*, 169–185.

Roomi, M., Ivanov, V., Kalinovsky, T., et al. (2006). Suppression of human cervical cancer cell lines HeLa and DoTc2 by a mixture of lysine, proline, ascorbic acid, and green tea extract. *Int J Gynecol Cancer, 16*, 1241–1247.

Rositch, A. F., Nowak, R. G., & Gravitt, P. E. (2014). Increased age and race-specific incidence of cervical cancer after correction for hysterectomy prevalence in the United States from 2000 to 2009. *Cancer, 120*, 2032–2038.

Scheurer, M. E., Danysh, H. E., Follen, M., & Lupo, P. (2014). Association of traffic-related hazardous air pollutants and cervical dysplasia in an urban multiethnic population: A cross-sectional study. *Environmental Health, 13*, 52.

TNM Classification of Malignant Tumours. (2002). In L. Sobin & C. Wittekind (Eds.), *UICC International Union Against Cancer* (6th ed., pp. 155–157). Geneva, Switzerland: UICC.

Tomljenovic, L., & Shaw, C. A. (2012). Too fast or not too fast: The FDA's approval of Merck's HPV vaccine Gardasil. *J Law Med Ethics, 40*, 673–681.

Tong, S.-Y., Kim, M. K., Lee, J. K., Lee, J. M., et al. (2011). Common polymorphisms in methylenetetrahydrofolate reductase gene are associated with risks of cervical intraepithelial neoplasia and cervical cancer in women with low serum folate and vitamin B12. *Cancer Causes Control, 22*, 63–72.

Trimble, E., Harlan, L., Gius, D., et al. (2008). Patterns of care for women with cervical cancer in the United States. *Cancer, 113*(4), 743–749.

Wright, T., Huh, W., Monk, B., et al. (2008). Age considerations when vaccinating against HPV. *Gynecol Oncol, 109*, S40–S47.

Zaohua, Z. (1987). Effect of acupuncture on 44 cases of radiation rectitis following radiation therapy for carcinoma of the cervix uteri. *J Trad Chin Med, 792,* 139–140.

Zhang, X., Dai, B., Zhang, B., & Wang, Z. (2012). Vitamin A and risk of cervical cancer: A meta-analysis. *Gynecol Oncol, 124,* 366–373.

Zhu, J., Wu, L., Kohlmeier, M., et al. (2013). Association between MTHFR C677T, MTHFR A1298C and MS A2756G polymorphisms and risk of cervical intraepithelial neoplasia II/III and cervical cancer: A meta-analysis. *Mol Med Rep, 8,* 919–927.

21

Breast Cancer Prevention and Treatment

DAWN LEMANNE

CASE STUDY

Shaniqua sits with her face in her hands, sobbing softly. The 43-year-old African American founder of a successful software company is usually impeccably dressed; today however, her blouse is misbuttoned and dirty.

A year ago Shaniqua presented with a tumor the size of a tangerine deep in her left breast. Biopsy revealed a "triple negative" invasive ductal carcinoma without hormone receptor expression or HER2/neu protein overexpression. With four cycles of neoadjuvant, or presurgical, chemotherapy the tumor shrank to the size of a peanut. Lumpectomy, radiation, and four more cycles of chemotherapy followed. Three months have passed since Shaniqua completed treatment. She is without any signs of cancer.

However, she forgets why she walked into a room, has difficulty reading dense material, and struggles to organize her professional reports. She sleeps 10 hours a night, and falls asleep at her desk. She feels her work quality is not what it used to be, and this embarrasses her. "I think I have chemo brain," she says.

Neuropsychiatric testing reveals intelligence, memory, and attention in the low normal range. Mood is normal. The interpretation: cancer-related cognitive impairment.

The neuropsychiatrist prescribes modafinil as needed, which Shaniqua finds useful for work projects requiring keenness of thought. A lapsed runner, she returns to jogging three times a week. She also signs up for a work-related class, begins a daily mindfulness meditation practice, and maintains a firm sleep-wake schedule.

Within six months of these lifestyle changes, Shaniqua reports that her brain is "almost back to normal." Repeat neuropsychiatric testing reveals superior intelligence, memory, and executive function.

Introduction

Breast cancer is common in the United States, striking one in eight women by age 80. Despite the high incidence, only one in every 36 women in the United States will eventually die of breast cancer. There are nearly three million breast cancer survivors in the United States alone, either cured of the disease, or living with it (Howlader et al., 2014; SEER, 2014).

As many as 75% of breast cancer patients use a combination of conventional and complementary treatments (Astin, Reilly, Perkins, & Child, 2006). Complementary modalities are primarily used to ameliorate side effects and to enhance treatment efficacy and survival.

RISK FACTORS

Breast cancer is not a single disease, but a collection of diseases with different etiologies and poorly understood risk factors. The strongest risk factors involve inherited defects in DNA repair capacity. Other risk factors involve signaling pathways related to sex steroids, inflammation, nutrient-sensing, and energy balance.

Risk factors are categorized by (1) the strength of their effect—major, moderate or minor; and (2) the degree to which that effect can be mitigated, that is, whether the risk factor is "modifiable" or "nonmodifiable." Major, moderate, and minor risk factors are listed in Table 21.1.

Moderate risk factors are often termed "reproductive risk factors," because of their connection to the female endocrine system. The effects of minor risk factors are apparent in large populations, but are difficult to quantify on the individual level, and degree of risk conferred may be modulated by individual genetic variation.

Table 21.1. Breast Cancer Risk Factors

Class	Comments and Possible Mitigations
Major	*2- to 10-fold risk increase*
Gender	incidence in female to male 100:1
Age	incidence peaks at age 70
BRCA1 deleterious mutation	"Triple negative" tumors associated w/BRCA1 Decrease incidence with:
BRCA2 deleterious mutation	• early and aggressive screening
Breast cancer in 1st-degree relative under 40	• prophylactic mastectomy • prophylactic tamoxifen or raloxifene • weight loss in early adulthood (esp. BRCA1)
Breast cancer in three or more close relatives of any age	• other lifestyle interventions? Other cancers common
Personal history of invasive breast cancer	
Personal history of DCIS, LCIS, or proliferative atypia	
Increased breast density on mammography	Unknown mitigations; effect of aggressive MRI/US screening under study
Moderate	**1.5- to 2-fold risk increase**
Early menarche and/or late menopause	Increased incidence of HR+ tumors
Older age at first pregnancy	Risk increase seen primarily in those with certain variants in insulin and angiogenesis genes
Lactation	Inverse association with HR+ tumors
Hormone replacement therapy, particularly equine estrogens and synthetic progestogens	Try TCM, hypnosis, exercise for menopausal symptoms
Minor	**Indeterminate risk increase**
Alcohol	Effect seen at 1 drink/day (Allen et al., 2009). Greater effect in premenopause (Poynter et al., 2013)
Race/ethnicity	In the United States, European heritage increases risk of hormone receptor-positive disease; African heritage increases risk of triple-negative disease (Howlader et al., 2014)
Environmental toxin exposure	Choose organic foods; avoid plastics, certain cosmetics, etc.

(continued)

Table 21.1. Continued

Class	*Comments and Possible Mitigations*
Major	*2- to 10-fold risk increase*
Physical activity	Population-wide incidence decreases with increasing activity levels (Lemanne et al., 2013)
Height, weight, fat distribution, and weight changes	Complex interactions with age, ethnicity, breast cancer subtype
Shift work (circadian disruption)	Interaction with certain genetic variants may lead to increased risk (Bracci et al., 2014)

Sources: Information in this table is derived from Allen et al. (2009); American Cancer Society (2014b); Bandera et al. (2013); Bracci et al. (2014); S. Chen & Parmigiani (2007); Dumalaon-Canaria et al. (2014); Grundy et al. (2013); Howlader et al. (2014); International Agency for Research on Cancer (2007); Juckett (2009); Lemanne et al. (2013); and Poynter et al. (2013).

Environmental Toxin Exposure

Animal studies show that over 200 commonly encountered chemicals have estrogenic effects and promote tumor growth. These chemicals are present in hundreds of everyday items (Dodson et al., 2012; Knower, To, Leung, Ho, & Clyne, 2014). A list of such products can be found on The Silent Spring website: http://www.silentspring.org/ resource/table-consumer-products-tested-endocrine- disruptors-and-asthma-associated-chemicals.

Adiposity and Risk

Obesity, as defined by body mass index (BMI) $\geq$ 30, is associated with increased risk of breast cancer in postmenopausal women (Munsell, Sprague, Berry, Chisholm, & Trentham-Dietz, 2014). In contrast, obesity is associated with decreased risk of breast cancer in premenopausal women of European descent. This effect is not seen in African American women (Bandera et al., 2013; Cecchini et al., 2012). However, fat deposited deep within the torso, termed central adiposity, has been shown to increase breast cancer risk in premenopausal women. This effect is most apparent in women of Asian descent, and is less pronounced in those of European or African heritage (Amadou et al., 2013). Central adiposity can be present in women of normal weight and BMI, and is a sign of insulin resistance.

Obesity is associated with worse survival after a breast cancer diagnosis, with the effect greater in premenopausal than in postmenopausal women (Pan &

Gray, 2014; Protani, Coory, & Martin, 2010). Whether weight loss after a breast cancer diagnosis improves survival is under investigation. Meanwhile, optimizing insulin sensitivity with nutrition, physical activity, and stress control is prudent for women at risk for breast cancer and for those recovering from the disease.

Alcohol

The LACE (Life After Cancer Epidemiology) study found that women drinking > 5 grams of alcohol per day had a hazard ratio (HR) of 1.35 of recurrence and 1.51 of death due to breast cancer, especially those who were postmenopausal and obese (Kwan et al., 2010). There was a compensatory decrease in cardiovascular mortality. Women with a history of breast cancer should not consume more than three or four drinks of alcohol per week.

EXERCISE IN BREAST CANCER PREVENTION AND SURVIVAL

Observational studies show the vigorous physical activity is strongly associated with a lower risk of breast cancer and with improved survival after diagnosis (Bradshaw et al., 2014; Lemanne, Cassileth, & Gubili, 2013).

SCREENING

Current breast cancer screening relies on mammography. Screening mammograms, however, miss about 20% of cancers. Therefore any woman who complains of a new lump or thickening in the breast should always be referred for further imaging and biopsy, even if mammographic imaging is normal (National Cancer Institute, 2014).

For asymptomatic women at average risk of breast cancer, screening recommendations vary. The US Preventive Services Task Force (USPSTF) (2009) gives a B level recommendation for screening mammography every other year between 50 and 74 years of age; the National Cancer Institute (NCI) recommends screening every one to two years in women over 40 (National Cancer Institute, 2014), while the American Cancer Society (ACS) recommends yearly mammograms in all women 40 and over (American Cancer Society, 2014a).

For asymptomatic women at high risk of breast cancer, defined as a 20% or greater lifetime risk, mammographic screening should be supplemented with

MRI or ultrasound (Mainiero et al., 2013). Women under 40 at high risk may opt for MRI screening alone (Yankaskas et al., 2010).

Interest in limiting radiation exposure has resulted in a search for other imaging techniques that can be applied to screening for breast cancer. Breast thermography detects only 25% of known breast cancers and at present should not be used for breast cancer screening or diagnosis (Fitzgerald & Berentson-Shaw, 2012). Tomosynthesis (3-D mammography), optical imaging, molecular breast imaging, and positron emission mammography are currently under investigation (American Cancer Society, 2014c).

Digital breast tomosynthesis or 3D tomosynthesis is technically similar to computed tomography (CT), but uses more advanced digital imaging processing algorithms that permit a lower radiation dose. At present, 3-D tomosynthesis is used only in combination with conventional mammography. The combination improves tumor detection rate and specificity, especially in women under 50, but increases radiation exposure (McCarthy et al., 2014). Rapid technical improvements are expected to make digital breast tomosynthesis a viable stand-alone breast cancer screening modality in the near future.

Molecular imaging and positron emission mammography can detect tumors by demonstrating increased metabolic activity. Current methods however, still result in radiation exposure that exceeds that of conventional mammography. At present these modalities find use as staging tools following a diagnosis of breast cancer (Drukteinis, Mooney, Flowers, & Gatenby, 2013).

Optical imaging of the breast uses various wavelengths of visible light to image the breast, and relies on the translucent properties of breast tissue, and on the difference in contrast between normal breast tissue and tumor tissue. Fluorescent dyes to enhance contrast are being explored. The advantages of optical imaging include no radiation exposure. However, optical imaging is still extremely experimental (Herranz & Ruibal, 2012).

Conventional Approach to Breast Cancer Treatment and Prevention

Staging is based on the size of the primary breast tumor, extent of any lymph node involvement, and the presence or absence of detectable metastatic disease. Staging guides the choice of appropriately restrained or aggressive treatment. Breast cancer tissue is always tested for expression of estrogen and progesterone receptors, and for HER2/neu protein overexpression. Positive results specify the targeted agents likely to be effective.

Breast-conserving therapy (BCT) involves surgical removal of the primary tumor along with a margin of normal tissue, and sampling of several nearby or "sentinel" lymph nodes. After surgery, the remaining portion of the breast is treated with radiation. Breast-conserving therapy followed by radiation leads to higher cure rates and better functional outcome than does mastectomy alone, and is therefore the standard of care (Agarwal, Pappas, Neumayer, Kokeny, & Agarwal, 2014).

Endocrine therapy is effective only in the prevention and treatment of hormone-receptor-positive breast cancer and is prescribed in the following circumstances: (1) prophylaxis in healthy women at high risk for breast cancer (discussed later), (2) adjuvant therapy in early stage breast cancer, and (3) treatment of metastatic breast cancer.

The aromatase inhibitors (AIs) prevent the peripheral conversion of steroids to estrogen, decreasing circulating levels of estrogen. The AIs are employed almost exclusively in the postmenopausal setting; if used in premenopausal women, concurrent ovarian suppression is required.

Selective estrogen receptor modulators (SERMs) competitively inhibit the estrogen receptor without decreasing circulating estrogen levels. A representative SERM is tamoxifen, commonly used in premenopausal breast cancer. Tamoxifen can be used in postmenopausal women intolerant of AIs. However, because AIs have better antitumor efficacy, they are preferred in postmenopausal women (Howell et al., 2005).

Chemotherapy drugs disable rapidly replicating cells, both normal and malignant. They are often used in combination, to take advantage of their complementary mechanisms of action. Monoclonal antibodies are a form of targeted therapy developed to treat breast cancer that overexpresses HER2/neu proteins. Several drugs have been developed and tested including trastuzumab (Herceptin), lapatinib (Tykerb), and pertuzumab (Perjeta). Although these drugs are extremely effective in HER2/neu-overexpressing breast cancers, prolonged treatment in the metastatic setting eventually leads to drug resistance. Trastuzumab-emtansine (T-DM1), a conjugate of trastuzumab and the cytotoxic agent maytansine 1, has recently gained approval for use in such cases (Giordano et al., 2014).

"Triple-negative" breast cancers lack estrogen or progesterone receptors, and do not overexpress the HER2/neu protein. Thus, targeted therapies are of no benefit. These tumors are often resistant to chemotherapy as well.

Neoadjuvant therapy is given before surgery, to reduce tumor size and simplify surgery. Most commonly chemotherapy is used, but neoadjuvant treatment can include any combination of chemotherapy, targeted therapy, or endocrine therapy. One of the benefits of neoadjuvant therapy is that it allows evaluation of the effectiveness of a particular drug regimen while a tumor is still present and its dimensions measurable.

Adjuvant therapy, in contrast, is given after surgery, when no remaining disease is evident. The rationale for its use is to eradicate micrometastatic deposits throughout the body, thereby preventing clinical recurrence.

Metastatic breast cancer commonly involves bones, liver, lungs, and brain. Systemic treatment can control symptoms and prolong life. Radiation and stabilizing surgery are used when metastases threaten long bones or the spinal cord.

Conventional and Integrative Approaches to Breast Cancer Prevention

Prophylactic bilateral mastectomy is offered to women at high risk of breast cancer. Alternatively, a 5-year course of endocrine therapy with tamoxifen or a similar drug can be used to decrease risk.

Limiting alcohol consumption, avoidance of weight gain after age 20, and physical activity can also play a role in breast cancer prevention, and are discussed in detail later.

Conventional and Integrative Approaches to Treatment Sequelae

Many women report side effects from the conventional treatment of breast cancer. Integrative medicine offers potential benefit to women when side effects are mitigated and women are able to finish conventional treatment, as completing treatment is associated with better outcomes.

HOT FLASHES

Hot flashes (vasomotor symptoms) affect up to 65% of women treated for breast cancer, and 30% of women taking tamoxifen rate their hot flashes as "severe" (Day, 2001). Hot flashes are a major reason that women discontinue endocrine therapy for breast cancer (Cella & Fallowfield, 2008). Therapy is therefore indicated for moderate or severe hot flashes.

Nonhormonal drugs effective against hot flashes include venlafaxine and citalopram. Fluoxetine and paroxetine decrease hot flashes, but can alter tamoxifen metabolism and therefore are contraindicated (L'Esperance, Frenette, Dionne, & Dionne, 2013), as are other treatments that increase estrogen or progesterone levels.

Melatonin

A 4-month placebo-controlled study of 95 postmenopausal women with a history of breast cancer found that 3 mg melatonin significantly improved sleep quality, even though reduction in hot flashes was not significantly different from placebo (W. Chen et al., 2014).

Supplemental Soy Isoflavones

Supplemental soy isoflavones significantly reduce hot flash frequency and severity, particularly those that provide a minimum of 18 mg/day of genistein (Taku, Melby, Kronenberg, Kurzer, & Messina, 2012). While there is no definite evidence of interaction, it is possible that higher doses of soy isoflavones (>100 mg/day) may interfere with antiestrogen therapy (Fritz et al., 2013).

Black Cohosh (Cimicifuga racemosa, Actaea racemosa)

Black cohosh is safe to use after a breast cancer diagnosis, however effectiveness is equal to placebo for most women (Fritz et al., 2014). Black cohosh should be avoided during chemotherapy because of potential drug interactions (Rockwell, Liu, & Higgins, 2005).

Acupuncture

Acupuncture is a safe treatment for hot flashes in women with breast cancer. Studies report mixed results. A controlled study demonstrated relief with acupuncture, and reported that the benefit persisted for several months (Frisk, Hammar, Ingvar, & Spetz Holm, 2014).

Aerobic Exercise

The data are mixed as to whether exercise can relieve vasomotor symptoms. A review of more than 30 studies found that half showed no effect on hot flashes, with the majority of the balance showing an inverse relationship between exercise and hot flashes and three studies reporting increased vasomotor symptoms with high levels of exercise (Sternfeld & Dugan, 2011). Because exercise enhances overall health, recommending it to women suffering from hot flashes seems prudent.

Hypnosis

Hypnosis reduces self-reported hot flashes among breast cancer survivors. Sixty female breast cancer survivors with hot flashes were randomized to receive five hypnosis sessions per week or no treatment. Hot flash scores decreased 68% from baseline to end point in the hypnosis arm. There were also significant improvements in self-reported anxiety, depression, interference of hot flashes on daily activities, and sleep in the hypnosis group (Elkins et al., 2008).

Yoga

A small ($N = 14$), uncontrolled trial found that eight weekly sessions of restorative yoga were helpful in decreasing the frequency of hot flashes (Cohen et al., 2007). A recent review of five randomized controlled trials found evidence that yoga improves psychological symptoms in menopausal women (Cramer Lange, Klose, Paul, & Dobos, 2012). Yoga can be safely recommended to women with hot flashes. Although effectiveness against hot flashes may vary, psychological benefit may still accrue.

Neurologic Sequelae of Breast Cancer and Their Treatment

Many chemotherapy drugs commonly used in treatment of breast cancer are neurotoxic, and damage the central and peripheral nervous systems. Deficits can involve attention, language, memory, and executive function. Symptoms may be flagrant or subtle, stable or progressive, temporary or permanent. Vigorous attention should be given to complaints of cognitive difficulties or peripheral neuropathy in breast cancer patients. Integrative approaches are helpful in recovery.

CANCER-RELATED COGNITIVE IMPAIRMENT: "CHEMO BRAIN"

Cancer-related cognitive impairment (CRCI) occurs in 30% of cancer patients prior to chemotherapy (Ahles et al., 2008). This timing implies a causative role for the cancer itself, possibly due to increased levels of proinflammatory cytokines. Cancer-related cognitive impairment affects up to 75% of cancer patients during treatment, and 35% of patients note continued problems after treatment (Janelsins, Kesler, Ahles, & Morrow, 2014).

Brain imaging studies in CRCI demonstrate atrophy, microstructural changes, and altered cerebral metabolism and blood flow (Pomykala, de Ruiter, Deprez, McDonald, & Silverman, 2013).

Conventional and Integrative Approaches to Cancer-Related Cognitive Impairment

Cognitive complaints in a breast cancer patient without evidence of central nervous system metastasis should prompt neuropsychiatric testing. With confirmation of the diagnosis of CRCI, formal cognitive and occupational rehabilitation should be prescribed.

Aerobic exercise

In rodent models, aerobic exercise stimulates neurogenesis in the hippocampus, and counteracts chemotherapy-induced damage (Winocur, Wojtowicz, Huang, & Tannock, 2014). In women with breast cancer, aerobic exercise during chemotherapy also reduces cancer-related fatigue (Zou, Yang, He, Sun, & Xu, 2014).

Mind–Body Approaches

A small controlled study has reported benefit in breast cancer patients with CRCI who undertake a meditation program (Milbury et al., 2013). In addition, several studies suggest yoga may be helpful in CRCI (Culos-Reed, Carlson, Daroux, & Hatley-Aldous, 2006; Galantino et al., 2012). The largest yoga study to date randomized 200 breast cancer survivors to 12 weeks of twice-weekly, 90-minute classes and home practice with DVDs, or to a wait list control. The practice of yoga was associated with less fatigue and higher levels of vitality, and markers for inflammation were 10%–15% lower (Kiecolt-Glaser et al., 2014).

Herbs

Though not tested in CRCI, herbs used in traditional Chinese medicine, such as *Panax ginseng* (Ginseng), *Rhodiola rosea* (Rhodiola or Hong Jing Tian), and *Schisandra chinensis* (Wu Wei Zi), and in Ayurvedic medicine, such as *Bacopa monnieri* (Bacopa), may be helpful for patients with cognitive complaints (Chan, 2012; Neale, Camfield, Reay, Stough, & Scholey, 2013). Although safe in most settings, these herbs should be avoided during chemotherapy, as they interact with multiple drug-metabolizing enzymes. *Ginkgo biloba* (Ginkgo) and *Hypericum perforatum* (St. John's Wort), often used for cognitive and mood complaints, must also be avoided during chemotherapy because they too interfere with drug metabolism (Shord, Shah, & Lukosa, 2009).

PERIPHERAL NEUROPATHY

Chemotherapy-induced peripheral neuropathy (CIPN) is common in breast cancer patients on chemotherapy. Symptoms are dose-dependent, worsen with treatment duration, and can be irreversible. Chemotherapy-induced peripheral neuropathy can interfere with activities of daily living, and decreases quality of life.

Integrative Approaches to Peripheral Neuropathy

Neuroprotective strategies tried in CIPN include administration of calcium/magnesium infusion, vitamin E, glutathione, glutamine, acetyl L-carnitine, and erythropoietin (Beijers, Jongen, & Vreugdenhil, 2012). Results are mixed as to efficacy, with vitamin E effective mainly in patients treated with cisplatin. Two studies found that intravenous glutathione given before an oxaliplatin infusion decreased risk of CIPN. Because these studies suffered from a high dropout rate and lack of long-term follow-up, further research is needed to confirm these findings (Schloss et al., 2013).

In contrast, a phase II trial showed that acetyl L-carnitine exacerbates CIPN when given with taxane therapy (Hershman et al., 2013).

A concern with all of these agents is that they may protect cancerous, as well as neuronal tissue, from chemotherapy-induced damage. Antioxidants such as vitamin E and N-acetyl cysteine (NAC), and the drug erythropoietin can promote tumor growth (Sayin et al., 2014; Zhou et al., 2014).

Note: Glutamine supplementation is commonly recommended to prevent chemotherapy-induced neuropathy. However, metabolic studies have shown that glutamine supports the growth of some breast cancers (McGuirk et al., 2013; Wise et al., 2008). Until testing of tumors for glutamine sensitivity is routine, glutamine loads should be avoided in patients with known malignancy.

Acupuncture

Acupuncture can ameliorate CIPN symptoms. A controlled study demonstrated reversal of nerve damage in the acupuncture treated group, as measured by nerve conduction (Schroeder, Meyer-Hamme, & Epplée, 2012).

LYMPHEDEMA

Sentinel lymph node sampling has largely replaced axillary dissection in the staging of breast cancer in early stage breast cancer. This has led to a decrease in the number of patients suffering from postoperative lymphedema, swelling of the arm caused by surgical removal of the axillary contents and resultant loss of lymphatic drainage from the arm (McLaughlin et al., 2008).

Dietary Patterns and Breast Cancer

Three large trials have investigated the use of low-fat and high-vegetable/fruit diets to reduce the risk of recurrence of breast cancer. In the Women's Health Initiative, a low-fat dietary pattern with five daily servings of vegetables and fruit and six daily servings of grains did not result in a statistically significant reduction in invasive breast cancer risk over an 8-year follow-up. However, it came close with a p value of .07; the study was likely underpowered, as just 31% of the women met the decreased fat goal (20%) in year one and only 14% met goal by year six (Prentice et al., 2006). The Women's Intervention Nutrition Study (WINS) had a goal of 15% fat diet. Women had difficulty complying and after a median follow-up of 5 years, there was only an 8% difference in energy from fat between the intervention and control groups. Overall, there was a 24% reduction in the relative risk of recurrence for the women on the low-fat diet, and a subgroup analysis found that breast cancer survival was significantly improved in women whose tumors were the difficult-to-treat ER negative/PR negative phenotype, with an HR of 0.36 (Chlebowski, 2006, 2008). Another notable trial revealed that when a low-fat diet resulted in weight loss survival improved (Blackburn & Wang, 2007).

Finally, the Women's Healthy Eating and Living (WHEL) study was a randomized trial designed to assess the role of a low-fat, high-produce, high-fiber dietary intervention on breast cancer recurrence. 1537 women in the intervention group and 1551 in the control group were evaluable after a mean followup of 7.3 years. The authors concluded that the study provided "no evidence that adoption of a dietary pattern very high in vegetables, fruit, and fiber, and low in fat vs a five-a-day fruit and vegetable diet prevents breast cancer recurrence or death among women with previously treated early stage breast cancer." (Pierce, et al., 2007).

The WHEL results conflicted with the similar WINS trial mentioned above. Possible reasons include the longer followup period in the WHEL trial, allowing time for more breast cancer-related events to occur. In addition, later subgroup analyses showed that women who did not report hot flashes at baseline, presumably because of higher estrogen levels, did benefit (Pierce, 2009). Also, women on tamoxifen whose baseline intake of cruciferous vegetables was above the median and who were also within the highest tertile of total vegetable intake had half the risk of recurrence (HR 0.48) (Thomson, 2011).

In terms of breast cancer prevention, genetic variability appears to play a role in determining what dietary pattern will benefit a particular woman. For example, the Women's Health Initiative (WHI) trial found that women who carried a particular variant of the fibroblast growth factor receptor 2 gene and who switched from a high-fat to a low-fat diet nearly halved their risk of being diagnosed with invasive breast cancer over 8 years of follow-up, lowering their odds ratio to 0.49–0.59. Approximately 40% of women in the WHI cohort carried this genetic variant (Prentice et al., 2010).

FATS AND FATTY ACIDS

Women concerned about breast cancer are frequently advised to avoid dietary saturated fats (Farvid, Cho, Chen, Eliassen, & Willett, 2014). However, replacing animal fat with vegetable oils leads to worsening of atherosclerosis in 35% of women with coronary artery disease (CAD), an effect associated with genetic variation in fatty acid metabolism (Kalantarian, Rimm, Herrington, & Mozaffarian, 2014). Because for most women, the risk of death from coronary artery disease is many-fold higher than the risk of death from breast cancer (American Heart Association Statistical Fact Sheet, 2014), women at risk for CAD and breast cancer should be cautioned not to replace saturated fat with polyunsaturated vegetable oils, nor with refined carbohydrates. A healthy diet can contain some saturated fats, but should emphasize omega-3 fatty acids and monounsaturated fatty acids. Trans fats should be avoided.

A meta-analysis of 21 studies concluded that higher consumption of dietary marine omega-3 fatty acids is associated with a lower risk of breast cancer (Zheng, Hu, Zhao, Yang, & Li, 2013.) In addition, research shows that women with higher consumption of eicosapentaenoic acid (EPA) and docosahexaenoic acid (DHA) from food, but not from fish oil supplements, have reduced rates of breast cancer recurrence and reduced mortality (Patterson et al., 2011). Women should be counseled to eat low-mercury fish two-to-three times per week.

CARBOHYDRATES

The Women's Healthy Eating and Living (WHEL) trial found that carbohydrate restriction was associated with a striking fivefold reduction in breast cancer recurrence in 50% of subjects, specifically those whose tumors expressed the insulin-like growth factor-1 (IGF-1) receptor. Carbohydrate restriction was of no benefit to the 50% of women whose tumors were IGF-1 receptor negative (Emond et al., 2014). Unfortunately, IGF-1 testing of tumors is not yet a routine clinical practice.

CALORIC RESTRICTION AND FASTING

Numerous animal studies have shown that reducing caloric intake inhibits cancer initiation and progression (Hursting, Dunlap, Ford, Hursting, & Lashinger, 2013). A small interventional study in Russia found that decreasing caloric intake by 15% during the three years following mastectomy and chemotherapy was associated with an unusually low breast cancer recurrence rate of only 7%. In contrast, the control group experienced a more typical 25% recurrence rate (Sopotsinskaia et al., 1992).

Intermittent fasting is superior to chronic caloric restriction in preventing chemically induced breast cancer in animals (Cleary & Grossman, 2011). In young women, extreme curtailment of calories for two days a week is superior to chronic caloric restriction in reducing obesity and other biomarkers of breast cancer risk (Harvie et al., 2011).

Repeated short fasting cycles are as effective as chemotherapeutic agents in delaying progression of several tumor types in animals. In animal models, fasting plus chemotherapy, but not either treatment alone, can result in long-term cancer-free survival (C. Lee et al., 2012). Preliminary human studies suggest that short fasts during chemotherapy are safe and help mitigate the side effects of chemotherapy, however controlled randomized studies are needed to determine the effect of fasting on clinical outcomes (Safdie et al., 2009).

SPECIFIC DIETARY ELEMENTS AND SUPPLEMENTS

Cruciferous Vegetables

A 2013 meta-analysis found an inverse relationship between cruciferous vegetable consumption and breast cancer (Liu & Lv, 2013). Not all women benefit equally in terms of this risk reduction; the Shanghai Breast Cancer Study found that high intake of cruciferous vegetables lowered breast cancer risk, but only in a subset of premenopausal women with a glutathione-S transferase polymorphism that increases urinary excretion of isothiocyanates (S. Lee et al., 2008). However, testing for this variant is not routinely available, and as cruciferous vegetables are beneficial to overall health, it is prudent to advise all women to routinely include cruciferous vegetables in the diet.

B Vitamins

Dietary intake and higher blood levels of folate, methionine, and pyridoxal 5'-phosphate (PLP), may decrease the risk of breast cancer, but only in postmenopausal women (Wu, Kang, & Zhang, 2013). The effect of these nutrients on breast cancer risk varies somewhat by age and ethnicity. In premenopausal African American women, natural food folate was associated with a significant decrease in breast cancer risk, an association not seen in European American women. In both groups, synthetic folate or folic acid from fortified foods was associated with an increased risk of breast cancer, and the association was stronger in European Americans. Methionine was associated with decreased risk in premenopausal African American women and postmenopausal European Americans (Gong et al., 2014).

Vitamin D

Numerous studies show that low serum vitamin D levels at the time of breast cancer diagnosis predict a worse outcome. Whether correcting a low vitamin D level after diagnosis improves survival is currently under investigation (Li et al., 2014). Meanwhile, it is prudent to achieve and maintain 25-hydroxyvitamin D levels in the normal range, both in healthy women and after a cancer diagnosis, by means of supplementation with vitamin D3.

Dairy

A large study found no association between dairy consumption and breast cancer risk in African American women (Genkinger, Makambi, Palmer, Rosenberg, & Adams-Campbell, 2013). However, high-fat, but not low-fat, dairy consumption is associated with worse outcome after breast cancer diagnosis (Printz, 2013).

Soy

Soy intake in childhood may be protective against breast cancer (Korde et al., 2009). Dietary soy in culinary amounts is safe and possibly beneficial in breast cancer (Fritz et al., 2013). In the LACE trial there was a 60% reduction in risk of breast cancer recurrence in women taking tamoxifen who were in the highest quintile of soy intake (Guha et al., 2009). Similar findings occurred in the Shanghai Breast Cancer Survival Study (Xiao et al., 2009).

Flaxseed

A systematic review found that five observational studies suggest that flaxseed intake may reduce risk of breast cancer and may improve survival following diagnosis (Flower et al., 2013). Lignans, a type of phytoestrogen found in flaxseed, appear to mediate this effect, which is seen with only ½ teaspoon of flaxseed per day (Cotterchio, Boucher, Kreiger, Mills, & Thompson, 2008). Flaxseed should be ground immediately before consumption, as the oils within the seed become rancid shortly after exposure to air.

Medicinal and Culinary Mushrooms

In Japan, PSK, an extract of turkey tail mushroom (*Coriolus versicolor*), is used routinely as part of cancer therapy (Takahashi, Mai, & Nakazato, 2005). Efficacy in human breast cancer is unknown. Because raw mushrooms, including the common button mushroom and shiitake, contain heat-labile toxins, including carcinogens (Ricar, Pizinger, & Cetkovsha, 2013; Toth & Erickson, 1986), mushrooms should be cooked.

Stress and Cancer, Integrative Approach

While stress does not cause cancer, there is growing evidence that chronic stress can promote the growth of tumors that are already present. Studies clearly demonstrate that social isolation and depression promote tumor growth (Lutgendorf & Sood, 2011). Thus, establishment of robust social support should be part of every breast cancer recovery program.

Excess sympathetic tone caused by emotional stress can decrease cancer survival (De Couck, van Brummelen, Schallier, De Grève, & Gidron, 2013). Observational studies have found decreased breast cancer mortality associated with use of beta-adrenergic receptor blockade, which decreases sympathetic tone, with propanolol more effective than atenolol (Barron, Connolly, Sharp, Bennett, & Visvanathan, 2011). Clinical trials of beta-blockade in metastatic breast cancer have been initiated.

That beta-blockade is associated with decreased breast cancer mortality suggests that nonpharmacologic interventions that improve autonomic balance, such as manual therapies, aerobic exercise, meditation, yoga, and heart-rate variability (HRV) training, may also be helpful for women with breast cancer. Manual therapies shown to increase vagal tone include myofascial trigger point massage and foot reflexology (Delaney, Leong, Watkins, & Brodie, 2002; Lu, Chen, & Kuo, 2011).

Heart-rate variability is used to assess autonomic balance (Malliani, 2005). Safe, enjoyable, HRV feedback devices such as HeartMath can teach patients how to control HRV using simple breathing maneuvers, although their effectiveness has not been validated.

Conclusion

Principles behind the integrative approach to breast cancer prevention and recovery include minimizing insulin resistance, decreasing inflammation, avoiding exposure to environmental toxins, and controlling stress. Whole foods, judicious use of supplements and herbs, regular exercise, and use of mind–body therapies can help women accomplish this.

Using evidence-based complementary modalities to diminish the side effects from chemotherapy and hormonal manipulation can empower patients to complete conventional treatment. Using lifestyle interventions to avoid weight gain after diagnosis may improve both overall, and breast-cancer-specific, survival.

REFERENCES

Agarwal, S., Pappas, L., Neumayer, L., Kokeny, K., & Agarwal, J. (2014). Effect of breast conservation therapy vs mastectomy on disease-specific survival for early-stage breast cancer. *JAMA Surg, 149*, 267–274.

Ahles, T. A., Saykin, A. J., McDonald, B. C., et al. (2008). Cognitive function in breast cancer patients prior to adjuvant treatment. *Breast Cancer Res Treat, 110*, 143–152.

Allen, N. E., Beral, V., Casabonne, D., et al. (2009). Moderate alcohol intake and cancer incidence in women. *J Natl Cancer Inst, 101*, 296–305.

Amadou, A., Ferrari, P., Muwonge, R., et al. (2013). Overweight, obesity and risk of premenopausal breast cancer according to ethnicity: A systematic review and dose-response meta-analysis. *Obes Rev, 14*, 665–678.

American Cancer Society. (2014a). *American Cancer Society recommendations for early breast cancer detection in women without breast symptoms*. Retrieved June

30, 2014, from http://www.cancer.org/cancer/breastcancer/moreinformation/breastcancerearlydetection/breast-cancer-early-detection-acs-recs

American Cancer Society. (2014b). *What are the risk factors for breast cancer?* Updated Jan 2014. Retrieved May 15, 2014, from http://www.cancer.org/cancer/breastcancer/detailedguide/breast-cancer-risk-factors

American Cancer Society. (2014c). *Other breast imaging methods.* Retrieved May 20, 2014, from http://www.cancer.org/treatment/understandingyourdiagnosis/examsandtestdescriptions/mammogramsandotherbreastimagingprocedures/mammograms-and-other-breast-imaging-procedures-newer-br-imaging-tests

American Heart Association Statistical Fact Sheet. (2014). *Update: Women and cardiovascular diseases.* Retrieved May 15, 2014, from http://www.heart.org/idc/groups/heartpublic/@wcm/@sop/@smd/documents/downloadable/ucm_462030.pdf

Astin, J. A., Reilly, C., Perkins, C., & Child, W. L. (2006). Breast cancer patients' perspectives on and use of complementary and alternative medicine: A study by the Susan G. Komen Breast Cancer Foundation. *J Soc Integr Oncol, 4,* 157–169.

Bandera, E. V., Chandran, U., Zirpoli, G., et al. (2013a). Body fatness and breast cancer risk in women of African Ancestry. *BMC Cancer, 13,* 475.

Bandera, E. V., Chandran, U., Zirpoli, G., et al. (2013b). Body size in early life and breast cancer risk in African American and European American women. *Cancer Causes Control, 24,* 2231–2243.

Barron, T. I., Connolly, R. M., Sharp, L., Bennett, K., & Visvanathan, K. (2011). Beta blockers and breast cancer mortality: A population-based study. *J Clin Oncol, 29,* 2635–2644.

Beijers, A. J. M., Jongen, J. L. M., & Vreugdenhil, G. (2012). Chemotherapy-induced neurotoxicity: The value of neuroprotective strategies. *Neth J Med, 70,* 18–25.

Blackburn, G. L., & Wang, K. A. (2007). Dietary fat reduction and breast cancer outcome: Results from the Women's Intervention Nutrition Study (WINS) 1–4. *Am J Clin Nutr, 86*(Suppl), 878S–881S.

Bradshaw, P. T., Ibrahim, J. G., Khankari, N., et al. (2014). Post-diagnosis physical activity and survival after breast cancer diagnosis: The Long Island Breast Cancer Study. *Breast Cancer Res Treat, 145,* 735–742.

Bracci, M., Manzella, N., Copertaro, A., et al. (2014). Rotating-shift nurses after a day off: Peripheral clock gene expression, urinary melatonin, and serum 17-β-estradiol levels. *Scand J Work Environ Health, 40,* 295–304.

Cecchini, R. S., Costantino, J. P., Cauley, J. A., et al. (2012). Body mass index and the risk for developing invasive breast cancer among high-risk women in NSABP P-1 and STAR breast cancer prevention trials. *Cancer Prev Res, 5,* 583–592.

Cella, D., & Fallowfield, L. J. (2008). Recognition and management of treatment-related side effects for breast cancer patients receiving adjuvant endocrine therapy. *Breast Cancer Res Tr, 107,* 167–180.

Chan, S.-W. (2012). *Panax ginseng, Rhodiola rosea* and *Schisandra chinenesis. Int J Food Sci Nutr, 63*(S1), 75–81.

Chen, S., & Parmigiani, G. (2007). Meta-analysis of BRCA1 and BRCA2 penetrance. *J Clin Oncol, 25*, 1329–1333.

Chen, W. Y., Giobbie-Hurder, A., Gantman, K., et al. (2014). A randomized, placebo-controlled trial of melatonin on breast cancer survivors: Impact on sleep, mood, and hot flashes. *Breast Cancer Res Treat, 145*, 381–388.

Chlebowski, R. T., Blackburn, G. L., Hoy, M. K., et al. (2008). Survival analyses from the Women's Intervention Nutrition Study (WINS) evaluating dietary fat reduction and breast cancer outcome (Abstract). *J Clin Oncol, 26*, 522.

Chlebowski, R. T., Blackburn, G. L., Thomson, C. A., et al. (2006). Dietary fat reduction and breast cancer outcome: Interim efficacy results from the Women's Intervention Nutrition Study. *J Natl Cancer Inst, 98*, 1767–1776.

Cleary, M. P., & Grossmann, M. E. (2011). The manner in which calories are restricted impacts mammary tumor cancer prevention. *J Carcinog, 10*, 21.

Cohen, B. E., Kanaya, K. M., Macer, J. L., Shen, H., Chang, A. A., & Grady, D. (2007). Feasibility and acceptability of restorative yoga for treatment of hot flashes: A pilot trial. *Maturitas, 56*, 198–204.

Cotterchio, M., Boucher, B. A., Kreiger, N., Mills, C. A., & Thompson, L. U. (2008). Dietary phytoestrogen intake—lignans and isoflavones—and breast cancer risk (Canada). *Cancer Causes and Control, 19*, 259–272.

Cramer, H., Lange, S., Klose, P., Paul, a, & Dobos, G. (2012). Yoga for breast cancer patients and survivors: a systematic review and meta-analysis. *BMC Cancer, 12*, 423: http://www.biomedcentral.com/1471-2407/12/412

Culos-Reed, S. N., Carlson, L. E., Daroux, L. M., & Hatley-Aldous, S. (2006). A pilot study of yoga for breast cancer survivors: Physical and psychological benefits. *Psychooncology, 15*, 891–897.

Day, R. (2001). Quality of life and tamoxifen in a breast cancer prevention trial: A summary of findings from the NSABP P-1study. National Surgical Adjuvant Breast and Bowel Project. *Ann NY Acad Sci, 949*, 143–150.

De Couck, M., van Brummelen, D., Schallier, D., De Grève, J., & Gidron, Y. (2013). The relationship between vagal nerve activity and clinical outcomes in prostate and non-small cell lung cancer patients. *Oncol Rep, 30*, 2435–2441.

Delaney, J. P., Leong, K. S., Watkins, A., & Brodie, D. (2002). The short-term effects of myofascial trigger point massage therapy on cardiac autonomic tone in healthy subjects. *J Adv Nurs, 37*, 364–371.

Dodson, R. E., Nishioka, M., Standley, L. J., Perovich, L. J., Green Brody, J. G., & Rudel, R. A. (2012). Endocrine disruptors and asthma-associated chemicals in consumer products. *Environ Health Perspect, 120*, 935–943.

Drukteinis, J. S., Mooney, B. P., Flowers, C. I., & Gatenby, R. A. (2013). Beyond mammography: New frontiers in breast cancer screening. *Am J Med, 126*, 472–479. http://dx.doi.org/10.1289/ehp.1104052

Elkins, G., Marcus, J., Stearns, V., et al. (2008). Randomized trial of a hypnosis intervention for treatment of hot flashes among breast cancer survivors. *J Clin Oncol, 26*, 5022–5026.

Emond, J., A., Pierce, J. P., Natarajan, L., et al. (2014). Risk of breast cancer recurrence associated with carbohydrate intake and tissue expression of IGF-1 receptor. *Cancer Epidemiol, Biomarkers Prev,* doi: 10.1158/1055-9965. EPI-13-1218.

Farvid, M. S., Cho, E., Chen, W. Y., Eliassen, A. H., & Willett, W. C. (2014). Premenopausal dietary fat in relation to pre- and post-menopausal breast cancer. *Breast Cancer Res Treat, 145,* 255–265.

Fitzgerald, A., & Berentson-Shaw, J. (2012). Thermography as a screening and diagnostic tool: A systematic review. *New Zeal Med J, 125,* 80–91.

Flower, G., Fritz, H., Balneaves, L. G., et al. (2013). Flax and breast cancer: A systematic review. *Integrative Cancer Therapies, 13,* 181–192.

Frisk, J. W., Hammar, M. L., Ingvar, M., & Spetz Holm, A. C. (2014). How long do the effects of acupuncture on hot flashes persist in cancer patients? *Support Care Cancer, 22,* 1409–1415.

Fritz, H., Seely, D., Flower, G., et al. (2013). Soy, red clover, and isoflavones and breast cancer: A systematic review. *PLoS One, 8,* e81968.

Fritz, H., Seely, D., McGowan, J., et al. (2014). Black cohosh and breast cancer: A systematic review. *Integr Cancer Ther, 13,* 12–29.

Galantino, M. L., Greene, L., Daniels, L., Dooley, B., Muscatello, L., & O'Donnell, L. (2012). Longitudinal impact of yoga on chemotherapy-related cognitive impairment and quality of life in women with early stage breast cancer: A case series. *Explore, 8,* 127–135.

Genkinger, J. M., Makambi, K. H., Palmer, J. R., Rosenberg, L., & Adams-Campbell, L. L. (2013). Consumption of dairy and meat in relation to breast cancer risk in the Black Women's Health Study. *Cancer Causes Control, 24,* 675–684.

Giordano, S. H., Temin, S., Kirshner, J. J., et al. (2014). Systemic therapy for patients with advanced human epidermal growth factor receptor 2-positive breast cancer: American Society of Clinical Oncology clinical practice guideline. *J Clin Oncol, 32,* 2078–2099.

Gong, Z., Ambrosone, C. B., McMann, S. E., et al. (2014). Associations of dietary folate, vitamins B6 and B12 and methionine intake with risk of breast cancer among African American and European American women. *Int J Cancer, 134,* 1422–1435.

Grundy, A., Richardson, H., & Burstyn, I. (2013). Increased risk of breast cancer associated with long-term shift work in Canada. *Occup Environ Med, 70,* 831–838.

Guha, N., Kwan, M. L., Quesenberry, C. P., Jr., Weltzien, E. K., Castillo, A. L., & Caan, B. J. (2009). Soy isoflavones and risk of cancer recurrence in a cohort of breast cancer survivors: The Life After Cancer Epidemiology study. *Breast Cancer Res Treat, 118,* 395–405.

Harvie, M. N., Pegington, M., Mattson, M. P., et al. (2011). The effects of intermittent or continuous energy restriction on weight loss and metabolic disease risk markers: A randomized trial in young overweight women. *Int J Obes (Lond), 35,* 714–727.

Herranz, M., & Ruibal, A. (2012). Optical imaging in breast cancer diagnosis: The next evolution. *J Oncology,* Article ID 863747.

Hershman, D. L., Unger, J. M., Crew, K. D., et al. (2013). Randomized double-blind placebo-controlled trial of acetyl-L-carnitine for the prevention of taxane-induced neuropathy in women undergoing adjuvant breast cancer therapy. *J Clin Oncol, 31*, 2627–2633.

Howell, A., Cuzick, J., Baum, M., et al. (2005). Results of the ATAC (arimidex, tamoxifen, alone or in combination) trial after completion of 5 years' adjuvant treatment for breast cancer. *Lancet, 365*, 60–62. http://www.silentspring.org/resource/table-consumer-products-tested-endocrine-disruptors-and-asthma-associated-chemicals

Howlader, N., Altekruse, S. F., Li, C. I., et al. (2014). US incidence of breast cancer subtypes defined by joint hormone receptor and HER2 status. *J Natl Cancer Inst, 106*.

Howlader, N., Noone, A. M., Krapcho, M., et al. (2014). *SEER cancer statistics review, 1975–2011*. Based on November 2013 SEER data submission. National Cancer Institute. Bethesda, MD. http://seer.cancer.gov/csr/1975_2011/

Hursting, S. D., Dunlap, S. M., Ford, N. A., Hursting, M. J., & Lashinger, L. M. (2013). Calorie restriction and cancer prevention: A mechanistic perspective. *Cancer and Metabolism, 1*, 10. www.cancerandmetabolism.com/content/1/1/10

International Agency for Research on Cancer (IARC). (2007). *Shiftwork*. Monograph 98, 562–764. Retrieved May 15, 2014, from http://monographs.iarc.fr/ENG/Monographs/vol98/mono98-8.pdf

Janelsins, M. C., Kesler, S. R., Ahles, T. A., & Morrow, G. R. (2014). Prevalence, mechanisms and management of cancer-related cognitive impairment. *Int Rev Psychiatry, 26*, 102–113.

Juckett, D. A. (2009). A 17-year oscillation in cancer mortality birth cohorts on three continents—Synchrony to cosmic ray modulations one generation earlier. *Int J Biometeor, 53*, 487–499.

Kalantarian, S., Rimm, E. B., Herrington, D. M., & Mozaffarian, D. (2014). Dietary macronutrients, genetic variation, and progression of coronary atherosclerosis among women. *Am Heart J, 167*, 627–635.

Kiecolt-Glaser, J. K., Bennett, J. M., Andridge, R., et al. (2014). Yoga's impact on inflammation, mood, and fatigue in breast cancer survivors: A randomized controlled trial. *JCO, 32*, 1040–1049.

Knower, K. C., To, S. Q., Leung, Y. K., Ho, S. M., & Clyne, C. D. (2014). Endocrine disruption of the epigenome: A breast cancer link. *Endocr Relat Cancer, 21*, T33–55.

Korde, L. A., Wu, A. H., Fears, T., et al. (2009). Childhood soy intake and breast cancer risk in Asian American women. *Cancer Epidemiol, Biomarkers Prev, 18*, 1050–1059.

Kwan, M. L., Kushi, L. H., Weltzien, E., et al. (2010). Alcohol consumption and breast cancer recurrence and survival among women with early-stage breast cancer: The Life After Cancer Epidemiology study. *J Clin Oncol, 28*, 4410–4416.

L'Espérance, S. J. Y. (2013). Pharmacological and nonhormonal treatment of hot flashes in breast cancer survivors: CEPO review and recommendations. *Support Care Cancer, 21*, 1461–1474.

Lee, C., Raffaghello, L., Brandhorst, S., et al. (2012). Fasting cycles retard growth of tumors and sensitize a range of cancer cell types to chemotherapy. *Sci Transl Med, 4*, 124ra27.

Lee, S. A., Fowke, J. H., Lu, W., et al. (2008). Cruciferous vegetables, the GSTP1 Ile105Val genetic polymorphism, and breast cancer risk. *Am J Clin Nutr*, *87*, 753–760.

Lemanne, D., Cassileth, B., & Gubili, J. (2013). The role of physical activity in cancer prevention, treatment, recovery, and survivorship. *Oncology*, *27*, 580–585.

Li, M., Chen, P., Li, J., et al. (2014). Review: The impacts of circulating 25-hydroxyvitamin d levels on cancer patient outcomes: A systematic review and meta-analysis. *J Clin Endocrinol Metab*, *99*, 2327–2336.

Liu, X., & Lv, K. (2013). Cruciferous vegetables intake is inversely associated with risk of breast cancer: A meta-analysis. *Breast*, *22*, 309–313.

Lu, W. A., Chen, G. Y., & Kuo, C. D. (2011). Foot reflexology can increase vagal modulation, decrease sympathetic modulation, and lower blood pressure in healthy subjects and patients with coronary artery disease. *Altern Ther Health Med*, *17*, 8–14.

Lutgendorf, S. K., & Sood, A. K. (2011). Biobehavioral factors and cancer progression: Physiological pathways and mechanisms. *Psychosom Med*, *73*, 724–730.

Mainiero, M. B., Lourenco, A., Mahoney, M. C., et al. (2013). ACR appropriateness criteria breast cancer screening. *J Am Coll Radiol*, *10*, 11–14.

Malliani, A. (2005). Heart rate variability: From bench to bedside. *Eur J Intern Med*, *16*, 12–20.

McCarthy, A. M., Kontos, D., Synnestvedt, M., et al. (2014). Screening outcomes following implementation of digital breast tomosynthesis in a general-population screening program. *Journal of the National Cancer Institute*, *106*.

McGuirk, S., Gravel, S.-P., Deblois, G., et al. (2013). PGC-1 alpha supports glutamine metabolism in breast cancer. *Cancer Metab*, *1*, 22. http://www.cancerandmetabolism.com/content/1/1/22

McLaughlin, S. A., Wright, M. J., Morris, K. T., et al. (2008). Prevalence of lymphedema in women with breast cancer 5 years after sentinel lymph node biopsy or axillary dissection: Objective measurements. *J Clin Oncol*, *26*, 5213–5219.

Milbury, K., Chaoul, B., Biegler, K., et al. (2013). Tibetan sound meditation for cognitive dysfunction: Results of a randomized controlled pilot trial. *Psychooncology*, *22*, 2354–2363.

Munsell, M. F., Sprague, B. L., Berry, D. A., Chisholm, G., & Trentham-Dietz, A. (2014). Body mass index and breast cancer risk according to postmenopausal estrogen-progestin use and hormone receptor status. *Epidemiol Rev*, *36*, 114–136.

National Cancer Institute. (2014). *Mammograms*. Retrieved May 20, 2014, from http://www.cancer.gov/cancertopics/factsheet/detection/mammograms

Neale, C., Camfield, D., Reay, J., Stough, C., & Scholey, A. (2013). Cognitive effects of two nutraceuticals Ginseng and Bacopa benchmarked against modafinil: A review and comparison of effect sizes. *Br J Clin Pharmacol*, *75*, 728–737.

Pan, H., & Gray, R. G. (2014). Effect of obesity in premenopausal ER+ early breast cancer: EBCTCG data on 80,000 patients in 70 trials. *J Clin Oncol*, *32*, 5s.

Patterson, R. E., Flatt, S. W., Newman, V. A., et al. (2011). Marine fatty acid intake is associated with breast cancer prognosis. *J Nutr*, *141*, 201–206.

Pierce, J. P. (2009). Diet and breast cancer prognosis: Making sense of the WHEL and WINS trials. *Currr Opin Obstet Gynecol* 21(1), 86–91.

Pierce, J. P., Natarajan, L., Caan, B. J., et al. (2007). Influence of a diet very high in vegetables, fruit, and fiber and low in fat on prognosis following treatment for breast cancer: The Women's Healthy Eating and Living (WHEL) randomized trial. *JAMA, 298*, 289–298.

Pomykala, K. L., de Ruiter, M. B., Deprez, S., McDonald, B. C., & Silverman, D. H. (2013). Integrating imaging findings in evaluating the post-chemotherapy brain. *Brain Imaging Behav, 7*, 436–452.

Poynter, J. N., Inoue-Choi, M., Ross, J. A., Jacos, D. R., Jr., & Robien, K. (2013). Reproductive, lifestyle and anthropometric risk factors for cancer in elderly women. *Cancer Epidemiol Biomark Prev, 22*, 681–687.

Prentice, R. L., Caan, B., Chlebowski, R. T., et al. (2006). Low-fat dietary pattern and risk of invasive breast cancer: The Women's Health Initiative Randomized Controlled Dietary Modification Trial. *JAMA, 295*, 629–642.

Prentice, R. L., Huang, Y., Hinds, D. A., et al. (2010). Variation in the FGFR2 gene and the effect of a low-fat dietary pattern on invasive breast cancer. *Cancer Epidemiol Biomarkers Prev, 19*, 74–79.

Printz, C. (2013). Link between high fat dairy consumption and poor breast cancer survival. *Cancer, 119*, 2517.

Protani, M., Coory, M., & Martin, J. H. (2010). Effect of obesity on survival of women with breast cancer: Systematic review and meta-analysis. *Breast Cancer Res Treat, 123*, 627–635.

Ricar, J., Pizinger, K., & Cetkovsha, P. (2013). Shiitake dermatitis: A distinct clinical entity. *Int J Derm, 52*, 1620–1621.

Rockwell, S., Liu, Y., & Higgins, S. A. (2005). Alteration of the effects of cancer therapy agents on breast cancer cells by the herbal medicine black cohosh. *Breast Cancer Res Treat, 90*, 233–239.

Safdie, F. M., Dorff, T., Quinn, D., et al. (2009). Fasting and cancer treatment in humans: A case series report. *Aging, 1*, 988–1007.

Sayin, V. I., Ibrahim, M. X., Larsson, E., Nilsson, J. A., Lindahl, P., & Bergo, M. (2014). Antioxidants accelerate lung cancer progression in mice. *Sci Transl Med, 6*, 221ra15.

Schloss, J. M., Colosimo, M., Airey, C., Masci, P. P., Linnane, A. W., & Vitetta, L. (2013). Nutraceuticals and chemotherapy induced peripheral neuropathy (CIPN): A systematic review. *Clin Nutr, 32*, 888–893.

Schroeder, S., Meyer-Hamme, G., & Epplée, S. (2012). Acupuncture for chemotherapy-induced peripheral neuropathy (CIPN): A pilot study using neurography. *Acupunct Med, 30*, 4–7.

SEER Stat Fact Sheets. (2014). *Breast cancer*. Retrieved June 10, 2014, from http://seer.cancer.gov/statfacts/html/breast.html

Shord, S. S., Shah, K., & Lukosa, A. (2009). Drug-botanical interactions: A review of the laboratory, animal, and human data for 8 common botanicals. *Integr Cancer Ther, 8*, 208–227.

Sopotsinskaia, E. B., Balitskiĭ, K. P., Tarutinov, V. I., et al. (1992). [Experience with the use of a low-calorie diet in breast cancer patients to prevent metastasis] (in Russian). *Vopr Onkol, 38,* 592–599.

Sternfeld, B., & Dugan, S. (2011). Physical activity and health during the menopausal transition. *Obstet Gynecol Clin North Am, 38,* 537–566.

Takahashi, Y., Mai, M., & Nakazato, H. (2005). Preoperative CEA and PPD values as prognostic factors for immunochemotherapy using PSK and 5-FU. *Anticancer Res, 25,* 1377–1384.

Taku, K., Melby, M. K., Kronenberg, F., Kurzer, M. S., & Messina, M. (2012). Extracted or synthesized soybean isoflavones reduce menopausal hot flash frequency and severity: Systematic review and meta-analysis of randomized controlled trials. *Menopause, 19,* 776–790.

Thomson, C. A., Rock, C. L., Thompson, P. A., Caan, B. J., Cussler, E., Flatt, S. W., & Pierce, J. P. (2011). Vegetable intake is associated with reduced breast cancer recurrence in tamoxifen users: A secondary analysis from the Women's Healthy Eating and Living Study. *Breast Cancer Res Treat, 125,* 519–527.

Toth, B., & Erickson, J. (1986). Cancer induction in mice by feeding of the uncooked cultivated mushroom of commerce *Agaricus bisporus. Cancer Res, 46,* 4007–4011.

US Preventive Services Task Force. (2009). Screening for breast cancer: US Preventive Services Task Force recommendation statement. *Ann Intern Med, 151,* 716–726.

Winocur, G., Wojtowicz, J. M., Huang, J., & Tannock, I. F. (2014). Physical exercise prevents suppression of hippocampal neurogenesis and reduces cognitive impairment in chemotherapy-treated rats. *Psychopharmacology, 231,* 2311–2320.

Wise, D. R., DeBerardinis, R. J., Mancuso, A., et al. (2008). Myc regulates a transcriptional program that stimulates mitochondrial glutaminolysis and leads to glutamine addiction. *Proc Natl Acad Sci USA, 105,* 18782–18787.

Wu, W., Kang, S., & Zhang, D. (2013). Association of vitamin B6, vitamin B12 and methionine with risk of breast cancer: A dose-response meta-analysis. *Br J Cancer, 109,* 1926–1944.

Xiao, O. S., Zheng, Y., Cai, H., et al. (2009). Soy food intake and breast cancer survival. *JAMA, 302,* 2437–2443.

Yankaskas, B. C., Haneuse, S., Kapp, J. M., Kerlikowske, K., Geller, B., & Buist, D. S. M. (2010). Performance of first mammography examination in women younger than 40 years. *J Natl Cancer Inst, 102,* 692–701.

Zheng, J. S., Hu, X. J., Zhao, Y. M., Yang, J., & Li, D. (2013). Intake of fish and marine n-3 polyunsaturated fatty acids and risk of breast cancer: Meta-analysis of data from 21 independent prospective cohort studies. *BMJ, 346,* f3706.

Zhou, B., Damrauer, J. S., Bailey, S. T., et al. (2014). Erythropoietin promotes breast tumorigenesis through tumor-initiating cell self-renewal. *J Clin Invest, 124,* 553–563.

Zou, L. Y., Yang, L., He, X. L., Sun, M., & Xu, J. J. (2014). Effects of aerobic exercise on cancer-related fatigue in breast cancer patients receiving chemotherapy: A meta-analysis. *Tumor Biol.* Published online 26 Feb 2014.

PART IV

Common Conditions in Women

22

Hypothyroidism

MARIA BENITO

CASE STUDY

Rebecca came to see me when she was 13 weeks pregnant with her second child. She had been diagnosed with hypothyroidism in her early teens and wanted to see what else she could do to improve her condition. Rebecca's first pregnancy had been complicated by gestational diabetes mellitus, and she required insulin during the third trimester. Her diet included no fish because her husband was allergic, she was lactose intolerant, and she cooked with (noniodized) sea salt. She had been taking a selective serotonin reuptake inhibitor (SSRI) up to the time of conception because of atypical depression and she was about to resume. She was taking generic levothyroxine (thyroxine, or T4) and a prenatal vitamin. But she did not feel well. She complained of brain fog, depression, and fatigue.

Will the addition of 3,5,3'-triodothyronine (T3) relieve her symptoms? How about dessicated thyroid? Are there any supplements she could add to her regimen? What about eating kale or other cruciferous vegetables? Will these foods cause a goiter? These questions are commonplace in my practice, whether the patient is a woman or a man and whether the woman is pregnant or not. But her history presented some challenges. First, Rebecca was pregnant, she had had gestational diabetes mellitus during a prior pregnancy, and she was possibly iodine deficient. She likely had hypothyroidism on an autoimmune basis. Her symptoms were nonspecific but common to patients with thyroid disorders.

This chapter presents an integrative approach to the general treatment of hypothyroidism, and the treatment of Hashimoto's thyroiditis specifically, and reviews the role of iodine, potential coexisting nutritional deficiencies, and goitrogens on thyroid function.

Hypothyroidism

PREVALENCE AND ETIOLOGY

Hypothyroidism is the most frequent disorder of thyroid function. In the United States, 4.3% of the population over the age of 12 years is hypothyroid (Hollowell et al., 2002), with an increased prevalence in women and older age. Subclinical hypothyroidism occurs in 3% of men and 8% of women (up to 5% during pregnancy, and up to 10% during postmenopausal years) (Cooper & Biondi 2012).

Hypothyroidism is classified as either primary or secondary. Primary hypothyroidism denotes a dysfunction of the thyroid gland and is covered in this chapter. In Western countries still considered iodine sufficient, such as the United States, the most likely etiology of primary hypothyroidism is autoimmunity (Hashimoto's thyroiditis), characterized by positive thyroid peroxidase (TPO) and/or antithyroglobulin antibodies. But worldwide, the most common etiology of hypothyroidism is iodine deficiency.

Other etiologies of primary hypothyroidism include postradiation, postsurgical removal of the thyroid gland and, less commonly, infiltrative diseases and antithyroid drugs. Occasionally, hypothyroidism is transient, such as in subacute thyroiditis, during the recovery phase of nonthyroidal illness and after withdrawal of thyroid hormone.

DIAGNOSIS

There is no one symptom that is sensitive or specific enough to make the diagnosis of hypothyroidism clinically. In general, symptoms are more apparent when hypothyroidism is severe and the development acute. However, symptoms also depend on how sensitive the individual is to thyroid hormone deficiency. In the Colorado Thyroid Disease Prevalence Study, the main symptoms of subclinical hypothyroidism (over euthyroid subjects) were dry skin, poor memory, slow thinking, weak muscles, fatigue, muscle cramps, cold intolerance, deep and hoarse voice, puffy eyes, and constipation. When several of these symptoms are present, hypothyroidism should be suspected and laboratory evaluation should ensue (Canaris, Manowitz, Mayor, & Ridgway, 2000).

The best laboratory test to diagnose primary hypothyroidism is a third- or fourth-generation thyroid-stimulating hormone (TSH), because of the log-linear relationship between TSH and serum-free thyroid hormone (Baloch et al. 2003).

An elevated TSH and low free T4 (later also a low T3) denote overt hypothyroidism; an elevated TSH and a free T4 within the reference range denote subclinical hypothyroidism. The reference range for TSH is 0.4 to 4.5 mIU/L in most laboratories. When excluding those with thyroid antibodies, the reference range for TSH shifts to the left, between 0.4 and 2.5 mIU/L (Wartofsky & Dickey, 2005).

Thirty percent of people over the age of 70 have an elevated TSH concentration but no signs of thyroid disease or thyroid antibodies (Surks & Hollowell, 2007). Therefore, mild elevations in TSH might reflect a physiologic adaption to aging, especially after age 80, and not subclinical thyroid disease. And "normal" TSH, within the reference range, might reflect early thyroid dysfunction.

MEASURING THYROID HORMONE

Most often the measurement of TSH and free T4 is sufficient to determine whether someone is hypothyroid. T3 can be measured when trying to determine whether the dose of L-T4 and L-T3 is adequate. However, measuring T3 is not recommended routinely in the diagnosis of hypothyroidism because it is neither specific nor sensitive enough. During hypothyroidism, T3 will be maintained in the normal reference range until severe hypothyroidism ensues due to enhanced T4 to T3 conversion. During nonthyroidal illness and situations of caloric deprivation, T3 concentration is low.

EVALUATION

The evaluation of hypothyroidism should include a repeat of thyroid function tests to determine whether the abnormal TSH is transient or permanent, as well as clinical and laboratory tests to determine the cause. Clinicians should inquire about previous neck surgery or radiation, history of pituitary or hypothalamic disease, medications, previous history of thyroid disease including postpartum thyroiditis in a woman, and family history.

Laboratory evaluation should include thyroid antibodies and urine iodine, if the clinical and dietary history is suggestive of iodine deficiency. Thyroid antibodies to thyroglobulin (Tg) and TPO occur in up to 95% of cases of Hashimoto's thyroiditis. However, up to 20% of patients with autoimmune thyroid disease have negative antibodies but evidence of autoimmune thyroiditis morphologically (abnormal ultrasound characterized by a hypoechoic pattern).

Treatment

WHOM TO TREAT AND WHEN TO TREAT

Treatment is indicated when there is overt hypothyroidism (high TSH, low T4 or free T4) or goiter and Hashimoto's thyroiditis even in cases of euthyroidism. There is no consensus regarding treatment of subclinical hypothyroidism (high TSH but normal T4 or free T4). The American Association of Clinical Endocrinologists (AACE) and the American Thyroid Association (ATA; Garber et al., 2012) do not endorse the treatment of subclinical hypothyroidism unless TSH is >10 mIU/L, or the woman is pregnant (TSH > 2.5 mIU/L and positive TPO antibody) because there is no clinical outcome data outside of those situations. The European Thyroid Association (ETA) has established an algorithm for the treatment of subclinical hypothyroidism depending on age, symptoms of hypothyroidism, and significant cardiovascular risk (Pearce et al., 2013). These recommendations are summarized in Table 22.1.

The ATA has issued guidelines for the management of hypothyroidism during pregnancy. Thyroid-stimulating hormone should be monitored every

Table 22.1. Recommendations for the Treatment of Subclinical Hypothyroidism by Several Medical Societies.

Organization		TSH >10	TSH 4.5–10	TSH 2.5–4.5
AACE/ATA (2012)		Yes	No recommendations	If pregnant, yes
ETA (2013)	Age <70	Yes	L-T4 trial if symptoms	No recommendations
	Age >70	If sxs or CV risk	Monitor	No recommendations

Note: Sxs, symptoms; CV, cardiovascular.

4 weeks during the first 20 weeks of pregnancy and every 6 weeks thereafter; it should be maintained at <2.5 mIU/L during the first trimester, <3.0 mIU/L during the second trimester, and <3.5 mIU/L during the third trimester. For those with subclinical hypothyroidism who are not pregnant, the ETA recommends a TSH in the lower half of the reference range (0.4–2.5 mIU/L) with a higher target (1–5 mIU/L) for those over the age of 70–75. The ATA/AACE recommend keeping TSH within the normal range, or 0.45–4.12 mIU/L, during the treatment of hypothyroidism. If free T4 is used for monitoring patients taking levothyroxine, patients should be advised to have their blood drawn before taking their daily dose because free T4 concentration remains elevated (up to 20%) for up to 9 hours after dosing.

HOW TO TREAT (L-THYROXINE ALONE VERSUS COMBINATION THERAPY)

Synthetic levothyroxine sodium (L-thyroxine or L-T4) preparations are the mainstay of treatment as recommended by the AACE, ATA, and ETA. It is not clear whether current bioequivalent studies truly ensure that various preparations (tablets, liquid-containing capsules) are interchangeable, and therefore, endocrinologists usually recommend the use of a consistent (e.g., brand-name) L-thyroxine preparation to minimize variability from refill to refill. The available brands of synthetic L-thyroxine preparations include:

- Synthroid by Abbot,
- Levoxyl by Pfizer,
- Tirosint by Akrimax. This is a liquid gel capsule with gelatin, glycerin, and water as inactive ingredients. This formulation seems to be less dependent on gastric pH for absorption, which along with the fact that there are no dyes or other fillers has made it an attractive option for practitioners and patients alike.
- Unithroid by Gemini.

The dose of L-T4 should be based on weight, and can be started at the full replacement dose (1.5 mcg/kg/day) in most adults except in patients with cardiac history or in the elderly. For best absorption, it is usually recommended to take L-T4 first thing in the morning on an empty stomach. However, a recent study has challenged this notion; taking L-T4 before bedtime led to an improved TSH and T3 (Bolk et al., 2010).

Some foods and medicines can interfere with the absorption of thyroid hormone, so in general these should be taken 4 hours apart from thyroid hormone.

Some examples include milk (due to its calcium content), soy (unclear mechanism), coffee, papaya, iron, calcium, antacids (including H2-receptor blockers, sucralfate, and proton pump inhibitors), cholestyramine, and raloxifene.

MAKING THE CASE FOR T3

Most hypothyroid patients achieve biochemical and clinical euthyroidism while taking levothyroxine. But between 5 and 15% of hypothyroid patients continue to report symptoms, including neurocognitive defects, despite a TSH within the reference range, even when TSH is maintained within a narrow range (median TSH 1.25-range 0.3–2.9 mIU/L) (Panicker et al., 2009).

Polymorphisms in the deiodinase enzyme type 2 gene (responsible for the conversion of T4 to T3) and in thyroid hormone transport have been implicated in the pathogenesis of a poor response to treatment with L-T4 alone. Favorable outcome with L-T4/L-T3 combination in patients with a rarer form of one such polymorphism has lent support to using L-T3 in selected patients who do not achieve clinical euthyroidism while taking levothyroxine alone (Bianco & Casula, 2012; Panicker et al., 2009).

But most single clinical studies and two meta-analyses have not shown significant benefit with the L-T4/L-T3 combination in patients with hypothyroidism. In spite of a lack of benefit in one meta-analysis and a suggestion of benefit in psychological and physical well-being in another (Grozinsky-Glasberg et al., 2006; Ma et al., 2009), several studies have noted patient preference for combination therapy (Escobar-Morreale et al., 2005; Nygaard et al., 2009).

Although current clinical practice guidelines by the AACE and ATA do not support the routine use of combination T4 and T3 therapy in hypothyroidism (Garber et al., 2012), the same authors recognize that there are "still-unresolved issues raised by studies that reported some patients prefer and some patient subgroups may benefit from a combination of L-thyroxine and L-triiodothyronine." The ETA (Wiersinga, Duntas, Fadeyev, Nygaard, & Vanderpump, 2012) has proposed that for patients who after evaluation and exclusion of other autoimmune disorders and counseling, remain feeling unwell, a 3-month trial of L-T4/L-T3 combination might be recommended. If at the end of 3 months, provided achievement of a normal TSH and appropriate FT4:FT3 ratio, symptoms have not improved, the trial should be considered futile and a return to L-T4 monotherapy should ensue.

Who might benefit from L-T4/L-T3 combination is still a clinical decision, as plasma T3 concentrations do not correlate with tissue T3 either pre- or posttreatment, even in those subjects with polymorphisms in the deiodinase 2 gene who responded clinically to L-T4/L-T3 combination. At present, there is no available clinical testing for this polymorphism, which occurs in approximately 16% of the population studied.

It is likely that a slow-release form of T3 would be more physiological than current forms of L-T3 (Hennemann, Docter, Visser, Postema, & Krenning, 2004), but currently there is no commercial preparation of slow-release T3. (It is possible to have a pharmacy compound a slow-release T3.)

PRACTICAL GUIDELINES

How to Start and Titrate T4/T3 Combination

In order to achieve a physiological human ratio, the ETA (Wiersinga et al., 2012) recommends using separate L-T4 and L-T3 preparations, L-T4 in a single daily dose and L-T3 in two daily doses, because of the short half-life of L-T3. Commercial porcine thyroidal secretion occurs in a T4:T3 ratio of 4:1, whereas human thyroidal secretion occurs in a ratio of 16:1.

Armour thyroid, Naturethroid, and West-throid are brands of dessicated porcine thyroid that contain a combination of T4 and T3. A synthetic form of L-T4/L-T3 is not currently available. Clinicians may opt for dessicated thyroid, replacement of synthetic L-T4 and L-T3 as separate prescriptions, or compounding.

There are several methods to calculate a starting L-T4/L-T3 regimen for someone receiving L-T4 monotherapy who wishes to transition to combination therapy.

1. Start by finding the daily dose of L-T4 that has normalized TSH. Calculate the dose of L-T3 by dividing the L-T4 monotherapy dose by 17 (because the thyroidal secretion of T4:T3 is 16:1; so for any given dose of L-T4, 16 parts will be L-T4 and one part will be the L-T3 dose).
2. Then, calculate the dose of L-T4 by multiplying the newly calculated dose of L-T3 by 3 (because the therapeutic equivalence of L-T4 to L-T3 has been found to be 3:1) and subtract that amount from the L-T4 monotherapy dose. So, if your patient is taking 88 mcg of levothyroxine, has a normal TSH, and you decide to change to L-T4/L-T3, you first divide 88 by 17 to calculate the T3 dose: 5.17. Then, to calculate the new dose of L-T4, multiply 5.17 times 3 (15.51), and then subtract it from 88 (88 − 15.51 = 72.49). So, the new doses (rounded off) are 5 mcg of L-T3 and 75 mcg of L-T4.

3. The normal serum free-T4:free-T3 ratio is around 3.3 in healthy controls, whereas the ratio usually obtained with L-T4 monotherapy is 4:5.5.
4. To ensure an adequate ratio, measure free T4 and free T3 and adjust as necessary.

Researchers and thyroid experts have postulated that persistent symptoms might be due to the inadequacy of hormone treatment, to the autoimmune process, to the coexistence of other autoimmune conditions, or to the presence of a chronic disease (Wiersinga et al., 2012). Therefore, a patient with Hashimoto's thyroiditis who has a TSH within the reference range but does not feel well deserves an evaluation for other autoimmune conditions including celiac disease, autoimmune gastritis, pernicious anemia, and Addison's disease.

In addition to considering coexisting autoimmune conditions and adding L-T3, nutrition, botanicals, dietary supplements, and yoga might be used as part of the integrative treatment of hypothyroidism. The following is a summary of the evidence for each one of these areas.

Hashimoto's Thyroiditis: Integrative Approaches

Hashimoto's thyroiditis is an important topic in women's health because, as in other autoimmune conditions, there is an increased female preponderance (approximately an 8:1 female to male ratio). Although Hashimoto's thyroiditis is the main etiology of hypothyroidism in Western countries, not all patients with Hashimoto's thyroiditis present with hypothyroidism. Hashimoto's thyroiditis is an organ-specific autoimmune condition, where genetic influences explain 70% of the development and environmental factors the remaining 30%. The TPO antibody correlates with the degree of lymphocytic infiltration. Studies by independent researchers noted a positive association between quality of life and TPO antibody level (Ott et al., 2011; Watt et al., 2012), including an association with dysphoric mood during pregnancy and postpartum but not with thyroid function (Groer & Vaughan, 2013). Some potential integrative strategies for affecting TPO antibody levels are discussed in what follows.

DIETARY INTERVENTION

Although there are no studies to determine the role of any particular diet in patients with Hashimoto's thyroiditis, gluten-free and paleo diets and the avoidance of goitrogenic foods are commonplace among patients.

Gluten-Free Diet

Celiac disease coexists with Hashimoto's thyroiditis in a significant number of patients. It is estimated that up to 5% of those with Hashimoto's thyroiditis have celiac disease (and up to 30% of those with celiac disease will develop autoimmune thyroid disease, or AITD). In addition, patients with AITD often present with subclinical celiac disease (Ch'ng, Keston Jones, & Kingham, 2007). There are no established guidelines to help decide how often to test, but clinicians should evaluate patients with Hashimoto's thyroiditis for celiac disease at diagnosis and in cases of increased requirement of L-T4 beyond what is expected (Virili et al., 2012); in the presence of gastrointestinal symptoms (such as irritable bowel syndrome); iron, folate, or vitamin B12 deficiency; and chronic fatigue.

In patients with biopsy-proven celiac disease, the following has been observed after gluten withdrawal: (1) improved absorption, including that of thyroid hormone (Valentino et al., 1999), (2) elimination or decrease in thyroid antibodies (Ventura et al., 2000), and (3) a potential reversal of subclinical hypothyroidism (whether patients had positive thyroid antibodies or not) (Sategna-Guidetti et al., 2001).

A gluten-free diet does not appear to protect from developing thyroid autoimmunity in adult patients with celiac disease (Metso et al., 2012), but may earlier in life (childhood and adolescence). At present, there are no data as to whether a gluten-free diet in a nonceliac patient may alter the natural course of Hashimoto's thyroiditis and the development of hypothyroidism. If a gluten-free diet is chosen as part of an integrative treatment plan, 1 year of treatment is recommended.

Anti-Inflammatory Diet

If Hashimoto's thyroiditis is an inflammatory, autoimmune condition characterized by high oxidative stress (Rostami, Aghasi, Mohammadi, & Nourooz-Zadeh, 2013), it follows that dietary strategies that dampen inflammation might improve its course. While there are no clinical studies on the effect of an anti-inflammatory diet or the inclusion (or exclusion) of specific foods on the course of Hashimoto's or hypothyroidism, in my experience many patients do feel better.

Paleolithic (Paleo) Diet

While there are numerous definitions of what constitutes the "Paleo" diet, in general one avoids processed foods, legumes, peanuts, and grains. Although there are no clinical data to support these recommendations, some of my patients feel better following a Paleo diet, in particular those who suffer from glucose intolerance.

Goitrogens

A goitrogen is a food substance that blocks thyroid hormone synthesis and can exacerbate the effect of iodine deficiency. Therefore goitrogens are covered under iodine deficiency, later in this chapter. The effect of goitrogens on the thyroid is dose dependent for some and age dependent, with a decreased effect noted with aging. None of the goitrogens have specifically been studied in patients with Hashimoto's thyroiditis.

Other

Cellular and humoral response mechanisms are implicated in the pathogenesis of Hashimoto's thyroiditis, with hypothetical improvement from maneuvers that enhance Th2 response and dampen Th1 and T helper type 17 (Th17) lymphocytes (D. Li et al., 2013). Several potential treatments that decrease Th1 and Th17 lymphocytes, such as berberine, an alkaloid present in plants such as goldenseal (*Hydrastis canadensis*) or Oregon Grape root (*Berberis aquifolium*) (Qin et al., 2010) , are intriguing. However, there are no studies or firm recommendations that can be made for specific foods or supplements.

IODINE

Of the environmental triggers of Hashimoto's thyroiditis, iodine excess is well established. In genetically susceptible individuals, such as those with positive antibodies or a family history, exposure to excessive dietary iodine (doses ≥ 1 mg) triggers autoimmune thyroiditis and may cause hypothyroidism. The effect of iodine on chronic autoimmune thyroiditis seems to be due to an increase in the iodination of thyroglobulin (Y. Li et al., 2008). Iodine restriction may restore normal thyroid function in those with positive TPO antibodies and subclinical hypothyroidism, especially when urine iodine is elevated and TSH mildly elevated (Yoon et al., 2003; Reinhardt et al., 1998).

While iodine is necessary for thyroid hormone synthesis, too much iodine may trigger autoimmunity or hypothyroidism. Therefore, I follow the recommended daily allowance (RDA) for iodine set forth by the Food and Nutrition Board at the Institute of Medicine for patients with Hashimoto's thyroiditis. For those 19 years and older who are not pregnant or breast-feeding, this is 150 mcg per day. In my view, having enough iodine not only ensures normal thyroid function but also likely prevents the entry into the thyroid gland of endocrine disruptors and goitrogens that work by competitive inhibition with the sodium iodine symporter. When iodine supplementation is necessary, I recommend iodized salt (1/2 tsp per day) or supplemental iodine in the form of potassium iodide. Kelp has variable amounts of iodine and should not be recommended as the preferred way to restore iodine stores. Note: Not all seaweeds contain large amounts of iodine. Dulse, nori, and wakame are perfectly safe as part of a varied diet (Mussig, et al., 2006)

SELENIUM

Selenium is an essential trace element with antioxidative and anti-inflammatory effects that is necessary for the function of two enzymes, glutathione peroxidase and thioredoxin reductase—that are responsible for protecting the thyroid from oxidative damage—and an additional three enzymes (the iodothyronine deiodinases types I, II, and III) responsible for thyroid hormone homeostasis. The mechanism of action of selenium supplementation in patients with Hashimoto's thyroiditis seems to be modulated by an antioxidative effect and perhaps by suppressing autoimmune activity.

Selenium supplementation slows the activity of autoimmune thyroiditis (decreases TPO, improves ultrasound morphology) in patients with Hashimoto's and hypothyroidism better than placebo, as supported by the majority of the 13 published trials on the topic (Toulis et al., 2010).

The doses recommended are at least 100 mcg/day of selenium, although most studies used 200 mcg/day and one used 80 mcg/day (a more physiological dose) over a longer period (Duntas, 2010). To put this in perspective, the RDA for selenium is 55–70 mcg/day and the tolerable upper limit has been set at 400 mcg/day for >14 years of age (Office of Dietary Supplements, 2013).

The response to selenium is not uniform; low selenium concentration and high TPO antibodies prior to treatment are associated with better outcomes. It is important to note that the effects last only while selenium is being administered. The organic forms (e.g., selenomethionine or SeMet, and yeast) are safer and more bioavailable than the inorganic form (e.g., sodium selenite) and in one study were associated with better results.

What is not known is whether selenium supplementation can delay or prevent the development of hypothyroidism and the need for thyroid hormone in patients with Hashimoto's who are euthyroid. A study in euthyroid children noted decreased thyroid volume after 6 months but no change in thyroid antibodies after 3 months of 50 mcg of L-selenomethionine supplementation (Onal, Keskindemirci, Adal, Ersen, & Korkmaz, 2012).

When selenium is consumed in excessive amounts, selenosis (selenium toxicity) ensues, which is characterized by diarrhea, fatigue, hair loss, and fingernail discoloration. Although the data are mixed, most studies of selenium supplementation show an increased risk of type 2 diabetes (Akbaraly et al., 2010; Bleys, Navas-Acien, & Guallar, 2007; Rajpathak et al., 2005; Stranges et al., 2007; Stranges et al., 2010), particularly when the baseline selenium concentration is in the highest tertile (about 122 mcg/L) or the amount of dietary selenium in the highest quintile. It has been suggested that the relationship between diabetes and selenium might follow a U-shaped curve with increased risk of diabetes at low and high selenium intakes. And selenium supplementation has also been linked to the development of glaucoma.

To assess selenium status, several biomarkers may be used, including plasma, whole blood, erythrocyte (red blood cell, or RBC), and selenoprotein P (Ashton, Hooper, & Harvey, 2009). Selenium in plasma and whole blood indicate recent selenium presence, whereas selenium in RBCs is more sensitive for long-term assessment. Some authors consider selenoprotein P the most reliable marker of selenium status. From selenium supplementation studies, it appears that selenium concentration plateaus in the first 3 months and does not increase afterward (Rayman, 2012). However, individual requirements may vary due to selenoprotein polymorphisms.

Clinical Pearl

In my practice, when a patient has Hashimoto's thyroiditis, I ask about personal or family history of diabetes. If there is a positive history, and I think that selenium supplementation is indicated, I discuss the potential association with diabetes and measure plasma selenium to ensure the level is below 122 mcg/L. For those patients at high risk of diabetes, I usually have them eat three Brazil nuts daily as their source of selenium. In fact, Brazil nuts are often my preferred form of selenium supplementation and selenium methionine or yeast-derived my second tier of treatment. I monitor plasma selenium at least once 3 months after starting Brazil nuts or supplementation and aim to keep plasma selenium between 130 and 150 mcg/L.

VITAMIN D

Some studies have found a relative vitamin D insufficiency in adults with Hashimoto's thyroiditis (Kivity et al., 2011), and polymorphisms in the vitamin D receptor gene have been associated with an increased risk of thyroid autoimmunity (Feng, Li, Cheng, Li, & Zhang, 2013). Others have not found an association between low vitamin D and autoimmune thyroid disease (Effraimidis, Badenhoop, Tijssen, & Wiersinga, 2012). There is, however, no available data on the effects of vitamin D supplementation on Hashimoto's thyroiditis.

IMMUNE AMPHOTERIC AND IMMUNOREGULATORY HERBS

Amphoterics in herbal medicine refer to those herbs that normalize function whether the organ is hyper or hypofunctioning. In the case of the immune system, mushrooms such as reishi (*Ganoderma lucidum*) and maitake (*Grifola frondosa*) are thought to be amphoteric. Other herbs, such as turmeric (*Curcuma longa*) are classified as immune regulators, helping to dampen excessive immune response. The herbal treatment of a patient with Hashimoto's thyroiditis may include the use of immune amphoterics and immune regulators; while there are no clinical data, the risk for adverse effects when consumed as part of the diet is low (as long as there are no allergies) and given their potential benefits, it is reasonable to include mushrooms and turmeric as part of the integrative management of Hashimoto's thyroiditis.

LEAKY GUT AND PROBIOTICS

Alterations in the intestinal microbiome and increased intestinal permeability have been postulated as the missing link in the increased incidence of autoimmune conditions seen in developed nations (Canche-Pool et al., 2008). Although researchers have suggested the presence of a "leaky gut" in Hashimoto's thyroiditis, the association between Hashimoto's and altered human microflora has not been studied extensively and the use of probiotics has not been evaluated clinically (Mori, Nakagawa, & Ozaki, 2012).

OTHER

Low-Dose Naltrexone

In thyroid forums, there are individual cases of improvement with low-dose naltrexone in patients with Hashimoto's thyroiditis. A literature search revealed preliminary data in patients with Crohn's disease and patients with fibromyalgia but no studies in patients with Hashimoto's. So, at this time, no valid recommendations can be made with regards to this off-label use.

Dehydroepiandrosterone

In patients with Hashimoto's thyroiditis, one study noted that dehydroepiandrosterone sulfate (DHEA-S) decreased natural killer cell activity (Solerte, et al., 2005). Although DHEA has been found to be clinically beneficial in other autoimmune conditions, such as systemic lupus erythematosus, to date, DHEA has not been evaluated clinically in patients with Hashimoto's.

There are herbal treatments touted to improve hypothyroidism; not all are specific for Hashimoto's.

Botanicals

Ashwagandha (*Withania somnifera*) from the Ayurvedic tradition is used as a calming adaptogen (e.g., herb purported to help the body withstand environmental and physiologic stressors), anti-inflammatory, and immunomodulator. In mice, at doses of 1.4 g/kg, ashwagandha administered through lavage increased T4 and T3 concentrations in one study and only T4 in another (Panda & Kar, 1999b; Panda & Kar, 1998a) without effects on T4 to T3 conversion. There is one poorly documented case report of a woman with chronic fatigue who developed thyrotoxicosis while taking ashwagandha and whose thyrotoxicosis resolved after discontinuing the preparation (Van der Hooft, Hoeskstra, Winter, de Smet, & Stricker, 2005). Although we cannot exclude the possibility that ashwagandha caused thyrotoxicosis in this woman, the constituents of the preparation she was taking were never determined. Therefore, we cannot exclude adulteration with thyroid hormone. My recommendation is that if you use ashwagandha, monitor T4 and T3 6 weeks after initiation of therapy and every 3 to 6 months afterward. In my practice, I use ashwagandha root in patients who have Hashimoto's and anxiety and have noted significant clinical improvement, without detrimental effects on thyroid tests.

Bacopa (*Bacopa monnieri*) is an herb with nootropic properties. In a single animal study, 200 mg/kg of bacopa leaf extract stimulated the production of T4 (Kar, Panda, & Bharti, 2002). There are no human trials of bacopa and no studies in hypothyroid animals.

Bladderwrack (*Fucus vesiculosus*), or sea kelp, is a type of seaweed and source (albeit variable) of iodine. So, it might be of help in cases of hypothyroidism caused by low iodine. For those with Hashimoto's thyroiditis, taking excess iodine, as in bladderwrack, might cause hypothyroidism (see earlier section on iodine and Hashimoto's thyroiditis).

Coleus (*Coleus forskohlii*) has been used in Ayurvedic medicine to treat asthma, heart disease, and hypothyroidism. Forskolin, a diterpene compound, has been found to stimulate adenylate cyclase in thyroid tissue (Ealey, Kohn, Marshall, & Ekins, 1985). However, a randomized, double-blind, placebo-controlled 12-week trial failed to document any change in body composition or thyroid hormones in mildly overweight women taking 250 mg per day of Coleus extract (10% forskolin) (Henderson et al., 2005). Coleus induces CYP3A4, so caution is advised if using with medications metabolized through this system.

Guggul (*Commiphora mukul*) is a shrub common to northern India and revered in Ayurvedic medicine for its anti-inflammatory and anti-obesity effects. (Z)-guggulsterone, a ketosteroid, is one of the active constituents derived from its oleo-resin. (Z)-guggulsterone stimulates thyroid function in rats (Tripathi et al., 1988), and an alcoholic extract of the resin (guggulu) stimulates liver T3 production in mice (Panda & Kar, 1999a) and ameliorates drug-induced hypothyroidism in mice (Panda & Kar, 2005). However, there are no studies evaluating the thyroidal effects in humans.

Haizao Yuhu is a traditional Chinese medicine formula containing hijiki seaweed (*Sargassum fusiforme*) and licorice root (*Glycyrrhiza uralensis*), among others. A recent evaluation of the bioactives in Haizao Yuhu in a rat model of autoimmune thyroiditis revealed the potential effects of hijiki and licorice on immunomodulation (Song et al., 2011). While hijiki contains high amounts of iodine and the expected effect in Hashimoto's thyroiditis would be one of goiter or hypothyroidism induction, other metabolites within the formula may inhibit the growth of the thyroid gland caused by excess iodine and improve immune function.

Holy basil (*Ocimum sanctum*) is frequently found in nutritional supplements engineered to support thyroid function, even though a mouse study using 500 mg/kg of the aqueous extract found a reduction in serum thyroxine (T4) concentrations (Panda & Kar, 1998b). No data are available regarding any direct effects of holy basil on the thyroid gland or thyroid function. Holy basil is considered an anti-stress herbal remedy with hypoglycemic effects, and has been found to have antioxidant effects. At this point, there is not enough data to determine whether holy basil has a significant effect on thyroid function.

Note: Issues of Adulteration. In a recent study, nine of ten tested "thyroid supplements" contained T4 or T3, some in enough quantities as to cause hyperthyroidism (Kang et al., 2013). Therefore when advising patients regarding the use of supplements, caution is recommended.

Endocrine-Disrupting Chemicals

Endocrine-disrupting chemicals (EDCs) encompass chemicals that interfere with hormone action. Most are designed for industrial purposes, others are found in some natural foods and may be more concentrated in processed foods or can contaminate foods during processing or storage.

Among the potential environmental triggers of Hashimoto's thyroiditis are chemicals such as bromine, polyhalogenated biphenyls—which include polychlorinated biphenyls (PCB) and polybrominated biphenyls (PBB)—and polyaromated hydrocarbons (pollutants produced from coal) (Burek & Talor, 2009). The challenges inherent to EDCs include that susceptibility, exposure, half-life, and persistence are highly individual; latency between exposure and clinical disorders occurs often; and as opposed to toxic exposures, chronic exposure to low amounts of a mixture of EDCs is common.

The EDCs can be classified according to their mechanism of action; those that act through the sodium iodine symporter (the sodium-potassium pump) can potentially be eliminated or mitigated by including dietary iodine.

Sodium Iodine Symporter Inhibition

Perchlorate, thiocyanate, and nitrate are anions that competitively inhibit the sodium iodine symporter (NIS) and, thus, decrease the transport of iodide into the thyroid. Exposure to all three NIS inhibitors occurs both through natural and anthropogenic sources. Prolonged inhibition of NIS is thought to cause thyroid hypertrophy or hyperplasia, and hypothyroidism, a similar effect to that of mild to moderate iodine deficiency (Tarone, Lipworth, & McLaughlin, 2010).

Perchlorate sources in the United States include drinking and irrigation water, tobacco, alfalfa, tomato, cow's milk, cucumber, lettuce, soybeans, eggs, and multiple vitamins (including prenatal vitamins). The effect is through a potent, competitive inhibitor of sodium iodine symporter in thyroid and lactating breast. Perchlorate occurs naturally worldwide at low levels and has been detected at very low levels in the US food supply. It has also been detected in some US water sources as a result of industrial uses of perchlorate as a component of rocket fuel, munitions, and fireworks.

There are mixed data regarding an association with thyroid levels. Although most studies do not support an association between perchlorate and thyroid function, two studies have (Blount, Pirkle, Osterloh, Valentin-Blasini, & Caldwell, 2006, Cao et al., 2010; E. Pearce et al., 2010). Of note, subjects had similar urine perchlorate levels in two contradictory studies, suggesting that other factors may be at play.

Cigarette smoke is a major source of thiocyanate, a metabolite of cyanide, and weak inhibitor of the NIS. Although thiocyanate is about 15 times less potent than perchlorate as a NIS competitor, there are positive studies showing an association between current smoking during pregnancy and lower free T4 in the first trimester (E. Pearce et al., 2008), and smoking and low iodine in breast milk in women with iodine deficiency (Laurberg, Nøhr, Pedersen, & Fuglsang, 2004). Thiocyanate has a longer half-life (~6 days) than perchlorate or nitrate (~6–8 hours or 5 hours, respectively).

Nitrate is ubiquitous in foods, either naturally as in greens or added as a preservative in processed meats. Nitrate is also common in water sources, primarily due to nitrate fertilizer in agriculture. Nitrate is about 240 times less potent than perchlorate as a competitive inhibitor of NIS. In areas of high nitrate the following has been observed: thyroid dysfunction in pregnant women (Gatseva & Argirova, 2008) and goiter and subclinical hypothyroidism in children from an iodine-sufficient area (Tajtakova et al., 2006).

Phthalates are found in plasticizers, adhesives, and solvents. The effect on the thyroid is via inhibition of the sodium iodine symporter (Meeker & Ferguson, 2011).

Endocrine-Disrupting Chemicals Acting via Other Mechanisms

Bisphenol A (BPA) can be found in epoxy resins in food cans, some plastics, and dental sealants. It is thought that BPA exerts its effect by altering thyroid signaling, as it binds to the thyroid receptor. Although there are no human data for BPA, in rats BPA causes a clinical picture similar to the thyroid resistance syndrome.

Triclosan, often found in antibacterial soaps and other products, may interfere with thyroid function. There are no human data, but in a rat model, triclosan decreased thyroxine levels.

Polychlorinated biphenyls (PCBs) affect deiodinase activity and bind to the thyroid receptor. While PCBs were outlawed in the United States in 1979, and their levels have decreased, they persist and remain widespread in the environment and the food chain. Human PCB exposure is primarily through food sources, especially fish. Their biological half-life in humans is up to 7 years. The structure of PCBs is similar to thyroid hormone, and they bind the thyroid hormone receptor, acting as either agonist or antagonist. In 334 pregnant women in California, PCB exposure was inversely correlated with serum free T4 (Chevrier, Eskenazi, Holland, Bradman, & Barr, 2008). Prenatal exposure to PCBs is associated with decreased cognitive function in children. The theory is that PCB exposure induces a state of relative hypothyroidism in the brain.

Some experts feel that our exposure to endocrine disruptors is a likely cause of the increase in autoimmune thyroid disease. Although there are inherent difficulties in determining the effect of any single endocrine disruptor because we are exposed to many, individuals at risk for autoimmune disease should limit their exposure as able. Educating patients about BPA-free cans, testing well water, and reducing the exposure to chemicals in the work environment is good practice (Brent, 2010). Recommending regular sufficient iodine (to reduce the effect of toxins that compete with iodine uptake) while avoiding excessive iodine is a plus.

STRESS AND THE MIND–BODY CONNECTION

Although stress has been postulated as a risk factor for the development of autoimmune thyroid disease, especially Graves' disease (and the recovery from stress potentially with Hashimoto's thyroiditis), clear evidence is lacking. In one study (Effraimidis, Tijssen, Brosschot, & Wiersinga, 2012), subjects with a high familial predisposition to autoimmune thyroid disease were followed and stressful events recorded. No difference in stress exposure was found between those who developed thyroid antibodies and those who did not.

Few studies have explored the effects of yogic practices in patients with hypothyroidism. Yoga practiced 1 hour daily for a month improved quality of life in hypothyroid women who were taking thyroid hormone (Singh, Singh, Dave, & Udainiya, 2011).

HYPOTHALAMIC-PITUITARY-ADRENAL AXIS DYSFUNCTION AND ATYPICAL DEPRESSION

Atypical depression is characterized by lethargy, fatigue, hypersomnia, hyperphagia, and a down-regulated hypothalamic-pituitary-adrenal (HPA) axis and corticotropin-releasing hormone (CRH) deficiency (Gold, & Chrousos, 2002).

Some of these symptoms are present and persist in hypothyroid patients with underlying Hashimoto's regardless of treatment. Although hypothyroidism is known to cause a dysfunction of the HPA axis with CRH deficiency, it is not known if Hashimoto's is as well. Whether the use of adaptogens or mind–body techniques might be beneficial in this situation has not been studied. In my practice, I frequently add an adaptogen and/or breathing and other relaxation techniques to the integrative treatment of a patient with Hashimoto's thyroiditis.

Iodine Deficiency and Other Nutrients Important for Thyroid Function

Some patients will present with an elevated TSH and or goiter but negative antibodies and no family or personal history suggestive of thyroid disease. Others might present with abnormal thyroid function tests, such as an elevated reverse T3. In these patients one should evaluate iodine and other potential coexisting nutritional deficiencies.

IODINE

Iodine deficiency and insufficiency are increasingly being recognized in countries once thought to be iodine sufficient, such as the United States, United Kingdom, and Australia. At particular risk are subpopulations, such as vegans (Leung et al., 2011), pregnant women (Perrine et al., 2010), and young adolescents (Vanderpump et al., 2011). Therefore, it is important to be aware of the potential for iodine deficiency, to know when and how to evaluate for iodine deficiency, and how to treat with iodine.

Iodine is an essential nutrient required for thyroid hormone synthesis. It is primarily absorbed in the gastrointestinal tract as the anion iodide. Iodide is actively transported into the thyroid gland by the sodium-iodide symporter as the first step in thyroid hormone formation. Iodine requirements increase during pregnancy and lactation. Normal thyroid function in the fetus (and breast-fed infant) depends on adequate maternal dietary intake of iodine.

The spectrum of iodine deficiency disorders varies depending on the life stage when iodine deficiency occurs. During pregnancy, iodine deficiency is associated with pregnancy loss, prematurity, cretinism, and mild neurocognitive defects in the fetus. Mild to moderate iodine deficiency during pregnancy has been associated with a higher incidence of ADHD (Vermiglio et al., 2004), lower IQ in the offspring, and goiter in mother and fetus. Increasing evidence links thyroid function during pregnancy and neuropsychological development in children. Supplementation with 300 mcg/day of potassium iodide starting in the first trimester resulted in children with better psychomotor assessment at 3–18 months than children whose mothers were not supplemented until the last month of pregnancy (Velasco et al., 2009).

Biochemically, a diet very low in iodine causes a decrease in intrathyroidal iodine content, an increase in the ratio of T3 to T4, decrease in the secretion of T4, and an increase of TSH. In school-age children, iodine deficiency causes learning disability, poor growth, and diffuse goiter. In adults, the resulting syndrome is one of goiter, high iodine uptake, hypothyroidism, and low T4 secretion. Serum T3 measurement is useful for investigating iodine deficiency because the same 5'deiodinase that converts T4 to T3 in peripheral tissues is also found in the thyroid gland. When iodine deficiency is present, this enzyme may increase the amount of T3 excreted by the gland, and therefore iodine deficiency is characterized by low T4 /high T3 ratio. If reverse T3 (rT3) is measured, it tends to be low.

Iodine supplementation must be instituted for a long enough period to allow the pituitary thyroid axis to fully equilibrate (weeks to months) and offer best protection against gestational maternal goiter (Glinoer, 2001). Because iodine deficiency when correctly diagnosed is easily treatable with iodine supplementation (iodized salt or potassium iodide) and does not necessitate thyroid hormone treatment, it is imperative that clinicians be aware of this condition. The role of iodine supplementation in those already taking thyroid hormone has been studied, and an increase in serum T4 on days 1 and 14 and a decrease of serum TSH on day 1 observed (Philippou, Koutras, Piperingos, Souvatzoglou, & Moulopoulos, 1992).

GOITROGENS

A goitrogen is a food substance that blocks thyroid hormone synthesis and can exacerbate the effect of iodine deficiency. There are several types of goitrogens, perhaps the most commonly mentioned are those belonging to the Cruciferae family. The following is a list of goitrogens and the foods where they are found:

- Thiocyanate and isothiocyanate are goitrogens found in members of the Cruciferae family (cabbage, broccoli, cauliflower, Brussels sprouts).
- Goitrin (antithyroid) in yellow turnips and Brassica seeds.

- Cyanoglucosides (precursors of thiocyanate) in cassava, sweet potato, maize, lima beans, and almond seeds.
- Flavonoids exert an antithyroid effect, inhibit TPO and the peripheral metabolism of thyroid hormones, and prevent TSH action. Soy isoflavones inhibit thyroid peroxidase activity.
- C-glycosylflavones and thiocyanate in pearl millet.
- Phlorogucinol and polyhydroxyphenols are potent antithyroid compounds found in seaweeds of the genera Laminaria.
- Aliphatic disulfides from onion and garlic exert thiourea-like antithyroid activity in the rat.

Several Factors to Consider

1. Malnutrition enhances the action of goitrogens.
2. Significant consumption, in addition to iodine deficiency, seems necessary for some. For example, epidemiologic evidence suggests that ingestion of millet plays a role in the genesis of endemic goiter in areas of Africa and Asia in the semiarid tropics. Goiter is more prevalent in rural villages of the Darfur province in Sudan, where as much as 74% of dietary energy is derived from millet, than in an urban area, where millet provides only 37% of calories, even though the degree of iodine deficiency is similar in the two areas (Gaitan, 1990).

The following is a summary of the known effects of goitrogens on thyroid function.

Thiocyanate

There is higher urinary thiocyanate in vegans but no demonstrable correlation with thyroid function in spite of low urine iodine in vegans (subjects had no history of thyroid disease). The lack of correlation is perhaps due to low concentration of thiocyanate in cruciferous vegetables (Leung, Lamar, He, Braverman, & Pearce, 2011). However, the effect on subjects with thyroid autoimmunity or subclinical hypothyroidism is unknown. The thiocyanate content is low and by itself unlikely to be of clinical relevance unless in area of severe iodine deficiency or in a "cabbage-only diet." Thiocyanate is a weak competitive inhibitor of the sodium iodine symporter, therefore the goitrogenic activity can be overcome by iodine administration.

Isothiocyanate

Isothiocyanate not only uses the thiocyanate metabolic pathway but also forms derivatives with an antithyroid (thiourea-like) effect. The thionamide or thiourea-like goitrogens interfere in the thyroid gland with the organification of iodine and formation of the active thyroid hormones, and their action usually cannot be antagonized by iodine. However, cooking foods with isothiocyanate at > 118 degrees F substantially decreases the bioavailability of isothiocyanate.

Soy

Isoflavones, primarily genistein and daidzein, inhibit TPO-catalyzed iodination and coupling, therefore inhibiting thyroid hormone formation. In subjects with subclinical hypothyroidism, 30 g/day of soy providing 16 mg/day of isoflavones (representative of a vegetarian diet) for 8 weeks carried a three-fold increase in the development of overt hypothyroidism. The effects were not associated with TPO antibodies or due to iodine deficiency and were not reversible (Sathyapalan et al., 2011). Goiter has been reported in infants fed non-iodine-fortified soy formula. In contrast, a review of 14 prospective trials of the effects of soy isoflavones in healthy adult volunteers revealed either modest or no effect in 13 of the studies; one study showed marked effect (30 g/day soybeans for 1 to 3 months) (de Souza dos Santos, Goncalves, Vaisman, Ferreira, & de Carvalho, 2011). The effect might be dose mediated, and further studies are needed to help elucidate whether this is the case.

In summary, thiocyanate (such in cassava, tobacco, and cruciferous vegetables) has the potential to aggravate goiter in severely iodine-deficient areas, especially when foods that contain it are main diet staples. In the United States, most of these goitrogenic substances do not have a major clinical effect unless there is coexisting iodine deficiency. Therefore, avoiding iodine deficiency rather than these foods should be the goal. However, for those patients concerned with the potential effect of cruciferous vegetables on thyroid, cooking cruciferous vegetables at > 118 degrees F substantially decreases the bioavailability of isothiocyanate. Isoflavones at a dose of 16 mg/day seem to accelerate course to overt hypothyroidism in patients with subclinical hypothyroidism.

Iron

Iron forms part of the TPO enzyme, a heme protein necessary in thyroid hormone synthesis. The importance of iron in thyroid function is reflected in studies of children with iron deficiency who reside in areas of iodine deficiency. Treatment of both iodine and iron deficiencies improved goiter more than iodine alone in those children (Zimmermann, 2006).

Zinc

Although zinc is important for normal thyroid hormone production, studies have not found consistent results of the effects of zinc deficiency on thyroid metabolism. One study has shown an inverse relationship between levels of zinc and thyroid volume in patients with nodular goiter (Ertek et al., 2010). Zinc is a mineral found in yeast, whole grains, nuts (almonds, peanuts, soy nuts) and seeds (pumpkin, sunflower), tofu, legumes (lentils), oysters, beef, crab, seafood, and poultry.

Vitamin A

The effects of vitamin A on thyroid metabolism are multiple. Vitamin A deficiency has been associated with goiter, decreased thyroidal uptake of iodine, decreased intrathyroidal T4 and T3, and decreased T4 to T3 conversion. In African children with mild to moderate vitamin A deficiency and goiter, vitamin A supplementation decreased goiter, TSH, and thyroglobulin. It is not clear from current data whether the effects of vitamin A supplementation are additive to the effects of iodine when both vitamin A and iodine deficiency coexist (Zimmermann et al., 2007). In the United States, vitamin A deficiency occurs in low-income children and pregnant women (World Health Organization, 2009) or those with fat malabsorption; and if goiter is found in those populations, measuring vitamin A might be cost-effective. Otherwise, the US population is considered vitamin A replete. In my practice, I think of vitamin A status when seeing a patient with borderline thyroid function (high TSH), negative antibodies, and normal iodine intake; especially when T3 is in the low range and reverse T3 is elevated. I measure vitamin A prior to treating patients if I am concerned about true nutritional deficiency or malabsorption.

B vitamins

Excess vitamin B6 has been associated with low TSH in humans (Sworczak 2011). In general, no consistent data are available regarding vitamin B status and thyroid function and there are no studies evaluating the effects of vitamin B supplementation on thyroid function.

Selenium

Deficiency of selenium may be linked to an increase in the incidence of thyroiditis by decreasing the activity of deiodinase isoenzymes, causing an elevated T4 and low T3. Deficiency of selenium exacerbates the consequences of iodine deficiency. When iodine and selenium deficiency coexist, iodine deficiency should be restored first. Otherwise, one risks worsening thyroid function.

In North American regions, selenium is abundant, and most US adults consume roughly 100 mcg of selenium as part of their daily diet. Several populations have been identified at risk for selenium deficiency; those with Crohn's disease, cystic fibrosis, pancreatic insufficiency, liver disease, cholestasis, and biliary atresia, and those living in regions of low selenium in their soil: Denmark, Finland, New Zealand, Russia, and some areas of China.

Tyrosine

Tyrosine is a nonessential amino acid, which is either derived from phenylalanine or consumed in the diet. Tyrosine forms part of the thyroglobulin molecule and is essential in thyroid hormone synthesis. Tyrosine residues receive iodine, and once iodinated, when coupled together, give rise to T3 and T4. Tyrosine is found in soy products, chicken, turkey, fish, peanuts, almonds, avocados, bananas, milk, cheese, yogurt, cottage cheese, lima beans, pumpkin seeds, and sesame seeds. There are no published studies on the effects of tyrosine supplementation on thyroid function. Therefore, at this time, my recommendation is to ensure a tyrosine-rich diet for adequate thyroid hormone synthesis.

> Rebecca was evaluated for coexisting autoimmune conditions. She showed biochemical evidence of celiac disease, vitamin D deficiency, and iron deficiency without anemia. She was referred to a gastroenterologist and dietitian and started a gluten-free diet. I reviewed with her how iodine deficiency increases vulnerability to certain endocrine disruptors. During the remainder of her pregnancy, she took a brand formulation of levothyroxine. She was instructed to take iron, vitamin D, and a daily prenatal vitamin with 150 mcg of potassium iodine. After delivery, she

discontinued brand levothyroxine and began a trial of L-T4/L-T3 combination. The L-T4/L-T3 was titrated until serum TSH and free-T4/free-T3 ratio were optimal. She incorporated Brazil nuts to her diet as her source of selenium. Three months later, selenium concentration was optimal and therefore, she continued to take Brazil nuts. She began practicing a breathing technique twice daily. I saw her 6 months later, and she reported feeling significantly better. She has maintained a gluten-free diet, L-T4/L-T3 combination, vitamin D, Brazil nuts, and a prenatal vitamin with potassium iodine. Iron has been discontinued and iron studies have been normal since she adopted a gluten-free diet.

Conclusion

In summary, for a patient with Hashimoto's thyroiditis who does not feel well in spite of having a normal thyroid function, possible coexisting autoimmune conditions should be evaluated, including celiac disease, pernicious anemia, iron-deficiency anemia, and Addison's disease. Consideration should be made to treating with L-T3 in addition to L-T4 and to include strategies targeting autoimmunity, such as selenium and vitamin D supplementation, and diet. The use of herbal therapy should be individualized and the practitioner aware of potential herb–drug interactions and quality control issues. And for those with a persistently elevated TSH, but no evidence of Hashimoto's thyroiditis, clinical and biochemical evaluation for nutritional deficiencies should be evaluated. Helping patients understand the effects of goitrogens in the context of iodine sufficiency ensures our patients are able to make informed decisions. Guiding our patients toward the prevention of exposure to endocrine disrupting chemicals may have important consequences for them and future generations.

REFERENCES

Akbaraly, T. N., Arnaud, J., Rayman, M. P., et al. (2010). Plasma selenium and risk of dysglycemia in an elderly French population: Results from the prospective Epidemiology of Vascular Ageing Study. *Nutr Metab (Lond)*, *7*, 21.

Ashton, K., Hooper, L., & Harvey, L. J. (2009). Methods of assessment of selenium status in humans: A systematic review. *Am J Clin Nutr*, *89*, 2025S–2039S.

Baloch, Z., Carayon, P., Conte-Devolx, B., et al. (2003). Guidelines Committee, Laboratory Medicine Practice Guidelines: Laboratory support for the diagnosis and monitoring of thyroid disease. *Thyroid*, *13*, 3–126.

Bianco, A. C., & Casula, S. (2012). Thyroid hormone replacement therapy: Three "simple" questions, complex answers. *Eur Thyroid J, 1*, 88–98.

Bleys, J., Navas-Acien, A., & Guallar, E. (2007). Selenium and diabetes in U.S. adults. *Diabetes Care, 30*, 829–834.

Blount, B. C., Pirkle, J. L., Osterloh, J. D., Valentin-Blasini, L., & Caldwell, K. L. (2006). Urinary perchlorate and thyroid hormone levels in adolescent and adult men and women living in the United States. *Environ Health Perspect, 114*, 1865–1871.

Bolk, N., Visser, T. J., Nijman, J., et al. (2010). Effects of evening vs. morning levothyroxine intake: A randomized double-blind crossover trial. *Arch Intern Med, 170*, 1996–2003.

Brent, G. (2010). Environmental exposures and autoimmune thyroid disease. *Thyroid, 20*, 755–761.

Burek, C. L., & Talor, M. V. (2009). Environmental triggers of autoimmune thyroiditis. *J Autoimmun, 33*, 183–189.

Cao, Y., Blount, B. C., Pirkle, J. L., Osterloh, J. D., Valentin-Blasini, L., & Caldwell, K. L. (2006). Goitrogenic anions, thyroid stimulating hormone, and thyroid hormone in infants. *Environ Health Perspect, 118*, 1332–1337.

Canaris, G. J., Manowitz, N. R., Mayor, G., & Ridgway, E. C. (2000). The Colorado thyroid disease prevalence study. *Arch Intern Med, 160*, 526–534.

Canche-Pool, E. B., Cortez-Gomez, R., Flores-Mejia, R., et al. (2008). Probiotics and autoimmunity: An evolutionary perspective. *Medical Hypotheses, 70*, 657–660.

Ch'ng, C. L., Keston Jones, M., & Kingham, J. G. C. (2007). Celiac disease and autoimmune thyroid disease. *Clinical Medicine and Research, 5*, 184–192.

Chevrier, J., Eskenazi, B., Holland, N., Bradman, A., & Barr, D. B. (2008). Effects of exposure to polychlorinated biphenyls and organochlorine pesticides on thyroid function during pregnancy. *Am J Epidemiol, 168*, 298–310.

Cooper, D. S., & Biondi, B. (2012). Subclinical thyroid disease. *Lancet, 379*, 1142–1154.

de Souza dos Santos, M. C., Goncalves, C. F., Vaisman, M., Ferreira, A. C., & de Carvalho, D. P. (2011). Impact of flavonoids on thyroid function. *Food and Chemical Toxicology, 49*, 2495–2502.

Duntas, L. H. (2010). Selenium and the thyroid. *J Clin Endocrinol Metab, 95*, 5180–5185.

Ealey, P. A., Kohn, L. D., Marshall, N. J., & Ekins, R. P. (1985). Forskolin stimulation of naphthylamidase in guinea pig thyroid sections detected with a cytochemical bioassay. *Acta Endocrinol (Copenhag), 108*, 367–371.

Effraimidis, G., Badenhoop, K., Tijssen, J. G., & Wiersinga, W. M. (2012). Vitamin D deficiency is not associated with early stages of thyroid autoimmunity. *Eur J Endocrinol, 167*, 43–48.

Effraimidis, G., Tijssen, J. G., Brosschot, J. F., & Wiersinga, W. M. (2012). Involvement of stress in the pathogenesis of autoimmune thyroid disease: A prospective study. *Psychoneuroendocrinology, 37*, 1191–1198.

Ertek, S., Cicero, A. F. G., Caglar, A., et al. (2010). Relationship between serum zinc levels, thyroid hormones, and thyroid volumes following successful iodine supplementation. *Hormones, 9*, 263–268.

Escobar-Morreale, H. F., Botella-Carretero, J. I., Gomez-Bueno, M., et al. (2005). Thyroid hormone replacement therapy in primary hypothyroidism: A randomized trial comparing L-thyroxine plus liothyronine with L-thyroxine alone. *Ann Intern Med, 142,* 412–424.

Feng, M., Li, H., Cheng, S. F., Li, W. F., & Zhang, F. B. (2013). Polymorphisms in the vitamin D receptor gene and risk of autoimmune thyroid disease: A meta-analysis. *Endocrine, 43,* 318–326.

Gaitan, E. (1990). Goitrogens in food and water. *Ann Rev Nutr, 10,* 21–39.

Garber, J. R., Cobin, R. H., Gharib, H., et al. (2012). Clinical practice guidelines for hypothyroidism in adults: Cosponsored by the American Association of Clinical Endocrinologists and the American Thyroid Association. *Endocrine Practice, 18,* 988–1028.

Gatseva, P. D., & Argirova, M. D. (2008). High-nitrate levels in drinking water may be a risk factor for thyroid dysfunction in children and pregnant women living in rural Bulgarian areas. *Int J Hyg Environ Health, 211,* 555–559.

Glinoer, D. (2001). Pregnancy and iodine. *Thyroid, 11,* 471–481.

Gold, P. W., & Chrousos, G. P. (2002). Organization of the stress system and its dys-regulation in melancholic an atypical depression: High vs low CRH/NE states. *Molecular Psychiatry, 7,* 254–275.

Groer, M. W., & Vaughan, J. H. (2013). Positive thyroid peroxidase antibody titer is associated with dysphoric moods during pregnancy and postpartum. *J Obstet Gynecol Neonatal Nurs, 42,* E26–E32.

Grozinsky-Glasberg, S., Fraser, A., Nahshoni, E., et al. (2006). Thyroxine-triiodothyronine combination therapy versus thyroxine monotherapy for clinical hypothyroid-ism: Meta-analysis of randomized controlled trials. *J Clin Endocrinol Metab, 91,* 2592–2599.

Henderson, S., Magu, B., Rasmussen, C., et al. (2005). Effects of coleus forskohlii supplementation on body composition and hematological profiles in mildly over-weight women. *J Int Soc Sports Nutr, 2,* 54–62.

Hennemann, G., Docter, R., Visser, T. J., Postema, P. T., & Krenning, E. P. (2004). Thyroxine plus low dose, slow-release triiodothyronine replacement in hypothy-roidism: Proof of principle. *Thyroid, 14,* 271–275.

Hollowell, J. G., Stachling, N. W., Flanders, W. D., et al. (2002). Serum TSH, T(4), and thyroid antibodies in the United States population (1988 to 1994); National Health and Nutrition Examination Survey (NHANES III). *J Clin Endocrinol Metab, 87,* 489–499.

Kang, G. Y., Parks, J. R., Fileta B, Chang, A., Abdel-Rahim, M. M., Burch, H. B., & Bernet, V. J. (2013). *Thyroid, 23,* 1233–1237.

Kar, A., Panda, S., & Bharti, S. (2002). Relative efficacy of three medicinal plant extracts in the alteration of thyroid hormone concentrations in male mice. *J Ethnopharmacol, 81,* 281–285.

Kivity, S., Agmon-Levin, S., Zisappl, M., et al. (2011). Vitamin D and autoimmune thy-roid diseases. *Cellular and Molecular Immunology, 8,* 243–247.

Laurberg, P., Nøhr, S. B., Pedersen, K. M., & Fuglsang, E. (2004). Iodine nutrition in breast-fed infants is impaired by maternal smoking. *J Clin Endocrinol Metab, 89,* 181.

Leung, A. M., Lamar, A., He, X., Braverman, L. E., & Pearce, E. N. (2011). Iodine status and thyroid function of Boston-area vegetarians and vegans. *J Clin Endocrinol Metab*, *96*, E1303–E1307.

Leung, A. M., LaMar, A., He, X., et al. (2011). Iodine status and thyroid function of Boston-area vegetarians and vegans. *J Clin Endocrinol Metab*, *96*, e1303–e1307.

Li, D., Cai, W., Gu, R., et al. (2013). Th17 cell plays a role in the pathogenesis of Hashimoto's thyroiditis in patients. *Clin Immunol*, *149*, 411–420.

Li, Y., Teng, D., Shan, Z., et al. (2008). Antithyroid peroxidase and antithyroglobulin antibodies in a five-year follow-up survey of populations with different iodine intakes. *J Clin Endocrinol Metab*, *93*, 1751–1757.

Ma, C., Xie, J., Huang, X., et al. (2009). Thyroxine alone or thyroxine plus triiodothyronine replacement for hypothyroidism. *Nucl Med Commun*, *30*, 586–593.

Meeker, J. D., & Ferguson, K. K. (2011). Relationship between urinary phthalate and bisphenol A concentrations and serum thyroid measures in US adults and adolescents from NHANES 2007–2008. *Environ Health Perspect*. *119*(10), 1396–1402

Metso, S., Hyytiä-Ilmonen, H., & Kaukinen, K., et al. (2012). Gluten-free diet and autoimmune thyroiditis in patients with celiac disease. A prospective controlled study. *Scand J Gastroenterol*, *47*, 43–48.

Mori, K., Nakagawa, Y., & Ozaki, H. (2012). Does the gut microbiota trigger Hashimoto's thyroiditis? *Discov Med*, *14*, 321–326. PMID: 23200063.

Mussig, K., Thamer, C., Bares, R., Lipp, H. P., Haring, H. U., & Gallwitz, B. (2006). Iodine-induced thyrotoxicosis after ingestion of kelp-containing tea. *J Gen Intern Med*, *21*, C11–C14.

Nygaard, B., Jensen, E. W., Kvetny, J., et al. (2009). Effect of combination therapy with thyroxine (T4) and 3,5.3'-triiodothyronine versus T4 monotherapy in patients with hypothyroidism, a double-blind, randomized cross-over study. *Eur J Endocrinol*, *161*, 895–902. PMID: 19666698.

Selenium. Dietary Supplement Fact Sheet. Office of Dietary Supplements. National Institutes of Health (2013).

Onal, H., Keskindemirci, G., Adal, E., Ersen, A., & Korkmaz, O. (2012). Effects of selenium supplementation in the early stage of autoimmune thyroiditis in childhood: An open-label pilot study. *J Pediatr Endocrinol Metab*, *25*, 639–644.

Ott, J., Promberger, R., Kober, F., Neuhold, N., Tea, M., Huber, J. C., & Hermann, M. (2011). Hashimoto's thyroiditis affects symptom load and quality of life unrelated to hypothyroidism: A prospective case-control study in women undergoing thyroidectomy for benign goiter. *Thyroid*, *21*, 161–167.

Panda, S., & Kar, A. (1998a). Changes in thyroid hormone concentrations after administration of aswagandha root extract to adult male mice. *J Pharm Pharmacol*, *50*, 1065–1068.

Panda, S., & Kar, A. (1998b). Ocimum sanctum leaf extract in the regulation of thyroid function in the male mouse. *Pharmacological Res*, *38*, 107–110.

Panda, S., & Kar, A. (1999a). Gugulu (*Commiphora mukul*) induces triiodothyronine production: Possible involvement of lipid peroxidation. *Life Sciences, 65,* PL137–PL141.

Panda, S., & Kar, A. (1999b). *Withania somnifera* and *Bauhinia purpurea* in the regulation of circulating thyroid hormone concentrations in female mice. *J Ethnopharmacol, 67,* 233–239.

Panda, S., & Kar, A. (2005). Guggulu (*Commiphora mukul*) potentially ameliorates hypothyroidism in female mice. *Phytother Res, 19,* 78–80.

Panicker, V., Evans, J., Bjoro, T., Asvold, B. O., Dayan, C. M., & Bjerkeset, O. (2009). A paradoxical difference in relationship between anxiety and depression and thyroid function in subjects on and not on T4: Findings from the HUNT study. *Clin Endocrinol, 71,* 574–580.

Panicker, V., Saravanan, P., Vaidya, B., Evans, J., Hattersley, A. T., Frayling, T. M., & Dayan, C. M. (2009). Common variation in the DIO2 gene predicts baseline psychological well-being and response to combination thyroxine plus triiodothyronine therapy in hypothyroid patients. *J Clin Endocrinol Metab, 94,* 1623–1629.

Pearce, E. N., Lazarus, J. H., Smyth, P. P. A., et al. (2010). Perchlorate and thiocyanate exposure and thyroid function in first-trimester pregnant women. *J Clin Endocrinol Metab, 95,* 3207–3215.

Pearce, E. N., Oken, E., Gillman, M. W., Lee, S. L., Magnani, B., Platek, D., & Braverman, L. E. (2008). Association of first-trimester thyroid function test values with thyroperoxidase antibody status, smoking, and multivitamin use. *Endocr Pract, 14,* 33–39.

Pearce, S. H. S., Brabant, G., Duntas, L. H., Monzani, F., Peeters, R. P., Razvi, S., & Wemeau, J. L. (2013). ETA guideline: Management of subclinical hypothyroidism. *Eur Thyroid J* 2, 215–228.

Perrine, C. G., Herrick, K., Serdula, M. K., et al. (2010). NHANES data: Some subgroups of reproductive age women in the United States may be at risk for iodine deficiency. *J Nutr, 140,* 1489–1494. PMID: 20554903.

Philippou, G., Koutras, D. A., Piperingos, G., Souvatzoglou, A., & Moulopoulos SD. (1992). The effect of iodide on serum thyroid hormone levels in normal persons, in hyperthyroid patients, and in hypothyroid patients on thyroxine replacement. *Clin Endocrinol, 36,* 573–578.

Qin, X., Guo, B. T., Wan, B., et al. (2010). Regulation of Th1 and Th17 cell differentiation and amelioration of experimental autoimmune encephalomyelitis by natural product compound berberine. *J Immunol, 185,* 1855–1863.

Rajpathak, S., Rimm, E., Morris, J. S., et al. (2005). Toenail selenium and cardiovascular disease in men with diabetes. *J Am Coll Nutr, 24,* 250–256.

Rayman, M. P. (2012). Selenium and human health. *Lancet, 379,* 1256–1268.

Reinhardt, W., Luster, M., Rudorff, K. H., et al. (1998). Effect of small doses of iodine on thyroid function in patients with Hashimoto's thyroiditis residing in an area of mild iodine deficiency. *Eur J Endocrinol, 139,* 23–28.

Rostami, R., Aghasi, M. R., Mohammadi, A., & Nourooz-Zadeh, J. (2013). Enhanced oxidative stress in Hashimoto's thyroiditis: Inter-relationships to biomarkers of thyroid function. *Clinical Biochemistry, 46,* 308–312.

Sategna-Guidetti, C., Volta, U., Ciacci, C., et al. (2001). Prevalence of thyroid disorders in untreated adult celiac disease patients and effect of gluten withdrawal: An Italian multicenter study. *Am J Gastroenterol, 96,* 751–757.

Sathyapalan, T., Manuchehri, A. M., Thatcher, N. J., Rigby, A. S., Chapman, T., Kilpatrick, E. S., & Atkin, S. L. (2011). The effect of soy phytoestrogen supplementation on thyroid status and cardiovascular risk markers in patients with subclinical hypothyroidism: A randomized, double-blind, crossover study. *J Clin Endocrinol Metab, 96,* 1442–1449.

Singh, P., Singh, B., Dave, R., & Udainiya, R. (2011). The impact of yoga upon female patients suffering from hypothyroidism. *Complementary Therapies in Clinical Practice, 17,* 132–134.

Solerte, S. B., Precerutti, S., Gazzaruso, C., et al. (2005). Defect of a subpopulation of natural killer immune cells in Graves' disease and Hashimoto's thyroiditis: Normalizing effect of dehydroepiandrosterone sulfate. *European Journal of Endocrinology, 152,* 703–712.

Song, X. H., Zan, R. Z., Yu, Z. H., et al. (2011). Effects of modified Haizao Yuhu decoction in experimental autoimmune thyroiditis in rats. *Journal of Ethnopharmacology, 135,* 321–324.

Stranges, S., Marshall, J. R., Natarajan, R., et al. (2007). Effects of long-term selenium supplementation on the incidence of type 2 diabetes: A randomized trial. *Ann Intern Med, 147,* 217–223.

Stranges, S., Sieri, S., Vinceti, M., et al. (2010). A prospective study of dietary selenium intake and risk of type 2 diabetes. *BMC Public Health, 10,* 564.

Surks, M. I., & Hollowell, J. G. (2007). Age-specific distribution of serum thyrotropin and antithyroid antibodies in the U.S. population: Implications for the prevalence of subclinical hypothyroidism. *J Clin Endocrinol Metab, 92,* 4575–4582.

Sworczak, K. (2011). The role of vitamins in the prevention and treatment of thyroid disorders. *Pol J Endocrinol, 62,* 340–344.

Tajtakova, M., Semanova, Z., Tomkova, Z., et al. (2006). Increased thyroid volume and frequency of thyroid disorders signs in schoolchildren from nitrate polluted area. *Chemosphere, 62,* 559–564.

Tarone, R. E., Lipworth, L., & McLaughlin, J. K. (2010). The epidemiology of environmental perchlorate exposure and thyroid function: A comprehensive review. *J Occup Environ Med, 52,* 653–660.

Toulis, K. A., Anastasilakis, A. D., Tzellos, T. G., et al. (2010). Selenium supplementation in the treatment of Hashimoto's thyroiditis: A systematic review and a meta-analysis. *Thyroid, 20,* 1163–1173. PMID: 20883174.

Tripathi, Y. B., Tripathi P, Malhotra, O. P., et al. (1988). *Planta Med, 54,* 271–277. PMID: 3222368.

Valentino, R., Savastano, S., Tommaselli, A. P., et al. (1999). Prevalence of coeliac disease in patients with thyroid autoimmunity. *Horm Res, 51,* 124–127.

Van der Hooft, C. S., Hoekstra, A., Winter, A., de Smet, P. A., & Stricker, B. H. (2005). Thyrotoxicosis following the use of Ashwagandha. *Ned Tijdschr Geneeskd, 149,* 2637–2638. PMID: 1635578.

Vanderpump, M. P., Lazarus, J. H., et al. (2011). Iodine status of UK school-girls: A cross-sectional survey. *Lancet, 377*, 2007–2012.

Velasco, I., Carreira, M., Santiago, P., et al. (2009). Effect of iodine prophylaxis during pregnancy on neurocognitive development of children during the first two years of life. *J Clin Endocrinol Metab, 92*, 3234–3241. PMID: 19567536.

Ventura, A., Neri, E., Ughi, C., et al. (2000). Gluten-dependent diabetes-related thyroid-related autoantibodies in patients with celiac disease. *J Pediatr, 137*, 263–265.

Vermiglio, F., Lo Presti, V. P., Moleti, M., et al. (2004). Attention deficit and hyperactivity disorders in the offspring of mothers exposed to mild-moderate iodine deficiency: A possible novel iodine deficiency disorder in developed countries. *J Clin Endocrinol Metab 89*, 6054–6060, 2004. PMID: 15579758.

Virili, C., Bassotti, G., Santaguida, M. G, et al. (2012). Atypical celiac disease as cause of increased need for thyroxine: A systematic study. *J Clin Endocrinol Metab, 97*, E419–E422.

Wartofsky, L., & Dickey, R. A. (2005). The evidence for a narrow TSH range is compelling. *J Clin Endocrinol Metab, 90*, 5483–5488.

Watt, T., Hegedus, L., Bjorner, J. B., Groenvold, M., Bonnema, S. J., Rasmussen, A. K., & Feldt-Rasmussen, N. (2012). Is thyroid autoimmunity per se a determinant of quality of life in patients with autoimmune hypothyroidism? *Eur Thyroid J, 1*, 186–192.

Wiersinga, W. M., Duntas, L., Fadeyev, V., Nygaard, B., & Vanderpump, M. P. J. (2012). ETA guidelines: The use of LT4 + LT3 in the treatment of hypothyroidism. *Eur Thyroid J, 1*, 55–71.

World Health Organization. (2009). Global prevalence of vitamin A deficiency in populations at risk 1995–2005. WHO Global Database on Vitamin A Deficiency. Geneva, Switzerland: Author.

Yoon, S. J., Choi, S. R., Kim, D. M., et al. (2003). The effect of iodine restriction on thryoid function in patients with hypothyroidism due to Hashimoto's thyroiditis. *Yonsei Medical Journal, 44*, 227–235.

Zimmermann, M. B. (2006). The influence of iron status on iodine utilization and thyroid function. *Ann Rev Nutr, 26*, 367–389.

Zimmermann, M. B., Jooste, P. L., Mabapa, N. S., Schoeman, S., Biebinger, R., Mushaphi, L. F., & Mbhenyane, X. (2007). Vitamin A supplementation in iodine-deficient African children decreases thyrotropin stimulation of the thyroid and reduces the goiter rate. *Am J Clin Nutr, 86*, 1040–1044.

23

Anxiety

ROBERTA LEE

CASE STUDY

April is a patient that I have worked with for 3 years. At 49 years, she had seen her share of difficult times. We had spent the last 3 months unraveling the significance of her difficulties on her health. A year ago, this mother of three robust children with a very supportive husband lost her youngest child to leukemia. The loss came suddenly. Her healthy son began experiencing illness after a viral illness, then chronic fatigue, and finally a devastating bone marrow cancer. The cancer was very aggressive and he failed chemotherapy, an unusual outcome. She felt very guilty about his death. In her family, she was the major wage earner, spending an average of 30% of her time traveling as a business executive in sales. It was not a surprise to hear her express guilt concerning her absences in her son's life and this was compounded by profound grief—all very normal reactions for such a difficult situation. Early on, we decided that she and her family would benefit greatly in airing the feelings they were struggling with by having a family therapist. She continued these sessions but experienced many challenging symptoms despite her active involvement in making sense of this loss. The primary feeling she experienced was anxiety. She had reoccurring thoughts that she might lose one of her other children to cancer. When this dread surfaced, she noticed a particular order of sensations. The day before she would be irritable, that night she would have difficulty sleeping and wake up from what seemed like hot flashes—and it all was much more dramatic on her travel away from home. When this happened, she also had a tougher time with her periods and her cycles seemed heavier. Often she would notice very dramatic bloating, cramping, and irritability several days before her period started. When I asked her what her diet was like—she sheepishly admitted that desserts and pasta were becoming a reward food on her travels—her weight was beginning to climb. She was "too tired" to keep up her walking routine and stopped her 45-minute walks, which she had done with a friend 4 days a week. I had her take the Hamilton Anxiety Rating test. April's score was 23 (range mild anxiety: 18+, moderate anxiety: 25+: severe anxiety: 30+). Her focus was "home and work, work and home"—gone were any lunches or even much conversation with her girlfriends. Much as she hated to admit it—she felt "imprisoned" by the routine. Lately, it was difficult to focus on work—she was simply too agitated.

Her treatment involved a full medical workup to exclude any medical diagnosis that would mimic these symptoms, for example, undiagnosed hypothyroidism or hypercortisolism. The next objective was to "rebalance her lifestyle routines." We put together a sleep ritual that included no e-mails or other electronic communication 1 hour prior to retiring, a hot bath and use of the essential oil of lavender (five drops in the tub). Her bedroom was cluttered and thus on one weekend, she made a commitment to remove all work-related things in the bedroom. Next, we established a general time of going to bed and waking up when at home. Her work life demanded frequent meals out and travel. We looked at her typical menus and selected potential food choices that were healthier. An exercise plan was formulated using a pedometer to assess distances achieved. She was able to initiate 10,000 steps 4 days a week. Several micronutrients were low on her lab tests: vitamin B12, magnesium, and vitamin D (25-hydroxy cholecalciferol). She was advised to start the following supplements: magnesium glycinate 200 mg/day, vitamin D3 2000 IU/day, and vitamin B12 1,000 μg/day sublingually. We reconstructed her diet and made a menu plan with the objective that she would stick to a Mediterranean diet increasing the use of olive oil, fish, whole grains, fruits, and vegetables. We blocked out her schedule so she had time to communicate regularly either in phone or in person with friends at least once a week. In 4 months, her HAM-A scale dropped to 10 (normal).

Introduction

Anxiety disorders affect approximately 40 million American adults or 18% of the population in a given year (Kessler, Chiu, Demler, & Walters, 2005). Anxiety disorders are categorized into subtypes: panic disorder, obsessive-compulsive disorder (OCD), posttraumatic stress disorder (PTSD), social phobia, specific phobia, and generalized anxiety disorder (GAD). Each anxiety disorder has different symptoms, but all share a commonality of excessive dread and irrational fear. According to prevalence estimates, women are twice as likely as men to suffer from generalized anxiety, panic disorder, social phobias, and so on. This chapter focuses on GAD.

The estimated lifetime prevalence of GAD is 4.1%. In a primary care setting, the prevalence of GAD is approximately 5%–8% (Kessler, Berglund, et al., 2005). Patients with GAD predominantly present with somatic symptoms (Hettema, Prescott, Myers, Neale, & Kendler, 2005).

In the National Comorbidity survey, patients with GAD were also shown to have a number of comorbid psychiatric diagnoses including social phobia, specific phobia, panic disorder, and major depression (Wittchen, Zhao, Kessler, & Eaton, et al., 1994; Table 23.1).

Approximately 40% of people with GAD have no comorbid conditions, but many develop another disorder as time evolves (Schweitzer, 1995). Psychiatric overlap is common. In fact, concurrent or coexistent organic or psychiatric disease is the rule rather than the exception in patients with GAD (Wittchen et al., 2011). For example, panic disorder is common among patients with irritable bowel syndrome (Solmaz, Kavuk, & Sayar, 2003). Anxiety disorders and depression frequently coincide—either can trigger the other. In the case of coexisting major depression, treatment of the depression is the primary objective. Subsequent visits will reveal whether the anxiety is relieved by addressing the depression. Many persons coping with anxiety use alcohol or drugs to mask their distress. About 30% of people with panic disorder abuse alcohol, while roughly 17% use drugs (Bradya, Haynes, Hartwell, & Killeen, 2013).

Table 23.1. Medical Conditions Often Associated with the Symptoms of Anxiety

Cardiovascular	Hematologic
Acute myocardial infarction	Anemia
Angina pectoris	Chronic immune disease
Arrhythmias	*Neurologic*
Congestive heart failure	Brain tumor
Hypertension	Delirium
Ischemic heart disease	Encephalopathy
Mitral valve prolapse	Epilepsy
Endocrine	Parkinson disease
Carcinoid syndrome	Seizure disorder
Cushing's disease	Vertigo
Hyperthyroidism	Transient ischemic attack
Hypoglycemia	*Respiratory*
Parathyroid disease	Asthma
Pheochromocytoma	Chronic obstructive pulmonary disease
Porphyria	Pulmonary embolism
Electrolyte imbalance	Dyspnea
Gastrointestinal	Pulmonary embolism
Irritable bowel syndrome	
Gynecologic	
Menopause	
Premenstrual syndrome	

Source: Adapted from Rakel (2012).

Pathophysiology

Generalized anxiety disorder is characterized by maladaptive responses to stressful stimuli and is multifactorial in etiology. Proposed theories include hypothalamic-pituitary-adrenal axis abnormalities with some link to the gut-brain neuropeptide cholecystokinin (Rotzinger & Vaccarino, 2003). An imbalance of neurotransmitters—norepinephrine, serotonin, gamma-aminobutyric acid (GABA)—has also been postulated (Stewart et al., 2001). The amygdala is part of the limbic system and plays a primary role in the processing and memory of emotional reactions. The memories of danger and fear stored in the amygdala appear to be indelible, thus creating a pathophysiologic phenomenon that may progress to GAD (Stewart et al., 2001).

Genetic factors have a modest link in GAD. Some studies suggest a 30% heritability of GAD. Studies indicate genetic concordance with certain genetic loci that produce functional serotonin polymorphisms (Osher, Javer, & Benjamin, 2000). The early environment also represents an important influence that affects genetic expression. One study reported that childhood adversity was associated with the emergence of GAD. Witnessing trauma in childhood was also linked with the development of GAD later in life (McFarlane, Groff, O'Brien, & Watson, 2003).

Medical causes may also be the primary reason for an anxiety state and should be excluded. These include hyperthyroidism and premenstrual syndrome (see Table 23.1) among others. In addition, assess for and discontinue medications that cause overstimulation such as albuterol, caffeine, pseudoephedrine, methylphenidate, phentermine, sibutramine, haloperidol, and acetazolamide, to name a few.

Diagnosis

The diagnostic criteria for GAD as defined by most psychiatric references requires the following (Williams et al., 2014):

- Excessive anxiety and worry about a number of events or activities, occurring more days that not for at least 6 months, worry is difficult to control,
- The anxiety and worry are associated with three (or more) of the following six symptoms (with at least some symptoms present for more days than not for the past 6 months):
  - Restlessness
  - Easy fatiguability
  - Difficulty concentrating
  - Irritability
  - Muscle tension
  - Sleep disturbance

Integrative Treatment

The following four steps are recommended for initial management of patients with GAD in conjunction with cognitive-behavioral therapy (CBT); use of either conventional medications or dietary supplements and botanicals. The approach focuses on addressing the mind–body–spirit continuum within the context of integrative care:

1. Remove exacerbating factors.
   Review of current medications and supplements that could contribute to anxiety (i.e., over-the-counter stimulants, botanical products designed for weight loss or "energy" enhancement). Caffeine and alcohol should be avoided.
2. Screen for diseases that mimic anxiety.
   Screening for underlying medical conditions that produce anxiety—for instance, hyperthyroidism or a withdrawal syndrome—should be done.
3. Institute physical activity.
   Physical activity (aerobic or anaerobic), at least 5 days out of 7 for 40 minutes, that is enjoyable to the patient.
4. Improve nutrition.
   Nutritional support such as with omega-3 fatty acid supplementation (two to three servings of cold water fish per week, or flaxseed oil 2 tablespoons a day or 1,000 mg of flaxseed oil in a capsule) is recommended.

EXERCISE

Numerous studies assessing the effects of exercise on anxiety have been published. The majority of these studies measured the effects of exercise on the presence of signs and symptoms of anxiety rather than with use of a diagnostic system like that of the DSM (Paluska & Schwenk, 2000). Nonetheless, most studies generally show a reduction in symptoms with increased physical activity.

Aerobic exercise programs produced a larger treatment effect than activities such as weight-training and flexibility regimens, although both demonstrate effectiveness in the improvement of mood (Paluska & Schwenk, 2000). The duration of physical activity is relevant. In one study, programs exceeding 12 minutes for a minimum of 10 weeks were required to achieve significant anxiety reduction. The beneficial effect appeared to be maximal with 40 minutes per session (Paluska & Schwenk, 2000), and the benefits were lasting.

Why exercise improves mood is not completely understood. However, increased physical activity has been correlated with changes in brain levels of norepinephrine, dopamine, and serotonin, which may account for improved mood (Anderson & Shivarkumar, 2013; Dunn & Dishman, 1991). Many studies have shown significant endorphin secretion with increased exercise, with beneficial effects on state of mind. But blockade of endorphin elevation with antagonists such as naloxone during exercise does not correlate with decreased mental health benefits (Anderson & Shivarkumar, 2013; Dunn & Dishman, 1991). This suggests that other factors may also be influential in mood improvement. Another neurotransmitter or neurotrophin, brain-derived neurotrophic factor (BDNF), has been linked to both anxiety and depression. Brain-derived neurotrophic factor is one of the most abundant neurotrophins in the brain and is found to be at low levels in the hippocampus in both anxiety and depression. In animal studies, with sustained exercise BDNF increases, and it has been proposed as an alternate mechanism accounting for improvement of mood with exercise (Duman & Monteggia, 2006).

The low incidence of side effects, low cost, and general availability make exercise a crucial component of integrative management. The level of exertion and specific exercise prescription should be determined by the patient's level of fitness, interests in specific physical activities, and health concerns. Working with a healthcare practitioner is advised if a patient is initiating an exercise prescription and is sedentary.

NUTRITION

In addition to recommending a wholesome diet, it is important to remove any foods or beverages that can exacerbate anxiety. The two primary offenders are caffeine and alcohol. Americans, on average, consume one or two cups of coffee a day, which contain approximately 150–300 mg of caffeine. People who are prone to feeling stress have reported that they experience increased anxiety from even small amounts of caffeine. Another source of caffeine and a growing problem with regard to excessive caffeine use are energy drinks. The content of caffeine can range from 50 mg to 550 mg per container. Screening for consumption of these beverages should also be considered in assessing nutritional sources exacerbating anxiety (Reissig, Strain, & Griffiths, 2009; Wolk, Ganetsky, & Babu, 2012). Whatever the source with long-term use, caffeine has been linked with anxiety as well as depression (Winston, Hardwick E., & Jaberi, 2005). Similarly, with regular and chronic consumption, alcohol has been found to diminish levels of serotonin and catecholamines. Discontinuation of alcohol consumption is therefore suggested (Lovinger, 1997).

Omega-3 Fatty Acids

Epidemiologic data suggest that omega-3 fatty acid deficiency correlates with increased anxiety. In animal studies, levels of polyunsaturated fats and cholesterol metabolism have been shown to influence neuronal tissue synthesis, membrane fluidity, and serotonin metabolism (Moriguchi, Greiner, & Salem, 2000). Studies in patients with major depressive disorder suggest that correction of the ratio of omega-6 to omega-3 consumption may improve mood. Given the evidence concerning neuronal tissue synthesis and serotonin metabolism, increased supplementation with omega-3 fatty acids seems reasonable as a dietary intervention (Su, Huang, Chiu, & Shen, 2003). Recommending consumption of cold water fish (sardines, mackerel, tuna, salmon, herring) at least two or three times a week, taking a fish oil supplement (eicosapentaenoic acid 1 g/day), freshly ground flaxseed (2 tablespoons daily), or flaxseed oil supplement (1,000–2,000 mg) would be appropriate.

DIETARY SUPPLEMENTS

B Vitamins

Deficiency of a number of vitamins, including the B vitamins, has been linked with mood disorders. Vitamin B6 (pyridoxine) and B12 (cobalamin) are important for the synthesis of S-adenosyl methionine (SAMe), the primary methyl donor in the production of brain neurotransmitters. Vitamin B6 is important for the production of serotonin and has been linked with improvement in mood disorders, including anxiety, when supplemented (McCarty, 2000). Although large-scale clinical studies are lacking, a trial of a B-complex supplement seems advisable, especially in the elderly and persons taking medications that may deplete these vitamins (e.g., oral contraceptives; Murray et al., 1999). Folic acid is a water-soluble B vitamin found in fruits, legumes, and green leafy vegetables. Folate is essential for normal brain function. Patients with low levels of folic acid do not respond well to selective serotonin reuptake inhibitors (SSRIs) (Alpert et al., 2000; Bottiglieri et al., 2000; Qureshi, 2013).

Dosage
The B complex vitamin should provide 100 mg of vitamin B6, 100 μg vitamin B12, and 400–600 μg folic acid (Natural Medicines Comprehensive Database, 2014).

Precautions

High doses of folic acid have been reported to cause altered sleep patterns, exacerbation of seizure frequency, gastrointestinal (GI) disturbances, and a bitter taste in the mouth. Serum vitamin B12 levels should be checked if folic acid supplementation is used, especially if megaloblastic anemia is noted in laboratory tests, as B12 deficiency can be masked by folic acid supplementation. The upper tolerable limit for vitamin B6 is 100 mg per day, as higher doses may be associated with neurological harm.

S-Adenosyl Methionine

S-adenosyl methionine is a biomolecule involved in the methylation of monoamines, neurotransmitters, and phospholipids such as phosphatidylcholine and phosphatidylserine. Synthesis of SAMe appears to be hampered in depressed patients. As depression is often a comorbid condition accompanying anxiety, SAMe may be considered an adjunctive addition in the treatment of anxiety.

Dosage

A total of 1,200–1,600 mg per day in divided doses is often used. Start with 200 mg twice daily for several days then increase to 400 mg twice daily for several days then 400 mg three times a day for several days and then, if necessary, increased to 400 mg four times a day (Natural Medicines Comprehensive Database, 2014).

Precautions

Nausea is reported in some patients with initial use. Also, SAMe is contraindicated in those with bipolar depression, as it can induce mania. Insomnia is a significant side effect, and some patients with predominantly anxiety and not depression may complain of increased agitation and irritability.

5-Hydroxytryptophan

5-hydroxytryptophan (5-HTP) is an amino acid that serves as a precursor to serotonin. 5-HTP easily crosses the blood-brain barrier and effectively increases central nervous system (CNS) synthesis of serotonin, which may improve mood, anxiety, and sleep. Definitive, large-scale studies of efficacy and safety have not been conducted for 5-HTP, though small studies suggest that it superior to placebo in the treatment of depression.

Dosage
100–300 mg/day (Natural Medicines Comprehensive Database, 2014).

Precautions
Years ago, L-tryptophan was linked to multiple cases of eosinophilic myalgia syndrome, a serious medical condition that involves the muscles, skin, blood, and other organs. It was thought that the cause of this rare syndrome was due to a bacterial contaminant in the production process rather than the amino acid itself.

BOTANICAL MEDICINE

Kava (Piper methysticum)

In the realm of botanical medicine, kava is considered as a therapeutic option for the treatment of GAD in the United States and Europe. It is derived from the pulverized lateral roots of a subspecies of a pepper plant, *P. methysticum*, and is indigenous to many Pacific islands. Several reviews of clinical trials evaluating kava as an anxiolytic found that kava was superior to placebo in the symptomatic treatment of GAD (Pittler & Ernst, 2000; Sarris, Laporte, & Schweitzer, 2011).

The pharmacologically active constituents are the kava lactones, which have a chemical structure similar to that of myristicin, found in nutmeg (Shulgin, 1973). These lipophilic lactone structures are present in the highest concentration in the lateral roots. Of the 15 isolated kava lactone structures, six are concentrated maximally in the root and vary depending on the variety of *P. methysticum* (Lebot et al., 1992). Kava's mechanism of action has not been completely elucidated, although the action seems similar to that of benzodiazepines.

Benzodiazepines exert their actions by binding to GABA and benzodiazepine receptors in the brain; animal studies analyzing kava's anxiolytic action, however, show mixed and minor effects at both sites. Other studies indicate the kava constituents produce anxiolytic effects by altering the limbic system, especially at the amygdala and hippocampus (Pepping, 1999). Other documented uses of kava have been as a muscle relaxant, anticonvulsant, anesthetic, and anti-inflammatory agent.

Indication
Mild to moderate generalized anxiety.

Dosage

For anxiety, use a product that provides 50–70 mg kava lactones three times daily. For products with a standardized kava lactone concentration of 30%, this would be equivalent to 100–250 mg of dried root (Natural Medicines Comprehensive Database, 2014).

Precautions

Kava has been reported to cause acute hepatitis. Case reports occurred in those using predominantly ethanol and acetone kava extracts. Although underlying mechanisms are not well established or understood, common sense dictates that kava should not be used in individuals who have liver problems or who drink alcohol on a daily basis (Blumenthal, 2001; Natural Medicines Comprehensive Database, 2014). Liver tests should be routinely done in individuals who use kava on a daily basis, and patients should be counseled on the signs and symptoms of hepatotoxicity (jaundice, malaise, and nausea). Furthermore, kava should be discontinued from daily use after approximately 4 months. Kava interacts with many medications due to inhibition of CYP450 isozymes: CYP1A2 (56% inhibition), 2C9 (92%), 2C19 (86%), 2D6 (73%), 3A4 (78%), and 4A9/11. Inhibition of CYP450 isozymes is believed to be the most likely factor in causing kava-mediated adverse drug reactions via inhibition of drug metabolism (Mathews et al., 2005).

Anecdotal reports have noted excessive sedation when kava is combined with other sedative medications (Almeida & Grimsley, 1996; Natural Medicines Comprehensive Database, 2014). Extrapyramidal side effects in four patients using two different preparations of kava were reported. Kava should be avoided in those with Parkinson syndrome (Schelosky, Raffaulf, Jendroska, & Poewe, 1995). With heavy kava consumption, a yellow, ichthyosiform condition of the skin known as kava dermopathy has been observed. This condition is reversible with discontinuation of the kava (Norton, & Ruze, 1994). The overdose potential appears low. In many cases, the rash, ataxia, redness of the eyes, visual accommodation difficulties, and yellowing of the skin reported in the literature from Australia and the Pacific region emerged after ingestion of up to 13 L/day, equivalent to 300–400 g of dried root per week. It should be noted that this amount represents a dose 100 times that of the recommended therapeutic dose (Blumenthal, 2001; Schultz, Hansel, & Tyler, 1998).

Pregnancy and Lactation

There are insufficient data to determine safety during pregnancy, thus it is best avoided. Kava is present in the milk of lactating mothers; therefore, use is discouraged during breastfeeding (Brinker & Stodart, 1998). Avoid use with other sedative medications.

*Valerian (*Valeriana officinalis*)*

Valerian is another botanical that may be used for the treatment of GAD. The clinical efficacy of valerian has been evaluated mostly for treating sleep disturbances; fewer clinical studies assessing its use in anxiety are available. Nevertheless, it has been used in Europe for more than 1,000 years as a tranquilizer and calmative. Valerian in combination with passionflower (*Passiflora incarnata*) or St. John's Wort (*Hypericum perforatum*) has been studied in small clinical trials for anxiety. One study compared valerian root and passionflower (100 mg of valerian root with 6.5 mg of passionflower extract) with chlorpromazine hydrochloride (Thorazine 40 mg/day) over a period of 16 weeks. In this study, 20 patients were randomly assigned to the two treatment groups after being identified as suffering from irritation, unrest, depression, and insomnia. Electroencephalographic changes in both groups consistent with relaxation were comparable; two psychological scales measuring these qualities demonstrated scores consistent with reduction in anxiety (Schellenberg, Schwartz, & Schellenberg, 1994). Another study evaluated anxiety in 100 patients receiving either a combination of 50 mg of valerian root plus 90–100 mg of standardized St. John's Wort for 14 days or 2 mg of diazepam twice daily in the first week and up to two capsules twice daily in the second week. The results showed reduction of anxiety in the botanical treatment group to levels in healthy persons. Patients in the diazepam treatment group still had significant anxiety score (Panijel, 1985).

Indication
Mild to moderate anxiety.

Dosage
For adults with anxiety, a dose of 150–400 mg valerian extract in the morning and another dose of 400–800 mg in the evening using a product standardized to 0.8% valerenic acid can be taken. Combinations with lemon balm (*Melissa officinalis*) and hops (*Humulus lupulus*) may also be considered. A combination of valerian and lemon balm was shown effective in treating restlessness and insomnia in children (Müller & Klement, 2006) and alleviated anxiety in a double-blind randomized controlled trial of healthy volunteers subjected to laboratory-induced stress (Kennedy, Little, Haskell, & Scholey, 2006). Studies using the combination of valerian and hops suggest it is beneficial for improving sleep (Dimpfel & Suter, 2008; Koetter, Schrader, Käufeler, & Brattström, 2007; Morin, Koetter, Bastien, Ware, & Wooten, 2005; Natural Medicines Comprehensive Database, 2014; Reichert, 1998).

Precautions

Valerian root is not suitable for the treatment of acute insomnia, as it takes several weeks before a beneficial effect is obtained. An alternative that gives a more rapid response should be taken when valerian root initiated (DiLorenzo et al., 1999). There are occasional reports of headache and gastrointestinal complaints.

MIND–BODY MEDICINE

Relaxation Techniques

Relaxation training, stress-reduction techniques, and breath work are of proven benefit. In fact, imaginal exposure is used as a tactic for repeated exposure to induce anxiety (in a gradual way). Patients learn through repeated exposure to cope with and manage their anxiety rather than eliminate it. A meta-analysis of relaxation techniques such as Jacobson's progressive relaxation, autogenic training, applied relaxation, and meditation were evaluated. Twenty-seven studies were included, and the results showed consistent and significant efficacy of these modalities in reducing anxiety (Manzonie, Pagnigni, Castelnuovo, & Molinari, 2008). Another meta-analysis published in 2012 of 36 randomized-controlled studies comparing the effects of meditation on anxiety also showed modest improvement over controls. However, the authors noted that the studies measured improvements in anxiety symptoms but did not assess outcomes of anxiety disorders as clinically diagnosed (Chen et al., 2012).

Clinical Pearl

I often encounter patients who admit to their anxiety and are willing to confront and learn to cope with it but lack the ability to completely relax. Depending on their preferences, I help them choose a relaxation technique that reinforces a sense of calm. Therapies that can be used for this purpose are massage, sound therapy, aromatherapy, guided interactive imagery, and hypnosis. Because many patients have somatic sensations that accompany their anxiety, a complementary therapy that imparts a "remembrance" of a deeply relaxed state should also be reinforced on a more somatic-kinesthetic level.

OTHER THERAPIES TO CONSIDER

Acupuncture

Traditional medical systems such as traditional Chinese medicine can be another option for the treatment of anxiety (Romili & Giommi, 1993). Several small trials showed a reduction of anxiety symptoms in patients using auricular acupuncture (Breier, Albus, & Pickar, 1987). A study of 185 women with anxiety, depression, and substance abuse found that 21 days of auricular therapy provided significant reduction in anxiety and physical cravings for substances (Courbasson, De Sorkin, Dullerd, & Van Wyk, 2007). Although the mechanisms are not well elucidated, these systems may somehow interface favorably with the autonomic nervous system (Kawakita & Okada, 2014; Pilkington, Kirkwood, Rampes, Cummings, & Richardson, 2007).

Yoga

Yoga, a physical and contemplative therapy, can be very calming for anxious individuals. A systematic review evaluated eight studies of yoga for the treatment of anxiety. While the results were encouraging, suggesting a benefit of yoga on reducing anxiety symptoms, the authors could not make any firm conclusions about effectiveness (Kirkwood, Rampes, Tuffrey, Richardson, & Pilkington, 2005). A study of 130 subjects with moderate stress either underwent 10 weeks of 2-hour weekly yoga sessions or relaxation therapy. Yoga was more effective in improving mental health, but at the end of a 6-week follow-up both modalities were comparable in reducing stress (Smith, Hancock, Blake-Mortimer, & Eckert, 2007).

Massage

Touch is a universal stimulus that can bring about great relaxation. Most of us have memories of touch that soothed us as children. Thirty-nine subjects with nausea, anxiety, and depression undergoing chemotherapy for breast cancer received massage treatment for 20 minutes on five occasions. The findings indicated reduction of nausea and anxiety (Billhult, Berbom, & Stener-Vitorin, 2007). Another review assessing the physiological effects of massage on stress showed reductions in diastolic blood pressure but was inconclusive and mixed in consistently demonstrating reductions in catecholamines and urinary cortisol mostly because the studies were small and lacked enough scientific rigor to make a definitive conclusion (Moraska, Pollini, Boulanger, Brooks, & Teitlebaum, 2008).

Drug Therapy

Consideration of drug therapy depends on the degree of agitation and anxiety. A number of randomized trials have demonstrated the efficacy of antidepressants in the treatment of GAD, however, only a few have FDA approval for this condition. Venlafaxine (Effexor) is the only serotonin-norepinephrine reuptake inhibitor approved for GAD.

Agents approved for panic disorder, social phobia, and PTSD are listed in Table 23.2 (Baldwin, Stein, & Hermann, 2014). Tricyclic antidepressants are an appropriate therapeutic option but are associated with significant anticholinergic, cardiovascular, and sedative effects. Most experts recommend a trial of at least 4 to 6 weeks to determine efficacy. As less cardiotoxicity is associated with SSRIs, they may represent a better choice for patients with heart disease. Serotonin reuptake inhibitors have been reported to reduce libido, though the actual incidence of sexual dysfunction is not clear. Strategies for reducing sexual dysfunction include lowering the dose, switching to another SSRI or non-SSRI, or recommending a drug holiday.

Anxiolytics, particularly benzodiazepines, are commonly used for acute treatment of GAD. However, the risk of abuse and habituation must be carefully weighed when prescribing. The anxiolytic buspirone (BuSpar) lacks the problematic issue of drug dependence and excessive sedation (Baldwin et al., 2014) and may be a better option.

Psychotherapy

The combination of psychotherapy in conjunction with supplements, botanicals, or prescription anxiolytic or antidepressant, is highly recommended, especially in GAD.

Two clinically proven and frequently used forms are behavioral therapy and CBT (Hunot, Churchill, Silva de Lima, & Teixeira, 2007). Behavioral therapy focuses on changing the specific unwanted actions by using techniques to stop the undesired behavior. In addition, both behavioral therapy and CBT help patients understand their thinking patterns so that they can react differently to situations that make them anxious.

Table 23.2. Selected Drug Recommendations for Treatment of Anxiety

Drug	Initial Dose (in mg) (Range)	Frequency
Tricyclics		
Amitriptyline (Elavil)	25–50 (100–300)	qd
Desipramine (Norpramin)	25–50 (100–300)	qd
Imipramine (Tofranil)	25–50 (25–50)	qd
Nortriptyline (Pamelor)	25 (50–200)	qd
Selective Serotonin Reuptake Inhibitors and Mixed Reuptake Blockers		
Fluoxetine (Prozac)	10–20 (10–80)	qd
Fluvoxamine (Luvox)	50 (50–300)	qd
Paroxetine (Paxil)	10 (10–60)	qd
Sertraline (Zoloft)	50 (50–200)	qd
Others		
Venlafaxine (Effexor)	75 (75–375)	bid
Nefazodone (Serzone)	200 (200–600)	bid
Bupropion (Wellbutrin)	100 (200–450)	bid
Mirtazapine (Remeron)	15–45 mg	qhs
Buspirone (Buspar)	5 (15–60)	bid

Source: Adapted from Depression Guideline Panel (1993).

A meta-analysis found CBT more effective in reducing symptoms in patients with GAD than treatment as usual or waiting list. A controlled study evaluating patients newly diagnosed with GAD found that brief supportive psychotherapy had comparable outcomes to those who initially received benzodiazepines at 3-and 6-month follow-up. Of note, visits to health are providers were not increased in the psychotherapy group. Outcomes were similar for CBT and supportive therapy (Baldwin et al., 2014).

Conclusion

In summary, GAD is a common complaint seen in primary care. The cause for GAD appears to be multifactorial, and an integrative approach is the most appropriate approach for most patients.

REFERENCES

Almeida, J. C., & Grimsley, E. W. (1996). Coma from the health food store: Interaction between kava and alprazolam. *Ann Intern Med, 125,* 940–941.

Alpert, J. E., Mischoulon, D., Nierenberg, A., & Fava, M. (2000). Nutrition and depression: The role of folate, methylation and monoamine metabolism in depression. *J Neurol Neurosurg Psychiatry 16,* 228–232.

Anderson, E., & Shivarkumar, G. (2013). Effects of exercise and physical activity on anxiety. *Front Psychiatry, 4,* 27.

Bottiglieri, T., Laundy, M., Crellin, R., Toone, B., Carney, M., & Reynolds, E. (2000). Nutrition and depression: The role of folate, methylation and monoamine metabolism in depression. *J Neurol Neurosurg Psychiatry,* 228–232.

Baldwin, D., Stein, M., & Hermann, R. (2014). *Overview of generalized anxiety disorder.* Last updated May 12, 2014. Retrieved July 13, 2014, from www.uptodate.com

Billhult, A., Berbom, I., & Stener-Vitorin, E. (2007). Massage relieves nausea in women with breast cancer who are undergoing chemotherapy. *J Altern Complement Med, 13,* 53–57.

Blumenthal, M. (1998). *The complete German Commission E monographs: Therapeutic guide to herbal medicines.* Austin, TX: American Botanical Council.

Blumenthal, M. (2001). *American Botanical Council announces new safety information on Kava.* ABC Safety Release. December 20.

Bradya, K., Haynes, L., Hartwell, K., & Killeen, T. (2013). Special issue: The role of social work in the prevention and treatment of substance use disorders. *Social Work in Public Health, 28,* 407–423.

Breier, A., Albus, M., & Pickar, D. (1987). Controllable and uncontrollable stress in humans: Alterations in mood and neuroendocrine and psychophysiological function. *Am J Psychiatry, 244,* 11.

Brinker, F., & Stodart, N. (1998). *Herbal contraindications and drug interactions* (2nd ed.). Sandy, OR: Eclectic Medical.

Chen, K., Berger, C., Manheimer, M., et al. (2012). Meditative therapies for reducing anxiety: A systematic review and meta-analysis of randomized controlled trials. *Depress Anxiety, 29,* 545–562.

Courbasson, C. M. A., De Sorkin, A. A., Dullerd, B., & Van Wyk, L. (2007). Acupuncture treatment for women with concurrent substance use and anxiety/depression: An effective alternative therapy? *Fam Community Health, 30,* 112–120.

Depression Guideline Panel. (1993). *Depression in primary care* (Vol. 2). AHCPR Publication No 93–0551, Rockville, MD: Author.

DiLorenzo T., Bargmana, E. P., Stucky-Roppa, R., Brassingtona, G. S., Frenscha, P. A., & LaFontaineb, T. (1999). Long-term effects of aerobic exercise on psychological outcomes. *Prev Med.;28,* 75–88.

Dimpfel, W., & Suter, A. (2008). Sleep improving effects of a single dose administration of a valerian/hops fluid extract: A double blind, randomized, placebo-controlled sleep-EEG study in a parallel design using electrohypnograms. *Eur J Med Res, 13,* 200–204.

Dunn, A., & Dishman, R. (1991). Exercise and the neurobiology of depression. *Exer Sport Sci Rev, 19*, 41–98.

Duman, R., & Monteggia, L. (2006). Neurotrophic model for stress-related mood disorders. *Biol Psychiatry, 59*, 1116–1127.

Lovinger, D. (1997). Serotonin's role in alcohol's effect on the brain. *Alcohol Health and Research World, 21.*

Hettema, J., Prescott, C., Myers, J., Neale, M., & Kendler, K. (2005). The structure of genetic and environmental risk factors for anxiety disorders in men and women. *Arch Gen Psych, 62*, 182–189.

Hunot, V., Churchill, R., Silva de Lima, M., & Teixeira, V. (2007). Psychological therapies for generalized anxiety disorder. *Cochrane Database Syst Rev*, CD001848.

Kawakita, K., & Okada, K. (2014). Acupuncture therapy: Mechanism of action, efficacy, and safety: A potential intervention for psychogenic disorders? *BioPsychoSocial Medicine, 8*, 4.

Kennedy, D. O., Little, W., Haskell, C. F., & Scholey, A. B. (2006). Anxiolytic effects of a combination of *Melissa officinalis* and *Valeriana officinalis* during laboratory induced stress. *Phytother Res, 20*, 96–102.

Kessler, R. C., Berglund, P., Demler, O., Jin, R., Merikangas, K. R., & Walters, E. E. (2005). Lifetime prevalence and age-of-onset distributions of DSM-IV disorders in the National Comorbidity Survey Replication. *Arch Gen Psychiatry, 62*, 593.

Kessler, R. C., Chiu, W. T., Demler, O., & Walters, E. E. (2005). Prevalence, severity, and comorbidity of twelve month DSM-IV disorders in the National Comorbidity Survey Replication (NCS-R). *Arch Gen Psychiatry, 626*, 617–627.

Kirkwood, G., Rampes, H., Tuffrey, V., Richardson, J., & Pilkington, K. (2005). Yoga for anxiety: A systematic review of the research evidence. *Br J Sports Med, 39*, 884–891.

Koetter, U., Schrader, E., Käufeler, R., & Brattström, A. (2007). A randomized, double blind, placebo-controlled, prospective clinical study to demonstrate clinical efficacy of a fixed valerian hops extract combination (Ze 91019) in patients suffering from non-organic sleep disorder. *Phytother Res, 21*, 847–s851.

Lebot, V., et al. (1992). *Kava: The pacific drug.* New Haven, CO: Yale University Press.

Lovinger, D. (1997). Serotonins role in alcohol's effect on the brain. *Alcohol Health and Research World, 21*, 114–120.

Moriguchi, T., Greiner, R. S., & Salem, N., Jr. (2000). Behavioral deficits associated with dietary induction of decreased brain docosahexaenoic acid concentration. *J Neurochem, 75*, 2563–2573.

Manzoni, G. M., Pagnigni, F., Castelnuovo, G., & Molinari, E. (2008). Relaxation training for anxiety: A ten-years systematic review with meta-analysis. *BMC Psychiatry, 8*, 41.

Mathews, J. M., Etheridge, A. S., Valentine, J. L., et al. (2005). Pharmacokinetics and disposition of the kavalactone kawain: Interaction with kava extract and kavalactones in vivo and in vitro. *Drug Metab Dispos, 33*, 1555–1563.

McCarty, M. F. (2000). High-dose pyridoxine in anti-stress strategy. *Med Hypotheses, 54*, 803–807.

McFarlane, J., Groff, J., O'Brien, J., & Watson, K. (2003). Behaviors of children who are exposed and not exposed to intimate partner violence: An analysis of 330 black, white, and Hispanic children. *Pediatrics, 112*, e202–207.

Moraska, A., Pollini, R., Boulanger, K., Brooks, M., & Teitlebaum, L. (2010). Physiological adjustments to stress measures following massage therapy: A review of the literature. *Evid Based Complement Alternat Med, 7*, 409–418.

Morin, C. M., Koetter, U., Bastien, C., Ware, J. C., & Wooten, V. (2005). Valerian-hops combination and diphenhydramine for treating insomnia: A randomized placebo-controlled clinical trial. *Sleep, 28*, 1465–1471.

Müller, S. F., & Klement, S. (2006). A combination of valerian and lemon balm is effective in the treatment of restlessness and dyssomnia in children. *Phytomedicine, 13*, 383–387.

Murray, M., et al. (1999). Affective disorders. In J. E. Pizzorno & M. T., Murray (Eds.), *Textbook of natural medicine.*(2nd ed.). Churchill Livingstone.

Natural Medicines Comprehensive Database. (2014). *Clinical management series, Natural medicines in the clinical management of anxiety.* Retrieved July 17, 2014, from www.naturaldatabase.com.

Norton, S. A., & Ruze, P. (1994). Kava dermopathy. *J Am Acad Dermatol, 31*, 89–97.

Osher, Y., Javer, D., & Benjamin, J. (2000). Association and linkage of anxiety related traits with a functional polymorphism of the serotonin transporter gene regulatory region in an Israeli sibling pair. *Mol Psychiatry, 5*, 216–219.

Paluska, S., & Schwenk, T. L. (2000). Physical activity and mental health: Current concepts. *Sports Med, 29*, 167–180.

Panijel, M. (1985). The treatment of moderate states of anxiety: Randomized double-blind study comparing the clinical effectiveness of a phytomedicine with diazepam. *Therapiwoche, 41*, 4659–4668.

Pepping, J. (1999). Alternative therapies: Kava: *Piper methysticum. Am J Health Syst Pharm, 56*, 957–960.

Pilkington, K., Kirkwood, G., Rampes, H., Cummings, M., & Richardson, J. (2007). Acupuncture for anxiety and anxiety disorders: A systematic literature review. *Acupunct Med, 25*, 1–10.

Pittler, M., & Ernst, E. (2000). Efficacy of kava extract for treating anxiety: Systematic review and meta-analysis. *J Clin Psychopharmacol, 20*, 84–89.

Rakel, D. (2012). Anxiety. In R. Lee (Ed.), *Integrative medicine* (3rd ed.). Philadelphia, PA: Saunders Elsevier.

Reichert, R. (1998). Valerian [clinical monograph]. *Q Rev Nat Med Fall*, 207–215.

Reissig, C. J., Strain, E., & Griffiths, R. (2009). Caffeinated energy drinks: A growing problem. *Drug Alcohol Depend, 99*, 1–10.

Romili, M., & Giommi, A. (1993). Ear acupuncture in psychosomatic medicine: The importance of Sanjiao (triple heater) area. *Acupunct Electrother Res, 18*, 185–194.

Rotzinger S., & Vaccarino, F. (2003). Cholecystokinin receptor subtypes: Role in the modulation of anxiety-related and reward-related behaviours in animal models *J Psychiatry Neurosci, 28*, 171–181.

Sarris, J., Laporte, E., & Schweitzer, I. (2011). Kava: A comprehensive review of efficacy, safety, and psychopharmacology. *Aust N Z J Psychiatry, 45,* 27–35.

Schellenberg, R., Schwartz, A., & Schellenberg, V. (1994). EEG-monitoring and psychometric evaluation of the therapeutic efficacy of Biral N in psychosomatic diseases. *Naturamed, 4, 9.*

Schelosky, L., Raffaulf, C., Jendroska, K., & Poewe, W. (1995). Kava and dopamine antagonism. *J Neurol Neurosurg Psychiatry, 58,* 639–640.

Schultz, V., Hansel, R., & Tyler, V. E. (1998). *Rational therapy: A physicians' guide to herbal medicine.* Berlin: Springer-Verlag.

Schweitzer, E. (1995). Generalized anxiety disorder: Longitudinal course and pharmacologic treatment. *Psychiatric Clin North Am.* 18:843–857.

Shulgin, A. T. (1973). The narcotic pepper: The chemistry and pharmacology of *Piper methysticum* and related species. *Bull Narc, 25,* 59–74.

Smith, C., Hancock, H., Blake-Mortimer, J., & Eckert, K. (2007). A randomized comparative trial of yoga and relaxation to reduce stress and anxiety. *Complement Ther Med, 15,* 77–83.

Solmaz, M., Kavuk, I., & Sayar, K., S. O. (2003). Psychological factors in the irritable bowel syndrome. *Eur J Med Res, 8,* 549.

Stewart, S. H., et al. (2001). Causal modeling of relations among learning history, anxiety sensitivity and panic attacks. *Behav Res Ther, 39,* 443–456.

Su, K., Huang, S., Chiu, C., & Shen, W. (2003). Omega-3 fatty acids in major depressive disorder: A preliminary double-blind, placebo-controlled trial. *Eur Neuropsychopharmacol, 213,* 267–71.

Qureshi, N., & Al-Bedah, A. M. (2013). Mood disorders and complementary and alternative medicine: A literature review. *Neuropsychiatr Dis Treat, 9,* 639–658.

Winston, A., Hardwick E., & Jaberi, N. (2005). Neuropsychiatric effects of caffeine *Advances in Psychiatric Treatment, 11,* 432–439.

Williams, B. A., et al. (2014). *Current diagnosis and treatment: Geriatrics* (2nd ed.). New York: McGraw-Hill Education.

Wittchen, H. U., Jacobi, F., Rehm, J., et al. (2011). *Eur Neuropsychopharmacol, 21,* 655–79.

Wittchen, H., Zhao, S., Kessler, R. C., & Eaton, W. W. (1994). DSM-III-R generalized anxiety disorder in the National Comorbidity Survey. *Arch Gen Psychiatry, 51,* 1216.

Wolk, B. J., Ganetsky, M., & Babu, K. M. (2012). Toxicity of energy drinks. *Curr Opin Pediatr, 24,* 243–51.

24

Depression

NAOMI LAM AND SUDHA PRATHIKANTI

CASE STUDY

Gloria is a 43-year-old married female who presented for treatment of a long-standing depression that had worsened in the 6 months prior to her initial visit. She complained of occasional crying spells, anxiety, sadness, insomnia, and difficulty in concentrating. She stated that she had been "stress eating" and had gained about 15 pounds in the past 6 months. She noted that she sometimes felt "paralyzed, not able to make decisions" and felt she was "constantly second-guessing myself." She denied suicidal thoughts and stated that she was "somehow" able to function relatively well at work and at home despite her symptoms, which were "worse than I've ever had."

Gloria had a full-time job managing a large sales office, was raising two active teenage children, and had recently been diagnosed with hypertension and borderline diabetes. She described herself as the "emotional safety net" not only of her close-knit, large extended family but also of her office staff. In addition to her commitments at work and with family, she was also very active in her church. She was devoted to all of her responsibilities but often felt "a lot of guilt" because she felt "drained, instead of nourished" by the many demands placed on her.

Gloria felt strongly that she would like to avoid using pharmaceuticals.

Although she had moderate symptoms of depression, as she had never experienced a decrease in functioning, denied suicidal ideation, was very motivated, and had a healthy support network, I felt comfortable to move ahead without recommending medication in the initial treatment plan. I did advise her that should her symptoms worsen, we would need to discuss the possibility of medication. She agreed, and after reviewing her history and medication list, we developed a plan that eventually included traditional Chinese medicine, aerobic exercise, dietary supplementation, and mind–body medicine.

Gloria started a trial of S-adenosyl methionine (SAMe) and tried her best to limit herself to three healthy meals per day with adequate hydration. I advised her to limit her caffeine intake. Always "on the go" but not a big fan of exercise, Gloria was curious about yoga. She attended a few beginning hatha yoga classes at her local gym but soon dropped out due to feeling that "it just wasn't for me." She tried tai chi as well, but felt "it takes too much patience." We then agreed that a short daily walk in her neighborhood would be a healthy initial exercise regimen.

One month later, Gloria noted that she had stopped having crying spells. She attributed this to the SAMe, which had caused some gastrointestinal (GI) upset during the first week of treatment, but which she subsequently tolerated well. She noted that her short-lived contact with yoga had had surprising results: Her insomnia had improved, with benefit from practicing savasana, or "corpse pose," at bedtime and when she awoke during the night. She was still having significant anxiety and some sadness during the day, and noted that her neck and shoulders were tight and painful. I recommended that she see an acupuncturist to address both the muscle pain and the mood symptoms. She began to lengthen her daily walks. I recommended that she try to increase her intake of fresh fruit and vegetables, and start taking omega-3 fatty acid supplements.

At her 8-week follow-up, Gloria felt that the SAMe was "definitely" helping with her mood. She also noted that with the changes she had made in diet and exercise, she had lost a couple of pounds, had more energy, and was sleeping better. Acupuncture had significantly decreased her muscle tension and pain, and she noted that the sessions were "incredibly healing and relaxing." We spoke in our sessions about the importance of self-care and about ways to reframe the guilt she felt about "spending so much time on me." She felt motivated to continue her treatment plan.

Four months into treatment, Gloria felt that her depression and anxiety had "mostly" resolved. She was eating and sleeping regularly, and took 1-hour walks approximately every other day. She had stopped seeing her acupuncturist but had incorporated a healthy diet and omega-3 fatty acid supplementation into her routine. We planned a gradual taper of SAMe. Her primary care doctor noted that her blood pressure and blood glucose had responded positively to these changes in her lifestyle. Gloria realized that she was gradually easing into a routine of self-care that helped her not only to stay healthy but also to function more effectively as a caregiver.

Introduction

Over a lifetime, major depression affects women approximately twice as frequently as it does men (Kessler, McGonagle, Swartz, Blazer, & Nelson, 1993). It is now the leading cause of disease-related disability among women worldwide (Kessler, 2001). The etiology of depression is unclear, but it appears to involve not only physiological and psychosocial but also genetic and environmental effects.

In addition to possible sex-hormone-related risk factors, psychosocial stressors play an important role in this increased vulnerability to depression. Women are more likely than men to live in poverty, which is in itself a chronic stressor, and they are thus more likely to be exposed to stressors such as violence and crime (Nolen-Hoeksema, 2000). Socialization into traditionally female roles, which tends to involve developing behaviors of nurturance, dependence, and passivity, is also postulated to have an impact on women's increased vulnerability to depression (Nolen-Hoeksema & Girgus, 1994).

Given the rich and complicated intra- and interpersonal environment in which depression arises, it seems prudent to approach treatment with a holistic and flexible mindset. Integrative medicine lends itself very well to this approach. This chapter presents brief descriptions of the diagnosis and conventional treatment of depression, and then focuses on specific integrative treatments for depression, presenting evidence for women where available.

Diagnosis

Currently, patients suspected of suffering from depression are diagnosed in accordance with criteria set forth in the *Diagnostic and Statistical Manual of Mental Disorders* (DSM-V) (American Psychiatric Association, 2013).

However, in the day-to-day treatment of primary care patients, providers see women presenting with depressive symptoms in a large range of severity. For women with mild-to-moderate symptoms, working with a caring primary care provider who has access not only to antidepressant medications but also to information about integrative treatments can be an incredibly positive experience. It is important to note, however, that those women presenting with moderate-to-severe depression, who are at risk for further decompensation, should be referred to a psychiatrist for specialized management of their symptoms.

Conventional Treatment

This chapter provides a brief overview of the many and varied conventional treatments for depression. Psychotropic medication (such as antidepressants, anxiolytics, and sedative/hypnotics), physiologic modalities such as electroconvulsive therapy (ECT) or transcranial magnetic stimulation (TMS), and psychotherapy are the major conventional treatments aimed at lessening depressive symptoms. For more detailed information, the Mayo Clinic website (www.mayoclinic.org) offers a succinct and thorough review of these conventional treatments. In addition, a practical introduction to the concept of psychotherapy can be found at www.psychcentral.com/lib/an-introduction-to-psychotherapy/00012.

As an integrative psychiatrist, I strive to optimize the balance between a woman's clinical need for medications, her attitudes and beliefs about medication, and her innate ability to cope with her feelings. I appreciate the value and benefits of pharmaceuticals and believe in their efficacy, especially in times of crisis. I also feel that if a woman does not believe that the medication will help, her depression may not respond optimally to this particular intervention. In the office, I take into consideration a woman's worries and concerns about taking medications and incorporate education about their risks and benefits into treatment planning. Formulating a strategy that is clinically appropriate, as well as sensitive to my patient's personal belief system, is of utmost importance to me.

Commonly prescribed antidepressant medications include those belonging to the selective serotonin reuptake inhibitor (SSRI) class such as fluoxetine (Prozac), paroxetine (Paxil), sertraline (Zoloft), citalopram (Celexa), and escitalopram (Lexapro). Other frequently prescribed antidepressants include mirtazapine (Remeron), bupropion (Wellbutrin), and venlafaxine (Effexor), which have mixed receptor action. Recently, a meta-analysis did show that pharmaceutical antidepressants are very effective for moderate-to-severe depression but are not often superior to placebo for treating mild-to-moderate depression (Fournier et al., 2010).

Sexual side effects of antidepressant medications are of concern to many women and may affect approximately 30%–40% of patients taking them. These side effects include decreased libido, delayed orgasm, and anorgasmia. Strategies to address this situation include decreasing the dosage, switching to another antidepressant medication, or adding an agent to decrease the sexual side effect. If a patient is having an otherwise robust positive response to the medication, I might recommend lowering the dose or augmenting before I would encourage a switch. Common augmentation strategies include addition of buproprion, which affects noradrenergic and dopaminergic receptors, or yohimbine, which acts on alpha-2 adrenergic receptors. Additional strategies can be found in the chapter "Sexuality." Of note, I find it vital to take a thorough history of the sexual side-effect symptoms and course, as depression itself can cause decreased libido.

Pharmacologic and physiologic treatment approaches are purely biologically based, but an interesting intersection between conventional and integrative medicine occurs in the realm of psychotherapy. This intersection exists because most psychotherapeutic models require the practitioner to have an understanding not only of a patient's symptoms but also of her life history, relationships, personality, coping skills, beliefs, and values, in order to provide effective treatment. There is a long-standing tradition within conventional psychiatry of valuing a patient's entire life story. Sadly, in the setting of today's fast-paced medication-management visits, and outside of psychotherapy treatment, that valuable part of the doctor–patient interaction is often absent. In my integrative psychiatric practice, I feel fortunate to be able to approach patients with an eye for their uniqueness. Life circumstances, personality traits, genetic tendencies, and past experiences all shape a person's experience of depressed mood. I think that each woman presents with a singular depression that is a phenomenon distinct from any other patient's. This subjectivity, in my opinion, makes integrative approaches extremely well suited to the treatment of depression. With integrative treatment in mind, I am able to formulate, together with my patients, individualized treatment plans that honor their particular strengths, interests, likes, and dislikes. This deeply personal way of supporting women through depression can provide a strong foundation on which to build future treatment success.

Integrative Approaches

NUTRITION

Nutritional deficiencies, such as in folate, vitamin B12, iron, and vitamin D, can contribute to depressive symptoms and can be easily corrected if detected by laboratory assessment. But there is also a burgeoning literature supporting the role of general diet and nutrition in treating depression, which fact echoes not only common sense, but also the medical traditions of ancient cultures (Low Dog, 2010). In particular, the benefits accrued by following a diet high in whole foods and low in processed foods appear substantial with respect to risk for depression (Akbaraly et al., 2009). The literature supporting a powerful connection between the inflammatory cascade and depression is also growing (Maes et al., 2012), and it is not coincidental that many nutritional approaches to depression are anti-inflammatory. Multiple inflammatory pathways, including cytokine-mediated cascades as well as oxidative and autoimmune responses, appear to be implicated (Moylan, Maes, Wray, & Berk, 2012). As well, simple sugars appear to contribute to inflammation and oxidative stress (Liu et al., 2002). Thus, along with encouraging my patients to choose fresh, whole foods whenever possible, I also recommend limiting simple sugar intake and cooking with herbs and spices rich in anti-inflammatory compounds such as turmeric, saffron, rosemary, garlic, bay leaf, cayenne, and cinnamon. Making dietary changes is difficult, particularly if one is in the throes of depression, so I try to make these recommendations at a slow and measured pace throughout the course of treatment, checking in often to assess my patient's level of enthusiasm or overwhelm.

DIETARY SUPPLEMENTS AND BOTANICALS

St John's Wort (Hypericum perforatum)

St. John's Wort is a flowering plant that is commonly used in western Europe for treatment of mild-to-moderate depression and anxiety. The herb is also extremely popular in the United States and is easy to find in drugstores, health food stores, and grocery stores.

Hypericin and hyperforin are regarded as probable active compounds in St. John's Wort and are thus often used as marker compounds for standardization. However, to date no consensus regarding the identity of the active compound(s) has been reached. Authors of a recent review (Butterweck & Schmidt, 2007) concluded that multiple compounds are most likely responsible for its pharmacologic activity.

St. John's Wort has been extensively studied as a possible treatment for depression. Meta-analyses have included trials comparing St. John's Wort to tricyclic antidepressants, maprotiline, and SSRIs in depression (Linde, Berner, Egger, & Mulrow, 2005; Linde et al., 1996; Roder, Schaefer, & Leucht, 2004; Whiskey et al., 2001). In these studies, the effect of St. John's Wort was equivalent to that of pharmacotherapy. Similarly, one randomized controlled trial (RCT) (Szegedi, Kohnen, Dienel, & Kieser, 2005) indicated that St John's Wort 1,800 mg/day was equivalent to paroxetine treatment in a group of patients with moderate-to-severe depression. Interestingly, in a large NIH-funded trial (Hypericum Depression Trial Study Group, 2002), neither St. John's Wort nor sertraline was found to be more effective than placebo in treatment-resistant patients with moderate-to-severe depression. In 2005, however, the Cochrane Library published a meta-analysis focusing on the highest quality literature available (Linde, Mulrow, Berner, & Egger, 2005). A subanalysis in this review suggested that the herb is effective in treating mild depression, but not effective in addressing moderate or severe depression. Taken together, the results of these studies seem to indicate that further research is needed to examine the efficacies of both herbal and pharmaceutical treatment of depression.

St. John's Wort may cause side effects similar to those of SSRIs including dry mouth, GI symptoms, anxiety, headache, fatigue, dizziness, or sexual dysfunction, though in clinical trials, it is better tolerated than SSRIs and the adverse effects are not significantly greater than placebo. St. John's Wort can also cause photosensitivity, and may increase the risk of serotonin syndrome when used in combination with serotonergic medications including antidepressants, migraine medications, certain opioid pain medications, lithium, cough medications containing dextromethorphan, and certain antinausea medications. It is a cytochrome P450 (CYP450) inducer, and thus can alter blood levels of multiple medications including oral contraceptives, cyclosporine, digoxin, warfarin, irinotecan, and antiretrovirals including indinavir and ritonavir. The standard dose is 300–600 mg of extract taken three times daily.

Note: The United States Pharmacopeia offers an online resource for those patients interested in finding dietary supplements manufactured to rigorous standards: www. uspverified.org

S-Adenosyl Methionine

S-adenosyl methionine (SAMe) is a ubiquitous biomolecule found in many metabolic pathways, including synthesis of monoamine neurotransmitters such as serotonin, dopamine, and norepinephrine. It has been used as an antidepressant in western Europe for over 30 years.

S-adenosyl methionine has been extensively studied. Meta-analyses (Bressa, 1994; Delle Chiaie et al., 2002) have shown that SAMe is superior to placebo and is equally effective as tricyclic antidepressants (TCAs) in the treatment of major depression. More recently, preliminary data (Papakostas, Mischoulon, Shyu, Alpert, & Fava, 2010) suggest that SAMe may have utility as an adjunctive treatment with SSRIs in patients with partial responses to pharmaceutical antidepressants.

S-adenosyl methionine has a side-effect profile similar to that of SSRIs and can cause symptoms including anxiety, agitation, dry mouth, GI disturbances, headache, insomnia, palpitations, dizziness, and sweating. However, it does not cause the sexual side effects so commonly found with SSRI treatment. Bipolar patients taking SAMe are at risk of switching into hypomania, so concomitant treatment with a mood stabilizer is strongly recommended. As with SSRI treatment, the potential for serotonin syndrome exists in patients also taking serotonergic medications (for examples of serotonergic medications, see earlier section on potential interactions with St. John's Wort).

S-adenosyl methionine is not covered by insurance and tends to be expensive. Thus, I have not found it useful to recommend to women on a limited income. However, I have seen positive results for those who can afford it and who do not experience continued GI side effects. I generally ask women to start at 200 mg PO QAM and increase by 200 mg every 2 to 3 days in a twice-a-day dosing schedule, as tolerated, up to a maximum dosage of 1,600 mg total per day (most people benefit from about 800 mg total per day). As SAMe can be activating, I advise taking the second dose in the midafternoon, no later than 2 pm. Gastrointestinal side effects can be mitigated by taking it with food.

Folate

Folate is a water-soluble B vitamin (vitamin B9) found in leafy green vegetables, fruits, and legumes. Epidemiological studies have found consistent associations between folate deficiency and depression. Theoretically, folate's action may be related to its role in the synthesis of SAMe (see earlier section), which is a precursor to the monoamine neurotransmitters, including serotonin. Folinic acid and methylfolate, which are active forms of folate, are preferred in oral supplementation, as they appear to be more bioavailable in certain populations, including those who drink alcohol and those with a genetic polymorphism in the methyltetrahydrofolate reductase (MTHFR) gene.

Several forms of folate appear to be safe and efficacious in individuals with major depressive disorder, but more information is needed about dosage and populations most suited to folate therapy. In a recent review article (Fava & Mischoulon, 2009), the 5-MTHF (5-methyltetrahydrofolate) form of folate demonstrated efficacy as adjunctive therapy or monotherapy in reducing depressive symptoms in patients with both normal and low folate levels. Adjunctive treatment with folinic acid reduced depressive symptoms in patients who were partially responsive or nonresponsive to SSRI medication.

Side effects are rare. Folate supplementation should be paired with vitamin B12 supplementation (1 mg PO qd), as exogenous folate can mask the symptoms of B12 deficiency. Study doses of folate typically range from 0.4 to 1 mg by mouth each day along with a standard antidepressant medication. Folate is usually continued for the duration of antidepressant therapy.

Note: High doses (1 mg/day) of folic acid have been shown to significantly increase the risk of colorectal and prostate cancer. Clinicians should take patient risk factors and past medical history into consideration before recommending higher doses of folic acid (Cole et al., 2007; Figueiredo et al., 2009).

Omega-3 Fatty Acids

Omega-3 fatty acids (eicosapentaenoic acid [EPA] and docosahexaenoic acid [DHA]) play many important roles in human metabolism, including that of supporting the growth and development of the nervous system. Epidemiological studies have linked low dietary consumption of omega-3s and increased prevalence of depression.

The literature concerning omega-3 fatty acids and depression is mixed, largely pointing to a relative dearth of large-scale, high-quality studies. A large review (Parker et al., 2006) included RCTs examining potential effects of omega-3 fatty acid supplementation on depressive disorders and showed benefits for depression due to augmentation of pharmacotherapy with omega-3 fatty acids. A more recent review (Bloch & Hannestad, 2012) included a meta-analysis of RCTs focused on omega-3 fatty acid mono therapy of major depressive disorder, and revealed no significant benefit.

Omega-3 fatty acids may exert their antidepressant effects by (1) contributing to neural cell stability and signal transduction by virtue of their integral role in neuronal membrane structure; (2) promoting secretion of brain-derived neurotrophic factor (BDNF), a peptide involved in promotion of neuronal longevity; and (3) dampening the inflammatory cascades, which are seen in severe depression and which can adversely affect neurotransmitter metabolism.

Side effects include GI disturbance and fishy-tasting burps, both of which can be reduced by using high-quality preparations and keeping daily doses below 5 grams per day. Omega-3 fatty acid supplementation, especially above 3 grams per day, can cause excessive anticoagulation, so patients taking warfarin should be monitored. There is a small risk of inducing hypomania in bipolar patients, so in these cases concurrent treatment with a mood stabilizer is indicated.

Studies examining omega-3 supplementation for depression have mainly used either EPA alone, or a combination of EPA/DHA wherein EPA was provided at a higher concentration. Study dosages for EPA range between 1 and 9 grams, with positive evidence for dosages at the lower end of this range, and some small positive studies at 1 g EPA/day (Freeman et al., 2006). I recommend omega-3 fatty acid augmentation therapy for my patients with major depressive disorder and also make it a part of my integrative treatment recommendations for patients with mild depression. I ask that patients start with about 500 mg EPA per day in a high-quality supplement containing both EPA and DHA, taken with a meal containing fat. Increase as tolerated by about 500 mg total omega-3's every 3 to 5 days in a twice-per-day divided dosing schedule, up to a maximum of 3 grams of total EPA+DHA per day.

5-Hydroxytryptophan

5-hydroxytryptophan (5-HTP) is the immediate metabolic precursor to serotonin. Up-regulation of serotonin biosynthesis is the potential mechanism of its antidepressant action. It is widely available in health food stores and online as a natural treatment for depression and insomnia. A 2002 Cochrane review (Shaw, Turner, & Del Mar, 2002) revealed only a small number of high quality studies and suggested that 5-HTP is superior to placebo in the treatment of depression. Another review (Turner, Loftis, & Blackwell, 2006) reported mixed data regarding the possible mood benefits of 5-HTP in depression. Of the 11 RCTs studied, only five yielded statistically significant positive results. Of the five positive trials, three used 5-HTP as adjunct therapy to conventional pharmacotherapy, one used it as monotherapy, and one tested a combination of 5-HTP and dopamine versus placebo.

Larger studies are needed in order to clarify the potential utility of 5HTP in the treatment of depression. If used, it is important to recommend a high-quality product, as there exists a theoretical risk of eosinophilic myalgia due to contamination. The recommended dosage of 5-HTP is 50–100 mg/day, though some studies have used up to 300 mg/day.

Inositol

Inositol, a naturally occurring isomer of glucose, is a key player in the second-messenger molecule system, which modulates cell surface receptors for serotonin and other neurotransmitters. It is found in a variety of foods including citrus fruit, nuts, whole-grain cereals, and blackstrap molasses. The theoretical mechanism of its antidepressant action is via facilitating cellular responses to serotonin. Inositol supplementation for mild depression has been part of European folk medicine for many years, but the formal medical literature concerning inositol is limited.

A Cochrane review (Taylor MJ, et al., 2005) yielded 4 small RCTs, with a combined 141 patients. This review indicated that while there were no significant benefits to inositol treatment of depressive disorder, there was also no evidence of adverse effects. Another, later meta-analysis identified and reviewed seven RCTs in depression (two bipolar depression studies, one bipolar and major depressive disorder [MDD] study, two MDD studies, and two premenstrual dysphoric disorder [PMDD] studies) and four RCTs in anxiety disorders (two obsessive-compulsive disorder studies, one panic disorder study, and one posttraumatic stress disorder study). These studies failed to note any statistically significant effects of inositol on depressive, anxiety, and obsessive-compulsive symptoms. However, all of the studies suffered from small sample size (Mukai, Kishi, Matsuda, & Iwata, 2014).

Taking into consideration the paucity of data available, the role of inositol in the treatment of depression remains unclear, and further study is needed.

Inositol is generally quite safe and well tolerated. Dosages typically used in studies are 10–12 g PO per day.

MIND–BODY APPROACHES

Meditation

The general medical literature focuses on two types of meditation for the treatment of depression, both of which are based in Eastern spiritual practices: concentration meditation and mindfulness meditation. There are little data addressing meditation as a primary treatment for major depression, rather existing studies investigated the benefits in medically ill patients with associated depressive symptoms and showed a potential positive effect (Goodale, Domar, & Benson, 1990; Irvin, Domar, Clark, Zuttermeister, & Friedman, 1996; Jayadevappa et al., 2007; Speca, Carlson, Goodey, & Angen, 2000). Two small studies of women with breast cancer (Targ & Levine, 2002) and fibromyalgia (Sephton et al., 2007) with associated depression also showed mood benefits for meditation. In one RCT (Sharma, Das, Mondal, & Goswampi, & Gandhi, 2005), depressed patients exhibited positive mood changes in response to concentration meditation as an adjunct to pharmacotherapy. Also, one review (Coelho, Canter, & Ernst, 2007) summarized data indicating that mindfulness-based cognitive therapy (MBCT), a psychotherapeutic model integrating meditation techniques with cognitive-behavioral therapy (CBT) techniques, has potential benefit as an adjunct treatment to reduce risk of relapse in major depression. Most recently, a review of RCTs evaluating the benefit of mindfulness meditation programs for the treatment of stress-related measures revealed positive evidence for treatment of depression (Goyal et al., 2014).

Meditation is postulated to exert its effects by modulating the sympathetic and parasympathetic nervous systems. When undertaken with an experienced teacher, health risks are few. However, meditation is not indicated for individuals with a history of psychosis, as meditative states can precipitate psychological crises in these patients. Where available, I have found it helpful to recommend beginning classes in mindfulness-based stress reduction (MBSR), MBCT, or vipassana meditation. For those who feel more comfortable learning about meditation on their own, I recommend the book *Peace Is Every Step*, a beautiful and accessible introduction to mindfulness meditation by the Vietnamese Buddhist monk Thich Nhat Hanh.

Yoga

Yoga, as practiced in the United States, involves breathing exercises (pranayama) and body postures (asanas). As yoga has entered mainstream American culture, many different types of yoga classes can now be found at local gyms and yoga centers. Some of these varieties include doing yoga in heated rooms, with or without vigorous pose changes. The medical literature is scant, but most available studies have focused on pranayama in combination with gentle and rhythmic pose shifts.

One review examined the effect of yoga practice in patients with major depression (Pilkington, Kirkwood, Rampes, & Richardson, 2005). Though the studies were found to have significant design problems, the authors concluded that yoga has mood benefits in comparison with control groups. Data on depressed women's responses to yoga are scant. A small study (Michalsen et al., 2005) indicated that Iyengar yoga improved depressive symptoms in a group of 24 female patients with "emotional distress," as quantified by the Center for Epidemiologic Studies Depression Scale.

Yoga is postulated to exert its effects by modulating the autonomic and central nervous systems. Performed under the guidance of an experienced teacher, it appears to be fairly safe. Beginning classes in hatha yoga or restorative yoga can be found at gyms, yoga centers, and sometimes temples or holistic health centers. In my experience, these forms of yoga are generally well tolerated by patients. Even a short course of classes can provide benefits, as breathing exercises and poses can be used at home to provide anxiolysis and to ease the transition into sleep.

Progressive Muscle Relaxation

Progressive muscle relaxation (PMR) is a behavioral technique that was developed by Dr. Edmund Jacobson in the 1930s. It involves a protocol of step-by-step voluntary muscular contraction and then relaxation with the goal of increased total body awareness and thus increased control over physical tension.

An interesting RCT (McLean & Hakstian, 1979) showed an equivalent antidepressant effect for PMR and pharmacologic treatment; it also revealed that both of these interventions were inferior to behavior therapy. Two more recent small studies showed value for PMR as an adjunct to pharmacotherapy (Bowers, 1990; Broota & Dhir, 1990). There is also more recent data suggesting that for patients with primary medical conditions and associated depression, PMR may provide mood benefits (Rodin et al., 2007; Stetter & Kupper, 2002; Stiefel & Stagno,

2004). A Cochrane Review (Jorm, 2008) examined controlled trials evaluating relaxation techniques including PMR as treatment for depression. It revealed that relaxation techniques were more effective than minimal or no treatment at decreasing self-rated depressive symptoms. More information on PMR, including step-by-step instructions for patients, can be found at http://www.guideto-psychology.com/pmr.htm. I have found that patients who are motivated, who have a strong sense of connection to their bodies, and who notice a direct relationship between mood and physical tenseness, respond well to this modality.

TRADITIONAL CHINESE MEDICINE

Acupuncture

Acupuncture involves the use of fine needles, and sometimes mild electrical current or lasers, to stimulate specific points on the body, which are postulated to regulate and balance the flow of *qi*, or life force. A treatment modality with thousands of years of history, acupuncture is a complex treatment that does not easily lend itself to conventional study design. Thus, the available medical literature is scant and of highly variable quality, as we see in what follows.

Data from RCTs examining the effects of acupuncture compared with wait-list control, sham acupuncture, and conventional treatment in patients with major depression have been analyzed in several review articles (Leo & Ligot, 2007; Mukaino, Park, White, & Ernst, 2005; Smith & Hay, 2005). The authors of these articles concluded that the studies were methodologically poor, and meta-analysis did not reveal statistically significant differences between treatment groups. A more recent 2012 review that included additional studies concluded that acupuncture is a potential effective monotherapy for depression, and a safe, well-tolerated augmentation in antidepressant partial responders and nonresponders. The authors, like previous reviewers, also noted that well designed studies are limited (Wu, Yeung, Schnyer, Wang, & Mischoulon, 2012).

Data supporting the use of acupuncture in women with depressive symptoms consists primarily of small studies. A pilot study of acupuncture in the treatment of menopause-related symptoms, including depression, in tamoxifen-treated women yielded some preliminary positive results (Porzio et al., 2002). Another RCT examining a group of women with chronic neck and shoulder pain with associated depression revealed benefits for mood and quality of life (He, Høstmark, Veiersted, & Medbø, 2005). As its benefits for analgesia and addiction are well known, and its healing effects for other conditions are becoming acknowledged, acupuncture is becoming more easily accessible. Those curious about the intervention can

484 COMMON CONDITIONS IN WOMEN

find out more information by going online to http://nccam.nih.gov/health/acupuncture/. Information on each state's licensure requirements can be found at http://acupuncture.com/statelaws/ statelaw.htm. Local healthcare providers, schools of traditional Chinese medicine, or integrative medicine clinics, if available, can be a helpful referral resource for women seeking acupuncture treatment. In my practice, I often refer patients for acupuncture to treat depression, as well as associated psychological and somatic symptoms.

Tai Chi/Qigong

Tai chi and qigong are elements of traditional Chinese medicine that involve not only prescribed movements but also regulated breathing and mental focus. For thousands of years, these approaches have been used in order to help rebalance the mind and body as well as enhance wellness. Studies available in English are few, but one RCT found positive results for depressed geriatric patients participating in a program of tai chi (Chou et al., 2004). Another RCT showed mood benefits from qigong in a group of depressed elderly patients (Tsang, Fung, Chan, Lee, & Chan, 2006). Interest in these approaches is growing rapidly, and one larger-scale review (Jahnke, Larkey, Rodgers, Etnier, & Lin, 2010) focused on the effects of both tai chi and qigong on multiple measures, including psychological wellness, bone density, cardiopulmonary effects, quality of life, and immune function. Positive results were found for both modalities. These meditative approaches tend to work best for those who prefer a gentle, nonhurried method of mind–body balancing, or those who have orthopedic issues that limit vigorous exercise. If available, local Chinese community centers or martial arts centers can be good resources for beginning tai chi and qigong classes.

OTHER INTEGRATIVE APPROACHES

Aerobic Exercise

Aerobic exercise is commonly recommended in treatment plans targeting general wellness, and the benefits of exercise in modulating mood and anxiety are widely accepted. Exercise is postulated to exert its antidepressant effects by increasing levels of monoamine neurotransmitters, up-regulating endogenous endorphin production, increasing social contact if done in groups, and possibly by derailing negative thought patterns.

The literature concerning exercise and its direct effects on depressive symptoms is fairly robust. An RCT (Blumenthal, et al., 2007) involved 202 depressed adults who were randomized among 4 groups: supervised exercise, home exercise, antidepressant medication, and placebo pills for 16 weeks. Study results indicated an equivalent response to exercise and antidepressants, which was higher than the response measured to placebo. A Cochrane Review (Cooney et al., 2013) examined 39 studies of varying quality that were published until March 2013 and included 2,326 patients. The review revealed that exercise does indeed reduce depressive symptoms and is no more effective than either medications or therapy. More research and higher-quality studies are needed in order to better quantify the positive effect that exercise has on mood.

> In my practice, I have found that enticing depressed people to exercise, if they are not already involved in regular activity, is quite difficult indeed. Often, the symptoms of decreased energy, psychomotor slowing, and decreased motivation are tenacious barriers. If my gentle suggestions are met with resistance, I will often wait until depression is partially treated before returning to this particular intervention. I then advise my patients to build an exercise routine slowly, sometimes even starting with stepping outside for 5 minutes.

Taking its efficacy into consideration not only for mood but also for general health and weight loss, I have been happy to see that patients often continue with regular exercise after their acute depression subsides.

Massage Therapy

Massage therapy involves the manual manipulation of soft tissue, using any of over 80 different techniques, with the goal of increasing relaxation and well-being. In the United States, classical Swedish massage is the most common form used, and involves the use of five distinct long and flowing strokes. Other common varieties include Shiatsu (a Japanese massage technique) and deep tissue massage.

There are little data available concerning massage therapy as treatment for major depression specifically, and a review of the scant data yielded inconclusive results (Coelho, Boddy, & Ernst, 2007), but authors of a meta-analysis of studies done on patients with primary medical conditions and associated depression concluded that a course of massage therapy may be as effective as a course of psychotherapy (Moyer, Rounds, & Hannum, 2004).

Massage therapy is proposed to exert its antidepressant action through modulation of the parasympathetic nervous system and/or by stimulating the release of endorphins or serotonin into the bloodstream via mechanical stimulation of tissue. In the hands of experienced practitioners, this intervention is quite safe. For those patients who experience pain from muscle tension, or those who notice that they "carry stress" in specific parts of the body, massage therapy can be incredibly healing. I recommend this modality to depressed patients who can tolerate touch without feeling more anxious or triggered. Finding high-quality referrals is important, and seeking these via integrative medicine clinics, your healthcare provider, or via national licensing agencies, is a good place to start.

Phototherapy

In the darker winter months, the brain's endogenous secretion of melatonin, a metabolic product of serotonin, is increased. Phototherapy suppresses melatonin secretion, which theoretically increases serotonin reserves, leading to an antidepressant effect. While phototherapy for seasonal affective disorder (SAD) is part of the conventional psychiatric armamentarium, this chapter examines the use of phototherapy in the treatment of nonseasonal depression.

A meta-analysis of three RCTs indicated that phototherapy alone provided significant reduction of depressive symptoms for nonseasonal major depression (Golden et al., 2005). An earlier review found positive effect from adjunctive phototherapy when meta-analysis was limited to RCTs of very high methodological quality (Tuunainen, Kripke, & Endo, 2004). A more recent review included 15 studies, revealing benefit for treatment of depression with phototherapy as augmentation alongside medications (Even, Schroder, Friedman, & Rouillon, 2008). Available data on phototherapy in depressed women was limited to a small RCT in which phototherapy showed benefit for patients with PMDD (Lam et al., 1999). All in all, these data appear to suggest that subpopulations of depressed patients respond differently to phototherapy and that further study is needed in order to clarify these subgroups.

Phototherapy appears to be most effective when patients are exposed to bright white light of 10,000 lux intensity for 30 minutes in the early morning, every day for at least 1 week. Side effects can include headache and eye irritation, and possible induction of hypomania in patients with bipolar disorder. Thus, close monitoring and concurrent treatment with a mood stabilizer is advised for bipolar patients. For those patients who can afford a light box, I recommend this treatment in cases where there is a direct correlation between less sun exposure and mood symptoms. There are many diverse phototherapy products available today, and I advise my patients to be aware and purchase equipment that provides the intensity and color spectrum mentioned above.

Summary

Depression, while relatively common, and especially so in women, is also a complex and infinitely variable disease entity. It is a true mind–body illness, marked by both physical and psychological manifestations, which are very well suited to integrative medicine approaches. Of paramount importance in treatment is the heartfelt desire of the practitioner to be helpful and to respect the uniqueness of each patient. This treatment philosophy has a deeply positive impact on depressed patients and on their course of illness.

REFERENCES

Akbaraly, T. N., Brunner, E. J., Ferrie, J. E., et al. (2009). Dietary pattern and depressive symptoms in middle age. *Br J Psychiatry*, *195*, 408–413.

American Psychiatric Association. (2013). *Diagnostic and statistical manual of mental disorders* (5th ed.). Washington, DC: American Psychiatric Association.

Blumenthal, J. A. (2007). Exercise and pharmacotherapy in the treatment of major depressive disorder. *Psychosom Med*, *69*, 587–596.

Bloch, M. H., & Hannestad, J. (2012). Omega-3 fatty acids for the treatment of depression: Systemic review and meta-analysis. *Molecular Psych*, *17*, 1272–1282.

Bowers, W. A. (1990). Treatment of depressed in-patients: Cognitive therapy plus medication, relaxation plus medication, and medication alone. *Br J Psychiatry*, *156*, 73–78.

Bressa, G. M. (1994). S-adenosyl-l-methionine (SAMe) as antidepressant: Meta-analysis of clinical studies. *Acta Neurol Scand Suppl*, *154*, 7–14.

Broota, A., & Dhir, R. (1990). Efficacy of two relaxation techniques in depression. *J Pers Clin Stud*, *6*, 83–90.

Butterweck, V., & Schmidt, M. (2007). St. John's Wort: Role of active compounds for its mechanism of action and efficacy. *Wien Med Wochenschr*, *157*, 356–361.

Chou, K. L., Lee, P. W., Yu, E. C., et al. (2004). Effect of tai chi on depressive symptoms amongst Chinese older patients with depressive disorders: A randomized clinical trial. *Int J Geriatr Psychiatry*, *19*, 1105–1107.

Coelho, H. F., Boddy, K., & Ernst, E. (2007). Massage therapy for the treatment of depression: A clinical review. *Int J Clin Practice*, *62*, 325–333.

Coelho, H. F., Canter, P. H., & Ernst, E. (2007). Mindfulness-based cognitive therapy: Evaluating current evidence and informing future research. *J Consult Clin Psychol*, *75*, 1000–1005.

Cole, B. F., Baron, J. A., Sandler, R. S., et al. (2007). Folic acid for the prevention of colorectal adenomas: A randomized clinical trial. *JAMA*, *297*, 2351–2359.

Cooney, G. M., Dwan, K., Greig, C. A., et al. (2013). Exercise for depression. *Cochrane Database Syst Rev.* doi: 10.1002/14651858.CD004366.pub6.

Delle Chiaie, R., Pancheri, P., Scapicchio, P., Delle Chiaie, R., Pancheri, P., & Scapicchio P. (2002). Efficacy and tolerability of oral and intramuscular S-adenosyl-L-methionine

1,4-butanedisulfonate (SAMe) in the treatment of major depression: Comparison with imipramine in 2 multicenter studies. *Am J Clin Nutr, 76*, 1172S–1176S.

Even, C., Schroder, C. M., Friedman, S., & Rouillon, F. (2008). Efficacy of light therapy in nonseasonal depression: A systematic review. *J Affect Disord, 108*, 11–23.

Fava, M., & Mischoulon, D. (2009). Folate in depression: Efficacy, safety, differences in formulations, and clinical issues. *J Clin Psych, 5*, 12–17.

Figueiredo, J. C., Grau, M. V., Haile, R. W., et al. (2009). Folic acid and risk of prostate cancer: Results from a randomized clinical trial. *J Natl Cancer Inst, 101*, 432–435.

Fournier, J. C., DeRubeis, R. J., Hollon, S. D., et al. (2010). Antidepressant drug effects and patient severity: A patient-level meta-analysis. JAMA, *303*, 47–53.

Freeman, M. P., Hibbeln, J. R., Wisner, K. L., et al. (2006). Omega-3 fatty acids: Evidence basis for treatment and future research in psychiatry. *J Clin Psychiatry, 67*, 1954–67.

Golden, R. N., Gaynes, B. N., Ekstrom, R. D., et al. (2005). The efficacy of light therapy in the treatment of mood disorders: A review and meta-analysis of the evidence. *Am J Psychiatry, 162*, 656–662.

Goodale, I. L., Domar, A. D., & Benson, H. (1990). Alleviation of premenstrual syndrome symptoms with the relaxation response. *Obstet Gynecol, 75*, 649–655.

Goyal, M., et al. (2014). Meditation programs for psychological stress and well-being: A systematic review and meta-analysis. *JAMA Intern Med, 174*, 357–368.

He, D., Høstmark, A. T., Veiersted, K. B., & Medbø, J. I. (2005). Effect of intensive acupuncture on pain-related social and psychological variables for women with chronic neck and shoulder pain: An RCT with six month and three year follow up. *Acupunct Med, 23*, 5.

Hypericum Depression Trial Study Group. (2002). Effect of Hypericum perforatum (St John's wort) in major depressive disorder: A randomized controlled trial. *JAMA, 287*, 1807–1814.

Irvin, J. H., Domar, A. D., Clark, C., Zuttermeister, P. C., & Friedman, R. (1996). The effects of relaxation response training on menopausal symptoms. *J Psychosom Obstet Gynaecol, 17*, 202–207.

Jahnke, R., Larkey, L., Rodgers, C., Etnier, J., & Lin, F. (2010). A comprehensive review of health benefits of qigong and tai chi. *Am J Health Promotion, 24*, e1–e25.

Jayadevappa, R., Johnson, J. C., Bloom, B. S., et al. (2007). Effectiveness of transcendental meditation on functional capacity and quality of life of African Americans with congestive heart failure: A randomized control study. *Ethn Dis, 17*, 72–77.

Jorm, A.F., Morgan, A.J., & Hetrick, S. E. Relaxation for depression. Cochrane Database of Systematic Reviews 2008, Issue 4. Art. No.: CD007142. doi: 10.1002/14651858. CD007142.pub2

Kessler, R. C. (2001). Epidemiology of women and depression. *J Affect Disord, 74*, 5–13.

Kessler, R. C., McGonagle, K. A., Swartz, M., Blazer, D. G., & Nelson, C. B. (1993). Sex and depression in the National Comorbidity Survey. I: Lifetime prevalence, chronicity and recurrence. *J Affect Disord, 29*, 85–96.

Lam, R. W., Carter, D., Misri, S., Kuan, A. J., Yatham, L. N., & Zis, A. P. (1999). A controlled study of light therapy in women with late luteal phase dysphoric disorder. *Psychiatry Res, 86*, 185–192.

Leo, R. J., & Ligot, J. S., Jr. (2007). A systematic review of randomized controlled trials of acupuncture in the treatment of depression. *J Affect Disord, 97*, 13–22.

Linde, K., Berner, M., Egger, M., & Mulrow, C. (2005b). St John's wort for depression: Meta-analysis of randomised controlled trials. *Br J Psychiatry, 186*, 99–107.

Linde, K., Mulrow, C. D., Berner, M., & Egger, M. (2005a). St John's wort for depression. *Cochrane Database Syst Rev,* 2:CD000448.

Linde, K., Ramirez, G., Mulrow, C. D., Pauls, A., Weidenhammer, W., & Melchart D. (1996). St John's wort for depression: An overview and meta-analysis of randomised clinical trials. *Br Med J, 313*, 253–258.

Liu, S., Manson, J. E., Buring, J. E., et al. (2002). Relationship between a diet with a high glycemic load and plasma concentrations of high-sensitivity C-reactive protein in middle-aged women. *Am J Clin Nutr, 75*, 492–498.

Low Dog, T. (2010). The role of nutrition in mental health. *Altern Ther Health Med, 16*, 42–46.

Maes, M., Berk, M., Goehler, L., et al. (2012).Depression and sickness behavior are Janus-faced responses to shared inflammatory pathways. *BMC Med, 10*, 66.

McLean, P. D., & Hakstian, A. R. (1979). Clinical depression: Comparative efficacy of outpatient treatments. *J Consult Clin Psychol, 47*, 818–836.

Michalsen, A., Grossman, P., Acil, A., et al. (2005). Rapid stress reduction and anxiolysis among distressed women as a consequence of a three-month intensive yoga program. *Med Sci Monitor, 11*, CR555–CR561.

Moyer, C. A., Rounds, J., & Hannum, J. W. (2004). A meta-analysis of massage therapy research. *Psychol Bull, 130*, 3–18.

Moylan, S., Maes, M., Wray, N. R., & Berk, M. (2012).The neuroprogressive nature of major depressive disorder: Pathways to disease evolution and resistance, and therapeutic implications. *Mol Psychiatry, 18*, 595–606.

Mukai, T., Kishi, T., Matsuda, Y., & Iwata, N. (2014). A meta-analysis of inositol for depression and anxiety disorders. *Hum Psychopharmacol, 29*, 55–63.

Mukaino, Y., Park, J., White, A., & Ernst, E. (2005). The effectiveness of acupuncture for depression: A systematic review of randomised controlled trials. *Acupunct Med, 23*, 70–76.

Nolen-Hoeksema, S. (2000). *The etiology of gender differences in depression, research trends and an integrative model.* Paper presented to the American Psychological Association Summit on Women and Depression, Wye River, MD, October 5–7.

Nolen-Hoeksema, S., & Girgus, J. S. (1994). The emergence of gender differences in depression during adolescence. *Psychol Bull, 115*, 424–443.

Parker, G., Gibson, N. A., Brotchie, H., Heruc, G., Rees, A. M., & Hadzi-Pavlovic, D. (2006). Omega-3 fatty acids and mood disorders. *Am J Psychiatry, 163*, 969–978.

Papakostas, G. I., Mischoulon, D., Shyu, I., Alpert, J. E., & Fava, M. (2010). S-adenosyl methionine augmentation of serotonin reuptake inhibitors for antidepressant non-responders with major depressive disorder: A double-blind, randomized clinical trial. *Am J Psychiatry, 167*, 942–948.

Pilkington, K., Kirkwood, G., Rampes, H., & Richardson, J. (2005). Yoga for depression: The research evidence. *J Affect Disord, 89*, 13–24.

Porzio, G., Trapasso, T., Martelli, S., et al. (2002). Acupuncture in the treatment of menopause-related symptoms in women taking tamoxifen. *Tumori, 88*, 128–130.

Roder, C., Schaefer, M., & Leucht, S. (2004). Meta-analysis of effectiveness and tolerability of treatment of mild to moderate depression with St. John's Wort. *Fortschr Neurol Psychiatr, 72*, 330–343.

Rodin, G., Lloyd, N., Katz, M., Green, E., Mackay, J. A., & Wong, R. K.; Supportive Care Guidelines Group of Cancer Care Ontario Program in Evidence-Based Care. (2007). The treatment of depression in cancer patients: A systematic review. *Support Care Cancer, 15*, 123–136.

Sephton, S. E., Salmon, P., Weissbecker, I., et al. (2007). Mindfulness meditation alleviates depressive symptoms in women with fibromyalgia: Results of a randomized clinical trial. *Arthritis Rheum, 57*, 77–85.

Sharma, V. K., Das, S., Mondal, S., & Goswampi, U., & Gandhi, A. (2005). Effect of Sahaj yoga on depressive disorders. *Indian J Physiol Pharmacol, 49*, 462–468.

Shaw, K., Turner, J., & Del Mar, C. (2002). Tryptophan and 5-hydroxytryptophan for depression. *Cochrane Database Syst Rev*, 1:CD003198.

Smith, C. A., & Hay, P. P. (2005). Acupuncture for depression. *Cochrane Database Syst Rev*, 2:CD004046.

Speca, M., Carlson, L. E., Goodey, E., & Angen, M. (2000). A randomized, wait-list controlled clinical trial: The effect of a mindfulness meditation-based stress reduction program on mood and symptoms of stress in cancer outpatients. *Psychosom Med, 62*, 613–622.

Stetter, F., & Kupper S. (2002). Autogenic training: A meta-analysis of clinical outcome studies. *Appl Psychophysiol Biofeedback, 27*, 45–98.

Stiefel, F., & Stagno D. (2004). Management of insomnia in patients with chronic pain conditions. *CNS Drugs, 18*, 285–296.

Szegedi, A., Kohnen, R., Dienel, A., & Kieser, M. 2005 Acute treatment of moderate to severe depression with hypericum extract WS 5570 (St John's wort): Randomised controlled double blind non-inferiority trial versus paroxetine. *BMJ, 330*, 503.

Targ, E. F., & Levine, E. G. (2002). The efficacy of a mind-body-spirit group for women with breast cancer: A randomized controlled trial. *Gen Hosp Psychiatry, 24*, 238–248.

Taylor, M. J., Wilder, H., Bhagwagar, Z., & Geddes J. (2004). Inositol for depressive disorders. *Cochrane Database Syst Rev*, 2:CD004049.

Tsang, H. W., Fung, K. M., Chan, A. S., Lee, G., & Chan, F. (2006). Effect of a qigong exercise programme on elderly with depression. *Int J Geriatr Psychiatry, 21*, 890–897.

Turner, E. H., Loftis, J. M., & Blackwell, A. D. (2006). Serotonin a la carte: Supplementation with the serotonin precursor 5-hydroxytryptophan. *Pharmacol Ther, 109*, 325–338.

Tuunainen, A., Kripke, D. F., & Endo, T. (2004). Light therapy for non-seasonal depression. *Cochrane Database Syst Rev*, 2:CD004050.

Whiskey, E., Werneke, U., & Taylor D. (2001). A systematic review and meta-analysis of *Hypericum perforatum* in depression: A comprehensive clinical review. *Int Clin Psychopharmacol, 16*, 239–252.

Wu, J., Yeung, A. S., Schnyer, R., Wang, Y., & Mischoulon, D. (2012). Acupuncture for depression: A review of clinical applications. *Can J Psychiatry, 57*, 397–405.

25

Urinary Tract Infections

PRISCILLA ABERCROMBIE

CASE STUDY

Rosemary is a 27-year-old college student who suffers from frequent bladder infections. She is worried about taking so many antibiotics. It seems like every time she goes home on vacation from school and has sex with her boyfriend she gets another infection. After she takes the antibiotics then she gets a yeast infection. She is wondering what she can do to prevent these infections and whether she can do it without taking antibiotics.

Introduction

More than 50% of all women will develop a urinary tract infection (UTI) in their lifetime (Fihn, 2003). Eighty percent to 90% of UTIs are caused by *Escherichia coli* (Fihn, 2003). Twenty-five percent of women will have a recurrence of their UTI in their lifetime (Franco, 2005).

DEFINITIONS

Acute lower UTI, also called acute bacterial cystitis, is characterized by urinary frequency, dysuria, and urgency. A combination of these symptoms without vaginal symptoms increases the diagnostic probability of UTI to more than 90% (Fihn, 2003). Other symptoms may include suprapubic pressure and gross hematuria.

Recurrent UTI is most commonly caused by reinfection with the same or different organism and occurs after resolution of a previously treated infection (Franco, 2005). Many possible modes of UTI recurrence have been proposed: the same UTI-causing strain of bacteria persists in the gut and reinoculates the bladder, a different strain is introduced into the gut and then colonizes the bladder, a quiescent bacteria residing in the bladder re-emerges, or a new strain of bacteria is introduced directly into the perineum (Silverman, Schreiber, Hooton, & Hultgren, 2013).

Interstitial cystitis (IC) is characterized by urinary frequency, urgency, and pelvic pain and is frequently misdiagnosed as recurrent UTI (Dell, 2007). Interstitial cystitis can be differentiated from recurrent UTI by the absence of pyuria or bacteria on urine culture in the setting of bladder pain. Standardized symptom surveys such as the Pelvic Pain and Urgency/Frequency (PUF) questionnaire have been used to identify women with IC, but the reliability of this tool has been questioned (Brewer, White, Klein, Klein, & Waters, 2007). Guidelines for the treatment of IC can be found at the American Urological Association website (Hanno et al., 2014). Interstitial cystitis remains a diagnosis made primarily by exclusion.

Women who present with fever, chills, and flank pain are more likely to have a complicated upper UTI or pyelonephritis, requiring more aggressive treatment and vigilant follow-up. The focus of this chapter is on the management of uncomplicated lower UTI.

Clinical Tip

In young women under age 23, infection with the sexually transmitted infections *Neisseria gonorrhoeae* or *Chlamydia trachomatis* urethritis should be ruled out. All women with vaginal symptoms including burning with urination on the external genitalia should be evaluated for vaginitis.

RISK FACTORS FOR URINARY TRACT INFECTION

The most common risk factor for acute and recurrent UTI in women of all ages is sexual intercourse. Other common risk factors include previous UTI, use of spermicide, diabetes, pregnancy, incontinence or voiding dysfunction, genetics, and female anatomy.

LABORATORY TESTING

Those with classic UTI symptoms should be treated empirically. A telephone consultation is an acceptable method of identifying and treating women with a UTI (Schauberger, Merkitch, & Prell, 2007). The presence of dysuria, frequency, hematuria, nocturia, and urgency increases the probability of a diagnosis of UTI, while the presence of vaginal discharge decreases the probability (Giesen, Cousins, Dimitrov, van de Laar, & Fahey, 2010). Women with a history of recent UTI, recurrent UTI, or symptoms of vaginitis or cervicitis should be seen for an evaluation.

A urine analysis by dipstick is sufficient for diagnosis in most cases. In a meta-analysis of clinical studies, a combination of clinical symptoms with nitrites on dipstick increased diagnostic accuracy (Giesen, Cousins, Dimitrov, van de Laar, & Fahey, 2010). In another meta-analysis, the presence of either nitrites or leukocytes on dipstick was the most reliable diagnostic tool and clinical symptoms were not helpful (Medina-Bombardo, & Jover-Palmer, 2011). All women with a positive dipstick with clinical symptoms should be treated. Patients with a negative urine dipstick, upper urinary tract symptoms, or with recurrent UTI should have a urine culture.

Management Strategies

Although evidence-based guidelines for the treatment of UTI are available from many organizations such as the Infectious Disease Society of America and the American College of Obstetricians and Gynecologists, many clinicians continue to conduct unnecessary tests and treat with inappropriate antimicrobials. One study conducted by the Mayo Clinic (Grover et al., 2007) found that only 30% of patients with UTI seen in a family medicine residency clinic setting were managed within clinical guidelines. Less than 25% of patients received empiric treatment; urine cultures were done despite positive dipsticks, and although trimethoprim-sulfamethoxazole is effective in most cases, it was prescribed less often than expected.

Clinical Management Guidelines

ACOG Practice Bulletin: Treatment of Urinary Tract Infections (American College of Obstetricians and Gynecologists [ACOG], 2008).

> International Clinical Practice Guidelines for the Treatment of Acute Uncomplicated Cystitis and Pyelonephritis in Women: A 2010 Update by the Infectious Diseases Society for Microbiology and Infectious Diseases (Gupta et al., 2011).

ANTIMICROBIALS

Three-day antimicrobial therapy is now the standard treatment regimen for acute UTI and is effective in over 90% of cases (ACOG, 2008). Trimethoprim-sulfamethoxazole (TMP-SMX) remains the treatment of choice for women with acute UTI. In community settings where there is a greater than 15%–20% resistance to TMP-SMX, other antimicrobials should be prescribed (ACOG, 2008). Recurrences can be treated with a 3-day or 7-day antimicrobial regimen. Women should be evaluated and counseled for risk factors for recurrence, such as sexual intercourse and the use of spermicides. Women with more than two UTIs in a year should be referred to a urologist or urogynecologist to rule out structural abnormalities. Prophylaxis with an antimicrobial (e.g., nitrofurantoin) once daily has been shown to reduce the risk of recurrence by 95% (Franco, 2005). A Cochrane analysis found that daily prophylaxis for 6 to 12 months successfully reduced recurrent UTIs compared with placebo (Albert et al., 2004). Of note, there were no differences between the groups when the antimicrobials were discontinued and an increase in side effects within the antimicrobial group. For women with recurrent UTI associated with sexual intercourse, a single dose of an antimicrobial after intercourse for prophylaxis has been found to be effective (Melekos et al., 1997). Health behaviors such as postcoital voiding, wiping pattern, and the wearing of pantyhose do not appear to reduce the recurrence of UTIs (Fihn, 2003). See Table 25.1 for a quick guide to antimicrobial treatment of UTIs.

Clinical Tip

The use of certain antimicrobials may adversely affect normal genital flora such as *Lactobacilli*, leading to an increase in the colonization of uropathogens (Franco, 2005). Trimethoprim and nitrofurantoin are thought to have less effect on normal genital flora than amoxicillin and beta-lactam antibiotics. Spermicides have been found to alter the vaginal microflora, increasing the risk of UTI (Gupta, Hillier, Hooton, Roberts, & Stamm, 2000).

Table 25.1. Quick Guide: Treatment of Uncomplicated UTIs

	Drug	*Dose*
Acute UTI	Trimethoprim—sulfamethoxazole (TMP-SMX)	One twice a day for 3 days, category C for pregnancy and breastfeeding
	Trimethoprim	100 mg, twice daily for 3 days
	Ciprofloxacin	250 mg twice daily for 3 days, do not use in pregnancy or breastfeeding
Recurrent UTI	Ciprofloxacin	250 mg twice daily for 3 or 7 days
	Nitrofurantoin	100 mg twice daily for 7 days
Prophylaxis	Nitrofurantoin	100 mg once daily for 6 to 12 months
	Nitrofurantoin	100 mg once daily after intercourse

ACOG Guidelines (ACOG, 2008).

ESTROGEN IN POSTMENOPAUSAL WOMEN

Vaginal estrogen increases antimicrobial peptides, improves tissue integrity, and promotes the growth of healthy microflora (Luthje, Hirschberg, & Brauner, 2014), which may suggest a potential role in the prevention of UTI in the postmenopausal woman. While a Cochrane review (Perrotta, Aznar, Mejia, Albert, & Ng, 2008) concluded that the use of oral estrogen did not reduce the risk of recurrent UTI in the four RCTs reviewed, two small RCTs found that vaginal estrogen successfully reduced the number of UTIs in postmenopausal women with recurrent UTIs (Perrotta, Aznar, Mejia, Albert, & Ng, 2008).

Nonconventional Approaches to Urinary Tract Infection

Some women prefer not to take antibiotics for the treatment of UTI. In a prospective cohort study, 137 women were asked to delay antibiotic treatment, 37% agreed (Gagyor et al., 2012). After 1 week, 55% had not used antibiotics and 71% of these women had clinical improvement or resolution of their symptoms. In qualitative interviews, most women said they welcomed the opportunity to delay the use of antibiotics, many wished to avoid side effects;

they liked being offered "natural" alternatives and felt validated by being offered a prescription in case symptoms persisted (Leydon, Turner, Smith, & Little, 2010).

PROBIOTICS

Lactobacilli are probiotics thought to play a role in the prevention of UTIs. A variety of *Lactobacilli* strains, particularly those that are hydrogen producing, prevent the growth of uropathogens and promote the restoration of normal genitourinary microflora. A decrease in hydrogen peroxide–producing *Lactobacilli* is thought to increase risk of recurrent UTI by facilitating colonization of *E. coli* (Gupta et al., 1998). To date, numerous issues have plagued the clinical research of probiotics for genitourinary health: small sample size, lack of quantitative evidence of colonization of *Lactobacilli*, issues regarding product stability and quality, lack of knowledge regarding the role of specific *Lactobacilli* strains in the genitourinary ecosystem, and the need for validated dosing strategies (Barrons & Tassone, 2008). However, despite these shortcomings, the use of certain species of *Lactobacilli* for the prevention of recurrent UTI looks promising.

Until recently, only three strains, *L. rhamnosus* GR-1 and *L. reuteri* B-54 and RC-14, have been found effective in the treatment of UTIs (Barrons & Tassone, 2008). In a 12-month double-blinded double dummy noninferiority trial postmenopausal women with recurrent UTI were randomized to either 480 mg per day of TMP-SMX or *L. rhamnosis* GR-1 and *L. reuteri* RC-14 twice daily (Reid & Bruce, 2006). After 12 months, the antibiotic was found superior. An intention-to-treat analysis showed a between-treatment difference of 0.4 UTIs per year. Although the study showed a statistically significant difference between the groups, 0.4 UTIs per year may have little clinical significance. In addition, antibiotic resistance occurred as early as the first month in the TMP-SMX group, unlike the *Lactobacilli* group, which had a much lower development of resistance. The authors conclude that the use of *Lactobacilli* may be an acceptable alternative in women who prefer not to use antibiotics.

A fourth species, *L. crispatus* may also be effective (Beerepoot et al., 2012). In a randomized placebo controlled trial, premenopausal women who received intravaginal suppositories containing *L. crispatus* after antimicrobial treatment had a UTI recurrence rate significantly lower (15%) than the placebo group (27%). This study showed that high vaginal colonization rates of *L. crispatus* were associated with a significant reduction in recurrent UTI (Stapleton et al., 2011).

Clinical Tip

Currently, there is one over-the-counter product available in the United States, Fem-Dophilus by Jarrow, which contains 5 billion colony forming unit (CFU) *L. rhamnosus* GR-1 and *L. reuteri* RC-14 per capsule

UVA URSI (*ARCTOSTAPHYLOS UVA URSI*)

Uva ursi, or bearberry leaf, has a long history of traditional use for inflammatory conditions of the urinary tract. The primary active constituent of the leaf is the glycoside arbutin, which undergoes hepatic conjugation to form hydroquinone, which acts as an antiseptic and antimicrobial in the bladder. It was originally thought that the urine must be alkaline for the hydroquinone glucuronide to decompose sufficiently to release the hydroquinone and have its antimicrobial effect (Yarnell, 2002), although more recent research has not borne this out (Siegers, Bodinet, Ali, & Siegers, 2003). According to the German E Commission, uva ursi is active in vitro against common uropathogens such as *E. coli, Proteus vulgaris, Ureaplasma urealyticum,* and *Staphylococcus aureus* (Blumenthal, Bundesinstitut für Arzneimittel und Medizinprodukte, Commission E., 2000). There is additional evidence that uva ursi has antimicrobial activity against *S. aureus* (Snowden et al., 2014). Although uva ursi is traditionally used as a treatment for mild acute UTI, one double-blinded placebo-controlled trial demonstrated that the botanical could be successfully used as a preventive therapy (Larsson, Jonasson, & Fianu, 1993). Fifty-seven women with recurrent cystitis were randomized to receive either standardized uva ursi extract combined with dandelion leaf/root or placebo for 1 month. In the following year, there were no UTIs in the treatment group and 23% in the placebo group.

The German E Commission has approved uva ursi for the treatment, not prevention, of UTI. However, no clinical trials have been conducted to support its effectiveness for treating UTI. The recommended dose is that which provides 420 mg/day arbutin, divided into two to three doses. This is equivalent to 1.5–2.5 grams in infusion or cold aqueous extract or 2–4 mL of a tincture (1:5) three times/day. Most authorities recommend using uva ursi for no longer than 2 weeks at a time and no more than 5 times a year due to concerns about the safety of arbutin and hydroquinone. One case of Bull's eye maculopathy secondary to prolonged use of uva ursi was reported in the literature (Wang, &

Del Priore, 2004), and uva ursi is a known melanin inhibitor, used to treat hyperpigmentation of the skin (Arndt, & Fitzpatrick, 1965; Fitzpatrick, Arndt, el-Mofty, & Pathak, 1966). However, this limitation on use may be unnecessary given a recent review of experimental and human studies that found that uva ursi was safe when used at the aforementioned dose, even for prolonged periods of time (de Arriba, Naser, & Nolte, 2013). Given the lack of reproductive studies, uva ursi should not be recommended during these times. It is interesting to note there is some in vitro evidence that herbs with high polyphenol content like uva ursi may decrease the bactericidal action of some antimicrobials like ciprofloxacin and ampicillin against *E. coli* and increase susceptibility to antimicrobials in other cases (Samoilova, Smirnova, Muzyka, & Oktyabrsky, 2014). It may be prudent to avoid the use of uva ursi in conjunction with antibiotics.

CRANBERRY (*VACCINIUM MACROCARPON*)

Cranberry is used widely for the prevention, but not treatment, of UTI. It was originally thought that it worked by acidifying the urine, but subsequent studies have shown that the proanthocyanadins (PACs) present in the fruit inhibit the adherence of bacteria to the uroepithelial cells lining the urinary tract (Sobota, 1984). Studies show efficacy of cranberry against uropathogens such as *E. coli* (Sobota, 1984; Zafriri, Ofek, Adar, Pocino, & Sharon, 1989). Blueberry (*Vaccinium augustifolium*) and lingonberry (*Vaccinium vitis-idaea*), cousins of cranberry, have similar PACs and antiadhesion properties, but more research is needed to understand whether they may be used interchangeably or whether one is superior to another (Davidson, Zimmermann, Jungfer, & Chrubasik-Hausmann, 2014).

A 2008 Cochrane review (Jepson, & Craig, 2008) concluded that that cranberry juice was effective in reducing recurrent UTIs. Since then 14 more studies have been conducted and were included in a 2012 review (Jepson, Williams, & Craig, 2012). In this review, cranberry was not found to be effective in the prevention of UTI, though a couple of caveats should be kept in mind. First, three small studies found that cranberry was equally effective as antibiotics in preventing UTI. Second, there were high dropout rates in some studies, attributed to the participants' inability to drink large quantities of cranberry juice over extended periods of time. Cranberry tablets may be better tolerated and less expensive, but the dosage used in the studies reviewed was probably inadequate (Jepson, Williams, & Craig, 2012). Future studies and meta-analyses should focus on high-quality studies that use a sufficient dose to compare the effectiveness of cranberry extract found in pill or powder forms with antibiotics used in the prevention of UTI.

Cranberry is available as a sweetened and unsweetened juice and as a concentrated juice extract tablet with or without other ingredients. One well-designed study used Ocean Spray cranberry cocktail 300 mL/day (10 ounces). Recommended juice dosages vary from 250 to 500 mL/day. Capsules of concentrated juice extract in 300–500 mg can be given two to three times a day. Cranberry is safe to use during pregnancy and lactation.

Clinical Tip

For my patients at risk for recurrent UTI, I recommend the use of 500 mg of cranberry extract in tablet form one to three times a day. The tablets are more convenient, do not contain sugar, and are better tolerated than unsweetened cranberry juice. Supplements containing both cranberry and D-mannose are also available over-the-counter.

OTHER BOTANICALS

There are a few other botanicals that should be mentioned because of their long-standing traditional use. The leaves and oil of buchu (*Agathosma betulina*), a South African plant, have been used as a diurectic and to treat bladder infections (Simpson, 1998). Unfortunately, one study found buchu had very little antimicrobial activity against *E. coli* when tested in vitro (Lis-Balchin, Hart, & Simpson, 2001). Corn silk stigmata (*Zea mays*) have been found to have diuretic effects and were shown in vitro to interfere with the outer membrane proteins of *E. coli*, blocking adhesion to the bladder mucosa (Maksimovic, Dobric, Kovacevic, & Milovanovic, 2004; Masteikova et al., 2007; Rafsanjany, Lechtenberg, Petereit, & Hensel, 2013). Birch (*Betula pendula*) is recognized by the German Commission E monograph "for irrigation therapy in bacterial and inflammatory conditions of the lower urinary tract and renal gravel; as supportive treatment in rheumatic complaints" (Blumenthal, Bundesinstitut für Arzneimittel und Medizinprodukte, Commission E, 2000). One experimental study found that all tested concentrations of birch extract significantly decreased the growth of *E. coli* (Wojnicz et al., 2012).

D-MANNOSE

D-Mannose is a sugar found in fruit such as peaches, oranges, cranberries, and blueberries. It is also present in the epithelial cells that line the urinary tract. Unlike most sugars, it is excreted unchanged in the urine. In the urinary tract, D-mannose coats *E. coli*, essentially inactivating the bacteria, rendering it unable to attach to mannose receptors on uroepithelial cells (Wojnicz et al., 2012). D-Mannose has been shown to decrease bacturia due to *E. coli* in rats (Michaels, Chmiel, Plotkin, & Schaeffer, 1983). Numerous in vitro studies document the useful role D-mannose plays in the urinary tract, but only one clinical trial exists. In the randomized clinical trial of 308 women with history of recurrent UTI, both D-mannose 2 grams once daily and nitrofurantoin 50 mg once daily were equally effective in preventing recurrence compared to placebo over 6 months (Altarac, & Papes, 2014). The D-mannose group had significantly fewer side effects than the antibiotic group, though they were both well tolerated. Unfortunately, the antibiotic group was given half the normal dose of nitrofurantoin that is currently recommended.

ACUPUNCTURE

In a small randomized study, acupuncture was very effective in reducing recurrent UTI compared with sham acupuncture and a control group (Aune, Alraek, LiHua, & Baerheim, 1998). In a larger study of women randomized to acupuncture versus no treatment, there was a 50% reduction in recurrence among the women receiving acupuncture over 6 months (Alraek, Soedal, Fagerheim, Digranes, & Baerheim, 2002). Acupuncture shows promise, but more high-quality studies are needed, including a comparison study with antibiotics used to prevent recurrent UTI.

CASE STUDY

Let us revisit Rosemary, our college student with recurrent UTI related to sexual intercourse. What treatment options does she have? She could take a single dose of an antibiotic after each episode of intercourse; there is good evidence to support this. But Rosemary has expressed concern about using antibiotics. The research evidence is strongest for the use of probiotics for the long-term prevention of UTI. Other choices that may be helpful but have less evidence for effectiveness are D-mannose, cranberry, and acupuncture. Because Rosemary is a college student, she will want to consider which of her options is most likely to fit into her lifestyle and is the most affordable.

Summary

Antimicrobials remain the standard choice for the treatment of acute UTI because of the strong evidence for their effectiveness. Probiotics containing certain strains of *Lactobacilli* show promise in preventing recurrent UTI. Uva ursi, cranberry, D-mannose, and, in postmenopausal women, vaginal estrogen are alternative treatments, though their proven benefits have yet to be established. These alternative treatments pose few safety concerns and are well tolerated. Five strategies for the prevention of recurrent UTI were reviewed in a comparative effectiveness study evaluating clinical trials (Eells, Bharadwa, McKinnell, & Miller, 2014). The use of daily antibiotics was the most effective and the most expensive treatment strategy compared with daily estrogen, daily cranberry, acupuncture, and symptomatic self-treatment. For women with poor access to healthcare, alternative strategies may be more cost effective than antibiotics for the prevention of UTI.

REFERENCES

Albert, X., Huertas, I., Pereiro, I. I., Sanfelix, J., Gosalbes, V., & Perrota, C. (2004). Antibiotics for preventing recurrent urinary tract infection in non-pregnant women. *Cochrane Database Syst Rev*, 3:CD001209.

Alraek, T., Soedal, L. I., Fagerheim, S. U., Digranes, A., & Baerheim, A. (2002). Acupuncture treatment in the prevention of uncomplicated recurrent lower urinary tract infections in adult women. *Am J Public Health*, 92, 1609–1611.

Altarac, S., & Papes, D. (2014). Use of D-mannose in prophylaxis of recurrent urinary tract infections (UTIs) in women. *BJU Int*, 113, 9–10.

American College of Obstetricians and Gynecologists. (2008). ACOG practice bulletin no. 91: Treatment of urinary tract infections in nonpregnant women. *Obstet Gynecol*, 111, 785–794.

Arndt, K. A., & Fitzpatrick, T. B. (1965). Topical use of hydroquinone as a depigmenting agent. *JAMA*, 194, 965–967.

Aune, A., Alraek, T., LiHua, H., & Baerheim, A. (1998). Acupuncture in the prophylaxis of recurrent lower urinary tract infection in adult women. *Scand J Prim Health Care*, 16, 37–39.

Barrons, R., & Tassone, D. (2008). Use of lactobacillus probiotics for bacterial genitourinary infections in women: A review. *Clin Ther*, 30, 453–468.

Beerepoot, M. A., ter Riet, G., Nys, S., et al. (2012). Lactobacilli vs antibiotics to prevent urinary tract infections: A randomized, double-blind, noninferiority trial in post-menopausal women. *Arch Intern Med*, *172*, 704–712.

Blumenthal, M., Bundesinstitut für Arzneimittel und Medizinprodukte, Commission E. (2000). *Herbal medicine: Expanded commission E monographs* (1st ed.). Newton, MA: Integrative Medicine Communications.

Brewer, M. E., White, W. M., Klein, F. A., Klein, L. M., & Waters, W. B. (2007). Validity of pelvic pain, urgency, and frequency questionnaire in patients with interstitial cystitis/painful bladder syndrome. *Urology*, *70*, 646–649.

Davidson, E., Zimmermann, B. F., Jungfer, E., & Chrubasik-Hausmann, S. (2014). Prevention of urinary tract infections with vaccinium products. *Phytother Res*, *28*, 465–470.

de Arriba, S. G., Naser, B., & Nolte, K. U. (2013). Risk assessment of free hydroquinone derived from arctostaphylos uva-ursi folium herbal preparations. *Int J Toxicol*, *32*, 442–453.

Dell, J. R. (2007). Interstitial cystitis/painful bladder syndrome: Appropriate diagnosis and management. *J Womens Health (Larchmt)*, *16*, 1181–1187.

Eells, S. J., Bharadwa, K., McKinnell, J. A., & Miller, L. G. (2014). Recurrent urinary tract infections among women: Comparative effectiveness of 5 prevention and management strategies using a Markov chain Monte Carlo model. *Clin Infect Dis*, *58*, 147–160.

Fihn, S. D. (2003). Clinical practice: Acute uncomplicated urinary tract infection in women. *N Engl J Med*, *349*, 259–266.

Fitzpatrick, T. B., Arndt, K. A., el-Mofty, A. M., & Pathak, M. A. (1966). Hydroquinone and psoralens in the therapy of hypermelanosis and vitiligo. *Arch Dermatol*, *93*, 589–600.

Franco, A. V. (2005). Recurrent urinary tract infections. *Best Pract Res Clin Obstet Gynaecol*, *19*, 861–873.

Gagyor, I., Hummers-Pradier, E., Kochen, M. M., Schmiemann, G., Wegscheider, K., & Bleidorn, J. (2012). Immediate versus conditional treatment of uncomplicated urinary tract infection: A randomized-controlled comparative effectiveness study in general practices. *BMC Infect Dis*, *12*, 146-2334-12-146.

Giesen, L. G., Cousins, G., Dimitrov, B. D., van de Laar, F. A., & Fahey, T. (2010). Predicting acute uncomplicated urinary tract infection in women: A systematic review of the diagnostic accuracy of symptoms and signs. *BMC Fam Pract*, *11*, 78-2296-11-78.

Grover, M. L., Bracamonte, J. D., Kanodia, A. K., et al. (2007). Assessing adherence to evidence-based guidelines for the diagnosis and management of uncomplicated urinary tract infection. *Mayo Clin Proc*, *82*, 181–185.

Gupta, K., Hillier, S. L., Hooton, T. M., Roberts, P. L., & Stamm, W. E. (2000). Effects of contraceptive method on the vaginal microbial flora: A prospective evaluation. *J Infect Dis*, *181*, 595–601.

Gupta, K., Hooton, T. M., Naber, K. G., et al. (2011). International clinical practice guidelines for the treatment of acute uncomplicated cystitis and pyelonephritis in women: A 2010 update by the Infectious Diseases Society of America and the European Society for Microbiology and Infectious Diseases. *Clin Infect Dis, 52,* e103–e120.

Gupta, K., Stapleton, A. E., Hooton, T. M., Roberts, P. L., Fennell, C. L., & Stamm, W. E. (1998). Inverse association of H2O2-producing lactobacilli and vaginal *Escherichia coli* colonization in women with recurrent urinary tract infections. *J Infect Dis, 178,* 446–450.

Hanno, P., Burks, D., Clemens, J., et al. (2014). *Diagnosis and treatment of interstitial cystitis/bladder pain syndrome.* American Urological Association website. Retrieved June 13, 2014, from http://www.auanet.org/education/guidelines/ ic-bladder-pain-syndrome.cfm

Jepson, R. G., & Craig, J. C. (2008). Cranberries for preventing urinary tract infections. *Cochrane Database Syst Rev,* 1:CD001321.

Jepson, R. G., Williams, G., & Craig, J. C. (2012). Cranberries for preventing urinary tract infections. *Cochrane Database Syst Rev,* 10:CD001321.

Larsson, B., Jonasson, A., & Fianu, S. (1993). Prophylactic effect of uva-E in women with recurrent cystitis: A preliminary report. *Current Therapeutic Research, 53,* 441–443.

Leydon, G. M., Turner, S., Smith, H., & Little, P.; UTIS team. (2010). Women's views about management and cause of urinary tract infection: Qualitative interview study. *BMJ, 340,* c279.

Lis-Balchin, M., Hart, S., & Simpson, E. (2001). Buchu (*Agathosma betulina* and *A. crenulata,* rutaceae) essential oils: Their pharmacological action on guinea-pig ileum and antimicrobial activity on microorganisms. *J Pharm Pharmacol, 53,* 579–582.

Luthje, P., Hirschberg, A. L., & Brauner, A. (2014). Estrogenic action on innate defense mechanisms in the urinary tract. *Maturitas, 77,* 32–36.

Maksimovic, Z., Dobric, S., Kovacevic, N., & Milovanovic, Z. (2004). Diuretic activity of maydis stigma extract in rats. *Pharmazie, 59,* 967–971.

Masteikova, R., Klimas, R., Samura, B. B., et al. (2007). An orientational examination of the effects of extracts from mixtures of herbal drugs on selected renal functions. *Ceska Slov Farm, 56,* 85–89.

Medina-Bombardo, D., & Jover-Palmer, A. (2011). Does clinical examination aid in the diagnosis of urinary tract infections in women? A systematic review and meta-analysis. *BMC Fam Pract, 12,* 111-2296-12-111.

Melekos, M. D., Asbach, H. W., Gerharz, E., Zarakovitis, I. E., Weingaertner, K., & Naber, K. G. (1997). Post-intercourse versus daily ciprofloxacin prophylaxis for recurrent urinary tract infections in premenopausal women. *J Urol, 157,* 935–939.

Michaels, E. K., Chmiel, J. S., Plotkin, B. J., & Schaeffer, A. J. (1983). Effect of D-mannose and D-glucose on *Escherichia coli* bacteriuria in rats. *Urol Res, 11,* 97–102.

Perrotta, C., Aznar, M., Mejia, R., Albert, X., & Ng, C. (2008). Oestrogens for preventing recurrent urinary tract infection in postmenopausal women. *Cochrane Database Syst Rev,* 2:CD005131.

Rafsanjany, N., Lechtenberg, M., Petereit, F., & Hensel, A. (2013). Antiadhesion as a functional concept for protection against uropathogenic *Escherichia coli*: In vitro studies with traditionally used plants with antiadhesive activity against uropathognic *Escherichia coli*. *J Ethnopharmacol*, *145*, 591–597.

Reid, G., & Bruce, A. W. (2006). Probiotics to prevent urinary tract infections: The rationale and evidence. *World J Urol*, *24*, 28–32.

Samoilova, Z., Smirnova, G., Muzyka, N., & Oktyabrsky, O. (2014). Medicinal plant extracts variously modulate susceptibility of *Escherichia coli* to different antibiotics. *Microbiol Res*, *169*, 307–313.

Schauberger, C. W., Merkitch, K. W., & Prell, A. M. (2007). Acute cystitis in women: Experience with a telephone-based algorithm. *WMJ*, *106*, 326–329.

Siegers, C., Bodinet, C., Ali, S. S., & Siegers, C. P. (2003). Bacterial deconjugation of arbutin by *Escherichia coli*. *Phytomedicine*, *10*(Suppl 4), 58–60.

Silverman, J. A., Schreiber, H. L., 4th, Hooton, T. M., & Hultgren, S. J. (2013). From physiology to pharmacy: Developments in the pathogenesis and treatment of recurrent urinary tract infections. *Curr Urol Rep*, *14*, 448–456.

Simpson, D. (1998). Buchu: South Africa's amazing herbal remedy. *Scott Med J*, *43*, 189–191.

Snowden, R., Harrington, H., Morrill, K., et al. (2014). A comparison of the anti-staphylococcus aureus activity of extracts from commonly used medicinal plants. *J Altern Complement Med*, *20*, 375–382.

Sobota, A. E. (1984). Inhibition of bacterial adherence by cranberry juice: Potential use for the treatment of urinary tract infections. *J Urol*, *131*, 1013–1016.

Stapleton, A. E., Au-Yeung, M., Hooton, T. M., et al. (2011). Randomized, placebo-controlled phase 2 trial of a lactobacillus crispatus probiotic given intravaginally for prevention of recurrent urinary tract infection. *Clin Infect Dis*, *52*, 1212–1217.

Wang, L., & Del Priore, L. V. (2004). Bull's-eye maculopathy secondary to herbal toxicity from uva ursi. *Am J Ophthalmol*, *137*, 1135–1137.

Wojnicz, D., Kucharska, A. Z., Sokół-Łętowska, A., et al. (2012). Medicinal plants extracts affect virulence factors expression and biofilm formation by the uropathogenic *Escherichia coli*. *Urol Res*, *40*, 683–697.

Yarnell, E. (2002). Botanical medicines for the urinary tract. *World J Urol*, *20*, 285–293.

Zafriri, D., Ofek, I., Adar, R., Pocino, M., & Sharon, N. (1989). Inhibitory activity of cranberry juice on adherence of type 1 and type P fimbriated *Escherichia coli* to eucaryotic cells. *Antimicrob Agents Chemother*, *33*, 92–98.

26

Irritable Bowel Syndrome

IRINA LISKER AND KATHIE MADONNA SWIFT

CASE STUDY

Sarah, a 36 year-old business woman and mother of three, presented with depression, anxiety, and chronic headaches for an integrative medicine consultation after unsuccessful treatment with conventional interventions for irritable bowel syndrome (IBS). Her main symptoms include abdominal pain and frequent bloating associated with periods of constipation. She regularly has IBS flares several days prior to menses. When Sarah was first diagnosed 5 years ago, she tried lactose- and gluten-free diets, without noticeable symptom improvement. This was later followed by antispasmodics, laxatives, antidepressants, and probiotics without long-term symptom relief. She struggles with stress management due to the demands of being a full-time professional and parent; however, she sees a psychologist on a weekly basis, which she has found helpful.

Introduction

Irritable bowel syndrome is a functional gastrointestinal (GI) disorder characterized by abdominal pain and irregular bowel movements. The condition has been recognized since ancient times, Hippocrates defining it as abdominal distress and irregular bowel movements accompanied by bloating and rectal urgency (Hanaway, 2012). The prevalence of IBS is 8%–20% in North America, depending on the criteria used to make the diagnosis

(Manning versus Rome criteria). Diarrhea-predominant IBS (IBS-D) represents 50% of the IBS cases in North America. Women are affected more than men, with a ratio of 1.2:3.1 in Western countries and 0.8:2.1 in developing ones. Because women are more likely to seek medical attention, the ratio in primary care settings tends to be 3:1 (Rey & Talley, 2009).

Irritable bowel syndrome costs have been on the rise, with $200 billion in direct and indirect medical costs in the United States (Inadomi, Fennerty, & Bjorkman, 2003), where it is the most common diagnosis among gastroenterologists, and 3.5 million annual doctor visits per year (Everhart & Renault, 1991).

The comorbidities that occur in more than half of those with IBS include fibromyalgia, chronic fatigue syndrome, chronic back pain, chronic pelvic pain, chronic headache, depression, and anxiety. Moreover, IBS patients with these comorbidities tend to have more severe symptom patterns than people without IBS. Irritable bowel syndrome patients report lower quality-of-life ratings and experience a higher frequency of invasive procedures including surgery (Canavan, West, & Card, 2014). Irritable bowel syndrome patients with higher self-reported food intolerances tend to have lower quality of life in sleep, energy, physical activity, diet, and social functioning domains (Böhn, Störsrud, Törnblom, Bengtsson, & Simrén, 2013).

Pathophysiology

The pathophysiology of IBS is complex, with many contributing factors including GI dysmotility, visceral hypersensitivity, stress and the gut–brain relationship, inflammation, genetics, altered gut microbiota, and ovarian hormones.

GASTROINTESTINAL DYSMOTILITY AND VISCERAL HYPERSENSITIVITY

Dysmotility describes the frequent colonic contractions characterized by high-amplitude propagated contractions (HAPCs) that result in abnormal bowel movements in patients with IBS-D. Visceral hypersensitivity is another contributing factor to IBS. This hypersensitivity manifests as abdominal pain and dysmotility producing changes in bowel movements (diarrhea or constipation). There is a direct relationship between stress and sensitivity and an inverse one between food intake and sensitivity (Lee & Park, 2014).

Mast cells appear to be involved in visceral hypersensitivity. Upon activation they release tryptase, which in turn activates proteinase-activated receptor-2

(PAR2), a transmembrane protein, on afferent GI neurons. Once the PAR2 is activated it stimulates GI neurons, resulting in pain (Katiraei & Bultron, 2011).

STRESS AND THE GUT–BRAIN RELATIONSHIP

Corticotropin-releasing hormone (CRH) and corticotropin-releasing factor (CRF) are key factors in the dynamic relationship between the brain and the gut. During stressful periods, CRH is produced, causing increased colonic motility, visceral hypersensitivity, and mood dysregulation (Lee & Park, 2014). A peptide produced in both the central nervous system and peripheral tissues, CRF is also activated during stress, stimulating colonic mast cells and altering the intestinal epithelium and mucosal barrier. Gastrointestinal neurons release substance P and calcitonin gene-related peptide (CGRP), also activating mast cells resulting in TNF-α release. All of this further promotes intestinal permeability and inflammation (Katiraei & Bultron, 2011).

Animal studies indicate that these stress-related cascades of events continue even after the stressor is eliminated. Stress-induced inflammation alters future epithelial response to stress signals, making the GI tract more prone to stress by altering mast cells' shape and contents. After the GI inflammatory response is triggered, mast cells directly produce CRF. Corticotropin-releasing factor causes another inflammatory cascade—stimulating lymphocyte proliferation and macrophage release of TNF-a, IL-1, and IL-6 (pro-inflammatory cytokines). Once these cells are activated they cause more CRF release and this further perpetuates mast cell activation. Due to persistent inflammation in IBS patients, compared with healthy controls, they have higher concentrations of macrophages, enterochromaffin cells (EC), lymphocytes, neutrophils, and eosinophils (Katiraei & Bultron, 2011).

Enterochromaffin cells play an integral role, particularly in IBS-D subtype. They release serotonin (5-HT) in the gut. The gut has a variety of 5-HT receptors (5-HT1, 5-HT2, 5-HT3, 5-HT4, and 5-HT7; compared with 5-HT5, 5-HT6, and 5-HT7 that are in the brain). Serotonin binds to the gut receptors and contributes to visceral hypersensitivity, as well as dysmotility (Katiraei & Bultron, 2011).

INFLAMMATION

Irritable bowel syndrome patients have high levels of active immunocompetent cells (T-lymphocytes, mast cells, neutrophils) in the intestinal mucosa. Moreover, there is evidence of postinfectious (i.e., postgastroenteritis) low-grade inflammation as a factor in IBS pathogenesis. A patient can develop new-onset IBS after recovering from a GI infection (infection diagnosed by meeting two or more of these symptoms: fever, diarrhea, vomiting, or positive bacterial stool culture). Patients who develop IBS after a GI infection tend to have more proinflammatory cytokines, higher IL-1β mRNA expression in the rectal mucosa, and flagellin antibodies. This suggests that triggering a luminal immune response contributes to IBS development (Lee & Park, 2014).

GENETICS

Although there is mixed evidence of genetics' role in IBS due to the varying IBS presentation, differing study protocol, and or study recruitment process, genetics is still a factor to consider. For example, monozygotic twins surveyed in Norway showed a higher concordance for IBS than dizygotic twins. Genetics also appears to play a role in mucosal inflammation and neurotransmitters (Lee & Park, 2014).

GUT MICROBIOTA

People with IBS tend to suffer from dysbiosis or disruption in the composition of gut microbiota composition. It has been noted that people suffering from small intestinal bacterial overgrowth (SIBO) exhibit IBS symptoms that resolve once the SIBO has been treated. Fecal bacteria differ in IBS groups, a situation that can be exploited for targeted treatment (Simrén, 2014). Patients with IBS-D have less *Lactobacilli* and *Bifidobacterium* spp. than those with IBS-C, while those with IBS-C have more *Veillonella* spp. than healthy people. The fact that probiotics and the antibiotic rifaximin improve IBS symptoms of flatulence and abdominal distention further supports the idea that the intestinal flora of IBS patients is disrupted (Lee & Park, 2014).

OVARIAN HORMONES

Currently, it is thought that estrogen and progesterone contribute to IBS symptoms because IBS is commonly diagnosed in premenopausal females in their teens through their forties. Women have higher pain sensitivity and worsening GI motility during the late luteal phase when estrogen/progesterone are declining and reach their nadir. Differences in pain sensitivity appear to be due to the length and level of hormone exposure; less hormone is associated with greater sensitivity. In terms of motility, progesterone decreases gastric emptying by reducing the strength of muscle contractions in the colon, supporting the higher prevalence of IBS-C in women (Roisinblit, 2013). In general, during life stages when hormone levels are lower, such as menopause, women's bowel symptoms and visceral hypersensitivity tend to worsen. In contrast, during pregnancy, where progesterone/estrogen are high, pain sensitivity and other associated IBS symptoms (except for constipation) improve. Interestingly, postmenopausal women on hormone replacement therapy (HRT) have a higher IBS prevalence and continue to have IBS symptoms much longer than other women their age not on HRT. Women post-oophorectomy often experience IBS exacerbations (Mulak, Taché, & Larauche, 2014).

Bloating is more prevalent among women than men, which is possibly related to female hormones, as many women experience bloating around and during menstruation. Bloating is also commonly associated with uterine cramping and breast soreness in perimenopausal women. The higher prevalence of bloating in women may indicate that there are differences in sensory processes, autonomic responses, and/or cognitive hypervigilance (Ringel, Williams, Kalilani, & Cook, 2009).

Integrative Diagnosis

Irritable bowel syndrome is a clinical diagnosis based primarily on the patient's history and physical exam. It is characterized by chronic abdominal pain with altered bowel movements. The American College of Gastroenterology (ACG) recommends using the Manning or Rome III criteria to make the diagnosis (Table 26.1). Per the Manning criteria, the more symptoms exhibited, the greater the chance of having IBS (Wald, Talley, & Grover, 2013).

There are four IBS subtypes: (1) IBS-C: hard/lumpy stools ≥25% or loose/watery stools <25% of bowel movements. (2) IBS-D: loose/watery stools ≥25% or hard/lumpy stools <5% of bowel movements. (3) Mixed IBS (IBS-M): hard/lumpy stools ≥25% or loose/watery stools ≥25% of bowel movements. (4) Unsubtyped IBS: inconsistent stool variety that does not fall into the other subtypes. Women tend to present with IBS-C and abdominal pain, men with IBS-D. Women often have accompanying dysphagia, chronic pain conditions (i.e., chronic pelvic pain), migraine headaches, fibromyalgia, and/or cystitis. A woman's colon is typically longer than a man's (155 cm compared with 145 cm), which may play a role in constipation. The transverse colon extends into the true pelvis in 62% of women versus 26% of men, possibly explaining the worsening of IBS symptoms during menstruation and the association of IBS and chronic pelvic pain (Mulak et al., 2014).

Table 26.1. Manning and Rome Diagnostic Criteria.

Manning Criteria	Rome III Criteria
• Pain alleviated with defecation • Increased stool frequency at pain onset • Looser stools at pain onset • Observable abdominal distention • Mucus in stool • Feeling of incomplete evacuation	Recurring abdominal pain/ discomfort* that started 6 months, lasting at least three days/month in the past three months with at least two of the symptoms below: • Pain improves with defection • Pain onset related to change in stool frequency • Pain onset related to change stool appearance

* Discomfort refers to an uncomfortable sensation not described as pain^^

^^ Longstreth GF, Thompson WG, Chey WD, Houghton LA, Mearin F, Spiller RC. Functional bowel disorders. *Gastroenterology*. 2006;130(5):1480–91.

Wald A, Talley NJ, Grover S. Clinical manifestations and diagnosis of irritable bowel syndrome in adults. *UpToDate*. 2013. Available at: www.uptodate.com. Accessed June 22, 2014.

There is no definitive test for IBS, and the ACG does not recommend routine testing (e.g., complete blood count, chemistries, thyroid studies, stool ova and parasites) or imaging for typical IBS presentation with no alarm signs (e.g., weight loss, fever, blood in stool, nighttime/worsening abdominal pain, laboratory abnormalities). The ACG advises testing for celiac disease in cases of IBS-D and IBS-M. For patients with IBS who are over age 50, the ACG recommends colonoscopy to rule out colorectal cancer (American College of Gastroenterology Task Force on Irritable Bowel Syndrome, 2009). Additionally, if one suspects lactose maldigestion even after dairy elimination, then lactose breath testing should be considered (Ringel et al., 2009).

NOVEL BIOMARKERS

Compromised intestinal barrier integrity, low-grade inflammation, and immune activation have been demonstrated in IBS and may be more prevalent in IBS subtypes such as IBS-D. Whether this is a cause or an effect remains a matter of debate. Assessing intestinal permeability in IBS patients by analyzing the ratios of sugars, such as lactulose and rhamnose (L/R) or lactulose and mannitol (L/M), in the urine may serve as a useful tool in diagnosis and therapeutic intervention (Mujagic et al., 2014).

A dsybiotic environment contributes to alterations in the metabolic activities of gut bacteria, creating metabolic signatures or "marker" metabolites in different biological fluids that may help elucidate disease-related mechanisms and candidate therapies (DePreter & Verbeke, 2013). For example, distinct changes in patterns of fecal volatile organic metabolites (VOMs) in IBS patients versus healthy controls have been observed. This may lead to the future development of a simple sensor technique to assess organic metabolites that could provide a reliable diagnostic and monitoring tool for various gastrointestinal disorders (Ahmed, Greenwood, Costello, Ratcliffe, & Probert, 2013). Advances in "omics" and microbiome-based technologies may also shift the diagnostic landscape and therapeutic management of IBS in the not-so-distant future.

Evaluation of nutritional biomarkers is another emerging area of interest. Compromised GI function can impact dietary intake and nutritional status in patients with IBS. Essential fatty acid deficiency, especially of long-chain omega-3 fatty acids, has been demonstrated in patients with IBS. Comprehensive nutritional profiling including vitamin and mineral levels, fatty acids, amino acids, and other biomarkers may someday be standard of care for the patient with IBS (Solakivi et al., 2011).

Diet

Diet has traditionally been considered to play a minor role in the treatment and pathogenesis of IBS. However, most women with IBS report symptom exacerbations associated with intake of specific foods (Eswaran, Tack, & Chey, 2011). Many women report experimenting with an array of dietary therapies, including restricting certain foods, to alleviate symptoms and improve their quality of life (Böhn, Störsrud, Törnblom, Bengtsson, & Simrén, 2013). Although there are limited studies on the role of diet in IBS, the contribution of adverse food reactions to IBS pathogenesis and management is gaining momentum in the scientific and medical community.

Digestion is a complex process. Patients with IBS have been noted to have alterations in the autonomic nervous system, including increased sympathetic nervous system activity and changes in secretion of gut hormones and neurotransmitters, such as serotonin (Hayes, Fraher, & Quigley, 2014). Food contains mixtures of chemicals that may drive a low-grade inflammation in the microenvironment of intestinal neurons. In addition, food components can induce changes in the gut that lead to luminal distension and visceral hypersensitivity (Gibson & Shepherd, 2012).

Some foods and food components that have been implicated in IBS include milk, wheat, gluten, caffeine, spicy foods, and fatty foods. Alcohol intolerance is also commonly reported in patients with IBS and can be a cofactor in precipitating or exacerbating adverse reactions. Traditional dietary advice has often focused around fiber manipulation of the diet, although no discernible differences comparing high and low fiber intake have been found. Recently, attention has focused on elimination diets; avoidance of certain carbohydrates rich in fermentable oligo-, di-, and monosaccharides and polyols (FODMAPs); gluten elimination; and the exclusion of various food chemicals.

FOOD ALLERGY AND INTOLERANCE

Adverse food reactions are now recognized as an emerging problem in adults, and their presentation in conditions such as IBS often involve reactions to a wide number of foods alongside cofactors such as stress, exercise, and medications (Skypala, 2011). Food allergy is mediated by immunogluboulin E (IgE), and there is no consistent evidence for this type of allergic response in IBS (El-Salhy, Ostgaard, Gundersen, Hatlebakk, & Hausken, 2012). However, a slower onset of food allergy that involves IgE, T-lymphocytes, eosinophils, mast cells, and mucosal cells may cause IBS symptoms in a subset of patients with atopy (El-Salhy et al., 2012). Some researchers propose that IgG may play a role in IBS (Atkinson, Sheldon, Shaath, & Whorwell, 2004; Drisko, Bischoff, Hall, & McCallum, 2006). Elimination-directed diets based on test results for IgE and IgG antibodies have shown some benefit in a few small studies, although the data are unclear and controversial. The gold standard for identifying adverse food reactions remains an elimination diet that is based on a personalized nutrition assessment and diet history (Swift & Lisker, 2012).

FODMAPS

FODMAPs is the collective term for carbohydrates that share similar physiological effects and cause luminal distension and IBS symptoms due to increased osmotic activity and rapid fermentation by bacteria. The principle sources of FODMAPs (lactose, fructose, fructans, galacto-oligosaacharides, and polyols) are outlined in Table 26.2. Researchers in Australia first described the low-FODMAP diet in 2005, and the evidence base for efficacy includes observational studies, comparative studies, challenge/rechallenge studies, and

Table 26.2. Foods and Food Additives High in FODMAPs

FODMAP	Food & Food Additives
Free Fructose	Apple, cherry, mango, pear, watermelon; artichoke, asparagus, sugar snap peas; honey and high fructose corn syrup
Lactose	Cow, goat and sheep milk and all milk products (yogurt, soft cheeses, ice cream, whipping cream, etc.)
Fructans	Peach, watermelon; artichoke, beetroot, Brussels sprout, chicory, garlic, leek, onion, peas; wheat, rye, barley; pistachios; legumes, lentils, chickpeas, chicory beverages; inulin and FOS
Galacto-oligosaccharides	Legumes, lentils, chickpeas
Polyols	Apple, apricot, avocado, blackberries, cherry, nectarine, plum, prune; cauliflower, mushroom, snow peas; food additives: isomalt, maltitol, mannitol, sorbitol, xylitol

Gibson PR, Shepherd SJ. Food choice as a key management strategy for functional gastrointestinal symptoms. *Amer J Gastroenterol* 2012;107:657–666.

Barrett JS, Gibson PR. Fermentable oliogsaccharides, disaccharides, monosaccharides and polyols (FODMAPs) and nonallergic food intolerance: FODMAPs or food chemicals. *Ther Adv Gastroenterol.* 2012;5(4):261–268.

http://www.med.monash.edu/cecs/gastro/fodmap/iphone-app.html

randomized controlled trials (Gibson & Shepherd, 2012). Not all of FODMAP foods will cause symptoms in everyone, because there are individual differences in small intestinal absorptive patterns. Dietary intolerance of fructose and fructan, both members of the FODMAP family, can cause unexplained GI symptoms, and restriction of these components independently of other FODMAPs requires further investigation (Fedewa & Rao, 2014).

The cumulative dose of FODMAP foods is often a critical factor in tolerance. The FODMAP diet is usually recommended for 4 to 8 weeks, followed by a rechallenge period. Because FODMAPs have prebiotic effects due to the production of short-chain fatty acids, long-term exclusion may pose detrimental effects on the gut microbiota. Thus, it is important that women are guided in the practical application of a low-FODMAP approach with the support of a skilled clinician, in order that the diet is not overly restrictive and nutritional integrity is not compromised. Additional research is needed to determine the influence of a low-FODMAP diet on nutrient intake, dietary diversity, and impact on gut microbiota and the colonic environment (Staudacher, Irving, Lomer, & Whelan, 2014).

GLUTEN

The interest in gluten, the main protein complex in wheat, rye, and barley, as a causative agent in IBS began more than a decade ago, when researchers showed that more than one-quarter of patients (66/300) with IBS had positive serology for celiac, though the majority (43/66) had normal duodenal biopsy (Sanders et al., 2001). Some investigators estimate that a diagnosis of celiac disease is four times more likely in a patient with IBS. It is now recognized that reactions to gluten are not limited to celiac disease. Some evidence suggests that IBS patients respond with symptom resolution on a gluten-free diet (Gibson & Shepherd, 2012).

The existence of nonceliac gluten sensitivity (NCGS) has been increasingly recognized as a predisposing factor for IBS-like symptoms in people for whom celiac disease has been excluded. A recent report of Asian patients with IBS found that 18% (34/186) were positive for IgA deamidated gliadin peptide (DGP), and all improved on a gluten exclusion diet (Lu et al., 2014).

Mechanisms for the gluten-induced gut symptoms in nonceliacs remain to be elucidated. It is interesting to note that wheat contains chains of fructo-oligosaccharides (fructans), and other fermentable oligo- and dimono-saccharides and polyols, members of the FODMAP family. Some argue that symptom induction might be wheat-specific rather than a gluten-specific phenomenon, which may also be dose-related.

FOOD CHEMICALS

Food contains complex mixtures of bioactive molecules that may induce or worsen IBS symptoms. Food chemicals, including salicylates, amines, and glutamates, widely distributed in whole, unprocessed (e.g., fruits and vegetables) and processed foods (e.g., deli meats) have been investigated for their role in asthma, headaches, urticaria, and anaphylactoid reactions mediated via nonimmune mechanisms. It is theorized that food chemicals induce gut symptoms by stimulating nerve endings in hypersensitive individuals, resulting in pain and discomfort (Barret & Gibson, 2012; Gibson & Shepherd, 2012). Withdrawal of the offending chemicals may lead to reduction in visceral hypersensitivity and subsequent resolution of IBS symptoms. An elimination diet for food chemicals can be highly restrictive and generally excludes other additives and preservatives such as benzoates, BHA/BHT, propionate, sulfites, nitrites, sorbic acid, and colorings. The concept behind food chemical intolerance is a build-up effect, causing symptoms once a certain threshold has been reached (Barret & Gibson, 2012). Dietary support may be needed to assist the patient on this strict elimination diet and rechallenge period to ascertain the impact of food chemicals on IBS symptoms.

Attention to diet and nutrition should be a first-line therapy in women suffering from IBS. A food and symptom journal is a critical clinical tool for the integrative practitioner to outline a roadmap of dietary investigation that can lead to dramatic symptom reduction or resolution. Referral to an integrative dietitian/nutritionist/clinician, skilled in elimination diet protocols is essential to support the patient during this process.

Integrative Treatment Options

PHARMACEUTICALS

Medications should be considered in patients whose IBS significantly impacts their quality of life. The IBS subtype and symptoms should guide the medication choice.

Osmotic Laxatives

In patients with IBS-C who do not respond to fiber, osmotic laxatives are recommended starting with polyethylene glycol (PEG) and moving to lubiprostone if there is no improvement. Lubiprostone, most commonly used in women with IBS-C, activates chloride channels to promote fluid secretion (Roisinblit, 2013; Wald et al., 2013).

Antidepressants

Tricyclics (i.e., nortriptyline) are used in IBS-D, as they slow down GI transit time and decrease pain. Selective serotonin reuptake inhibitors (SSRIs) (i.e., fluoxetine, paroxetine, citalopram) help with abdominal pain and bloating. Antidepressants may be an appropriate choice for women with coexisting chronic conditions such as dysmenorrhea, chronic pelvic pain, fibromyalgia, and psychiatric illness (Roisinblit, 2013).

Antibiotics

Rifaximin, a poorly absorbed antibiotic, is used for patients presenting with IBS-C, bloating, and abdominal pain with postinfectious diarrhea caused by

Escherichia coli. Neomycin is recommended for IBS patients who concurrently have SIBO, as it lowers methane production and improves transit time (Roisinblit, 2013).

Antispasmodics

Antispasmodics are intended for short-term symptom relief of postprandial abdominal pain, gas, bloating, and fecal urgency. They can be taken in advance of known stressors or situations that will exacerbate IBS symptoms. Examples include dicyclomine and hyoscyamine, which bind to anticholinergic receptors to promote GI smooth muscle relaxation (Wald et al., 2013).

DIETARY SUPPLEMENTS

Peppermint Oil

Peppermint (*Mentha x piperita*) is one of the most widely studied botanicals for relieving IBS symptoms. A recent systematic review and meta-analysis of nine studies showed enteric-coated peppermint oil capsules are a safe and effective short-term treatment for IBS (Khanna, MacDonald, & Levesque, 2014). Menthol, a major constituent in peppermint, acts as an antispasmodic possibly blocking Ca^{2+} channels in the gut and decreasing smooth muscle contractions. The recommended dosage is 0.2 mL peppermint oil in enteric-coated capsules three times daily between meals. Possible side effects include perianal burning and heartburn or reflux, as it can relax the lower esophageal muscles (Natural Medicines Comprehensive Database, 2013), though this is less likely when properly enteric-coated.

Combination Herbals

STW5 is a mixture of plant extracts from chamomile flowers (*Matricaria recutita*), bitter candytuft (*Iberis amara*), peppermint leaves (*Mentha x piperita*), caraway fruit (*Carum carvi*), celandine herb (*Chelidonium majus*), licorice root (*Glycyrrhiza glabra*), lemon balm leaves (*Melissa officinalis*), angelica root (*Angelica archangelica*), and milk thistle fruit (*Silybum marianum*). A review of 12 clinical trials on the safety and efficacy of STW5 in functional GI disorders found significant benefits on GI symptoms (Ottillinger, Storr, Malfertheiner, & Allescher, 2013). The extract has been shown to exert various actions in the gastrointestinal tract including stimulating mucus secretion, reducing hypersensitivity of the enteric neurons and influencing the whole symptom complex of IBS (Krueger et al., 2009). A well-known brand of STW5 is Iberogast, and the common dosage is 20 drops mixed in water.

Traditional Chinese medicine (TCM) has been used in treating IBS. Herbal formulas should be individualized based on syndrome differentiation including liver stagnation and spleen deficiency, spleen-stomach weakness, and spleen-kidney yang deficiency, as well as cold and heat (Li, Yang, & Liu, 2013). Other herbal formulas including a complex Tibetan formula, Padma Lax, and Ayurvedic preparations have shown improvement in global symptoms of IBS, however, high-quality trials of these formulations are needed (Liu, Yang, Liu, Wei, & Grimsgaard, 2006).

Probiotics

Manipulation of the gut microbiota with probiotics is being intensively studied. In a large trial of women with IBS, *Bifidobacterium infantis* 35624 has been shown to be effective in reducing symptoms (Whorwell et al., 2006). Other studies have shown positive effects for *Bifidobacterium animalis*, *B. bifidum* MIMBb75, *E. coli Nissle*, *L. plantarum* 299v, *B. lactis Bi-07*, and VSL#3 (Magge & Wolf, 2013). There is a need for further studies to elucidate the specific probiotic strains and dosages that are of greatest benefit in IBS.

Fiber

Research on the addition of fiber supplements in IBS has been mixed. Some fibers, specifically insoluble fiber found in whole grains and nuts, may exacerbate IBS symptoms. Use of a soluble fiber supplement, such as ispaghula or psyllium seed husk, may be beneficial in some women with IBS-C (Eswaran, Tack, & Chey, 2011).When used, fiber should be introduced at a low dose and gradually titrated to the targeted amount. Adverse reactions to fiber supplements include abdominal distension, flatulence, constipation, and diarrhea.

Melatonin

Melatonin (N-acetyl-5-methoxytryptamine) is a hormone produced by the pineal gland and enterochromaffin cells of the digestive mucosa. Secretion of melatonin decreases with age, particularly in postmenopausal women. Melatonin exerts beneficial effects on the gut including analgesic effects and regulation of GI motility. Studies have consistently shown improvement in IBS symptoms with 3 mg melatonin at bedtime (Siah, Wong, & Ho, 2014).

MIND–BODY THERAPIES

Evidence supports the effectiveness of different forms of mind body and relaxation therapies including meditation, deep-breathing exercises, gut-directed hypnotherapy, biofeedback, mindfulness-based stress reduction (MBSR), cognitive-behavioral therapy (CBT), and other psychological techniques in reducing the symptoms and improving quality of life in women with IBS (Siah et al., 2014). Energy, manual medicine, and movement-based therapies including reflexology, massage, acupuncture, moxibustion, yoga, and qigong are also therapeutic options for IBS management (Grundmann, & Yoon, 2014).

Yoga

The form of yoga used for IBS incorporates both physical activity and relaxation techniques. This translates to consciously coordinating postures to specific breath work that brings one's attention to muscle contraction and relaxation. Yoga has specific postures that are beneficial for gut motility and abdominal pain perception. Although there are limited studies using yoga for IBS, those that have been conducted show positive results. Overall, yoga appears to decrease pain frequency and perception and improves IBS symptoms (Grundmann, & Yoon, 2014).

Hypnotherapy

Hypnotherapy involves guiding a patient into a tranquil and deeply relaxed state. Studies indicate that gut-directed hypnotherapy improves IBS symptoms as effectively as pharmaceuticals. Some have even demonstrated that the effects of hypnotherapy can last up to 10 months after patients discontinue therapy (Grundmann & Yoon, 2014).

Cognitive-Behavioral Therapy

Cognitive-behavioral therapy focuses on teaching patients to be more aware and conscious of their IBS symptoms in order to help them change their behavior and perspective on IBS. This type of conscious change has resulted in improving not only IBS symptoms but also chronic pain and depressive disorders. All in all, CBT increases quality-of-life metrics and decreases IBS symptom severity, particularly in the pain category (Grundmann & Yoon, 2014).

ACUPUNCTURE

In IBS, acupuncture may play a role in regulating serotonergic, cholinergic, and glutamatergic pathways and decreasing cortisol caused by stress. Acupuncture also increases endogenous opioids that in turn modulate pain and visceral hypersensitivity. Multiple studies show that acupuncture improves the quality of life and symptoms in patients with IBS (Grundmann & Yoon, 2014). It should be noted that rating acupuncture's effectiveness poses challenges due to inherent difficulties in study design (e.g., appropriate comparison group).

PHYSICAL ACTIVITY

Research has documented that regular exercise, whether it is mild, moderate, or vigorous, decreases IBS severity and improves IBS symptoms. The amount and level of activity recommended is based on the patient's ability. Specifically for women, exercise seems to improve fatigue symptoms when compared with inactive controls with IBS (Ringel et al., 2009). In general, exercise tends to relieve bloating and gas production and increase GI motility (Grundmann & Yoon, 2014).

Summary

Irritable bowel syndrome can significantly impact a woman's quality of life. An individualized integrative approach that addresses diet, lifestyle, and stress can be very helpful in improving symptoms and enhancing well-being. Sarah was better able to manage her IBS by experimenting with a combination of a low-FODMAP diet, enteric-coated peppermint oil supplementation, twice-weekly yoga class, and ongoing cognitive-behavioral therapy.

Electronic Resources

The Monash University Low FODMAP Diet

App by Monash University.
Guide with FODMAP foods and low FODMAP recipes.

My Food My Health

http://www.myfoodmyhealth.com/FODMAP/?id=home
Customized meal plans including FODMAP.

My Symptoms Food & Symptom Tracker

App by SkyGazer Labs Ltd.
Allows patients to track their food intake and symptoms and then analyzes the information.

IBS Diary

App by Boehringer Ingelheim Pharma.
Helps track food intake and IBS symptoms.

REFERENCES

Ahmed, I., Greenwood, R., Costello, B. D. L., Ratcliffe, N. M., & Probert, C. S. (2013). An investigation of fecal volatile organic metabolites in irritable bowel syndrome. *Plos One, 8*, e58204.

American College of Gastroenterology Task Force on Irritable Bowel Syndrome; Brandt, L. J., Chey, W. D., Foxx-Orenstein, A. E., et al. (2009). An evidence-based position statement on the management of irritable bowel syndrome. *Am J Gastroenterol* 104 Suppl 1:S1–S35.

Atkinson, W., Sheldon, T. A., Shaath, N., & Whorwell, T. J. (2004). Food elimination based on IgG antibodies in irritable bowel syndrome: A randomized controlled clinical trial. *Gut, 53*, 1459–1464.

Barret, J. S., & Gibson, P. R. (2012). Fermentable oligosaccharides, disaccharides, monosaccharides and polyols (FODMAPs) and nonallergic food intolerance: FODMAPs or food chemicals? *Ther Adv Gastroenterol, 5*, 261–268.

Böhn, L., Störsrud, S., Törnblom, H., Bengtsson, U., & Simrén, M. (2013). Self-reported food-related gastrointestinal symptoms in IBS are common and associated with more severe symptoms and reduced quality of life. *Am J Gastroenterol, 108*, 634–641.

Canavan, C., West, J., & Card, T. (2014). The epidemiology of irritable bowel syndrome. *Clin Epidemiol, 6,* 71–80.

DePreter, V., & Verbeke, K. (2013). Metabolomics as a diagnostic tool in gastroenterology. *World J Gastrointest Pharmacol Ther, 4,* 97–107.

Drisko, J., Bischoff, B., Hall, M., & McCallum, R. (2006). Treating irritable bowel syndrome with a food elimination diet followed by food challenge and probiotics. *J Am Coll Nutr, 25,* 514–522.

El-Salhy, M., Ostgaard, H., Gundersen, D., Hatlebakk, J. G., & Hausken, T. (2012). The role of diet in the pathogenesis and management of irritable bowel syndrome (Review). *International J Molec Med, 29,* 723–731.

Eswaran, S., Tack, J., & Chey, W. D. (2011). Food the forgotten factor in the irritable bowel syndrome. *Gastroenterol Clin N Am, 41,* 141–162.

Everhart, J. E., & Renault, P. F. (1991). Irritable bowel syndrome in office-based practice in the United States. *Gastroenterology, 100,* 998–1005.

Fedewa, A., & Rao, S. S. (2014). Dietary fructose intolerance, fructan intolerance and FODMAPs. *Curr Gastroenterol Rep, 16,* 370.

Gibson, P. R., & Shepherd, S. J. (2012). Food choice as a key management strategy for functional gastrointestinal symptoms. *Am J Gastroenterol, 107,* 657–666.

Grundmann, O., & Yoon, S. L. (2014). Complementary and alternative medicines in irritable bowel syndrome: An integrative view. *World J Gastroenterol, 20,* 346–362.

Hanaway, P. J. (2012). Irritable bowel syndrome. In D. Rakel (Ed.), *Integrative medicine* (3rd ed., pp. 392–399). Philadelphia, PA: Saunders.

Hayes, P., Fraher, M. H., & Quigley, E. M. M. (2014). Irritable bowel syndrome: The role of food in pathogenesis and management. *Gastroenterol and Hepatol, 10,* 164–174.

Inadomi, J. M., Fennerty, M. B., & Bjorkman, D. (2003). Systematic review: The economic impact of irritable bowel syndrome. *Aliment Pharmacol Ther, 18,* 671–682.

Katiraei, P., & Bultron, G. (2011). Need for a comprehensive medical approach to the neuro-immuno-gastroenterology of irritable bowel syndrome. *World J Gastroenterol, 17,* 2791–2800.

Khanna, R., MacDonald, J. K., & Levesque, B. G. (2014). Peppermint oil for the treatment of irritable bowel syndrome: A systematic review and meta-analysis. *J Clin Gastroenterol, 48,* 505–512.

Krueger, D., Gruber, L., Buhner, S., Zeller, F., et al. (2009). The multi-herbal drug STW 5 (Iberogast) has prosecretory action in the human intestine. *Neurogastroenterol Motil, 21,* 1203–e110.

Lee, Y. J., & Park, K. S. (2014). Irritable bowel syndrome: Emerging paradigm in pathophysiology. *World J Gastroenterol, 20,* 2456–2469.

Li, Q., Yang, G. Y., & Liu, J. P. (2013). Syndrome differentiation in Chinese herbal medicine for irritable bowel syndrome: A literature review of randomized trials. *Evid Based Complement Altern Med, 2013,* 232147.

Liu, J. P., Yang, G. Y., Liu, Y. X., Wei, M., & Grimsgaard, S. (2006). Herbal medicines for the treatment of irritable bowel syndrome. *Cochrane Database System Rev,* 1:CD004116.

Lu, W., Gwee, K. A., Ho Siah, K. T., Kang, J. Y., Lee, R., & Lai Ngan, C. C. (2014). Prevalence of anti-deamidated gliadin peptide antibodies in Asian patients with irritable bowel syndrome. *J Neurogastroenterol Motil*, *20*, 236–241.

Magge, S. S., & Wolf, J. L. (2013). Complementary and alternative medicine and mind-body therapies for treatment of irritable bowel syndrome in women. *Womens Health (Lond Engl)*, *9*, 557–567.

Mujagic, Z., Ludidi, S., Keszthelyi, D., et al. (2014). Small intestinal permeability is increased in diarrhea predominant IBS, while alterations in gastroduodenal permeability in all IBS subtypes are largely attributable to confounders. *Aliment Pharmacol Ther*, *40*(3), 288–297.

Mulak, A., Taché, Y., & Larauche, M. (2014). Sex hormones in the modulation of irritable bowel syndrome. *World J Gastroenterol*, *20*, 2433–2448.

Natural Medicines Comprehensive Database. (2013). *Peppermint monograph*. Retrieved June 28, 2014, from http://naturaldatabase.therapeuticresearch.com/home.aspx?cs=&s=ND

Ottillinger, B., Storr, M., Malfertheiner, P., & Allescher, H. D. (2013). STW 5 (Iberogast®): A safe and effective standard in the treatment of functional gastrointestinal disorders. *Wien Med Wochenschr*, *163*, 65–72.

Rey, E., & Talley, N. J. (2009). Irritable bowel syndrome: Novel views on the epidemiology and potential risk factors. *Dig Liver Dis*, *41*, 772–780.

Ringel, Y., Williams, R. E., Kalilani, L., & Cook, S. F. (2009). Prevalence, characteristics, and impact of bloating symptoms in patients with irritable bowel syndrome. *Clin Gastroenterol Hepatol*, *7*, 68–72.

Roisinblit, K. C. (2013). Irritable bowel syndrome in women. *J Midwifery Womens Health*, *58*, 15–24.

Sanders, D. S., Carter, M. J., Hurlstone, D. P., et al. (2001). Association of adult coeliac disease with irritable bowel syndrome: A case-control study in patients fulfilling ROME II criteria referred to secondary care. *Lancet*, *358*, 1504–1508.

Siah, K. T., Wong, R. K., & Ho, K. Y. (2014). Melatonin for the treatment of irritable bowel syndrome. *World J Gastroenterol*, *20*, 2492–2498.

Simrén, M. (2014). IBS with intestinal microbial dysbiosis: A new and clinically relevant subgroup? *Gut*. [Epub ahead of print]

Skypala, I. (2011). Adverse food reactions: An emerging issue for adults. *J Am Diet Assoc*, *111*, 1877–1891.

Solakivi, T., Kaukinen, K., Kunnas, T., Lehtimäki, T., Mäki, M., & Nikkari, S. T. (2011). Serum fatty acid profile in subjects with irritable bowel syndrome. *Scandinavian Journal of Gastroenterology*, *46*, 299–303.

Staudacher, H. M., Irving, P. M., Lomer, M. C., & Whelan, K. (2014). Mechanisms and efficacy of dietary FODMAP restriction in IBS. *Nat Rev Gastroenterol Hepatol*, *11*, 256–266.

Swift, K. M. S., & Lisker, I. (2012). The science and art of the elimination diet. *Altern Comp Ther*, *18*, 251–258.

Wald, A., Talley, N. J., & Grover, S. (2013). Clinical manifestations and diagnosis of irritable bowel syndrome in adults. *UpToDate*. Retrieved June 22, 2014, from www. uptodate.com

Whorwell, P. J., Altringer, L., Morel, J., et al. (2006). Efficacy of an encapsulated probiotic Bifidobacterium infantis 35624 in women with irritable bowel syndrome. *Am J Gastroenterol, 101*, 1581–1590.

27

Headaches

HILARY MCCLAFFERTY AND KELLY MCCANN

CASE STUDY

At 40, Justine entered perimenopause and developed debilitating menstrual migraines. She tried conventional pharmaceutical therapies, but preferred a more holistic approach in keeping with her lifestyle. An elimination diet was recommended as an initial approach, and she discovered that avoidance of alcohol and cheese reduced her migraine frequency. Lifestyle measures including sleep, exercise, and stress reduction were then addressed. She reported further reduction of migraine symptoms with a regular 9 hours of sleep and addition of a regular yoga practice. Riboflavin, magnesium, and butterbur were also added to her daily regimen. Acupuncture treatments prior to menses rounded out her integrative treatment plan. Her migraines continued to diminish in both frequency and intensity. Now at 52, her menstrual cycles have stopped, and her migraines have virtually disappeared. She continues to enjoy her healthy lifestyle as she moves into menopause.

Introduction

The 2010 Global Burden of Disease Study lists headache among the top 10 causes of disability (measured in years-lived with disability), with tension-type and migraine being the second and third most prevalent disorders in the world (Vos et al., 2012). The study identified migraine headache as the seventh most common cause of disability (Steiner, Stovner, & Birbeck, 2013). Although the majority of headaches are medically benign, in that they are treatable and not permanently disabling, the societal cost of headache is substantial in terms of overall reduced quality of life, impact on family, and lost work days (Linde et al., 2012; Schwedt & Shapiro, 2009).

An estimated 47% of adults globally have active headache disorder, with 38% reporting tension-type headache, 10%–12% reporting migraine, and 3%–4% with chronic headache that lasts for more than 15 days per month (Jensen & Stovner, 2008). Medication overuse headache, a subset of chronic headache, affects an estimated 1%–2% of the population. (It is characterized as headache occurring on 15 or more days per month due to overuse of acute symptomatic headache medication; International Classification of Headache Disorders 3rd beta edition [ICHD-IIIb]; Kristoffersen & Lundqvist, 2014.) Cluster headache is the least prevalent overall, impacting 0.1% of the general population, primarily men (Bahra & Goadsby, 2004).Women experience headache significantly more frequently than men, for example 21% versus 12% in a large European population-based survey of 8,271 adults (Andree et al., 2014; Table 27.1).

Aura is defined as a recurring disorder manifesting in attacks of reversible neurological symptoms (e.g., visual, sensory, dysphasic speech) that develop gradually over 5 to 20 minutes and last no more than 1 hour.

A thorough history and physical exam are essential in establishing the proper headache diagnosis and determining further evaluation and treatment plans. Questions should screen for space-occupying lesions, metabolic disturbance, and systemic disease. Some examples of conditions that may present with headache include infections, autoimmune temporal arteritis, posttraumatic headache, sinus conditions, temporomandibular joint dysfunction, and refractive errors. Barring an abnormal neurological exam, sudden onset of symptoms, or atypical features, imaging is not routinely indicated. Once an accurate diagnosis is reached, therapies are generally divided into two main categories: preventive and abortive.

Use of complementary medicine has been shown to be high in adult (Adams, Barbery & Lui, 2013; Wells et al., 2011) and pediatric patients with recurrent headaches (Bethell et al., 2013), often concurrent with conventional treatment. Inquiry about complementary and integrative therapies with each patient, at every visit, would ideally encourage an expanded approach to treatment options and help prevent potential drug–dietary supplement interactions. This chapter provides an overview of integrative approaches to migraine and tension-type headache, the two most prevalent types of headache affecting women.

Migraine Headache

BACKGROUND

Large population-based studies reflect a migraine headache prevalence range of 16.6%–22.7% in adults (Smitherman et al., 2013) with an increased prevalence of

Table 27.1. Characteristics of Common Headache Symptoms

Symptom	Migraine Headache	Tension Headache	Cluster Headache
Location	Unilateral in 60%–70%; global in 30%	Bilateral	Always unilateral, usually begins around the eye or temple
Characteristics	Gradual in onset; crescendo pattern; dull, deep and steady when mild to moderate; throbbing and pulsating when moderate to severe in intensity; aggravated by routine physical activity	Pressure or tightness which waxes and wanes	Pain begins quickly, reaches peak in minutes; pain is deep, continuous, excruciating, and explosive in quality
Patient appearance	Patient prefers resting in a dark, quiet room	Patient may remain active	Patient remains active
Duration	4 to 72 hours	Variable	30 minutes to 3 hours
Associated symptoms	Nausea, vomiting, photophobia, phonophobia; may have aura which is usually visual but may involve other senses	None	Ipsilateral lacrimation and eye redness; nasal congestion, rhinorrhea, pallor, sweating, and Horner's syndrome; focal neurologic symptoms are rare

Aura is deﬁ ned as a recurrent disorder manifesting in attacks of reversible neurological symptoms that develop gradually over 5–20 minutes and last for less than 60 minutes.

migraine seen in women (adjusted prevalence ratios ranging from 1.48 to 3.25) across the life span. Women also report more severe symptoms, higher headache-related disability, presence of aura, and greater use of healthcare resources (Buse et al., 2013). Before puberty the prevalence of migraine is essentially equal in boys and girls, but after menarche, girls have greater incidence, possibly due to fluctuating estrogen levels (Wober-Bingol, 2013).

Migraine burden has been shown to be highest in women 18–44 years, where the 3-month prevalence of migraine has been reported as 26.1% in national surveillance studies (Smitherman et al., 2013), reflecting the significant impact of migraine on women during their peak educational, professional, reproductive, and mothering years. Migraine has been found to have a prevalence of 25.3%–48.5% in university students (Smitherman, McDermott, & Buchanan, 2011; Souza-e-Silva & Rocha-Filho, 2011). detrimentally impacting class attendance and academic standing; it is prevalent in medical students as well, and in one school survey migraine was seen in 24.8% of 359 students (Johnson et al., 2014).

Despite its disabling nature, almost half of people with migraine are undiagnosed and many are not effectively treated. Results of a large population survey found that of 162,576 respondents, the prevalence of migraine was 17.1% in women and 5.6% in men. Only 56.2% of those who met the criteria for migraine had ever received a medical diagnosis, and 98% of the migraineurs relied on acute treatment for their migraine attacks. Only 12.4% of migraineurs indicated that they were taking any type of migraine preventive medication (Diamond et al., 2007).

MIGRAINE TRIGGERS

A migraine trigger is any factor that on exposure or withdrawal leads to the development of acute migraine. Mechanisms, exposure time, and frequency are individualized. Emotional stress has been shown to be a common migraine trigger, as has inadequate sleep. Multiple triggers are common (Andress-Rothrock, King, & Rothrock, 2010; Fraga et al., 2013). Dietary triggers have been associated with release of serotonin and norepinephrine that influence blood flow and neuronal functioning, although specific mechanisms remain unclear. Fasting is identified as a frequent trigger in some studies, possibly associated with reactive hypoglycemia (Finocchi & Sivori, 2012).

Although alcohol is frequently listed as a trigger, studies suggest it impacts only 10% of migraineurs as a trigger consistently (Panconesi, 2008). A headache diary is a useful tool to help identify triggers, which may take 24–48 hours to manifest (Table 27.2).

Table 27.2. Systematic History for Headache Evaluation

Frequency, intensity, duration of attack

Recent change in the pattern, frequency or severity of headaches

Worsening of headache despite appropriate therapy

Presence or absence of aura and prodrome

Age at onset (concern for development after age 40)

Number of headache days per month

Time and mode of onset (concern for development with cough, exertion or sexual activity)

Quality, site and radiation of pain

Associated symptoms and abnormalities

Family history of migraine

Precipitating and relieving factors

Effect of activity on pain and pain on activity

Relationship with food/alcohol

Relationship with pain medications

Response to any previous treatment

Any recent change in vision

Any recent changes in sleep, exercise, weight, or diet

State of general health

Associated psychological conditions, i.e., depression

Change in work or lifestyle (evaluating disability)

Change in method of birth control (women)

Environmental factors

Effects of menstrual cycle and exogenous hormones (women)

Widely recognized lifestyle recommendations for migraine patients include limiting caffeine but not abruptly stopping it, maintenance of regular restorative sleep, regular meals, and effective stress management.

ESTROGEN-ASSOCIATED MIGRAINE

Classic studies have shown that migraine becomes more prevalent in females after menarche, reaching peak prevalence by age 40 before declining in menopause (Waters & O'Connor, 1971). Literature review supports the finding that migraine is influenced by the timing of estrogen secretion, occurring less frequently before puberty and after menopause. It is often precipitated by significant drops in estrogen levels, as typically seen 2 days before to 3 days after the onset of menstrual bleeding. The exact mechanism for these menstrual migraines, also called catamenial migraine, remains an area of active study. Women may experience migraines at other times of the cycle, however menstrual migraines may be more severe, longer lasting, and less responsive to treatment (MacGregor et al., 2010).

Use of oral contraceptives can be successful in headache sufferers, but can precipitate migraine headache and may worsen symptoms in some migraineurs, especially in the hormone-free interval of the pill cycle. Although data exists supporting the use of hormone therapy and oral contraceptives for modulation of estrogen levels, definitive recommendations have not been published (Caserta et al., 2014; Chai, Peterlin, & Calhoun, 2014). Stroke risk and history of smoking further complicate this highly individualized issue (Machado et al., 2010). Caution is especially indicated in women with migraine with aura, as oral contraceptives have been associated with increased risk of stroke in this population (Silberstein, & Patel, 2014). A systematic review and meta-analysis of nine studies found that the pooled relative risk of ischemic stroke in women age < 45 years with migraine ± aura was 3.6, and the risk of ischemic stroke was further increased to 7.2 among women currently using oral contraceptives (Schurks et al., 2009). If clinicians choose to use an estrogen-containing oral contraceptive, using the lowest effective dose would be prudent. A review of headache in pregnancy by Nappi et al. (2011) suggests that a majority of women report improvement in their migraines during pregnancy, and that breastfeeding is associated with a protective effect post partum.

COMORBIDITIES IN MIGRAINE

Active migraine with aura has been associated with increased risk of major cardiovascular events, myocardial infarction, ischemic stroke, and death due to ischemic cardiovascular disease in women in large population based studies ($N = 27,840$). Active migraine without aura was not associated with any increased risk of cardiovascular event in this prospective study (Kurth et al., 2006). Younger women with migraine with aura have been shown to be at increased risk of overall recurrent vascular events and recurrent ischemic stroke, and in some studies migraine has been associated with infarct-like brain lesions by MRI imaging studies (Sacco & Kurth, 2014). Studies also suggest some increased risk of cardiovascular disease in adult female migraineurs primarily related to sedentary behavior, sleep disturbance, obesity with related increase in insulin resistance and elevation in HDL cholesterol (Rockett et al., 2013).

Migraine has been associated with obesity in female adolescents (Pinhas-Hamiel et al., 2008) and significantly associated with endometriosis in a population-based survey ($N = 20,220$) (odds ratio [OR], 1.70; 95% confidence interval [CI] [1.59, 1.82]; $p < .001$). An association with restless leg syndrome has also been identified, which in itself has a high correlation with depression (Szentkiralyi et al., 2014; Zanigni et al., 2014).

A series of three articles by Tietjen et al. (2010a, 2010b, 2010c), exploring the relationship between childhood maltreatment (physical, sexual, emotional) in 1,348 migraineurs (88% women, 40% of whom reported migraine with aura), raises awareness about the important link between chronic stress and migraine headache. The authors found a high prevalence of abuse in study participants (physical 21%, sexual 25%, emotional 38%, physical neglect 22%, emotional neglect 38%, combined physical, emotional, sexual 9%). All types of abuse in this cohort were strongly associated with depression and anxiety (OR = 6.91, 95% CI: 3.97–12.03) or either depression or anxiety (OR = 3.66, 95% CI: 2.28–5.88) as compared with controls. Transformation from episodic to chronic headache was also seen in 26%. Emotional abuse was associated with higher levels of headache-related disability and increased migraine-associated pain sensitivity. Childhood emotional abuse was also associated with younger age of migraine onset (16 versus 19 years; $p = .002$). Statistically significantly increased prevalence of chronic illness and chronic pain were also found, particularly irritable bowel syndrome, chronic fatigue syndrome, and arthritis in cases of emotional abuse, and arthritis with physical abuse.

CONVENTIONAL MIGRAINE TREATMENT: BRIEF OVERVIEW

Over-the-counter and prescription medications remain the cornerstone of conventional therapy to address pain, vomiting, and other headache-related disabilities. Treatment is approached in two ways, preventive and abortive.

Abortive Therapies

Acute management often begins with simple steps to reduce sensory stimuli (e.g., light, noise, odors). Sleep can be an effective abortive intervention for some migraineurs.

The risk-benefit ratio of each pharmaceutical should be carefully considered. Although an exhaustive medication review of abortive therapies is beyond the scope of the chapter, a comprehensive 2012 review by Kelley and Tepper provides a useful resource (Kelley & Tepper, 2012a, 2012b, 2012c). Selected oral medications that have shown benefit in acute migraine management are discussed in this section.

Acetaminophen (Paracetamol)

A 2013 Cochrane Database systematic review of 11 studies ($N = 2,942$) found acetaminophen 1,000 mg superior to placebo for moderate-to-severe migraine pain with minimal downside. However, the reviewers noted that the number needed to treat (NNT) of 12 for pain-free response at 2 hours is inferior to other commonly used analgesics. When 10 mg metoclopramide was added, efficacy in acute pain management equaled that of oral sumatriptan 100 mg at 2 hours. In conclusion, acetaminophen may be a useful first-line treatment, especially in those who cannot tolerate nonsteroidal anti-inflammatory drugs (NSAIDs) or aspirin (Derry & Moore, 2013).

Aspirin

A 2013 Cochrane Database systematic review of 13 studies (N = 4,222) found that aspirin 1,000 mg remains an effective treatment for acute migraine, with equivalency in pain relief with oral sumatriptan, at 50-mg or 100-mg doses, at 2 hours. Combined treatment with metoclopramide (10 mg) and aspirin (1,000 mg) offered effective pain relief and reduction of nausea and vomiting with minimal adverse effects (Kirthi, Derry, & Moore, 2013).

Fixed Combination of Acetaminophen, Aspirin, and Caffeine

Over-the-counter tablets with fixed combinations of acetaminophen, aspirin, and caffeine are widely available and frequently used in self-treatment of migraine and tension-type headache under brand names such as Excedrin and Thomapyrin.

These combination drugs have been shown to be generally safe and efficacious, although caution is indicated depending on the individual's health conditions, especially with the use of caffeine. A study of 179 patients with a range of headache diagnosis, including mild-to-severe migraine and tension-type headache, compared treatment with two tablets of a fixed combination of 250 mg acetylsalicylic acid + 200 mg acetaminophen + 50 mg caffeine versus placebo. Combination treatment resulted in statistically significant improvement over placebo (p = .0008) measured in time to 50% pain relief and by extent of impairment of daily activities (Diener, Peil, & Aicher, 2011).

An earlier multicenter, randomized controlled trial in 1,555 migraine patients showed superior efficacy (p < .03) of two tablets of acetaminophen 250 mg, aspirin 250 mg, and caffeine 65 mg (per tablet) over ibuprofen 400 mg (total dose) and placebo in mild-to-moderate migraine. Results were measured by time to meaningful pain relief and pain intensity reduction (Goldstein et al., 2006).

Nonsteroidal Anti-Inflammatory Agents

Ibuprofen. A 2010 Cochrane Database review of nine studies (N = 4,373) showed that 400 mg was significantly more effective than 200 mg ibuprofen in providing pain relief in acute migraine pain in approximately 50% of patients studied. The NNT for 2-hour pain free and 2-hour pain relief were 9.7 and 6.3, respectively. Liquid preparations of 400 mg ibuprofen provided more rapid relief. Minimal side effects were noted (Rabbie, Derry, & Moore, 2013).

Naproxen. A 2013 Cochrane review ($N = 1,241$) comparing 500 mg and 825 mg naproxen for acute migraine management found both superior to placebo, but positive response in fewer than 2 out of 10 patients led to conclusion that other over-the-counter analgesics have superior efficacy as stand-alone therapy for acute migraine (Law, Derry, & Moore, 2013a). Parenteral ketoralac has been used successfully in acute migraine where oral route is not feasible (Friedman et al., 2014). Usual precautions for NSAID use include monitoring for gastrointestinal bleeding and avoiding/minimizing use in renal or cardiovascular disease.

Triptans. The triptans are serotonin 1b/1d agonists and considered first-line abortive therapy for migraine, especially when used in the earliest symptom stages. There are seven FDA-approved triptans, which are thought to work by releasing vasoactive peptides from trigeminal neurons, promoting vasoconstriction, and activating pain inhibitory systems (Cologno et al., 2012; Dussor, 2014). Research is active around new agents that work centrally to block neurogenic inflammation, avoiding potential complications from vasoconstriction (Rizzoli, 2014).

Sumatriptan is one of the most studied triptans and comes in oral, intranasal, transdermal, rectal, and parenteral forms. A 2014 Cochrane review ($N = 52,236$) showed that subcutaneous administration of 6 mg sumatriptan was the most effective overall in acute migraine, although intranasal and rectal forms were most commonly used. Adverse effects of triptans are dose related and generally transient, although they can be of concern in patients with uncontrolled hypertension, vasospastic or ischemic heart disease, and in those at risk for coronary artery disease. Cost can be a limiting factor in parenteral use (Derry, Derry, & Moore, 2012a, 2014). Oral sumatriptan at 50 mg and 100 mg was shown to be better than placebo for acute pain relief in 37,250 patients, especially when used early in the migraine attack, and provided good pain relief at 24 hours compared to other triptans, acetaminophen, aspirin, NSAIDs, and ergotamine combination therapy. Relief of nausea, photophobia, and phonophobia was also seen. Adverse effects recorded were primarily transient and mild (Derry, Derry, & Moore, 2012b).

Combination oral sumatriptan (85 mg or 50 mg) plus naproxen (500 mg) was also studied and shown to be effective than either drug alone at equivalent dose, however, the conclusion was that naproxen added relatively little beneficial effect in acute migraine treatment (Law, Derry, & Moore, 2013b). However, a comparison study of 500 mg naproxen alone versus sumatriptan 85 mg plus 500 mg naproxen in a combination tablet (SumaRT/Nap) showed naproxen was associated with a statistically significant reduction in migraine headache at month 3 compared with the combination drug (combination drug was more efficacious at 2-hour pain relief). No symptoms of medication overuse head-ache were reported for either approach in this study group. Work is ongoing in this area (Cady et al., 2014).

Preventive Therapies

Preventive therapies are highly individualized and tailored to patient needs and underlying health conditions. Many commonly used preventive agents carry serious or unwanted side effects, strengthening the case for an open-minded approach to integrative treatments.

Some of the common pharmaceutical categories used for migraine prevention include:

- Antihypertensives: especially beta-blockers and calcium-channel blockers.
- Antidepressants: especially tricyclics, which down-regulate serotonin receptors and enhance exogenous opioid receptor activity
- Anticonvulsants: especially topiramate and valproic acid (Linde et al., 2013; Shamliyan, Kane, & Taylor, 2013).

INTEGRATIVE APPROACHES TO MIGRAINE

The multifactorial nature of migraine and its significant comorbidities present a powerful argument for the use of an integrative approach in women, especially in regard to migraine prophylaxis. Elements of an integrative approach can include:

- Nutrition: eliminate triggers, lower cardiovascular risk and inflammation
- Dietary supplements: abortives and preventives, anti-inflammatory and antioxidants
- Physical activity: overall fitness, stress management
- Mind–body therapies: stress management, reduction of anxiety, pain, and depression
- Relationships: assessment of social support, compassionate inquiry about prior abuse or trauma should be included in a full workup
- Environment: exposures to chemicals, light, noise, technology
- Whole medical systems: traditional Chinese medicine, homeopathy, naturopathy

An overview of selected integrative approaches to migraine is presented below.

Nutrition

Nutrition, especially the use of the Mediterranean (anti-inflammatory) diet is a cornerstone of integrative medicine. Nutrition is thought to influence many aspects of migraine, although individual variation and methodological challenges have prevented definitive research conclusions (Finkel, Yerry, & Mann, 2013; Hoffmann, & Recober, 2013; Panconesi, Bartolozzi, & Guidi, 2011). While there are no studies examining the effectiveness of the Mediterranean diet in migraine, one study of 57 adults comparing consumption of a high omega-3 fatty acid (anti-inflammatory) diet versus a (pro-inflammatory) omega-6 fatty acid diet on chronic headache (including chronic migraine and chronic tension-type headache) over a 12-week study period showed statistically significant improvement in headache severity ($p < .001$), reduction in headache hours per day ($p = 0.01$), and reduction in inflammatory markers ($p < .001$) (Ramsden et al., 2013). In addition to commonly mentioned potential triggers such as fasting, alcohol, cheese, and chocolate, caffeine withdrawal, processed foods, aspartame, and monosodium glutamate have been implicated as possible migraine triggers, supporting a general argument for a healthy, whole-food diet in migraine sufferers (Finocchi & Sivori, 2012). Partnering with patients to help them identify and avoid individual triggers is likely to be the most effective approach. Data on elimination diets to reduce migraine that are based on immunoglobulin G (IgG) antibodies to food antigens has been mixed and is not routinely recommended (Alpay et al., 2010; Mitchell et al., 2011). The ketogenic diet has garnered some interest in migraine therapy, although data is insufficient to recommend it at this time.

Dietary Supplements

Substantial research interest has focused on dietary supplements for migraine prophylaxis. The following section provides an overview on several with the strongest evidence.

Butterbur Root (*Petasites hybridus*)

Butterbur has a long history of use in both migraine and allergy treatment and is noted for its anti-inflammatory, vasodilatory, and smooth muscle–relaxant properties. Active components of butterbur, especially isopetasin, inhibit leukotriene synthesis. Mast cell activation is also reduced, which reduces systemic release of leukotrienes and histamine (Monograph, 2001). Butterbur has a Level A (highest) recommendation for migraine prophylaxis in adults from the American Academy of Neurology and the American Headache Society

(Holland et al., 2012) and is "strongly recommended" (highest category) for migraine prophylaxis in updated guidelines from the Canadian Headache Society (Pringsheim et al., 2012). These recommendations are the result of randomized, placebo-controlled, double-blind clinical studies showing dramatic reduction, up to 60% compared with baseline ($p < 0.05$), in migraine frequency in one study (Grossman & Schmidramsl, 2001) and 48% reduction compared with placebo ($p = .0012$) in another using butterbur extract 75 mg orally twice a day (Lipton et al., 2004). Butterbur has been well studied in children over 6 years and found to have a wide margin of safety (Utterback et al., 2014).

Adverse Effects, Cautions:
- Generally well tolerated, occasional eructation (burping).
- Use only standardized extracts containing ~7.5% petasin and free of pyrrolizidine alkaloids (hepatotoxic and carcinogenic).
- The German Health Authority (Commission E) endorses brand-name product Petadolex as nontoxic.
- Safety has not been established in pregnancy or lactation or for children younger than 6 years of age.
- Avoid concurrent use with anticholinergic medication.

Dose:
- 50–150 mg orally, total daily dosage. Generally divided twice a day.
- Start children on low range of dose and adjust as needed.

Magnesium
Magnesium is integral to a broad range of intracellular processes involving mitochondria, DNA and RNA synthesis, neuronal conduction, vasomotor tone, cardiac function, muscle contraction, and others. Deficiency has been associated with migraine, especially menstrual migraine. It carries a "strong recommendation" for migraine prophylaxis from the Canadian Headache Society and a Level B recommendation (probably effective) from the American Academy of Neurology and the American Headache Society based on results from randomized, double-blind, placebo-controlled trials (Holland et al., 2012; Pringsheim et al., 2012; Tarighat Esfanjani et al., 2012). A prospective study with 270 women with menstrual migraines, reported that the incidence of intracellular magnesium deficiency was 45% during menstrual attacks and 15% during nonmenstrual attacks. Serum magnesium levels were normal in the study, even though intracellular levels were low (Mauskop, Altura, & Altura, 2002). An earlier clinical study found that women with menstrual-related migraine reported a significant decrease in headache days and an improvement in the

Menstrual Distress Questionnaire Score after receiving treatment with oral magnesium (360 mg/day vs. placebo) for 2 months (Facchinetti et al., 1991).

Magnesium stores are held primarily in bone (~67%), intracellularly (31%), and in serum (<2%). Routine blood levels are the least reliable measurement (except in the face of severe deficiency). Ionized magnesium and red blood cell magnesium are more sensitive but less available tests, making research and recommendations in this area more challenging (Mauskop & Varughese, 2012; Nielsen, 2010; Volpe, 2013).

Intravenous magnesium (1 g) has shown some benefit in abortive treatment. One small study resulted in elimination of pain in 86.6% and 100% elimination of nausea and vomiting, versus 7% pain relief in the placebo group (Demirkaya et al., 2001).

There is some evidence to support the efficacy of IV magnesium (1 g) in migraine with aura, although more studies are needed before definitive recommendation could be made (Bigal et al., 2002).

Adverse Effects, Cautions:

- One of the benefits of magnesium is relatively low risk and affordable cost.
- Magnesium oxide may cause diarrhea, citrate or chelated forms may be better tolerated.
- Magnesium loading in any form is contraindicated in those with renal disease.
- Safe in pregnancy and lactation (Volpe, 2013).

Dose:

- Standardized recommendations do not currently exist. However, based on clinical trials and experience, many practitioners recommend 400–600 mg per day for healthy adults.
- Oral prophylaxis of 9 mg/kg/day was shown to be effective in one randomized controlled 16-week trial involving children ages 3–17 years (Wang et al., 2003). Another study in 81 patients, age 18–65 years, showed that 600 mg of trimagnesium dicitrate daily for 12 weeks reduced migraine frequency by 41.6% compared with 15.8% in the control group. Adverse effects were diarrhea and gastric irritation (Peikert, Wilimzig, & Kohne-Volland, 1996).
- It has been reported that dietary intake of magnesium is low in ~60% of US adults. Maintenance of adequate magnesium levels in food should be encouraged, although achieving the recommended daily allowance (RDA) for females (360 mg/day for 14- to 18-year-olds

to 320 mg/day for 31- to 70-year-olds) can be difficult to achieve in food alone. There is no one specific food that provides significant magnesium, although some food groups higher in magnesium include unrefined whole grains, spinach, nuts, legumes and tubers (USDA, 2011).

Riboflavin

A member of the B vitamin family, precursor in the mitochondrial electron transport chain, and a cofactor in the Krebs cycle, riboflavin (B2) contributes to cellular growth, enzyme function, and energy production. There is research to suggest that mitochondrial dysfunction may play a role in migraine in a subset of patients with abnormal phosphorylation of ADP to ATP (Sandor et al., 2000). Although studies are mixed with regard to effectiveness in migraine, with both positive and negative studies in adults using 400 mg/day riboflavin (Monograph, 2008), it has a "strongly recommended" recommendation from the Canadian Headache Society guidelines and a Level B from the American Academy of Neurology and American Headache Society.

Adverse Effects, Other Concerns:
- Generally well tolerated, inexpensive.
- Occasional reports of diarrhea and vomiting.
- Orange discoloration of urine is common.
- Safety in pregnancy and lactation is unknown.

Dose:
- 400 mg/day used in several adult trials.

Coenzyme Q10

Coenzyme Q10 (CoQ10) plays an important role in the electron transport chain in mitochondrial membranes. Deficiency in biosynthesis or in bioavailability has been linked to various disease states (Potgieter, Pretorius, & Pepper, 2013). It has been studied for effectiveness in migraine treatment, and has a "strong recommendation" for migraine prophylaxis from the Canadian Headache Society (Pringsheim et al., 2012), but only a Level C (possibly effective) rating from the American Academy of Neurology and American Headache Society based on mixed study results.

One randomized controlled trial of 42 patients found 100 mg CoQ10 orally three time a day for 3 months superior to placebo; 48% of subjects had 50% reduction in attack frequency, with a NNT of three (Sandor et al., 2005).

A larger study of 1,550 migraine patients, age 3–22 years (mean 13.3 years) found low CoQ10 levels in 33% of participants. Supplementation with CoQ10 (1–3 mg/kg) resulted in reduction of headache frequency and associated disability in patients whose levels of CoQ10 returned to normal reference range ($p < .001$) (Hershey et al., 2007).

Adverse Effects, Other Concerns:
- CoQ10 is generally well tolerated.
- Optimal absorption is found with a liquid gel-based capsule or as ubiquinol.
- Safety in pregnancy and lactation has not been determined.

Dose:
- Adults 100–300 mg/day.

Feverfew (*Tanacetum parthenium*)
Feverfew leaf, a member of the Asteracae family, was widely used as a folk medicine for migraines and has also been the subject of controlled trials. Earlier studies showed mixed benefit (Pittler & Ernst, 2004), but more recently a CO_2 extract of feverfew, MIG-99, has shown promise. One study in 170 migraine dosed patients with 6.25 mg MIG-99 three times daily for 16 weeks. Migraine frequency decreased by 1.9 attacks per month in the treatment group compared with 1.3 headaches in the placebo group ($p = .0049$). Adverse events were rare (Diener et al., 2005a). MIG-99 has a Level B rating from the American Academy of Neurology and the American Headache Society.

Adverse Events, Other Concerns:
- Occasional include sore mouth, oral ulcers, and gastrointestinal (GI) disturbance. Mouth sores may be primarily associated with chewing the fresh leaf.
- Feverfew should not be used in pregnant women because of possible inhibition of platelets and history of use as an abortifacient (Evans & Taylor, 2006).

Dose:
- Adults take 6.25 mg three times per day of standardized CO_2 extract

Ginger (*Zingiber officinale*)

Ginger has a long history of use for treatment of nausea and vomiting associated with migraine, and is used in some whole medical systems, such as Ayurveda, for neurologic conditions, including headache. Studies have evaluated ginger for both its preventive and abortive properties in headache treatment (Mustafa & Srivastava, 1990).

A recent randomized, double-blinded clinical trial of ginger powder versus sumatriptan therapy in 100 patients with acute migraine without aura showed equivalent efficacy of ginger powder to sumatriptan. Fewer adverse effects were seen in the ginger treatment group (Maghbooli et al., 2014).

Ginger has also been studied in sublingual form in combination with feverfew in acute migraine headache (Cady et al., 2005). Combination feverfew/ginger was found to be more effective than placebo in pain relief ($p = .002$) at hour 2 of treatment in 45 patients with a combined total of 163 treated migraine headaches. Authors concluded feverfew/ginger sublingually was an effective first-line treatment for migraineurs, especially those who experienced mild headache as an initial clinical finding prior to onset of severe headache (Cady et al., 2011).

Ginkgo (*Ginkgo biloba*)

There are some data examining the effectiveness of ginkgolide B, a constituent extracted from ginkgo leaf, for migraine prophylaxis. Its efficacy has been assessed in a combination product Migrasoll (60 mg *G. biloba* terpenes phytosome, 11 mg CoQ10, 8.7 mg vitamin B2) administered twice daily for 4 months in patients suffering from migraine with aura (D'Andrea et al., 2009). In the study, the number of migraine auras and their duration was significantly decreased ($p < .0001$).

A second open trial of the same combination product in 25 patients (16 female, mean age 39.7 years) evaluated effect treatment of acute migraine with aura. Aura duration measured in minutes was significantly reduced ($p < .001$), and in 18% of patients pain resolved completely. No adverse effects were reported (Allais et al., 2013). Ginkgo is considered generally considered of low toxicity when used at the doses typically seen in clinical trials.

Dose:

- The majority of research has been conducted on doses of 120–240 mg standardized extract standardized to 24–27% flavonol glycosides and 6–7% terpene lactones per dose, taken at once or in two divided doses.

Mind–Body Therapies

There is a strong role for mind–body therapies in treatment of migraine, in part because of the close correlation between emotional distress and migraine. Behavioral treatments (e.g., relaxation, biofeedback, and cognitive-behavioral therapy) possess the most evidence for successful headache management and have a substantial history of randomized trials showing efficacy. They are considered first-line preventive options, especially in those who have significant headache-related disability, comorbid mood or anxiety disorders, difficulty managing stress or other triggers, and medication overuse (Nicholson et al., 2011). Mind–body therapies can be especially useful in situations when medication may be contraindicated, such as during pregnancy and lactation. Various mind–body therapies can be combined, for example biofeedback with relaxation training (e.g., progressive muscle relaxation, autogenics), and have been shown to be more effective than solo therapy in reducing headache frequency, muscle tension, anxiety, depression, and medication usage in migraine patients (Nestoriuc & Martin, 2007). Increase in self-efficacy can be an added benefit in the successful use of mind–body therapies.

Multiple studies support the efficacy of clinical hypnosis in migraine treatment.

Many studies include self-hypnosis instruction or use of self-hypnosis recordings, resulting in significant reductions in frequency, duration, and intensity of headaches. Mindfulness-based stress reduction (MBSR) has been found to be effective in multiple studies of patients experiencing various types of chronic pain (Rosenzweig et al., 2010). An MBSR course was found to be safe and feasible in a small randomized controlled trial of 19 migraineurs. Small study size limited conclusive findings, although overall reduction in migraine frequency and severity was seen. Further study in warranted in this emerging area (Wells et al., 2014).

Exercise/Physical Activity

Enjoyable regular physical activity is fundamental to good health and can help decrease frequency, intensity, and duration of migraine headache (Narin et al., 2003). One study in 30 migraine patients showed significant improvement in self-rated pain and improvement in depression related symptoms after a 6-week, biweekly exercise program combined with relaxation training (Dittrich et al., 2008).

Yoga

Yoga combines physical and mindfulness practice, and has been shown to be helpful for headache relief in several studies. In one study, yoga therapy was contrasted with self-care for 72 randomized migraineurs over 3 months. Headache intensity, frequency, pain, medication use, and anxiety and depression scores were statistically lower in the yoga group ($p < .001$ all categories) (John et al., 2007).

Acupuncture

Strong supporting evidence exists for the use of acupuncture in migraine prophylaxis.

A 2009 Cochrane Database systematic review of 22 studies ($N = 4,419$) concluded "acupuncture is at least as effective as, or possibly more effective than, prophylactic drug treatment, and has fewer adverse effects. Acupuncture should be considered a treatment option for patients willing to undergo this treatment" (Linde et al., 2009). Very rare risks include infection, pneumothorax, and localized bleeding. Acupuncture in pregnancy should be administered by highly trained and experienced practitioners.

Craniosacral Therapy

Craniosacral therapy is a gentle hands-on therapy often used in conjunction with osteopathic treatment and massage therapy (Mann et al., 2008). Craniosacral therapy has been shown to alleviate migraine symptoms in one 4-week crossover study of 20 people with migraine receiving six treatments each (Arnadottir & Sigurdardottir, 2013).

Homeopathy

Homeopathy has been studied for both migraine treatment and prophylaxis, although the highly individualized treatment approach makes standardization difficult (Jonas, Kaptchuk, & Linde, 2003). A prospective multicenter study in 212 adults (89.2% women) with a 10- to 15-year history of migraine were evaluated over a 24-month period. Participants received individualized homeopathic remedies by trained physicians. Migraine severity and frequency decreased significantly, health-related quality of life improved significantly, and use of conventional and health services decreased substantially (Witt, Ludtke, & Willich, 2010). Adverse effects were rare.

Even with these positive studies, given the variability in methodology, reviews have concluded that there is insufficient evidence to support or refute the use of homeopathy in the management of migraine (Schiapparelli et al., 2010).

Sleep

Environmental factors such as irregular sleep patterns are common in headache patients and are known triggers for both migraines and tension-type headache (de Tommaso et al., 2014; Engstrom et al., 2014a). Sleep disturbance is associated with increased anxiety, insomnia, and daytime tiredness, and has been associated with chronic sleep deprivation in headache patients that may contribute to increased pain sensitivity and headache frequency (Engstrom et al., 2014b). Research reveals that migraineurs, especially women, have altered levels in melatonin overall and during migraine attacks (Brun et al., 1995; Masruha et al., 2008). Tryptophan serves as the precursor for melatonin (N-acetyl-5-methoxytryptamine) synthesis. Researchers are actively exploring melatonin's anti-inflammatory and antinociceptive (pain-blocking) properties (Srinivasan et al., 2012). Although an 8-week, randomized, double-blind, placebo-controlled crossover study in 48 men and women, age 18–65 years, using 2 mg extended-release melatonin 1 hour before bedtime failed to reduce migraine frequency as compared with placebo ($p = .497$) (Alstadhaug et al., 2010), other studies suggest that women with sleep disturbance and migraines may derive benefit from melatonin's effects. A recent study showed that the melatonin agonist agomelatine at a dose of 25 mg/day decreased frequency and duration of migraine attacks in study participants. More research is needed in this important area (Tabeeva, Sergeev, & Gromova, 2011). While there is general agreement that melatonin has a very good safety profile, safety during pregnancy and lactation has not been well established.

MIGRAINE SUMMARY

Treatment of migraine is complex and lends itself to a multifaceted integrative approach.

Precedent exists for educational programs on migraine that address both the cognitive and emotional aspects of headache management. In one educational program on migraine, 284 patients of whom 92% were women, showed a 50%

or greater reduction in headache frequency over a 12-month study period (p < .001) after participating in a program designed to provide patients tools to self-manage their migraines in conjunction with their healthcare teams. Patient materials included *The Migraineur's Guide to Migraine*, a headache diary, patient tip sheet, nutrition information, written and visual range-of-motion and stretching exercises, and biofeedback tapes. In addition to decrease in headache frequency, patients reported significantly increased satisfaction with headache care and decreased worry about headache. Sense of self-efficacy was also improved at 12 months in study participants (p < .001) (Smith, Nicholson, & Banks, 2010).

TENSION-TYPE HEADACHE

Phyllis suffered with tension-type headache for years. She had developed them when she was commuting 2 hours a day to a job she despised. Sometimes the headache episodes would come on just prior to a vacation. Over time they began to occur daily, for up to 10 weeks in a row. Conventional medications took the edge off the pain, but nothing seemed to resolve them. Eventually she began psychotherapy coupled with healthy lifestyle choices and acupuncture, which helped her decide to leave her job and return to school. She began to notice improvement in her headaches within the first 2 weeks of changing her routine.

TENSION-TYPE HEADACHE CLASSIFICATION AND EPIDEMIOLOGY

Tension-type headache has significant socioeconomic burden, and has been identified as the most prevalent headache disorder, with prevalence ranging from 20% to greater than 80% in various study populations. It is estimated to affect approximately 40% of Americans (Chu et al., 2014; Rosen, 2012).

Symptoms are often described as nonthrobbing headache with pain of mild-to-moderate intensity. Tension-type headaches are classified as infrequent episodic, occurring less than once monthly; frequent episodic, occurring between 1 and 14 days per month; and chronic tension-type headache, occurring more than 15 days a month. The overall 1-year prevalence was found to be 86% in a large Danish population-based twin study (N = 33,764, ages 12–41 years), with a prevalence of 92.5% among women and 78.9% in men. Women in this study had a significantly higher prevalence of frequent episodic and chronic tension-type headache than men. The risk and frequency of tension-type headache was significantly higher in those who also experienced migraine as opposed to people who had never experienced migraine (Russell et al., 2006).

Both peripheral (myofascial) and central mechanisms are thought to be involved, leading to recommendations of combined drug and nondrug therapy (such as relaxation therapies) for best outcome (Fumal & Schoenen, 2008). As in migraine, depression and anxiety have been associated with tension-type headache in some studies (Beghi et al., 2007).

TRIGGERS

Common triggers have been reported as stress, hunger, dehydration, and sleep deprivation, which would ideally be addressed proactively (Spierings, Ranke, & Honkoop, 2001). Preventive health lifestyle recommendations for migraine prevention also extend to tension-type headache and include healthy nutrition, effective stress management, restorative sleep, and regular physical activity. Although less evidence exists to suggest that specific foods trigger tension-type headache than migraine headache, an anti-inflammatory diet may provide overall benefit.

Other important potential sources of chronic secondary headache (as classified by the International Headache Society) include dental and temporomandibular joint disease. These conditions may require specialty consultation for accurate diagnosis if suspected (Bernstein et al., 2013).

CONVENTIONAL TREATMENT

Common conventional treatments for tension-type headache include NSAIDs such as aspirin and acetaminophen (Lecchi et al., 2014). Fixed combination drugs containing caffeine have also been shown to be widely used and generally safe in tension-type headache, although some individuals may have adverse reaction to caffeine (Anneken, Evers, & Husstedt, 2010; Diener et al., 2005b). The use of butalbital and codeine or other opiates is not recommended because of the propensity of overuse, which can transform episodic into chronic headaches (Silberstein & McCrory, 2001).

Lack of benefit for prophylactic treatment of uncomplicated tension-type headache with antidepressants, muscle relaxants, benzodiazepines, or vasomotor dilators has been shown in several studies (Fumal & Schoenen, 2008; Verhagen et al., 2010). Medication overuse headache is a frequent risk in this population (Valguarnera & Tanganelli, 2010). Botulinum toxin A has shown some positive preventive potential in patients with chronic migraine, although it has not been shown to be effective in patients with episodic migraine or tension-type headache (Ashkenazi & Blumenfeld, 2013).

INTEGRATIVE APPROACHES TO TENSION-TYPE HEADACHE

In addition to preventive lifestyle measures, some integrative approaches have shown promise in tension-type headache. An overview of selected therapies is reviewed below.

Mind–Body Medicine

Mind–body therapies have been reported as the most common type of complementary therapy used in headache patients, and are frequently used in adults with common neurological conditions. Deep-breathing exercises, meditation, and yoga were the most frequently reported therapies used in a 2007 National Health Interview Survey of 23,393 people (Erwin Wells, Phillips, & McCarthy, 2011). Hypnosis also has a long history of use in tension-type headache, and has been found to be effective, similar to its efficacy in migraine treatment (Hammond, 2007).

Electromyographic biofeedback has shown efficacy in tension-type headache, as have cognitive-behavioral therapy and relaxation training (autogenics, progressive muscle relaxation) (Bendtsen & Jensen, 2011; Nestoriuc et al., 2008; Sun-Edelstein & Mauskop, 2012). Mindfulness based stress reduction (MBSR) has shown promise in a pilot study of a six-week MBSR course in tension type headache patients who showed a significant decrease in headache frequency (Cathcart et al., 2014). Mindfulness-based cognitive therapy was also found to significantly reduce pain perception and improve sense of self-efficacy in a randomized controlled trial in patients with tension-type headache. Overall the therapy was found to be tolerable, feasible, and acceptable by the majority of study participants (Day et al., 2014). Behavioral strategies present a viable option for women who are pregnant, planning pregnancy, or breastfeeding.

Manual Therapy

A review of the effectiveness of any manual therapy in tension-type headache revealed significant variability in study design and outcome, although overall results were positive and reported side effects were mild and rare (Jull et al., 2002; Lozano Lopez et al., 2014). Osteopathic manipulative therapy has been assessed in a single-blind randomized placebo-controlled pilot study of 44 patients in the primary care setting. Treatments were tailored to the individual's needs, versus sham therapy over a 1-month time period. Treatment group (n = 21) showed a 40%, statistically significant reduction in headache frequency, which improved to 50% at 3-month follow-up (Rolle et al., 2014).

Although trigger point therapy has been evaluated in tension-type headache, further studies are needed before clear recommendations can be made (Alonso-Blanco, de-la-Llave-Rincon, & Fernandez-de-las-Penas, 2012).

A review of randomized controlled trials of therapeutic exercise in tension-type headache patients showed strong correlation with improvement in intensity, frequency, and duration of pain (Gil-Martinez et al., 2013; Hindiyeh, Krusz, & Cowan, 2013).

Research in the use of acupuncture in tension-type headache continues to accrue and shows promise, although its use is less clear-cut than in treatment of migraine headache.

Evidence in support of acupuncture for tension-type headache was considered insufficient in earlier Cochrane Database reviews. With accrual of more data, including six additional randomized trials, Linde et al. concluded that acupuncture could be a valuable nonpharmacological tool in patients with frequent episodic or chronic tension-type headaches (Linde et al., 2009). Acupuncture may also hold promise for patients who are unable to tolerate other therapies, and has a broad margin of safety when administered by a trained practitioner (Hao et al., 2013; Yancey, Sheridan, & Koren, 2014).

Essential Oils

Essential oils have been used for thousands of years to reduce anxiety and promote restful sleep. They are the focus of active medical research (Wu, 2014). Topical application of the essential oil from peppermint (*Mentha x piperita*) has been shown to have some efficacy in the treatment of tension-type headache, thought to be attributable to its antispasmodic effect (Kligler & Chaudhary, 2007).

An earlier study of peppermint and eucalyptus (*Eucalyptus globulus*) essential oils increased cognitive function and relaxed muscles in 32 healthy subjects but had little influence on pain sensitivity (Gobel, Schmidt, & Soyka, 1994). More research is needed before specific recommendations can be made for tension headache, but the margin of safety for the use of essential oils in both aerosolized and topical form is wide.

Summary

Migraine and tension-type headache are common conditions in women. An integrative approach that emphasizes preventive measures such as healthy nutrition, effective stress management, regular enjoyable physical activity, and restorative sleep has the potential to reduce headache frequency and severity. Research advances have identified butterbur, acupuncture, and mind–body medicine as therapies with special promise in integrative migraine treatment. Partnership with patients can assist them in identifying personal triggers and identify expanded treatment options. Integrative therapies may be used concurrently with or in place of conventional care in some patients, to improve approaches to preventing and managing headache.

REFERENCES

Adams, J., Barbery, G., & Lui, C. W. (2013) Complementary and alternative medicine use for headache and migraine: A critical review of the literature. *Headache, 53,* 459–473.

Allais, G., et al. (2013). The efficacy of ginkgolide B in the acute treatment of migraine aura: An open preliminary trial. *Neurol Sci, 34*(Suppl 1), S161–S163.

Alonso-Blanco, C., de-la-Llave-Rincon, A. I., & Fernandez-de-las-Penas, C. (2012). Muscle trigger point therapy in tension-type headache. *Expert Rev Neurother, 12,* 315–322.

Alpay, K., et al. (2010). Diet restriction in migraine, based on IgG against foods: A clinical double-blind, randomised, cross-over trial. *Cephalalgia, 30,* 829–837.

Alstadhaug, K. B., et al. (2010). Prophylaxis of migraine with melatonin: A randomized controlled trial. *Neurology, 75,* 1527–1532.

Andree, C., et al. (2014). Headache yesterday in Europe. *J Headache Pain, 15,* 33.

Andress-Rothrock, D., King, W., & Rothrock, J. (2010). An analysis of migraine triggers in a clinic-based population. *Headache, 50,* 1366–1370.

Anneken, K., Evers, S., & Husstedt, I. W. (2010). Efficacy of fixed combinations of acetylsalicyclic acid, acetaminophen and caffeine in the treatment of idiopathic headache: A review. *Eur J Neurol, 17,* 534–e25.

Arnadottir, T. S., & Sigurdardottir, A. K. (2013). Is craniosacral therapy effective for migraine? Tested with HIT-6 Questionnaire. *Complement Ther Clin Pract, 19,* 11–14.

Ashkenazi, A., & Blumenfeld, A. (2013). OnabotulinumtoxinA for the treatment of headache. *Headache, 53*(Suppl 2), 54–61.

Bahra, A., & Goadsby, P. J. (2004). Diagnostic delays and mis-management in cluster headache. *Acta Neurol Scand, 109,* 175–179.

Beghi, E., et al. (2007). Headache and anxiety-depressive disorder comorbidity: The HADAS study. *Neurol Sci, 28*(Suppl 2), S217–S219.

Bendtsen, L., & Jensen, R. (2011). Treating tension-type headache: An expert opinion. *Expert Opin Pharmacother, 12,* 1099–1109.

Bernstein, J. A., et al. (2013). Headache and facial pain: Differential diagnosis and treatment. *J Allergy Clin Immunol Pract, 1,* 242–251.

Bethell, C., et al. (2013). Complementary and conventional medicine use among youth with recurrent headaches. *Pediatrics, 132,* e1173–e1183.

Bigal, M. E., et al. (2002). Intravenous magnesium sulphate in the acute treatment of migraine without aura and migraine with aura: A randomized, double-blind, placebo-controlled study. *Cephalalgia, 22,* 345–353.

Brun, J., et al. (1995). Nocturnal melatonin excretion is decreased in patients with migraine without aura attacks associated with menses. *Cephalalgia, 15,* 136–139; discussion 79.

Buse, D. C., et al. (2013). Sex differences in the prevalence, symptoms, and associated features of migraine, probable migraine, and other severe headache: Results of the American Migraine Prevalence and Prevention (AMPP) Study. *Headache, 53,* 1278–1299.

Cady, R. K., et al. (2005). Gelstat Migraine (sublingually administered feverfew and ginger compound) for acute treatment of migraine when administered during the mild pain phase. *Med Sci Monit, 11,* PI65–PI69.

Cady, R. K., et al. (2011). A double-blind placebo-controlled pilot study of sublingual feverfew and ginger (LipiGesic M) in the treatment of migraine. *Headache, 51,* 1078–1086.

Cady, R., et al. (2014). SumaRT/Nap vs naproxen sodium in treatment and disease modification of migraine: A pilot study. *Headache, 54,* 67–79.

Caserta, D., et al. (2014). Combined oral contraceptives: Health benefits beyond contraception. *Panminerva Med, 56,* 233–244.

Cathcart, S., et al. (2014). Brief mindfulness-based therapy for chronic tension-type headache: A randomized controlled pilot study. *Behav Cogn Psychother, 42,* 1–15.

Chai, N. C., Peterlin, B. L., & Calhoun, A. H. (2014). Migraine and estrogen. *Curr Opin Neurol, 27,* 315–324.

Chu, M. K., et al. (2014). Field testing the alternative criteria for tension-type headache proposed in the third beta edition of the international classification of headache disorders: Results from the Korean headache-sleep study. *J Headache Pain, 15,* 28.

Cologno, D., et al. (2012). Triptans: Over the migraine. *Neurol Sci, 33*(Suppl 1), S193–S198.

D'Andrea, G., et al. (2009). Efficacy of ginkgolide B in the prophylaxis of migraine with aura. *Neurol Sci, 30*(Suppl 1), S121–S124.

Day, M. A., et al. (2014). Mindfulness-based cognitive therapy for the treatment of headache pain: A pilot study. *Clin J Pain, 30,* 152–161.

de Tommaso, M., et al. (2014). Sleep features and central sensitization symptoms in primary headache patients. *J Headache Pain, 15,* 64.

Demirkaya, S., et al. (2001). Efficacy of intravenous magnesium sulfate in the treatment of acute migraine attacks. *Headache, 41,* 171–177.

Derry, C. J., Derry, S., & Moore, R. A. (2012a). Sumatriptan (intranasal route of administration) for acute migraine attacks in adults. *Cochrane Database Syst Rev*, 2:CD009663.

Derry, C. J., Derry, S., & Moore, R. A. (2012b). Sumatriptan (oral route of administration) for acute migraine attacks in adults. *Cochrane Database Syst Rev*, 2:CD008615.

Derry, C. J., Derry, S., & Moore, R. A. (2014). Sumatriptan (all routes of administration) for acute migraine attacks in adults: Overview of Cochrane reviews. *Cochrane Database Syst Rev*, 5:CD009108.

Derry, S., & Moore, R. A. (2013). Paracetamol (acetaminophen) with or without an antiemetic for acute migraine headaches in adults. *Cochrane Database Syst Rev*, 4: CD008040.

Diamond, S., et al. (2007). Patterns of diagnosis and acute and preventive treatment for migraine in the United States: Results from the American Migraine Prevalence and Prevention study. *Headache*, 47, 355–363.

Diener, H. C., et al. (2005a). Efficacy and safety of 6.25 mg t.i.d. feverfew CO_2-extract (MIG-99) in migraine prevention: A randomized, double-blind, multicentre, placebo-controlled study. *Cephalalgia*, 25, 1031–1041.

Diener, H. C., et al. (2005b). The fixed combination of acetylsalicylic acid, paracetamol and caffeine is more effective than single substances and dual combination for the treatment of headache: A multicentre, randomized, double-blind, single-dose, placebo-controlled parallel group study. *Cephalalgia*, 25, 776–787.

Diener, H. C., Peil, H., & Aicher, B. (2011). The efficacy and tolerability of a fixed combination of acetylsalicylic acid, paracetamol, and caffeine in patients with severe headache: A post-hoc subgroup analysis from a multicentre, randomized, double-blind, single-dose, placebo-controlled parallel group study. *Cephalalgia*, 31, 1466–1476.

Dittrich, S. M., et al. (2008). Aerobic exercise with relaxation: Influence on pain and psychological well-being in female migraine patients. *Clin J Sport Med*, 18, 363–365.

Dussor, G. (2014). Serotonin, 5HT1 agonists, and migraine: New data, but old questions still not answered. *Curr Opin Support Palliat Care*, 8, 137–142.

Engstrom, M., et al. (2014a). Sleep quality and arousal in migraine and tension-type headache: The headache-sleep study. *Acta Neurol Scand Suppl*, 2014(198), 47–54.

Engstrom, M., et al. (2014b). Sleep quality, arousal and pain thresholds in tension-type headache: A blinded controlled polysomnographic study. *Cephalalgia*, 34, 455–463.

Erwin Wells, R., Phillips, R. S., & McCarthy, E. P. (2011). Patterns of mind-body therapies in adults with common neurological conditions. *Neuroepidemiology*, 36, 46–51.

Evans, R. W., & Taylor, F. R. (2006). "Natural" or alternative medications for migraine prevention. *Headache*, 46, 1012–1018.

Facchinetti, F., et al. (1991). Magnesium prophylaxis of menstrual migraine: Effects on intracellular magnesium. *Headache*, 31, 298–301.

Finkel, A. G., Yerry, J. A., & Mann, J. D. (2013). Dietary considerations in migraine management: Does a consistent diet improve migraine? *Curr Pain Headache Rep*, 17, 373.

Finocchi, C., & Sivori, G. (2012). Food as trigger and aggravating factor of migraine. *Neurol Sci, 33 Suppl 1,* S77–S80.

Fraga, M. D., et al. (2013). Trigger factors mainly from the environmental type are reported by adolescents with migraine. *Arq Neuropsiquiatr, 71,* 290–293.

Friedman, B. W., et al. (2014). Randomized trial of IV valproate vs metoclopramide vs ketorolac for acute migraine. *Neurology, 82,* 976–983.

Fumal, A., & Schoenen, J. (2008). Tension-type headache: Current research and clinical management. *Lancet Neurol, 7,* 70–83.

Gil-Martinez, A., et al. (2013). [Therapeutic exercise as treatment for migraine and tension-type headaches: A systematic review of randomised clinical trials]. *Rev Neurol, 57,* 433–443.

Gobel, H., Schmidt, G., & Soyka, D. (1994). Effect of peppermint and eucalyptus oil preparations on neurophysiological and experimental algesimetric headache parameters. *Cephalalgia, 14,* 228–234; discussion 182.

Goldstein, J., et al. (2006). Acetaminophen, aspirin, and caffeine in combination versus ibuprofen for acute migraine: Results from a multicenter, double-blind, randomized, parallel-group, single-dose, placebo-controlled study. *Headache, 46,* 444–453.

Grossman, W., & Schmidramsl, H. (2001). An extract of Petasites hybridus is effective in the prophylaxis of migraine. *Altern Med Rev, 6,* 303–310.

Hammond, D. C. (2007). Review of the efficacy of clinical hypnosis with headaches and migraines. *Int J Clin Exp Hypn, 55,* 207–219.

Hao, X. A., et al. (2013). Factors associated with conflicting findings on acupuncture for tension-type headache: Qualitative and quantitative analyses. *J Altern Complement Med, 19,* 285–297.

Hershey, A. D., et al. (2007). Coenzyme Q10 deficiency and response to supplementation in pediatric and adolescent migraine. *Headache, 47,* 73–80.

Hindiyeh, N. A., Krusz, J. C., & Cowan, R. P. (2013). Does exercise make migraines worse and tension type headaches better? *Curr Pain Headache Rep, 17,* 380.

Hoffmann, J., & Recober, A. (2013). Migraine and triggers: Post hoc ergo propter hoc? *Curr Pain Headache Rep, 17,* 370.

Holland, S., et al. (2012). Evidence-based guideline update: NSAIDs and other complementary treatments for episodic migraine prevention in adults: Report of the Quality Standards Subcommittee of the American Academy of Neurology and the American Headache Society. *Neurology, 78,* 1346–1353.

Jensen, R., & Stovner, L. J. (2008). Epidemiology and comorbidity of headache. *Lancet Neurol, 7,* 354–361.

John, P. J., et al. (2007). Effectiveness of yoga therapy in the treatment of migraine without aura: A randomized controlled trial. *Headache, 47,* 654–661.

Johnson, H., et al. (2014). Migraine in students of a US medical school. *Fam Med, 46,* 615–619.

Jonas, W. B., Kaptchuk, T. J., & Linde, K. (2003). A critical overview of homeopathy. *Ann Intern Med, 138,* 393–399.

Jull, G., et al. (2002). A randomized controlled trial of exercise and manipulative therapy for cervicogenic headache. *Spine (Phila Pa 1976), 27,* 1835–1843; discussion 1843.

Kelley, N. E., & Tepper, D. E. (2012a). Rescue therapy for acute migraine: Part 1. triptans, dihydroergotamine, and magnesium. *Headache, 52*, 114–128.

Kelley, N. E., & Tepper, D. E. (2012b). Rescue therapy for acute migraine: Part 2. neuroleptics, antihistamines, and others. *Headache, 52*, 292–306.

Kelley, N. E., & Tepper, D. E. (2012c). Rescue therapy for acute migraine: Part 3. opioids, NSAIDs, steroids, and post-discharge medications. *Headache, 52*, 467–482.

Kirthi, V., Derry, S., & Moore, R. A. (2013). Aspirin with or without an antiemetic for acute migraine headaches in adults. *Cochrane Database Syst Rev, 4*, CD008041.

Kligler, B., & Chaudhary, S. (2007). Peppermint oil. *Am Fam Physician, 75*, 1027–1030.

Kristoffersen, E. S., & Lundqvist, C. (2014). Medication-overuse headache: A review. *J Pain Res, 7*, 367–378.

Kurth, T., et al. (2006). Migraine and risk of cardiovascular disease in women. *JAMA, 296*, 283–291.

Law, S., Derry, S., & Moore, R. A. (2013a). Naproxen with or without an antiemetic for acute migraine headaches in adults. *Cochrane Database Syst Rev*, 10:CD009455.

Law, S., Derry, S., & Moore, R. A. (2013b). Sumatriptan plus naproxen for acute migraine attacks in adults. *Cochrane Database Syst Rev*, 10:CD008541.

Lecchi, M., et al. (2014). Pharmacokinetics and safety of a new aspirin formulation for the acute treatment of primary headaches. *Expert Opin Drug Metab Toxicol, 10*, 1381–1395.

Linde, et al. 2009.

Linde, K., et al. (2009). Acupuncture for migraine prophylaxis. *Cochrane Database Syst Rev*, 1:CD001218.

Linde, M., et al. (2012). The cost of headache disorders in Europe: The Eurolight project. *Eur J Neurol, 19*, 703–711.

Linde, M., et al. (2013). Topiramate for the prophylaxis of episodic migraine in adults. *Cochrane Database Syst Rev*, 6:CD010610.

Lipton, R. B., et al. (2004). *Petasites hybridus* root (butterbur) is an effective preventive treatment for migraine. *Neurology, 63*, 2240–2244.

Lozano Lopez, C., et al. (2014). Efficacy of manual therapy in the treatment of tension-type headache. A systematic review from 2000–2013. *Neurologia, 2014*, pii: S0213-4853(14)00011-5.

MacGregor, E. A., et al. (2010). Characteristics of menstrual vs nonmenstrual migraine: A post hoc, within-woman analysis of the usual-care phase of a nonrandomized menstrual migraine clinical trial. *Headache, 50*, 528–538.

Machado, R. B., et al. (2010). Epidemiological and clinical aspects of migraine in users of combined oral contraceptives. *Contraception, 81*, 202–208.

Maghbooli, M., et al. (2014). Comparison between the efficacy of ginger and sumatriptan in the ablative treatment of the common migraine. *Phytother Res, 28*, 412–415.

Mann, J. D., et al. (2008). Craniosacral therapy for migraine: Protocol development for an exploratory controlled clinical trial. *BMC Complement Altern Med, 8*, 28.

Masruha, M. R., et al. (2008). Low urinary 6-sulphatoxymelatonin concentrations in acute migraine. *J Headache Pain, 9*, 221–224.

Mauskop, A., Altura, B. T., & Altura, B. M. (2002). Serum ionized magnesium levels and serum ionized calcium/ionized magnesium ratios in women with menstrual migraine. *Headache, 42*, 242–248.

Mauskop, A., & Varughese, J. (2012). Why all migraine patients should be treated with magnesium. *J Neural Transm, 119*, 575–579.

Mitchell, N., et al. (2011). Randomised controlled trial of food elimination diet based on IgG antibodies for the prevention of migraine like headaches. *Nutr J 10*, 85.

Monograph. (2001). *Petasites hybridus. Altern Med Rev, 6*, 207–209.

Monograph. (2008). Riboflavin. *Altern Med Rev, 13*, 334–340.

Mustafa, T., & Srivastava, K. C. (1990). Ginger (*Zingiber officinale*) in migraine headache. *J Ethnopharmacol, 29*, 267–273.

Nappi, R. E., et al. (2011). Headaches during pregnancy. *Curr Pain Headache Rep, 15*, 289–294.

Narin, S. O., et al. (2003). The effects of exercise and exercise-related changes in blood nitric oxide level on migraine headache. *Clin Rehabil, 17*, 624–630.

Nestoriuc, Y., et al. (2008). Biofeedback treatment for headache disorders: A comprehensive efficacy review. *Appl Psychophysiol Biofeedback, 33*, 125–140.

Nestoriuc, Y., & Martin, A. (2007). Efficacy of biofeedback for migraine: A meta-analysis. *Pain, 128*, 111–127.

Nicholson, R. A., et al. (2011). Nonpharmacologic treatments for migraine and tension-type headache: How to choose and when to use. *Curr Treat Options Neurol, 13*, 28–40.

Nielsen, F. H. (2010). Magnesium, inflammation, and obesity in chronic disease. *Nutr Rev, 68*, 333–340.

Panconesi, A. (2008). Alcohol and migraine: Trigger factor, consumption, mechanisms: A review. *J Headache Pain, 9*, 19–27.

Panconesi, A., Bartolozzi, M. L., & Guidi, L. (2011). Alcohol and migraine: What should we tell patients? *Curr Pain Headache Rep, 15*, 177–184.

Peikert, A., Wilimzig, C., & Kohne-Volland, R. (1996). Prophylaxis of migraine with oral magnesium: Results from a prospective, multi-center, placebo-controlled and double-blind randomized study. *Cephalalgia, 16*, 257–263.

Pinhas-Hamiel, O., et al. (2008). Headaches in overweight children and adolescents referred to a tertiary-care center in Israel. *Obesity (Silver Spring), 16*, 659–663.

Pittler, M. H., & Ernst, E. (2004). Feverfew for preventing migraine. *Cochrane Database Syst Rev, 1*:CD002286.

Potgieter, M., Pretorius, E., & Pepper, M. S. (2013). Primary and secondary coenzyme Q10 deficiency: The role of therapeutic supplementation. *Nutr Rev, 71*, 180–188.

Pringsheim, T., et al. (2012). Canadian Headache Society guideline for migraine prophylaxis. *Can J Neurol Sci, 39*(2 Suppl 2), S1–S59.

Rabbie, R., Derry, S., & Moore, R. A. (2013). Ibuprofen with or without an antiemetic for acute migraine headaches in adults. *Cochrane Database Syst Rev, 4*: CD008039.

Ramsden, C. E., et al. (2013). Targeted alteration of dietary n-3 and n-6 fatty acids for the treatment of chronic headaches: A randomized trial. *Pain, 154*, 2441–2451.

Rizzoli, P. B. (2014). Emerging therapeutic options for acute migraine: Focus on the potential of lasmiditan. *Neuropsychiatr Dis Treat, 10*, 547–552.

Rockett, F. C., et al. (2013). Cardiovascular disease risk in women with migraine. *J Headache Pain, 14*, 75.

Rolle, G., et al. (2014). Pilot trial of osteopathic manipulative therapy for patients with frequent episodic tension-type headache. *J Am Osteopath Assoc, 114*, 678–685.

Rosen, N. L. (2012). Psychological issues in the evaluation and treatment of tension-type headache. *Curr Pain Headache Rep, 16*, 545–553.

Rosenzweig, S., et al. (2010). Mindfulness-based stress reduction for chronic pain conditions: Variation in treatment outcomes and role of home meditation practice. *J Psychosom Res, 68*, 29–36.

Russell, M. B., et al. (2006). Tension-type headache in adolescents and adults: A population based study of 33,764 twins. *Eur J Epidemiol, 21*, 153–160.

Sacco, S., & Kurth, T. (2014). Migraine and the risk for stroke and cardiovascular disease. *Curr Cardiol Rep, 16*, 524.

Sandor, P. S., et al. (2000). Prophylactic treatment of migraine with beta-blockers and riboflavin: Differential effects on the intensity dependence of auditory evoked cortical potentials. *Headache 40*, 30–35.

Sandor, P. S., et al. (2005). Efficacy of coenzyme Q10 in migraine prophylaxis: A randomized controlled trial. *Neurology, 64*, 713–715.

Schiapparelli, P., et al. (2010). Non-pharmacological approach to migraine prophylaxis: Part II. *Neurol Sci, 31*(Suppl 1), S137–139.

Schurks, M., et al. (2009). Migraine and cardiovascular disease: Systematic review and meta-analysis. *BMJ, 339*, b3914.

Schwedt, T. J., & Shapiro, R. E. (2009). Funding of research on headache disorders by the National Institutes of Health. *Headache, 49*, 162–169.

Shamliyan, T. A., Kane, R. L., & Taylor, F. R. (2013). *Migraine in adults: Preventive pharmacologic treatments*. Rockville (MD).

Silberstein, S. D., & McCrory, D. C. (2001). Butalbital in the treatment of headache: History, pharmacology, and efficacy. *Headache, 41*, 953–967.

Silberstein, S., & Patel, S. (2014). Menstrual migraine: An updated review on hormonal causes, prophylaxis and treatment. *Expert Opin Pharmacother, 15*, 2063–2070.

Smith, T. R., Nicholson, R. A., & Banks, J. W. (2010). Migraine education improves quality of life in a primary care setting. *Headache, 50*, 600–612.

Smitherman, T. A., et al. (2013). The prevalence, impact, and treatment of migraine and severe headaches in the United States: A review of statistics from national surveillance studies. *Headache, 53*, 427–436.

Smitherman, T. A., McDermott, M. J., & Buchanan, E. M. (2011). Negative impact of episodic migraine on a university population: Quality of life, functional impairment, and comorbid psychiatric symptoms. *Headache, 51*, 581–589.

Souza-e-Silva, H. R., & Rocha-Filho, P. A. (2011). Headaches and academic performance in university students: A cross-sectional study. *Headache, 51*, 1493–502.

Spierings, E. L., Ranke, A. H., & Honkoop, P. C. (2001). Precipitating and aggravating factors of migraine versus tension-type headache. *Headache, 41*, 554–558.

Srinivasan, V., et al. (2012). Melatonin in antinociception: Its therapeutic applications. *Curr Neuropharmacol, 10*, 167–178.

Steiner, T. J., Stovner, L. J., & Birbeck, G. L. (2013). Migraine: The seventh disabler. *J Headache Pain, 14*, 1.

Sun-Edelstein, C., & Mauskop, A. (2012). Complementary and alternative approaches to the treatment of tension-type headache. *Curr Pain Headache Rep, 16*, 539–544.

Szentkiralyi, A., et al. (2014). Multimorbidity and the risk of restless legs syndrome in 2 prospective cohort studies. *Neurology, 82*, 2026–2033.

Tabeeva, G. R., Sergeev, A. V., & Gromova, S. A. (2011). [Possibilities of preventive treatment of migraine with the MT1- and MT2 agonist and 5-HT2c receptor antagonist agomelatin (valdoxan)] (in Russian). *Zh Nevrol Psikhiatr Im S S Korsakova, 111*, 32–36.

Tarighat Esfanjani, A., et al. (2012). The effects of magnesium, L-carnitine, and concurrent magnesium-L-carnitine supplementation in migraine prophylaxis. *Biol Trace Elem Res, 150*, 42–48.

Tietjen, G. E., et al. (2010a). Childhood maltreatment and migraine: Part I. Prevalence and adult revictimization: A multicenter headache clinic survey. *Headache, 50*, 20–31.

Tietjen, G. E., et al. (2010b). Childhood maltreatment and migraine: Part II. Emotional abuse as a risk factor for headache chronification. *Headache, 50*, 32–41.

Tietjen, G. E., et al. (2010c). Childhood maltreatment and migraine: Part III. Association with comorbid pain conditions. *Headache, 50*, 42–51.

USDA. (2011). *National Nutrient Database for Standard Reference, Release 24*. Available from http://www.ars.usda.gov/ba/bhnrc/ndl

Utterback, G., et al. (2014). Butterbur extract: Prophylactic treatment for childhood migraines. *Complement Ther Clin Pract, 20*, 61–64.

Valguarnera, F., & Tanganelli, P. (2010). The efficacy of withdrawal therapy in subjects with chronic daily headache and medication overuse following prophylaxis with topiramate and amitriptyline. *Neurol Sci, 31*(Suppl 1), S175–S177.

Verhagen, A. P., et al. (2010). Lack of benefit for prophylactic drugs of tension-type headache in adults: A systematic review. *Fam Pract, 27*, 151–165.

Volpe, S. L. (2013). Magnesium in disease prevention and overall health. *Adv Nutr, 4*, 378S–383S.

Vos, T., et al. (2012). Years lived with disability (YLDs) for 1160 sequelae of 289 diseases and injuries 1990–2010: A systematic analysis for the Global Burden of Disease Study (2010). *Lancet, 380*, 2163–2196.

Wang, F., et al. (2003). Oral magnesium oxide prophylaxis of frequent migrainous headache in children: A randomized, double-blind, placebo-controlled trial. *Headache, 43*, 601–610.

Waters, W. E., & O'Connor, P. J. (1971). Epidemiology of headache and migraine in women. *J Neurol Neurosurg Psychiatry, 34*, 148–153.

Wells, R. E., et al. (2011). Complementary and alternative medicine use among adults with migraines/severe headaches. *Headache, 51*, 1087–1097.

Wells, R. E., et al. (2014). Meditation for migraines: A pilot randomized controlled trial. *Headache*,54(9), 1484–1495

Witt, C. M., Ludtke, R., & Willich, S. N. (2010). Homeopathic treatment of patients with migraine: A prospective observational study with a 2-year follow-up period. *J Altern Complement Med*, 16, 347–355.

Wober-Bingol, C. (2013). Epidemiology of migraine and headache in children and adolescents. *Curr Pain Headache Rep*, 17, 341.

Wu, J. J., et al. (2014). Modulatory effects of aromatherapy massage intervention on electroencephalogram, psychological assessments, salivary cortisol and plasma brain-derived neurotrophic factor. *Complement Ther Med*, 22, 456–462.

Yancey, J. R.,Sheridan, R., & Koren, K. G. (2014). Chronic daily headache: Diagnosis and management. *Am Fam Physician*, 89, 642–648.

Zanigni, S., et al. (2014). Association between restless legs syndrome and migraine: A population-based study. *Eur J Neurol*, 21, 1205–1010.

28

Fibromyalgia and Chronic Fatigue

MELINDA RING

CASE STUDY

Janet is a successful professor of literature at a Midwestern university. Several years ago she presented to her primary care physician with overwhelming fatigue. Janet underwent a thorough battery of tests, with no clear cause identified for her symptoms. She was referred for an evaluation at the Osher Center for Integrative Medicine at Northwestern University. After an in-depth history and physical exam, I felt her symptoms were consistent with chronic fatigue syndrome and recommended a regimen of supplements and complementary therapies. Her symptoms evolved to include the widespread pain characteristic of fibromyalgia, leading to adjustments in her treatment. Janet's progress has been gradual, with ups and downs in great part related to her life circumstances. However, within a few months of her original visit she was able to return to work and over the next 2 years she published a book of poetry. Throughout this chapter, comments from the Northwestern team of practitioners who care for Janet will show the benefits of an integrative team approach achieved by uniting diverse philosophies of health and moving beyond the Western view of disease.

Introduction

Fibromyalgia (FM) and chronic fatigue syndrome (CFS) are conditions that confound clinicians for many reasons. Patients present with a wide range of symptoms, and no confirmatory diagnostic test is currently available. There is no unanimous agreement on the etiology and management, and patient responses to interventions are inconsistent. In general, medical and nursing trainees receive minimal education about FM/CFS. As a result, many doctors discredit the diagnoses as psychosomatic or psychiatric conditions (Chew-Graham, Cahill, Dowrick, Wearden, & Peters, 2008).

Interestingly, these diseases are not new to this century. Similar symptomology was described in the literature as "little fever" in 1750 and "rheumatism" in the 16th century (Inanici & Yunus, 2004; Kim, 1994). We now know more about the underlying pathophysiology and effective management than ever before, as the evidence base grows through research. Combining this knowledge with a patient-centered approach, the integrative medicine practitioner is uniquely situated to help relieve suffering and reduce disability across the full spectrum of FM/CFS symptoms.

My sister-in-law was diagnosed with CFS when I was an internal medicine resident. Like many physicians, I had a poor understanding of her condition. She looked healthy; it was a challenge for my family to understand why she couldn't come to some gatherings because of her fatigue. Over the years, as I gained a better understanding of CFS, I appreciated her bravery and the struggle of battling not just her disease but also the misconceptions of everyone around her. I developed a deep appreciation for her willingness to engage in activities such as playing with my two boisterous young boys, knowing that the following day she may be too exhausted to do more than the minimum necessary activities. This personal experience helped nurture empathy toward my own patients with CFS. For many FM/CFS patients, finding a physician just willing to listen and acknowledge their condition without judgment provides significant relief and begins the healing process.

This chapter on FM/CFS offers an introduction to the symptoms, current hypotheses of the pathophysiology, and practical diagnostic algorithms, with special attention to issues specific to female patients. The remainder of the chapter explores the evidence for available treatment modalities, including conventional pharmacology and complementary therapies. Current research suggests that CFS and FM fall along a continuum of related disorders with common pathogenesis: 50%–70% of CFS and FM patients meet both diagnostic criteria (Aaron, Burke, & Buchwald, 2000; Goldenberg, Simms, Geiger, &

Komaroff, 1990). In this chapter the two diseases are discussed as such, with distinctions noted when relevant.

Definition and Symptomatology

The 1994 Centers for Disease Control (CDC) criteria for CFS and 1990 American College of Rheumatology (ACR) criteria for FM were developed primarily primarily for researchers needing to identify a uniform patient population (Box 28.1) (Fukuda et al., 1994; Wolfe et al., 1990). In practice, expanding beyond these definitions allows the physician to identify large numbers of patients with chronic fatigue and widespread pain, likely arising from similar immuno-logic and hormonal imbalances and appropriate for the same interventions (Harth & Nielson, 2007). Efforts are ongoing in both FM and CFS to refine the diagnostic criteria to make them more relevant to clinicians and patients. The ACR created a clinical case definition of fibromyalgia in 2010 that includes a widespread pain index and a symptom severity scale assessed through inter-view questions in place of a reliance on tender point examinations (Table 28.1; Clauw, Fitzcharles, & Wolfe, 2010). A reframing of the CFS diagnostic criteria to address the needs of health providers, patients, and their caregivers began in 2013 via an ad hoc committee of the Institute of Medicine. The group undertook

---

Box 28.1 Fibromyalgia and Chronic Fatigue

A case of chronic fatigue syndrome is defined by the presence of:

1. Clinically evaluated, unexplained, persistent or relapsing fatigue that is of new or definite onset; is not the result of ongoing exertion; is not alleviated by rest; and results in substantial reduction in previous levels of occupational, educational, social, or personal activities

   And

2. Four or more of the following symptoms that persist or recur during 6 or more consecutive months of illness and that do not predate the fatigue:
   Self-reported impairment in short-term memory or concentration
   Sore throat
   Tender cervical or axillary nodes
   Muscle painMultijoint pain without redness or swelling
   Headaches of a new pattern or severity
   Unrefreshing sleep
   Postexertional malaise lasting 24 hours

Table 28.1. Fibromyalgia Diagnostic Criteria

1990 American College of Rheumatology Criteria for Fibromyalgia	2010 American College of Rheumatology Preliminary Criteria for Fibromyalgia

≥3 months of widespread pain
 • Above and below the waist
 • Bilateral
 • In the axial skeleton
 	
 AND
 	
 Manual tender point examination
 • ≥11 of 18 specific tender points on digital palpation force: 4 kg/1.4 cm²
	Pain & symptoms for ≥3 months
	 AND
	 Widespread pain index (WPI) and symptom severity scale (SSS) scored by healthcare practitioner questionnaire totaling:
	    WPI ≥7 and SSS* ≥5
	    OR
	    WPI 3–6 and SSS ≥9
	 WPI,
	 In how many areas has the patient had pain over the last week? (Total score between 0 and 19)
	 Shoulder girdle, L and R (2)
	 Upper arm L and R (2)
	 Lower arm L and R (2)
	 Hip L and R (2)
	 Upper leg L and R (2)
	 Lower leg L and R (2)
	 Jaw L and R (2)
	 Chest
	 Abdomen—
	 Upper back
	 Lower back —
	 Neck
	
	 SSS:
	 Fatigue, Waking unrefreshed, Cognitive symptoms:
	 For each indicate the level of severity over the week,
	 0 no problem
	 1 slight or mild problems, generally mild or intermittent
	 2 moderate, considerable problems, often present
	 3 severe, pervasive continuous, life-disturbing problems
	
	 Considering somatic symptoms in general, *indicate if*
	 0 no symptoms
	 1 few symptoms
	 2 a moderate number of symptoms
	 3 a great deal of symptoms
	
	 SSS score (0-12) = severity of the 3 symptoms + somatic symptoms

Source: Based on Wolfe et al. (1990) and Wolfe et al. (2010).

an 18-month comprehensive evaluation of the current criteria for the diagnosis of myalgic encephalomyelitis/chronic fatigue syndrome (ME/CFS), including reviews of international consensus definitions, the 2007 National Institute for Health and Care Excellence (NICE) Clinical Guidelines and the ongoing CDC Multi-site Clinical study of CFS (http://www.iom.edu/Activities/Disease/DiagnosisMyalgicEncephalomyelitisChronicFatigueSyndrome.aspx).

The hallmark symptoms common to both FM/CFS patients include the following: overwhelming fatigue which is exacerbated post exertion, concentration issues (brain fog) and disequilibrium, nonrefreshing sleep and sleep disturbances, headaches, flu-like feelings, and myalgia. The physical examination is usually unremarkable except for tender points. Patients often have coexisting conditions such as irritable bowel syndrome, interstitial cystitis, dyspareunia, allergies, chemical sensitivities, and depression or anxiety.

Epidemiology

Chronic fatigue syndrome and FM are much more common in women than men. The prevalence of FM is estimated at 2%–4% in the general US population, with a breakdown of 3.4% of all women and only 0.5% of men (Wolfe et al., 1995). It is a challenge to ascertain the prevalence of CFS; one study of a primary care population estimates 8.5% of patients have debilitating fatigue lasting over 6 months, but as per the stricter CDC definition, less than 15% of these patients would be diagnosed with CFS (Bates et al., 1993). Both conditions have a modal age distribution, with most cases diagnosed from age 20 to 50; onset in childhood and postmenopausal occurs to a much lesser degree.

Pathophysiology

Research since the early 2000s has identified pathophysiologic abnormalities in multiple areas including central nervous system pain processing, neuroendocrine and autonomic nervous system function, neurotransmitter levels, and oxidative stress (Afari & Buchwald, 2003; Bradley, 2008). Current hypotheses suggest the manifestation of FM/CFS and related conditions are multifactorial, a complex interplay of environmental triggers, genetic susceptibility, and disordered biochemical functioning. Briefly, some of the documented risk factors and abnormalities that contribute to symptoms include the following:

- *Genetics:* Familial studies in both CFS and FM have identified a familial predisposition, with a greater than eight odds ratio of FM occurrence in first-degree relatives (Arnold, Hudson, et al., 2004). In FM the foremost genes include those that impact on neurotransmitter/monoamine levels, such as serotonin and dopamine receptors, and transporters (Cohen, Buskila, Neumann, & Ebstein, 2002; Offenbaecher et al., 1999). In CFS, 88 genes have differential expression compared with normal controls; those identified have links to hematological function, immunologic disease, cancer, cell death, immune response, and infection (Kerr, Petty, et al., 2008). One group identified seven genomically distinct subtypes, which may correlate with variable phenotypic expression (Kerr, Burke, et al., 2008).

- *Triggers*: A significant number of patients identify a triggering event prior to the onset of symptoms. Frequent offenders are physical trauma (e.g., motor vehicle accident), psychological stressors (e.g., grief, stressful life events), and infections (e.g., viral, gastroenteritis, Lyme disease). It is important for the treating physician to help patients understand that these events are considered triggers in someone with an underlying predisposition, rather than the ultimate etiology. Without this clarification, some patients seek costly and invasive testing to identify the perceived cause and pursue potentially harmful treatments.

- *Central Pain Augmentation*: Central sensitization causes hyperalgesia, allodynia, and referred pain, leading to chronic widespread pain. Fibromyalgia studies support the existence of triggers for sensitization: wind-up or temporal summation (pain augmentation at the dorsal horn neuron, whereby repeated pain stimuli lead to augmented pain response), dysregulated descending inhibitory pathways, and up-regulated facilitatory modulation (stimulated by behavioral and cognitive factors) (Meeus & Nijs, 2007). Objective central abnormalities noted include hyperexcitability of the spinal cord, decreased perfusion of pain-related brain structures on functional MRI, and high cerebrospinal fluid levels of substance P. Cognitive central sensitization can also derive from pain hypervigilance, maladaptive coping strategies, and catastrophizing often found on presentation.

- *Autonomic/Neuroendocrine Dysfunction:* A review of recent neuroendocrine studies reported that aberrations in the hypothalamic-pituitary-adrenal (HPA) axis and serotonin pathways have been identified in CFS, suggesting an altered stress response (Demitrack, 1997). About one-third of patients exhibit low cortisol, as well as decreased dehydroepiandrosterone-sulfate (DHEA-S) and insulin-like growth factor. Dysfunction of the HPA axis is also present in FM due to an apparent deficit in corticotropin-releasing hormone (CRH) released from the hypothalamus, as identified through irregular cortisol levels (McBeth et al., 2007).

- *Immune Dysfunction:* Multiple immune disturbances have been noted in CFS and FM patients. The impact of this dysregulation is unclear, with studies showing conflicting results in markers such as levels of circulating immunoglobulin and immune complexes, natural killer (NK) cells, and CD8 cells and altered NK cell function and interferon activity (Landay, Jessop, Lennette, & Levy, 1991; Mawle et al., 1997).

- *Oxidative Stress and Nitric Oxide:* Research has identified elevations in nitric oxide, oxidative stress, mitochondrial dysfunction, NF-kappa B activity, inflammatory cytokines activity, vanilloid activity, and N-methyl-D-aspartate (NMDA) activity. Some scientists postulate a paradigm known as the NOO/ONOO⁻ cycle as the underlying etiology of the aforementioned biochemical disorders and manifested symptoms (Pall, 2007). The NO/ONOO⁻ cycle describes a biochemical response in which an elevation in nitric oxide (NO) levels and its oxidant product, peroxynitrite (ONOO⁻), initiate a pathophysiologic response in the body's regulatory systems. It is postulated that symptoms results from both direct effects of the elevated NO/ONOO⁻ compounds and downstream increases in inflammatory molecules such as NF-kappa B and cytokines and activity of two transmitter systems active in many neuronal cells: the vanilloid receptors and the NMDA receptors. At this time it is unclear whether the oxidative stresses are incidental or causal.

Diagnostic Approach

As CFS and FM are diagnosed primarily based on history, and through exclusion of other causes for fatigue and pain, limited laboratory testing is recommended: complete blood count with differential, erythrocyte sedimentation rate, chemistry panel, a thyroid panel, 25-hydroxyvitamin D, DHEA-S, and cortisol. Other tests should be performed if indicated by physical exam and history.

Expensive immunologic tests and serologies are not recommended. Although infections may act as a trigger, a CDC epidemiologic study that evaluated more than 40 organisms found no consistent association (Mawle et al., 1995). Therefore, checking serologies for Epstein-Barr virus (EBV), cytomegalovirus (CMV), or Lyme disease in the absence of a high index of suspicion does not influence treatment recommendations (Straus et al., 1985). Although abnormalities have been noted in neuroimaging studies, they are of unclear significance and routine MRI and SPECT are not currently recommended

(Schwartz, Garada, & Komaroff, 1994). Finally, genetic panels are of great interest but are not yet validated as diagnostic tests for FM/CFS.

Primary Care

Factors such as general disability and a focus on managing fatigue and pain may lead women with FM/CFS to skip recommended screening tests. It is incumbent on the physician to incorporate age-appropriate screening for cervical, breast, and colon cancer. An additional challenge is treating common primary care issues such as hypertension, as patients with FM/CFS are often very sensitive to medication side effects and may require starting at low doses with gradual titration.

PREGNANCY

There are limited data of the impact of pregnancy on CFS/FM outcomes and vice versa. The few studies available suggest an equal number of patients felt no change, improvement, or worsening of symptoms during and after pregnancy (Schacterle & Komaroff, 2004). Many medications and supplements are not advised during pregnancy, necessitating a shift to safer therapies such as acupuncture, mind–body therapies, and homeopathy. High-quality prenatal vitamins and omega-3 fish oil should be recommended.

OVERVIEW OF PHARMACOLOGIC TREATMENT

Trials of medications for CFS/FM have increased over the past decade. These pharmacological therapies are often neuromodulatory agents that target cells involved in sleep regulation and pain signaling. Therapies are also available for the conditions associated with FM/CFS such as irritable bowel syndrome, interstitial cystitis, and dyspareunia, but these are addressed in other chapters and are not reviewed here.

Antiepileptic Drugs ($α_2δ$ Ligands)

Pregabalin (Lyrica) was the first FDA-approved drug for FM. Both pregabalin and gabapentin (Neurontin) bind to the $α_2δ$ subunit of voltage-gated calcium channels of neurons, thereby inhibiting release of neurotransmitters such as glutamate and substance P. In 2005 a 14-week randomized controlled trial (RCT) enrolled over 500 patients that met ACR criteria for FM, had a pain visual analog scale greater than 40 mm (0–100 mm), and mean numeric pain rating scale of at least four (0–10) (Crofford et al., 2005). Pregabalin was dosed at 150, 300, and 450 mg daily. Statistically significant improvements of more than 30% reduction in pain and sleep quality were seen beginning at week 1; higher doses also demonstrated improvement in global assessment and health status. The primary adverse effects leading to discontinuation were dizziness (6.4%) and somnolence (4%). Weight gain can be an issue at higher doses, often due to increased appetite and sugar cravings. A 6-month double-blind placebo-controlled trial of pregabalin used an initial open-label treatment; only those patients who responded with 50% or greater reduction in pain and scored as "much" or "very much" improved were eligible for randomization (Crofford et al., 2008). In responders, beneficial effects in pain reduction persisted in about two-thirds of patients over the 6-month study. Improvements in sleep and mental functioning and fatigue were also noticed. Gabapentin is not FDA approved for use in fibromyalgia, and a Cochrane review concluded that the amount and quality of evidence for gabapentin was insufficient to draw any definitive conclusions (Uceyler, Sommer, Walitt, & Hauser, 2013).

Antidepressants

In June 2008, duloxetine HCL (Cymbalta) became the second FDA-approved drug for FM. The approval was a result of two 3-month clinical trials with a total of 874 patients (Arnold, Lu, et al., 2004). In both studies, compared with placebo, duloxetine was associated with more than a 30% reduction in pain as measured by the Brief Pain Inventory (BPI). Onset of pain relief began during the first week of treatment. Approximately two-thirds of patients in the treatment groups reported improved overall functioning on duloxetine 60 mg/day. Discontinuation from adverse effects (nausea, dry mouth, constipation, decreased appetite, sleepiness, increased sweating, and agitation) was 20% versus 12% in the placebo group. Milnacipran (Savella) is another serotonin–norepinephrine reuptake inhibitor (SNRI) medication more recently approved for FM. A 2013 Cochrane meta-analysis reported a small incremental benefit over placebo: Pain was reduced by 50% in 29/100 people on medication versus 19/100 people on placebo. No substantial benefit in the areas of quality of life, fatigue, or sleep was noted (Hauser, Urrútia, Tort, Uçeyler, & Walitt, 2013).

Low-Dose Naltrexone

Administration of low-dose naltrexone (LDN) tricks the brain into producing more endorphins by blocking receptors; it also causes NK cell stimulation, B-cell inhibition, and microglial cell inhibition—inhibiting an overactive CNS immune response and reducing central and peripheral inflammation. It may be the first glial cell modulator useful as an anti-inflammatory agent for chronic pain management. Low-dose naltrexone, 4.5 mg, was effective in reducing symptoms by more than 30% and improving mechanical and heat pain thresholds in all 10 participants in a single-blinded pilot study. (Younger & Mackey, 2009) Interestingly, patients with higher inflammatory processes, identified by higher sedimentation rates, experienced the greatest reduction of symptoms. A follow-up blinded RCT, which increased duration and sample size, found similar results with a 28.8% reduction in baseline pain as well as improved mood and general life satisfaction compared with placebo (Younger, Noor, McCue, & Mackey, 2013). Treatment with LDN has minimal adverse side effects and is less expensive, with an average out-of-pocket cost of $35 per month versus $100 per month for FDA-approved prescription medications for FM. The FDA has not approved LDN as a treatment for fibromyalgia.

Other Medications

Other medications studied in FM/CFS with conflicting or negative results include galantine, intramuscular and intravascular immune globulin, acyclovir, fluoxetine, paroxetine, strong opioids, newer selective serotonin reuptake inhibitors (SSRIs: citalopram, escitalopram, desvenlafaxine), hydrocortisone, fludrocortisone, antivirals, and nonsteroidal anti-inflammatory drugs (NSAIDs) (Clauw, 2014). Cyclobenzaprine, amitriptyline, tramadol, older selective serotonin reuptake inhibitors (fluoxetine, sertraline, paroxetine), methylphenidate, and acetaminophen seem to provide some relief in FM (Bennett, Kamin, Karim, & Rosenthal, 2003; Tofferi, Jackson, & O'Malley, 2004) and methylphenidate in CFS.

Integrative Therapies

Unlike many conditions where complementary therapies are chosen to supplement conventional therapy, in FM and CFS the paucity of treatments or desire to avoid dependence on addictive medications draws high number of patients to complementary and alternative medicine (CAM) therapies regardless of the level of evidence. For many of these women, the severity of symptoms fluctuates; moments of relative "wellness" give hope of return to former levels of functioning. Helping our patients maintain that hope, while keeping them from potentially harmful practices, is crucial to their continued healing.

Integrative Medicine Perspective: Naturopathic Viewpoint

Naturopathic doctors strive to address the underlying individual cause, whether nutritional, environmental, or biochemical. From my experience, in FM/CFS symptoms arise when specific cells are unable to perform normal cellular function. The first step in a naturopathic approach is to combine homeopathic drainage (to aid in detoxification of cellular metabolites) with the removal of identified underlying causes (to prevent further damage). Cells are then in an optimal position to absorb the nutrients found lacking in the body. By addressing imbalances, the body is able to restore a balanced physiology.

—Judy Fulop, ND

BOTANICALS AND SUPPLEMENTS

A broad array of dietary supplements are employed in the management of FM/CFS. Very little research is available on the supplements used in FM/CFS, and small numbers, high dropout rates, and poor methodological quality limit most studies (Mannerkorpi & Henriksson, 2007). A few that show promise include the following:

D-Ribose

Based on the theory that mitochondrial energy is the core issue, D-ribose, a naturally occurring pentose carbohydrate, was given to 41 CFS/FM patients at a dose of 5 g three times daily for a total of 280 g. Sixty-six percent of patients showed a significant improvement in five visual analog scale (VAS) categories: energy, sleep, mental clarity, pain intensity, and well-being (Teitelbaum, Johnson, & St Cyr, 2006). Unfortunately, there are no other studies that have been conducted to evaluate the efficacy of D-ribose in CFS/FM.

L-Carnitine

This amino acid affects mitochondrial energy production by supporting free fatty acid transfer across mitochondrial membranes. Two studies on this compound and the related propionyl-L-carnitine, 2 g/day, are suggestive of benefit for general fatigue in CFS after 4 to 8 weeks of treatment (Plioplys & Plioplys, 1997; Vermeulen & Scholte, 2004). A 2007 study randomized 102 FM patients to 2 capsules/day of 500 mg acetyl L-carnitine (LAC) or placebo plus one intramuscular injection of either 500 mg LAC or placebo for 2 weeks. During the following 8 weeks the patients took 3 capsules daily containing either 500 mg LAC or placebo. At 10 weeks the LAC group compared with placebo had a significant decrease in number of positive tender points, and the sum of pain threshold (kg/cm^2 or "total myalgic score"), as well as statistically significant improvements in depression per the Hamilton depression scale and multiple measure on the Short Form 36 (Rossini et al., 2007).

Melatonin

Patients with CFS/FM often have delayed circadian rhythmicity, contributing to sleep disturbances. A pilot study of melatonin, a chronobiotic drug, 5 mg orally for 3 months resulted in significant improvement in scores for fatigue, concentration, and activity in 8/29 patients (van Heukelom, Prins, Smits, & Bleijenberg, 2006). An 8-week double-blind placebo controlled trial assessed melatonin dosage in combination with fluoxetine for FM treatment, finding a combination of 5 mg/day of melatonin with 20 mg/day of fluoxetine to reduce fibromyalgia impact questionnaire (FIQ) scores most significantly from pre-treatment values (Hussain, Al-Khalifa, Jasim, Gorial, 2011).

S-Adenosyl Methionine

S-adenosyl methionine (SAMe) has analgesic, anti-inflammatory, and antidepressant effects. A trial in FM patients comparing SAMe 800 mg/day versus placebo for 6 weeks, demonstrated statistically significant improvements in pain, fatigue, and morning stiffness but not in tender point score, isokinetic muscle strength, or mood evaluated by Beck Depression Inventory (Jacobsen, Danneskiold-Samsoe, & Andersen, 1991). A second crossover study of 17 patients with primary FM did show reduced number of trigger points and improved scores on both the Hamilton and SAD rating scales (Tavoni, Vitali, Bombardieri, & Pasero, 1987). A 10-day crossover trial in 34 patients with FM did not find any significant difference for 600 mg/day intravenous SAMe over placebo (Volkmann et al., 1997). Unfortunately, these studies are more than 15 years old and there are no additional studies for review. While SAMe is generally well tolerated, it should be used with caution in patients with bipolar disorder and Parkinson's Disease. S-adenosyl methionine may have hypoglycemic effects or impact blood pressure, so patients with diabetes and hypertension should be monitored. Patients should not use SAMe with MAO inhibitors.

5-Hydroxytryptophan

5-Hydroxytryptophan (HTP) is the precursor compound in the synthesis of serotonin. There is some promising data that 5-HTP, typically given in doses of 50–150 mg in the evening, can reduce the number of tender points and improve anxiety, pain, sleep, and fatigue (Caruso, Sarzi Puttini, Cazzola, & Azzolini, 1990; Nicolodi & Sicuteri, 1996; Puttini & Caruso, 1992). Episodes of eosinophilia-myalgia syndrome (EMS) in the 1980s from contaminated tryptophan, a very similar compound, have raised some safety concerns. The contaminant called Peak X has been identified in some 5-HTP supplements, and a small number of cases of EMS have been linked to 5-HTP (Johnson et al., 1999). As with any supplement, patients should be guided toward high-quality products from reputable manufacturers, and recommendations should include a discussion of the potential risks and benefits.

Dehydroepiandrosterone

The adrenal hormone dehydroepiandrosterone (DHEA) may regulate excitatory neurotransmission via the limbic system. In some people, low DHEA levels create memory impairment and decreased concentration, which improve after supplementation. Typical doses in female patients are 5–15 mg/day in the morning (Himmel & Seligman 1999; Kuratsune et al., 1998). Dehydroepiandrosterone is available both over the counter as a dietary supplement and via prescription through a compounding pharmacy. Levels of DHEA-S should be measured periodically to ensure therapeutic levels, and women should be monitored for adverse effects from increased androgen levels, such as acne or hirsutism.

Magnesium

Magnesium and malate, both needed for ATP formation, are sometimes recommended for FM/CFS, though limited data are available (Russell et al., 1995).

When low red blood cell magnesium is documented, intramuscular magnesium sulfate 1 g weekly may improve energy levels and mood and reduce pain (Cox, Campbell, & Dowson, 1991). Sixty premenopausal women diagnosed with FM were divided into three groups: magnesium citrate (300 mg/day), amitriptyline (10 mg/day), and combined magnesium citrate (300 mg/day) + amitriptyline (10 mg/day) treatment. While number of tender points, tender point index, fibromyalgia impact questionnaire (FIQ) and Beck depression scores decreased significantly with the magnesium citrate alone, the combined amitriptyline + magnesium citrate treatment also proved effective on pain intensity, pain threshold and Beck anxiety scores (Bagis et al., 2013).

Nicotinamide Adenine Dinucleotide Hydrate

Nicotinamide adenine dinucleotide hydrate (NADH) is a coenzyme essential to the production of ATP. In one study, some participants with CFS noted that 10 mg/day NADH taken for 4 weeks improved fatigue, other symptoms, and quality of life (Forsyth et al., 1999).

NUTRITION

Nutrition plays a large role in the regulation of symptoms in FM/CFS patients (Werbach, 2000). The most commonly recommended diets include the following.

Anti-Inflammatory Diet

Though FM is not related to inflammation, the principles of eating whole foods with high consumption of phytonutrient-rich fruits and vegetables and omega-3 rich protein sources is a healthy diet for all individuals.

Vegan Diet

A 3-month study in Finland of a vegan diet consisting of fruits, legumes, seeds, nuts, and vegetables with elimination of coffee, tea, alcohol, sugar, and salt concluded with improvement of symptoms in pain, sleep, and overall wellness (Kaartinen et al., 2000). However, symptoms returned to baseline with resumption of a full diet.

Elimination Diet

Food sensitivities can contribute to many CFS/FM symptoms such as fatigue, mental sluggishness, and gastrointestinal and genitourinary complaints. While many independent labs offer immunoglobulin G (IgG) testing for food sensitivities, the use of these tests is controversial. Alternatively, some providers recommend a trial of an elimination diet to identify the most frequent offending foods. An elimination diet may vary but often restricts sugar, alcohol, dairy products, wheat, eggs, citrus, soy, chocolate, coffee, and artificial sweeteners and additives. After a 3-week elimination, these foods are added back in, one at a time, every 4 days with monitoring for an exacerbation.

Avoidance of monosodium glutamate (MSG) and aspartame (NutraSweet) is recommended. Also found in labels as gelatin, hydrolyzed or textured protein, and yeast extract, MSG is digested into the excitatory amino acid glutamate. Glutamate activates the NMDA receptors involved in the central nervous system's wind-up sensitization, known to be a problem in FM patients. Aspartame is converted into aspartate, another excitatory amino acid that can induce pain-amplifying receptors. Other common offenders include nitrates, nitrites, sulfites, preservatives, and coloring/flavoring additives.

Candida Diet

Overgrowth of *Candida albicans*, or the "yeast syndrome," is a controversial diagnosis with scant scientific data. One study examined the impact of a low sugar, low yeast diet (LSLY) versus healthy eating diet in 52 individuals with CFS. Intention-to-treat analysis showed no statistically significant differences on levels of fatigue or quality of life (Hobday, Thomas, O'Donovan, Murphy, & Pinching, 2008).

PHYSICAL ACTIVITY

The fatigue and pain of FM/CFS often make it challenging for patients to engage in an active lifestyle, and counseling needs to be done with empathy for those limitations. Some patients are able to exercise at full intensity and duration from the outset, but others can do no more than 5 minutes at a stretch (Jones et al., 2006). Asking the patient her current maximal exertion and duration, and then working to increase that amount should be the starting goal. For deconditioned women or those with joint issues, an exercise physiologist or physical therapist with experience in FM/CFS can be invaluable. An association between physical activity and pain perception and modulation in patients with FM has been observed using functional magnetic resonance imaging (fMRI; McLoughlin, Stegner, & Cook, 2011). The application of a repeated heat stimuli in patients who were highly active versus those who were sedentary, showed positive correlations on fMRI in regions of the brain implicated in pain regulation along with concordant decreased self-reported pain ratings.

Aerobic Exercise

Graded exercise is an intervention reliably shown to have benefit in FM/CFS (Fulcher & White, 1997; Powell, Bentall, Nye, & Edwards, 2001). Research has shown reduced number of tender points, improved sleep and sense of well-being, increased serotonin, and reduced depression. A systematic review of RCTs including all forms of exercise concluded that aerobic-only exercise training at intensity levels as recommended by the American College of Sports Medicine has positive effects on global well-being and physical function, with possible additional relief of pain and tender points (Busch et al., 2008).

Muscle Strengthening

Strength training using free weights or elastic bands is associated with improvements in several measures including pain, number of tender points, and muscle strength as well as a decrease in the mean score on the Beck Depression Inventory (Busch et al., 2008; Jones et al., 2002). A small number of patients experienced worsening symptoms during the study.

Yoga/Tai Chi

Benefits of yoga for FM patients have been examined in small pilot studies. Eight weekly sessions of relaxing yoga showed improvement in pain and functional assessments over time (da Silva, Lorenzi-Filho, & Lage, 2007). Tai chi is a traditional Chinese discipline with both physical and mental components that appears to benefit varied chronic conditions such as rheumatoid arthritis. A randomized trial in FM reported clinically important improvements in the FIQ total score and quality of life, with maintenance at 24 weeks (Wang et al., 2010).

ACUPUNCTURE AND TRADITIONAL CHINESE MEDICINE

Integrative Medicine Perspective: Traditional Chinese Medicine

Janet's progress provides an excellent example of how acupuncture must be individualized for the specific patient. Although acupuncture is very effective in treating the symptoms of FM/CFS especially pain, insomnia, fatigue, anxiety, and depression, the body's ability to take correction with acupuncture is individual.

Each acupuncture treatment gives the person a measured push to promote healing and decrease symptoms. The pace and intensity varies with each individual. With Janet, this was a challenge because with CFS there is a thin line between what promotes healing and what can be too much.

—Virginia Burns, LAc and Ania Grimone, LAc

Within 2 years of diagnosis, one in five FM patients seek acupuncture treatment. A systematic review on the use of acupuncture for FM using nine trials, 395 patients, found low to moderate evidence of improvement in pain reduction and stiffness (Deare et al., 2013). Electroacupuncture was more effective than manual acupuncture for reducing pain, stiffness, and increasing overall well-being, sleep, and fatigue. Another systematic review in 2007 found only five RCTs meeting criteria for inclusion (Mayhew & Ernst, 2007). Two trials yielded negative results and three using electroacupuncture were positive. Well-conducted studies in peer-reviewed journals have conflicting results, with some claiming significant improvement in pain, fatigue, and energy and others showing no benefit (Assefi et al., 2005; Martin, Sletten, Williams, & Berger, 2006). Some of the differences may arise from difficulties inherent to acupuncture research, such as blinding techniques, and prescribed treatment protocols versus the more individual approach used in a clinical setting.

MIND–BODY MEDICINE

Integrative Medicine Perspective: Health Psychology

In my experience working with FM/CFS patients like Janet, it is important to maintain an overall biopsychosocial model of illness, while looking at the unique factors that are impacting the individual. Janet was experiencing a moderate reactive depression related to issues of competency and fears of lost capabilities. In addition, she had difficulty handling stresses when her needs competed with the demands of others. This conflict arose around her work, her personal creative endeavors, and in close interpersonal relationships. Our focus was on mind–body methods to reduce the resultant stress as well as cognitive approaches to managing the conflict and reaching a realistic balance around internal and external demands.

—Howard Feldman, PhD

Patients with FM/CFS often fear being labeled as having a psychosomatic condition. It is important for the physician recommending psychotherapy and mind–body therapies to clarify their role in the overall treatment plan, validating the true physical nature of the illness. A systematic review of mind–body therapies for FM by the Cochrane Collaboration identified 13 eligible trials on autogenic training, relaxation exercises, mindfulness meditation, cognitive-behavioral training (CBT), hypnosis, guided imagery, biofeedback, or education (Hadhazy, Ezzo, Creamer, & Berman, 2000). The conclusion was that there is strong evidence that mind–body therapy is effective for self-efficacy, moderate evidence for improved quality of life, and inconclusive evidence for other outcomes such as pain. A review focused solely on CBT concluded a small incremental benefit of CBT over control interventions in reducing pain, negative mood, and disability at the end of treatment (intervention ranged from 5 to 15 weeks, median 9) and long-term follow-up (range 2–48 months, median 6) (Bernardy et al., 2010). Similar positive results were noted for CBT and meditation-based stress reduction in CFS (Prins et al., 2001).

MANUAL AND MANIPULATIVE THERAPIES

Integrative Medicine Perspective: Bodyworker and Energy Healer

Initially, most patients with FM/CFS, including Janet, are in too much pain for even superficial massage techniques. Treatments such as cranial sacral therapy and Reiki have resulted in decreased pain and anxiety, improved energy, and greater relaxation. Both therapies are noninvasive and use very light touch.

—Chris Wilson, CMT

Current research suggests gentle massage may lower anxiety and benefit sleep quality in FM/CFS (Field et al., 2002). In addition, after 5 weeks of twice-weekly therapy, substance P levels decreased and the patients' physicians assigned lower disease ratings and noted fewer tender points. A study using mechanical deep tissue massage (LPG technique) also showed reduction in tender points after 15 treatments by a physical therapist (Gordon, Emiliozzi, & Zartarian, 2006). The deep tissue work of Rolfing showed benefit in one study, but for many patients the technique is too painful. In recommending manual therapies the physician should be aware that therapists vary considerably in technique, as well as knowledge about treating FM/CFS, making it imperative to refer to an experienced and well-qualified practitioner. In 2013 a systematic review of massage therapy for patients with FM showed that 5 weeks of treatment significantly improved pain, anxiety, and depression but did not significantly reduce sleep disturbances (Li, Wang, Feng, Yang, & Sun, 2014). Craniosacral therapy is a gentle, hands-on approach that purportedly can release tension and promote health through the release of restrictions in tissues influencing the craniosacral system and negatively impacting the motion of cerebrospinal fluid bathing the brain and spinal cord. One 20-week RCT of craniosacral therapy found a reduction in 13 of 18 tender points, with improvements persisting at 1 year post therapy (Castro-Snachez et al., 2011).

ENERGY HEALING

Qigong

The Traditional Chinese medicine energy therapy qigong was examined in a pilot study of 10 patients (Chen, Hassett, Hou, Staller, & Lichtbroun, 2006). Five to seven qigong treatments over 3 weeks led to complete recovery in two patients and improvements in pain, depression, and function in the remaining subjects.

Reiki

Reiki, the Japanese-based energy field therapy is promoted as helpful for pain, sleep, immune function, and anxiety/depression. A randomized, sham-controlled trial with 100 participants in private medical offices found no changes in subjective pain through a visual analog scale over 3 months of twice-weekly treatment. Furthermore, they observed no secondary outcome changes in physical and mental function, medical use, and health provider visits (Assefi, Bogart, Goldberg, & Buchwald, 2008).

Distance Healing

A European study of the effect of distance healing versus wait list on over 400 CFS patients did not demonstrate a statistically significant effect on mental and physical health (Walach & Bosch, 2008).

Conclusion

Although FM is the second most common condition seen by rheumatologists, only 20% of cases are cared for in specialty clinics, leaving the bulk of the management to primary care providers. The first step in the patient's healing is for the clinician to enter into the relationship with acceptance and empathy. Next, simply educating her about the current scientific understanding and real nature of the disease can provide significant relief. Finally, recognize that the disease course will be a journey that you and your patient will take together as you explore a variety of integrative therapeutic approaches to ease her pain and suffering.

REFERENCES

Aaron, L. A., Burke, M. M., & Buchwald, D. (2000). Overlapping conditions among patients with chronic fatigue syndrome, fibromyalgia, and temporomandibular disorder. *Arch Intern Med, 160,* 221.

Afari, N., & Buchwald, D. (2003). Chronic fatigue syndrome: A review. *Am J Psychiatry, 160,* 221–236.

Arnold, L. M., Hudson, J. I., Hess, E. V., et al. (2004). Family study of fibromyalgia. *Arthritis Rheum, 50,* 944.

Arnold, L. M., Lu, Y., Crofford, L. J., et al. (2004). A double-blind, multicenter trial comparing duloxetine to placebo in the treatment of fibromyalgia patients with or without major depressive disorder. *Arthritis Rheum, 50,* 2974.

Assefi, N., Bogart, A., Goldberg, J., & Buchwald, D. (2008). Reiki for the treatment of fibromyalgia: A randomized controlled trial. *J Altern Complement Med, 14,* 1115–1122.

Assefi, N. P., Sherman, K. J., Jacobsen, C., Goldberg, J., Smith, W. R., & Buchwald, D. (2005). A randomized clinical trial of acupuncture compared with sham acupuncture in fibromyalgia. *Ann Intern Med, 143,* 10.

Bagis, S., Karabiber, M., As, I., Tamer, L., Erdogan, C., & Atalay, A. (2013). Is magnesium citrate treatment effective on pain, clinical parameters and functional status in patients with fibromyalgia? *Rheumatol Int, 33,* 167–172.

Bates, D. W., Schmitt, W., Buchwald, D., et al. (1993). Prevalence of fatigue and chronic fatigue syndrome in a primary care practice. *Arch Intern Med, 153,* 2759.

Bennett, R. M., Kamin, M., Karim, R., & Rosenthal, N. (2003). Tramadol and acetaminophen combination tablets in the treatment of fibromyalgia pain: A double-blind, randomized, placebo-controlled study. *Am J Med, 114,* 537.

Bernardy, K., et al. (2013) Cognitive-behavioral therapies for fibromyalgia. *Cochrane Database Syst Rev,* 9:CD009796.

Bradley, L. A. (2008). Pathophysiologic mechanisms of fibromyalgia and its related disorders. *J Clin Psychiatry, 69*(Suppl 2), 6.

Busch, A. J., et al. (2008). Exercise for fibromyalgia: A Systematic Review. *J Rheum*, *35*, 1130–1144.

Caruso, I., Sarzi Puttini, P., Cazzola, M., & Azzolini, V. (1990). Double-blind study of 5-hydroxytryptophan versus placebo in the treatment of primary fibromyalgia syndrome. *J Int Med Res*, *18*, 201.

Castro-Sánchez, A. M., Matarán-Peñarrocha, G. A., Sánchez-Labraca, N., et al. (2011) A randomized controlled trial investigating the effects of craniosacral therapy on pain and heart rate variability in fibromyalgia patients. *Clin Rehab*, *25*, 25–35.

Chen, K. W., Hassett, A. L., Hou, F., Staller, J., & Lichtbroun, A. S. (2006). A pilot study of external qigong therapy for patients with fibromyalgia *J Altern Complement Med*, *12*, 851.

Chew-Graham, C. A., Cahill, G., Dowrick, C., Wearden, A., & Peters, S. (2008). Using multiple sources of knowledge to reach clinical understanding of chronic fatigue syndrome *Ann Fam Med*, *6*, 340.

Clauw, D. J. (2014). Fibromyalgia: A clinical review. *JAMA*, *311*, 1547–1555.

Cohen, H., Buskila, D., Neumann, L., & Ebstein, R. P. (2002). Confirmation of an association between fibromyalgia and serotonin transporter promoter region (5-HTTLPR) polymorphism, and relationship to anxiety-related personality traits. *Arthritis Rheum*, *46*, 845.

Cox, I. M., Campbell, M. J., & Dowson, D. (1991). Red blood cell magnesium and chronic fatigue syndrome. *Lancet*, *337*, 757.

Crofford, L. J., Mease, P. J., Simpson, S. L., et al. (2008). Fibromyalgia relapse evaluation and efficacy for durability of meaningful relief (FREEDOM): A 6-month, double-blind, placebo-controlled trial with pregabalin, *Pain*, *136*(3), 419–431.

Crofford, L. J., Rowbotham, M. C., Mease, P. J., et al. (2005). Pregabalin for the treatment of fibro-myalgia syndrome: Results of a randomized, double-blind, placebo-controlled trial. *Arthritis Rheum*, *52*, 1264.

da Silva, G. D., Lorenzi-Filho, G., & Lage, L. V. (2007). Effects of yoga and the addition of Tui Na in patients with fibromyalgia *J Altern Complement Med*, *13*, 1107.

Deare, J. C., Zheng, Z.,Xue, C. C., et al. (2013). Acupuncture for treating fibromyalgia. *Cochrane Database of Systematic Reviews*, Issue 5.

Demitrack, M. A. (1997). Neuroendocrine correlates of chronic fatigue syndrome: A brief review. *J Psychiatr Res*, *31*, 69.

Field, T., Diego, M., Cullen, C., Hernandez-Reif, M., Sunshine, W., & Douglas, S. (2002). Fibromyalgia pain and substance P decrease and sleep improves after massage therapy. *J Clin Rheumatol*, *8*, 72.

Forsyth, L. M., Preuss, H. G., MacDowell, A. L., et al. (1999). Therapeutic effects of oral NADH on the symptoms of patients with chronic fatigue syndrome. *Ann Allergy Asthma Immunol*, *82*, 185–191.

Fukuda, K., Straus, S. E., Hickie, I., et al. (1994). The chronic fatigue syndrome: A comprehensive approach to its definition and study. International Chronic Fatigue Syndrome Study Group. *Ann Intern Med*, *121*, 953.

Fulcher, K. Y., & White, P. D. (1997). Randomized controlled trial of graded exercise in patients with the chronic fatigue syndrome. *BMJ*, *314*, 1647.

Goldenberg, D. L., Simms, R. W., Geiger, A., & Komaroff, A. L. (1990). High frequency of fibromyalgia in patients with chronic fatigue seen in a primary care practice *Arthritis Rheum*, *33*, 381.

Gordon, C., Emiliozzi, C., & Zartarian, M. (2006). Use of a mechanical massage technique in the treatment of fibromyalgia: A preliminary study. *Arch Phys Med Rehabil*, *87*, 145–147.

Hadhazy, V. A., Ezzo, J., Creamer, P., & Berman, B. M. (2000). Mind-body therapies for the treatment of fibromyalgia: A systematic review *J Rheumatol*, *27*, 2911–2918.

Harth, M., & Nielson, W. R. (2007). The fibromyalgia tender points: Use them or lose them? A brief review of the controversy. *J Rheumatol*, *34*, 914.

Hauser, W., Urrútia, G., Tort, S., Uçeyler, N., & Walitt, B. (2013) Serotonin and noradrenaline reuptake inhibitors (SNRIs) for fibromyalgia syndrome. *Cochrane Database Syst Rev*, 1:CD010292.

Himmel, P. B., & Seligman, T. M. (1999). A pilot study employing dehydroepiandrosterone (DHEA) in the treatment of chronic fatigue syndrome. [Abstract] *J Clin Rheumatol*, *5*, 56.

Hobday, R. A., Thomas, S., O'Donovan, A., Murphy, M., & Pinching, A. J. (2008). Dietary intervention in chronic fatigue syndrome. *J Hum Nutr Diet*, *21*, 141.

Holton, K. F. (2012). Monosodium glutamate likely worsened fibromyalgia symptoms. *Clin Exp Rheumatol*, *30*, S10–S17.

Hussain, S. A., Al-Khalifa, I. I., Jasim, N. A., Gorial, F. I. (2011). Adjuvant use of melatonin for treatment of fibromyalgia. *J Pineal Research*, *50*, 267–271.

Inanici, F., & Yunus, M. B. (2004). History of fibromyalgia: Past to present *Curr Pain Headache Rep*, *8*, 369.

Jacobsen, S., Danneskiold-Samsoe, B., & Andersen, R. B. (1991). Oral S-adenosylmethionine in primary fibromyalgia: Double-blind clinical evaluation. *Scand J Rheumatol*, *20*, 294.

Johnson, K. L., Klarskov, K., Benson, L. M., Williamson, B. L., Gleich, G. J., & Naylor, S. (1999). Presence of peak X and related compounds: The reported contaminant in case related 5- hydroxy-L-tryptophan associated with eosinophilia-myalgia syndrome. *J Rheumatol*, *26*, 2714–2717.

Jones, K. D., Adams, D., Winters-Stone, K., & Burckhardt, C. S. (2006). A comprehensive review of 46 exercise treatment studies in fibromyalgia (1988–2005). *Health Qual Life Outcomes*, *4*, 67.

Jones, K. D., Burckhardt, C. S., Clark, S. R., et al. (2002). A randomized controlled trial of muscle strengthening versus flexibility training in fibromyalgia. *J Rheumatol*, *29*, 1041.

Kaartinen, K., Lammi, K., Hypen, M., Nenonen, M., Hanninen, O., & Rauma, A. L. (2000). Vegan diet alleviates fibromyalgia symptoms. *Scand J Rheumatol*, *29*, 308.

Kerr, J. R., Burke, B., Petty, R., et al. (2008). Seven genomic subtypes of chronic fatigue syndrome/myalgic encephalomyelitis: A detailed analysis of gene networks and clinical phenotypes. *J Clin Path*, *61*, 730.

Kerr, J. R., Petty, R., Burke, B., et al. (2008). Gene expression subtypes in patients with chronic fatigue syndrome/myalgic encephalomyelitis. *J Infect Dis, 197,* 1171.

Kim, E. (1994). A brief history of chronic fatigue syndrome *JAMA, 272,* 1070.

Kuratsune, H., Yamaguti, K., Sawada, M., et al. (1998). Dehydroepiandrosterone sulfate deficiency in chronic fatigue syndrome. *Int J Mol Med, 1,* 143.

Landay, A. L., Jessop, C., Lennette, E. T., & Levy, J. A. (1991). Chronic fatigue syndrome: Clinical condition associated with immune activation. *Lancet, 338,* 707.

Li, Y. H., Wang, F. Y., Feng, C. Q., Yang, X. F., Sun, Y. H. (2014). Massage therapy for fibromyalgia: A systematic review and meta- analysis of randomized controlled trials. *PloS One, 9,* e89304.

Mannerkorpi, K., & Henriksson, C. (2007). Non-pharmacological treatment of chronic widespread musculoskeletal pain *Best Pract Res Clin Rheumatol, 21,* 513.

Martin, D. P., Sletten, C. D., Williams, B. A., & Berger, I. H. (2006). Improvement in fibromyalgia symptoms with acupuncture: Results of a randomized controlled trial. *Mayo Clin Proc, 81,* 749.

Mawle, A. C., Nisenbaum, R., Dobbins, J. G., et al. (1995). Seroepidemiology of chronic fatigue syndrome: A case-control study. *Clin Infect Dis, 21,* 1386.

Mawle, A. C., Nisenbaum, R., Dobbins, J. G., et al. (1997). Immune responses associated with chronic fatigue syndrome: A case-control study. *J Infect Dis, 175,* 136.

Mayhew, E., & Ernst, E. (2007). Acupuncture for fibromyalgia: A systematic review of randomized clinical trials. *Rheumatology (Oxford), 46,* 801.

McBeth, J., Silman, A. J., Gupta, A., et al. (2007). Moderation of psychosocial risk factors through dysfunction of the hypothalamic-pituitary-adrenal stress axis in the onset of chronic widespread musculoskeletal pain: Findings of a population-based prospective cohort study. *Arthritis and Rheumatism, 56,* 360–371.

McLoughlin, M. J., Stegner, A. J., & Cook, D. B. (2011). The relationship between physical activity and brain responses to pain in fibromyalgia. *Journal of Pain, 12,* 640–651.

Meeus, M., & Nijs, J. (2007). Central sensitization: A biopsychosocial explanation for chronic widespread pain in patients with fibromyalgia and chronic fatigue syndrome. *Clin Rheumatol, 26,* 465.

Nicolodi, M., & Sicuteri F. (1996). Fibromyalgia and migraine, two faces of the same mechanism: Serotonin as the common clue for pathogenesis and therapy. *Adv Exp Med Biol, 398,* 373.

Offenbaecher, M., Bondy, B., de Jonge, S., et al. (1999). Possible association of fibromyalgia with a polymorphism in the serotonin transporter gene regulatory region. *Arthritis Rheum, 42,* 2482.

Pall, M. (2007). *Explaining "unexplained illnesses."* New York: Harrington Park Press.

Plioplys, A. V., & Plioplys, S. (1997). Amantadine and L-carnitine treatment of chronic fatigue syndrome. *Neuropsychobiology, 35,* 16.

Powell, P., Bentall, R. P., Nye, F. J., & Edwards, R. H. (2001). Randomized controlled trial of patient education to encourage graded exercise in chronic fatigue syndrome. *BMJ, 322,* 387.

Prins, J. B., Bleijenberg, G., Bazelmans, E., et al. (2001). Cognitive behaviour therapy for chronic fatigue syndrome: A multicentre randomised controlled trial. *Lancet*, *357*, 841.

Puttini, P. S., & Caruso, I. (1992). Primary fibromyalgia syndrome and 5-hydroxy-L-tryptophan: A 90-day open study. *J Int Med Res*, *20*, 182–189.

Rossini, M., Di Munno, O., Valentini, G., et al. (2007). Double-blind, multicenter trial comparing acetyl l-carnitine with placebo in the treatment of fibromyalgia patients. *Clin Exp Rheumatol*, *25*, 182–188.

Russell, I. J., Michalek, J. E., Flechas, J. D., et al. (1995). Treatment of fibromyalgia syndrome with Super Malic: A randomized, double blind, placebo controlled, cross-over pilot study. *J Rheumatol*, *22*, 953–958.

Schacterle, R. S., & Komaroff, A. L. (2004). A comparison of pregnancies that occur before and after the onset of chronic fatigue syndrome. *Arch Intern Med*, *164*, 401.

Schwartz, R. B., Garada, B. M., & Komaroff, A. L. (1994). Detection of intracranial abnormalities in patients with chronic fatigue syndrome: Comparison of MRI imaging and SPECT. *AJR Am J Roentgenol*, *162*, 935.

Straus, S. E., Tosato, G., Armstrong, G., et al. (1985). Persisting illness and fatigue in adults and evidence of Epstein-Barr virus infection. *Ann Intern Med*, *102*, 7.

Tavoni, A., Vitali, C., Bombardieri, S., & Pasero, G. (1987). Evaluation of S-adenosylmethionine in primary fibromyalgia. *Am J Med*, *83*(Suppl 5A), 107.

Teitelbaum, J. E., Johnson, C., & St Cyr, J. (2006). The use of D-ribose in chronic fatigue syndrome and fibromyalgia: A pilot study. *J Altern Complement Med*, *12*, 857.

Tofferi, J. K., Jackson, J. L., & O'Malley, P. G. (2004). Treatment of fibromyalgia with cyclobenzaprine: A meta-analysis. *Arthritis Rheum*, *51*, 9.

Uceyler, N., Sommer, C., Walitt, B., & Hauser, W. (2013). Anticonvulsants for fibromyalgia. *Cochrane Database Syst Rev*, 10:CD010782.

van Heukelom, R. O., Prins, J. B., Smits, M. G., & Bleijenberg, G. (2006). Influence of melatonin on fatigue severity in patients with chronic fatigue syndrome and late melatonin secretion *Eur J Neurol*, *13*, 55.

Vermeulen, R. C., & Scholte, H. R. (2004). Exploratory open label, randomized study of acetyl- and propionylcarnitine in chronic fatigue syndrome *Psychosom Med*, *66*, 276.

Volkmann, H., Norregaard, J., Jacobsen, S., et al. (1997). Double-blind, placebo-controlled cross-over study of intravenous S-adenosyl-L-methionine in patients with fibromyalgia. *Scand J Rheumatol*, *26*, 206–211.

Walach, H., & Bosch, H. (2008). Effectiveness of distant healing for patients with chronic fatigue syndrome: A randomised controlled partially blinded trial. *Psychother Psychosom*, *77*, 158.

Wang, C., Schmid, C. H., Rones, R., et al. (2010). A randomized trial of tai chi for fibromyalgia. *NEJM*, *363*, 743–754.

Werbach, M. R. (2000). Nutritional strategies for treating chronic fatigue syndrome. *Altern Med Rev*, *5*, 93.

Wolfe, F., Clauw, D. J., Fitzcharles, M. A., et al. (2010). The American College of Rheumatology preliminary diagnostic criteria for fibromyalgia and measurement of symptom severity. *Arthritis Care Res, 62*(5), 600-610.

Wolfe, F., Ross, K., Anderson, J., et al. (1995). The prevalence and characteristics of fibromyalgia in the general population. *Arthritis Rheum, 38,* 19.

Wolfe, F., Smythe, H. A., Yunus, M. B., et al. (1990). The American College of Rheumatology 1990 Criteria for the classification of fibromyalgia: Report of the Multicenter Criteria Committee. *Arthritis Rheum, 33,* 160.

Younger, J., Noor, N., McCue, R., & Mackey, S. (2013). Low-dose naltrexone for the treatment of fibromyalgia: Findings of a small, randomized, double-blind, placebo-controlled, counterbalanced, crossover trial assessing daily pain levels. *Arthritis Rheum, 65,* 529–538.

Younger, J., & Mackey, S. (2009). Fibromyalgia symptoms are reduced by low-dose naltrexone: A pilot study. *Pain Medicine, 10,* 663–672.

29

Rheumatoid Arthritis

NISHA MANEK

CASE STUDY

Teresa was rehearsing the dance routine for her role in a musi-
cal. The difficulty was that her ankles and feet were swollen,
painful, and stiff. She could barely move in the mornings, and
the first hour after she rose from bed was particularly difficult. She thought she had pushed too hard in her practice and
"sprained" her joints. She also felt more tired. In the last 2 weeks,
Teresa noticed her hands were swelling and she could no longer remove her wedding ring. Her hands felt numb and weak,
and today she dropped a cup of coffee. Her mother insisted that
Teresa see a physician as she had been complaining of painful
feet for 2 months.

Introduction

Since the publication of the first edition of this textbook, many developments have occurred in the treatment of rheumatoid arthritis (RA).
Among new concepts are the idea of active resolution of inflammation
by endogenous proteins termed "resolvins"; new understanding of the neural
control of inflammation that provides an understanding of the mind–body
therapeutics' mechanism of controlling inflammation; and the treat-to-target
paradigm of RA, which emphasizes remission of disease inflammation as
quickly and safely as possible with guidance from disease activity outcome
measures. Greater understanding of the immune system has opened the way

for development of targeted therapeutics; all this and more makes it an exciting time for rheumatology.

The Role of Integrative Medicine and Treatment of Rheumatoid Arthritis

With the remarkable progress in conventional therapeutics for RA, what can complementary and integrative medicine (CIM) offer the physician and patient? Rheumatologists appear to have an overall positive attitude toward CIM modalities used for osteoarthritis and back pain (Manek et al., 2010). The use of CIM in self-directed therapy for RA varies between 28% and 90%, and the desire for patients to be able to choose natural products for controlling arthritis remains strong (Kolasinski, 2012; Taibi & Bourguignon, 2003). The high rate of CIM usage among patients with RA reflects unmet needs (Efthimiou, Kukar, & Mackenzie, 2010; Quandt, Chen, Grzywacz, Bell, Lang, & Arcury, 2005; Saydah & Eberhardt, 2006; Verstappen & Symmons, 2011). Current conventional and biologic disease-modifying therapies sometimes fail or produce only partial responses. Furthermore, reliable predictive biomarkers of prognosis, therapeutic response, sustained remission, and toxicity are lacking (van den Broek, Visser, Allaart, & Huizinga, 2013). Personalized conventional medicine for RA treatment remains elusive at present, although there is much research into factors such as epigenetics and these may become more important in future healthcare delivery (Julia & Marsal, 2013; Szekanecz et al., 2013). Over time an integrative treatment approach appears to lead to less utilization of healthcare and less medical costs (Sharpe, Allard, & Sensky, 2008; Young, Bradley, & Turner, 1995). An integrative approach to treating inflammation may also change the inner terrain, reducing the expression of master switches of inflammation such as nuclear factor kappa-B (NF-kappa B) and averting or delaying development of the RA phenotype. For example, it is known that detectable anticitrullinated protein antibody (anti-CCP) predates the development of RA by several years (Klareskog, Ronnelid, Lundberg, Padyukov, & Alfredsson, 2008). Similarly, the anti–nuclear antibody test (ANA) predates SLE by up to 9 years (Arbuckle et al., 2003).

This chapter will review the epidemiology of RA, diagnosis and conventional management of RA, and address the gender bias of this disease with a focus on reproductive and hormonal issues. The goal is to provide the clinician with a framework to approach the woman with RA, create a treatment program and discuss the evidence for the more common integrative modalities that have been studied in RA.

Epidemiology

The incidence of RA in women appears to have increased during the time period from 1995 to 2007 in a well-described population residing in Olmstead County, Minnesota (Myasoedova, Crowson, Kremers, Therneau, & Gabriel, 2010). The reasons for this increase are unknown, but environmental factors are thought to play a role. A corresponding increase in the prevalence of RA was also observed (Myasoedova et al., 2010). The lifetime risk of RA developing in US adults has been estimated at 3.6% for women and 1.7% for men (Crowson et al., 2011).

Risk Factors for Rheumatoid Arthritis

Rheumatoid arthritis is a multifactorial disease resulting from interaction of genetic and environmental factors (Aho & Heliovaara, 2004; Karlson et al., 2013). The genetic basis is associated with human leukocyte antigen (HLA) class II alleles especially with subtypes DRB1 (Turesson, Weyand, & Matteson, 2004). Of the traditional lifestyle exposures, cigarette smoking has been associated with a consistently increased risk that might also apply to the passive inhalation of smoke (Aho & Heliovaara, 2004; Costenbader, Feskanich, Mandl, & Karlson, 2006; Turesson et al., 2004). The attributable risk of smoking in RA incidence approaches 20% (Criswell et al., 2002). That is, one of every five new cases of RA could potentially be prevented if smoking was taken out of the equation. Diet also appears to influence the risk, but a specific beneficial nutrient has not been identified (Choi, 2004; Karlson, Mandl, Aweh, & Grodstein, 2003). Obesity is associated with a modest risk for developing RA. Given the rapidly increasing prevalence of obesity, this has had a significant impact on RA incidence and may account for much of the recent increase in the incidence of RA (Crowson, Matteson, Davis, & Gabriel, 2013).

Of the many infections that have been speculated to play a role in RA risk, one that has attracted much attention recently is *Porphyromonas gingivalis*, a gram-negative bacterium associated with periodontitis (Bingham & Moni, 2013; Janssen, Vissink, de Smit, Westra, & Brouwer, 2013; Rutger Persson, 2012). *P. gingivalis* is known to express peptidylarginine deaminase, an enzyme responsible for the posttranslational conversion of arginine to citrulline (Janssen et al., 2013). With further epitope spreading, it is postulated that these bacterially mediated changes could ultimately result in expression of RA-specific autoantibodies. Immune responses to *P. gingivalis* are significantly associated with the expression of disease specific anti-CCP antibodies (Mikuls et al., 2014).

Newly emerging understanding of autoimmune diseases has focused on commensal microbial community; gut bacteria alter sex hormone levels and regulate autoimmune disease fate in individuals with high genetic risk for conditions such as diabetes (Markle et al., 2013). Recent research suggests that the developmental processes of sexual differentiation might render women more susceptible than men to similar levels of immune or inflammatory burden by virtue of sex-specific differences in body composition and structure (Kovacs & Olsen, 2011).

Making the Diagnosis

The diagnosis of RA is primarily a clinical one, requiring the collection of historical and physical features as well as an alert and informed clinician. Early consultation with a rheumatologist is recommended to help solidify the diagnosis. The American College of Rheumatology has defined new classification criteria for RA (Aletaha et al., 2010). The distribution of involved joints is an important clue to the underlying diagnosis. Most patients report involvement of small joints, classically the proximal interphalangeal (PIP), metacarpophalangeal (MCP), and metatarsophalangeal (MTP) joints followed by the wrists, knees, elbows, ankles, hips, and shoulders in roughly that order. Of particular importance, RA almost always spares the distal interphalangeal joint.

It is crucial not to mistakenly label osteoarthritis (OA) as RA. The DIP joints are spared in RA, but are involved in OA. In a woman with RA, DIP joints are spared unless she also has OA; both diseases are common and can coexist, particularly in the elderly patient. A careful history and joint examination to ascertain pattern of arthritis can help differentiate the two conditions.

Back to Teresa: She complained of painful balls of her feet, and she reported that it felt like she was "walking on marbles." She had metatarsalgia due to the subluxation of the MTP joints. Also, she was found to have clinical symptoms of carpal tunnel syndrome, which can be a presenting feature of RA.

Diagnostic Tests and Radiographic Findings

Rheumatoid factor (RF) is the most characteristic laboratory abnormality in RA. The RF will be positive in about 50% of cases at presentation, and about

20%–35% of cases will go on to become positive in the first 6 months after diagnosis. The RF is an antibody that recognizes immunoglobulin G (IgG) as its antigen. A positive RF test is associated with more severe joint disease, as well as extra-articular features.

Enzyme-linked immunosorbent assays (ELISA) for anti-CCP have nearly the same sensitivity (45% to 70%) as RF and are more specific for RA (>95%). Anti-CCP antibodies are found earlier in the disease course and predict a more severe outcome (van Venrooij, van Beers, & Pruijn, 2011).

Other laboratory tests that can be useful in supporting the diagnosis of RA include synovial fluid analysis, measurement of acute-phase reactants; erythrocyte sedimentation rate (ESR); C-reactive protein (CRP), and the complete blood count (CBC). Elevation in the ESR and/or CRP level provides a surrogate measure of active inflammation and may be useful in establishing a diagnosis, estimating the prognosis, and gauging the response to therapy. The most common abnormality in the CBC in patients with RA is a normochromic, normocytic anemia (anemia of chronic disease). The degree of anemia is in proportion to the activity of disease. Thrombocytosis may also be seen with uncontrolled inflammation. Nonspecific mild (twofold) elevation of alkaline phosphatase (ALP) is seen sporadically.

Imaging in early RA has undergone extraordinary change in recent years, and new techniques are now available to help the clinician diagnose and manage patients much more effectively. While established modalities such as plain radiography (X-ray) remain important, especially for detection of erosions and determining the progression of joint damage, there are many instances where ultrasound (US), magnetic resonance imaging (MRI) and computed tomography (CT) scanning provide added information. Clinicians now regularly use MRI and US to help diagnose RA in the preradiographic stage, as they offer improved visualization of joint erosions. They also have the potential to provide prognostic information as MRI bone edema/osteitis is linked to the later development of erosions. Power Doppler ultrasound (PDUS) joint positivity is also a predictor of joint damage (McQueen, 2013).

Reproductive and Endocrine Factors

The greater prevalence of RA among women argues for an effect of sex hormones on the disease. Women with RA report decreased joint pain during the postovulatory phase of the menstrual cycle and during pregnancy, when estradiol and progesterone levels are high (Ansar Ahmed & Penhale, 1985). In contrast, during the postpartum period, when estrogen and progesterone levels fall, RA symptoms usually flare. The first few months of the postpartum period are a time of increased risk for developing RA (Mathur, Mathur, Goust, Williamson, & Fudenberg, 1979). Nulliparity has been associated with an increased risk of developing RA (Ansar Ahmed & Talal, 1989; Cutolo & Lahita, 2005; Persellin, 1976), and in some studies oral contraceptives were protective against RA (Kay & Wingrave, 1983; Linos, Worthington, O'Fallon, & Kurland, 1983; Vandenbroucke et al., 1982). Previous studies, including those among women in the Nurses' Health Study, a prospective cohort study of 121,700 women, have yielded conflicting results regarding potential associations of postmenopausal hormones and risk of RA (Bijlsma, Huber-Bruning, & Thijssen, 1987; Hall, Daniels, Huskisson, & Spector, 1994; MacDonald, Murphy, Capell, Bankowska, & Ralston, 1994; Merlino, Cerhan, Criswell, Mikuls, & Saag, 2003).

Sexual Health, Fertility, and Pregnancy in Rheumatoid Arthritis

The burden imposed by RA on the patient and the family can be considerable, and intimate relationships can be strained because of chronic pain. It is important for husbands to understand RA and its cyclic nature and avoid underestimating consequences of RA in their wives (Kasle, Wilhelm, & Zautra, 2008; Sterba et al., 2008).

Infertility in women with RA is an underrecognized but remarkably common phenomenon. The causes of decreased fertility in this population likely revolve around chronic inflammation, increased age when conception is attempted, limited sexual function, and possibly medications limiting ovarian function. Contraception is necessary, especially if a woman of childbearing age is taking methotrexate or leflunomide, which are teratogenic. Although research continues into the underlying causes, physicians can discuss this topic and refer women to reproductive endocrinology when needed (Provost, Eaton, & Clowse, 2014).

Research is also needed to establish the safety of biologic agents in pregnancy and lactation. Remission of RA in pregnancy is achieved by up to 75% of women. This reverts in the postpartum period. Although tumor necrosis factor (TNF) inhibitors are classified as FDA pregnancy category B, few would disagree that TNF inhibitors should be avoided just before or during pregnancy until more data are available (Partlett & Roussou, 2011). However, many patients risk permanent functional and structural disability if untreated for a prolonged period. A reasonable compromise for women with severe arthritis is to allow continuation of TNF inhibitors until the time of conception, with short-term use of low-dose prednisone permitted, as required, during the pregnancy. Given the known teratogenicity of metho-trexate and leflunomide, TNF inhibitors might offer disease control during the period that conception is attempted which, for some, can be lengthy (Clowse, 2010).

Rheumatoid Arthritis as a Multisystem Disease

Rheumatoid arthritis is a disease of premature aging. This is thought to be due to senescence of the immune, endocrine, cardiovascular, muscular, and ner-vous systems. Senescence represents a biological model that may in part explain the excess mortality observed in RA (Crowson, Liang, Therneau, Kremers, & Gabriel, 2010; Myasoedova et al., 2010). The data from Olmsted County, Minnesota, suggest that, in terms of mortality rates, patients with seroposi-tive RA are effectively 2 years older at time of disease incidence, and thereafter age 11.4 effective years for each 10 years of calendar time (Crowson, Liang, et al., 2010). Most of the excess deaths are attributable to infection, cardiovas-cular disease, and respiratory diseases (Naz, Farragher, Bunn, Symmons, & Bruce, 2008). Seropositive patients younger than 55 years appear to be most at risk for cardiovascular disease, and women who fall in this group there-fore require particular attention in terms of disease and risk factor modifica-tion (Naz et al., 2008; Zhang et al., 2014). The increased mortality may stem from accelerated atherogenesis caused by RA-related chronic inflammation (Crowson, Liao, et al., 2013).

Heart Rate Variability and Rheumatoid Arthritis

The pioneering work of Tracy and colleagues has demonstrated that the vagus nerves have an important role in limiting the inflammatory response, a con-cept referred to as the cholinergic anti-inflammatory pathway (Tracey, 2002). Acetylcholine (ACh), the principal neurotransmitter of the vagal nerves, is a key mediator of the cholinergic anti-inflammatory pathway. Heart rate vari-ability (HRV) is a measure of beat-to-beat temporal changes in heart rate, and these changes, rather than being random noise, reflect the output of the central autonomic network. The reader is directed to resources to understand HRV in more detail, as it is beyond the scope of this chapter (Sloan et al., 2007; Task Force of the European Society of Cardiology and the North American Society of Pacing and Electrophysiology, 1996).

The importance of involvement of autonomic nervous system in the reg-ulation of immune function justifies the question as to whether autonomic dysfunction represents a consequence of the progression of autoimmune diseases or whether it may directly participate in the etiopathogenesis of autoimmune diseases (Mravec, 2007). Patients with RA have decreased vagus nerve activity, raising the possibility that they may be incapable of responding to cholinergic agonist-based therapy to control TNF production (Evrengul, Dursunoglu, Cobankara, et al., 2004). Evidence shows that HRV is an independent predictor of response to anti-TNF treatment in RA and psoriatic arthritis (A. Holman & Ng, 2008). Vagus nerve stimulation has the potential, theoretically, to halt or ameliorate RA (Das, 2011). The cholinergic anti-inflammatory pathway suggests the possibility of unconventional strategies to control inflammation, such as that seen in RA, and includes meditation and acupuncture, which have been shown to increase vagus nerve activity (Oke & Tracey, 2009; van Maanen, Vervoordeldonk, & Tak, 2009).

The Heart–Brain Connection in Rheumatoid Arthritis

Reduced resting-state HRV has important functional significance for motivation to engage in social situations, self-regulation, and psychological flexibility in the face of stressors (Kemp & Quintana, 2013). Depression, a risk factor for cardiovascular disease (CVD), is also highly prevalent in RA (Margaretten et al., 2009; Margaretten, Julian, Katz, & Yelin, 2011). A missing link in neuroimmunomodulation in CVD and depression is the cholinergic anti-inflammatory pathway. Living with RA requires that individuals manage symptoms, balance emotional states (Parker et al., 2003; VanDyke et al., 2004), adjust to changes in physical status and social activity (Morris, Yelin, Panopalis, Julian, & Katz, 2011), learn self-management strategies, and communicate with health professionals in a variety of disciplines (H. Holman & Lorig, 1997).

Pain, Fatigue, and Sleep Hygiene in Rheumatoid Arthritis

People with RA identify pain as their most important symptom, one that often persists despite optimal control of inflammatory disease. The American College of Rheumatology emphasizes a multidisciplinary approach to addressing pain (American College of Rheumatology, 2010). The pain of RA arises from multiple mechanisms involving inflammation and increased cytokine release (Rohleder, Aringer, & Boentert, 2012), peripheral and central pain processing, and, with disease progression, structural change within the joint. Consequently, RA pain has a wide range of characteristics—constant or intermittent, localized or widespread—and is often associated with psychological distress and fatigue (Walsh & McWilliams, 2014). Fatigue is also a common symptom; similarities and differences between men and women and their experience of this symptom, and the contribution from psychological distress may inform future interventions for RA-related fatigue (M. Davis, Okun, Kruszewski, Zautra, & Tennen, 2010; Lee et al., 2014; Treharne et al., 2008). A related issue with pain and fatigue is sleep hygiene. Patients with RA have increased sleep disturbance and diffuse pain sensitivity such as noted in central pain conditions like fibromyalgia (Lee et al., 2009; Taylor-Gjevre, Gjevre, Nair, Skomro, & Lim, 2011a). Sleep assessment should be considered. There are many available instruments for the practitioner (Omachi, 2011; Wells et al., 2009). Improved sleep efficiency is seen with adequate disease control (Taylor-Gjevre, Gjevre, Nair, Skomro, & Lim, 2011b).

Understanding Resolution of Inflammation

Accumulating evidence indicates that anti-inflammation and proresolution are distinct mechanisms for control of inflammation (Serhan, 2011). The actions of proresolution mediators are in sharp contrast to those of widely used anti-inflammatory therapeutics such as inhibitors of cyclooxygenase-2 (COX-2), which, ironically, disrupt the endogenous resolution mechanisms (Serhan, Chiang, & Van Dyke, 2008). This evidence has spurred a paradigm shift whereby the resolution of acute inflammation is a biochemically active process regulated in part by compounds derived from polyunsaturated fatty acids (PUFAs) (Fredman & Serhan, 2011). Among these are a novel genus of specialized proresolving mediators (SPMs) that comprise families of mediators including lipoxins, resolvins, and protectins. Compounds from eicosapentanoic acid (20:5[n-3], or EPA) are designated as resolvins of the E series, while those formed from the precursor docosahexaenoic acid (22:6[n-3], or DHA) are denoted as either resolvins or protectins ("neuroprotectins") of the D series. These lipid mediators have emerged as novel potent and stereoselective players that counter-regulate excessive inflammation and stimulate molecular and cellular events that define resolution (Spite & Serhan, 2010). It appears that disruption of acute resolution processing leads to uncontrolled inflammation such as seen in RA. Similarly, a failure in resolution of acute inflammation may also lead to transition from acute pain to chronic pain (Ji, Xu, Strichartz, & Serhan, 2011). Studies have shown antihyperalgesic effects of resolvin (RvE1; Ji et al., 2011).

Interestingly, the vagal anti-inflammatory pathway may be activated by dietary fatty acids such as EPA and DHA, and augment the formation of resolvins and protectins. Therefore two very different pathways of inflammation resolution, vagal activity and PUFAs, appear to come together in one final common pathway (O'Keefe, Abuissa, Sastre, Steinhaus, & Harris, 2006).

Clinical Implications for Omega-3 Fatty Acids

Given the high tolerability of fish oil supplements and the benefits of omega-3 fatty acid intake in cardiovascular disease, resolvins and protectins could take center stage as future biomarkers and well-tolerated therapies for inflammation (Calderon Artero, Champagne, Garigen, Mousa, & Block, 2012). Resolvins have also been found to improve salivary gland epithelial integrity, resolve inflammation in periodontitis, and reduce hyperalgesia (Keinan, Leigh, Nelson, De Oleo, & Baker, 2013). Resolvins have been found to reduce inflammation in ocular tissues and improve dry eye symptoms (Serhan & Petasis, 2011). Outstanding questions remain, however. For example, it remains unknown what minimum dietary requirements of EPA and DHA are needed to evoke endogenous resolvin biosynthesis and timely resolution of pain. Oral ingestion of fish oil will not automatically be metabolized to resolvins under normal conditions, partly because the biosynthetic enzymes have low expression in most tissues. Nevertheless, it is reasonable to promote omega-3 intake in patients with RA, and trials have used doses upward of 2,000 mg daily total of EPA and DHA (Proudman et al., 2013).

Housekeeping Issues for Rheumatoid Arthritis

Screening patients for hepatitis B and C infections, as well as tuberculosis, prior to starting biologic therapy is imperative (Rosen, 2011; Virgin, Wherry, & Ahmed, 2009). Additional clinical issues that need to be addressed include bone health and prevention of osteoporosis, age-appropriate screening of malignancies, and annual vaccinations (McCloskey, 2013; Perry, Winthrop, Curtis, 2014; Rubbert-Roth, 2012). A fracture risk assessment tool (FRAX) has been developed that includes clinical risk factors (Kanis, Johnell, Oden, Johansson, & McCloskey, 2008). Integrative care for patients with RA who have malignancies such as breast cancer is challenging and beyond the scope of this chapter.

Teresa's lipid panel is checked at least annually, and at every clinic visit her blood pressure is measured and recorded. The Centers for Disease Control (CDC) recommends screening of hepatitis C virus (HCV) in everyone born between 1945 and 1965. Teresa's HCV test by commercial ELISA was positive. However, the HCV RNA test was negative, indicating she had cleared the virus; therefore it is an old infection and reactivation is unlikely. In this setting, it would be reasonable to consider biologic therapy.

Treatment Program

The primary target for treatment of RA should be a state of clinical remission. Clinical remission is defined as the absence of signs and symptoms of significant inflammatory disease activity (Smolen et al., 2010). Treatment to target by measuring disease activity and adjusting therapy accordingly optimizes outcomes in RA (Smolen et al., 2010). Complementary and integrative medicine can be aligned with this current paradigm, as was shown in a recent trial examining fish oil in early onset RA that found supplemental fish oil reduced traditional Disease-modifying antirheumatic drug (DMARD) failure and higher rates of RA disease remission (Proudman et al., 2013). Additionally, mental and spiritual aspects are brought to the fore.

The author uses the Clinical Disease Activity Index (CDAI), as it is a rapid 28-joint count and does not require measurement of an acute-phase reactant (Aletaha & Smolen, 2009). The CDAI does include the patient global score in the final calculated score (Figure 29.1). Systematic monitoring of RA activity by CDAI provides a longitudinal view of treatment effects and outcomes, which greatly facilitates evaluation of success of the integrative approach (J. Davis & Matteson, 2012).

Integrative Therapies: A Review of the Evidence in Rheumatoid Arthritis

In the sections that follow, examination of the research trial data is presented for the various integrative therapies. Recommending a particular integrative modality must be done in the context of each individual woman's needs. Drug–nutrient–herb interactions must also be considered.

Clinical Disease Activity Index (CDAI)

Joint	Left		Right	
	Tender	Swollen	Tender	Swollen
Shoulder				
Elbow				
Wrist				
MCP 1				
MCP 2				
MCP 3				
MCP 4				
MCP 5				
PIP 1				
PIP 2				
PIP 3				
PIP 4				
PIP 5				
Knee				
Total	Tender:		Swollen:	

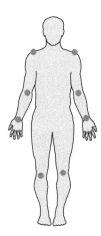

Patient Global Assessment of Disease Activity

Considering all the ways your arthritis affects you, rate how well you are doing on the following scale:

Very ○ Very
Well 0 0.5 1.0 1.5 2.0 2.5 3.0 3.5 4.0 4.5 5.0 5.5 6.0 6.5 7.0 7.5 8.0 8.5 9.0 9.5 10 Poor

Your Name _____ **Date of Birth** _____ **Today's Date** _____

Provider Global Assessment of Disease Activity

Very ○ Very
Well 0 0.5 1.0 1.5 2.0 2.5 3.0 3.5 4.0 4.5 5.0 5.5 6.0 6.5 7.0 7.5 8.0 8.5 9.0 9.5 10 Poor

How to Score the CDAI

Variable	Range	Value
Tender joint score	(0–28)	
Swollen joint score	(0–28)	
Patient global score	(0–10)	
Provider global score	(0–10)	
Add the above values to calculate the CDAI score	(0–76)	

CDAI Score Interpretation	
0.0–2.8	Remission
2.9–10.0	Low Activity
10.1–22.0	Moderate Activity
22.1–76.0	High Activity

FIGURE 29.1. Clinical Disease Activity Index (CDAI).

ACUPUNCTURE

A Cochrane review evaluated the evidence of acupuncture or electroacupuncture in patients with RA (Casimiro et al., 2005). Two randomized controlled trials (RCTs; $N = 84$), one of each for acupuncture and electroacupuncture were reviewed. For acupuncture, there were no significant differences in pain, number of swollen and tender joint account, disease activity, CRP, or amount of pain medication needed compared with sham procedure. A short-term reduction in knee pain was reported for the trial in electroacupuncture, however the authors of the review felt the trial was of low quality and may have overestimated effectiveness. Another pilot study ($N = 36$) reported promising results, which will lead to the design of a large-scale trial that may help clarify the role for acupuncture in RA (Tam, Leung, Li, Zhang, & Li, 2007). Overall, at this time, poor trial data precludes recommendation of acupuncture for RA (Macfarlane et al., 2012).

AYURVEDA

A systematic review assessed the evidence from RCTs on the effectiveness of Ayurvedic herbal medicines (Park & Ernst, 2005). Trials tested either Ayurveda herbal preparations against placebo or other Ayurvedic herbal formulations. In general, patient and physician global assessments on the severity of pain, and morning stiffness were used as end points (Park & Ernst, 2005). The existing RCTs failed to show convincingly that the chosen Ayurvedic herbal treatments are effective therapeutic options for RA (Park & Ernst, 2005).

An interesting development is the establishment of a consortium of academic institutions in India, and one of the charges of the New Millennium Technology Leadership Initiative (NMITLI) is to study Ayurvedic medicine rigorously with the goal of fostering global use. This initiative is tackling some of the complexity of traditional Indian herbal medicine by systematically assessing components commonly used for disorders such as RA to reveal the contributions of various components. Such an approach is more aligned with a disease-centric versus the traditional Ayurvedic patient-centered approach. Publications resulting from this endeavor satisfy a number of recommendations delineated for reporting trials of herbal interventions (Gagnier et al., 2006). The NMITLI investigators have reported that a standardized polyherbal mixture (*Tinospora cordifolia* and *Zingiber officinale* based) and monoherb (*Semecarpus anacardium*) were equivalent in efficacy to hydroxychloroquine for the treatment of moderately severe RA (Chopra et al., 2012). The ability of a well-characterized crude ginger extract to inhibit joint swelling in an animal model of rheumatoid arthritis, streptococcal cell wall–induced arthritis has been demonstrated and suggests significant joint-protective effect (Funk, Frye, Oyarzo, & Timmermann, 2009).

TRADITIONAL CHINESE MEDICINE

Another system of medical care in Asia, traditional Chinese medicine (TCM) has been compared with conventional "Western" care. Conventional care was more effective in the treatment of RA than TCM with regard to efficacy as measured by the American College of Rheumatology 20% improvement criteria (ACR20) (He, Lu, Zha, & Tsang, 2008; He et al., 2014). Symptoms including those not directly related to joints and those inquired about in TCM may have influence on the efficacy of therapy, and might merit further study to ascertain whether they can be helpful to guide specific therapy (He, Lu, et al., 2007). A frequently used TCM mushroom and herb combination of *Ganoderma lucidum* (lingzhi) and San Miao San (*Phellodendron chinense, Coix lacryma-jobi, Atractylodes lancea, Achyranthes bidentata*), with purported diverse health benefits including antioxidant properties in RA (Xi Bao et al., 2006), has been shown to have a significant effect in the number of trial patients achieving an ACR20 response (Li et al., 2007). Additionally, pain score and patient's global score improved significantly only in the TCM group. However, no significant antioxidant, anti-inflammatory, or immunomodulatory effects were demonstrated (Li et al., 2007).

BOTANICALS AND HERBAL MEDICINES

In addition to the therapies listed above, one of the first herbal therapies in the West to be assessed in the treatment of RA was gamma-linoleic acid (GLA) derived from several plant oils including blackcurrant, borage, and evening primrose seed oils. Although GLA is an essential fatty acid of the omega-6 series, its metabolite dihomo-gamma-linolenic acid (DGLA) is a source of anti-inflammatory eicosanoids (prostaglandins of series 1 and leukotrienes of series 3) (Belch & Hill, 2000). Gamma-linoleic acid and its metabolites also affect expression of various genes, thereby regulating the levels of gene products including matrix proteins. These gene products play a significant role in immune functions and also in cell death (apoptosis; Kapoor & Huang, 2006). Clinical trials using GLA in doses of 1,400 to 2,800 mg daily showed clinically relevant reductions in joint pain and morning stiffness as well as improvements in patient global assessment in RA (Cameron, Gagnier, & Chrubasik, 2011; Zurier et al., 1996). At doses used in this study, GLA appears to be well tolerated and could constitute adjunctive treatment for active RA. Long-term safety data, efficacy, and potential drug interaction remain unknown for GLA.

Curcumin (diferuloylmethane) is a polyphenol isolated from the rhizome of turmeric (*Curcuma longa*). In recent years, extensive in vitro and in vivo studies suggest curcumin has anticancer, antiarthritic, antiamyloid, and anti-inflammatory properties. The underlying mechanisms of these effects are diverse and appear to involve the regulation of various molecular targets, including transcription factors (such as NF-kappa B) (Funk et al., 2006; Goel,

Jhurani, & Aggarwal, 2008; Reuter, Gupta, Park, Goel, & Aggarwal, 2011). Translational studies support further clinical evaluation of turmeric dietary supplements in the treatment of RA (Funk et al., 2006). In periodontitis, curcumin effectively inhibited cytokine gene expression at mRNA and protein levels and dose-dependently inhibited activation of NF-kappa B in the gingival tissues (Guimaraes et al., 2011). Although curcumin is well tolerated, the in vivo bioavailability of curcumin is poor due to the hydrophobic nature of the molecule, poor absorption, and the metabolic biotransformation in intestine and liver. The use of adjuvants such as piperine, an alkaloid from black pepper, increases bioavailability by suppressing glucuronidation in the liver (Zhou, Beevers, & Huang, 2011).

Phytodolor, a German proprietary medicine containing a fixed combination of extracts from aspen leaves and bark (*Populus tremula*), common European ash bark (*Fraxinus excelsior*), and goldenrod herb (*Solidago virgaurea*) has been evaluated in clinical trials. Phytodolor is equally effective as standard nonsteroidal anti-inflammatory drugs (NSAIDs) in alleviating pain and improving joint function (Gundermann & Muller, 2007; von Kruedener, Schneider, & Elstner, 1995).

Tripterygium wilfordii Hook F (TwHF), better known as thunder god vine, is one of the most studied herbal interventions for RA. Root extracts of TwHF have been used in TCM to treat many inflammatory diseases; abundant diterpenoids, such as triptolide, are active components of TwHF (Mao, Tao, & Lipsky, 2000). An initial small trial of 35 patients with RA who had failed DMARD therapy, used a standardized extract of TwHF in low dose (180 mg daily), high dose (360 mg daily) and placebo over 20 weeks. The active groups had higher rates of ACR20, ACR50, and ACR70 responses, as well as reductions in ESR and CRP in the high dose group (Tao, Younger, Fan, Wang, & Lipsky, 2002). Another RCT evaluating TwHF against an active comparator indicated that TwHF might be superior to sulfasalazine (SSZ) (Goldbach-Mansky et al., 2009). In this study, 121 patients with RA were randomized to receive TwHF at 180 mg or SSZ at 2 grams daily. The adverse effects, which included nausea, vomiting, abdominal pain, and diarrhea, were similar in both groups. Interestingly, interleukin-6 (IL-6) levels rapidly and significantly decreased in the TwHF group (Goldbach-Mansky et al., 2009). Only 62% and 41% of patients continued receiving TwHF extract and SSZ, respectively, during the 24 weeks of the study. Questions linger about safety issues, as less standardized preparations of TwHF and the adverse effect profile make it an unappealing option given the efficacy and availability of biologics.

An extract of *Uncaria tomentosa* (cat's claw) was tested in 40 patients who were being treated with SSZ or hydroxychloroquine for their RA (Mur, Hartig, Eibl, & Schirmer, 2002). After 24 weeks of treatment, a modest reduction in number of painful joints with the extract was noted compared with placebo. Likewise, the evidence for the effectiveness of *Boswellia serrata* extracts in RA is encouraging but not compelling (Ernst, 2008). Oral feverfew (*Tanacetum parthenium*) and willow bark extract (*Salix* spp) do not appear to have beneficial effects in RA (Biegert et al., 2004; Pattrick, Heptinstall, & Doherty, 1989).

DIETARY FACTORS

The role of diet in the prevention and treatment of RA is a familiar question to most rheumatologists. Scientific data to illuminate this question are emerging. Pattison and colleagues (2004) reported the first prospective investigation of the association with meat intake and RA, and their data suggest a link between meat intake and the risk of inflammatory polyarthritis or RA, but this has not been confirmed in other studies (Benito-Garcia, Feskanich, Hu, Mandl, & Karlson, 2007). Many types of diets have been studied in RA. For example, the Mediterranean diet as a whole has been reported as a lifestyle factor reducing the risk of developing RA and protecting against severe course of the disease (Skoldstam, Hagfors, & Johansson, 2003). The role of dietary strategies such as fasting, followed by a vegetarian eating plan, vegan eating plans, and elimination diets as well as elemental eating plans remain uncertain, as high dropout rates and weight loss in the groups with dietary manipulation indicate potential adverse effects (Hagen, Byfuglien, Falzon, Olsen, & Smedslund, 2009; Smedslund, Byfuglien, Olsen, & Hagen, 2010). Some investigators suggest periods of modified fasting for 7 to 10 days may be beneficial in treatment of RA (Michalsen, 2013).

Other dietary factors of interest include the lack of an association between caffeinated coffee and daily caffeine intake and development of RA (Mikuls et al., 2002). However, interestingly, these investigators found that compared with those reporting no use, subjects drinking four or more cups per day of decaffeinated coffee were at increased risk of RA (relative risk [RR]: 2.58, 95% confidence interval [CI]: 1.63–4.06). In contrast, women consuming more than three cups per day of tea displayed a decreased risk of RA (RR: 0.39, 95% CI: 0.16–0.97) compared with women who never drank tea (Mikuls et al., 2002). Whether decaffeinated coffee contains an antigen or an immune-activating agent leading to autoimmunity or whether it is a confounder remains unknown (Bazzi, Portnoff, & Pischel, 2003). Green tea's active ingredient, epigallocatechin 3-gallate (EGCG), has gained significant attention among scientists. However, limitations of the dose, pharmacokinetics, and bioavailability of EGCG in experimental animals and EGCG–drug interaction require further preclinical studies before clinical trials can be undertaken in joint diseases (Ahmed, 2010).

Recently, vitamin D has been recognized as important for numerous extraskeletal functions, including immune function (Khazai, Judd, & Tangpricha, 2008). Available data suggest an inverse association between vitamin D intake (both dietary and supplemental) and risk of RA (highest versus lowest tertile RR: 0.67, 95% CI: 0.44–1.00, p-trend = .05) (Merlino et al., 2004). Greater intakes (highest tertile (>251 mg daily vs. lowest, <145 mg daily) of supplemental vitamin C (RR: 0.70, 95% CI: 0.48, 1.09; p-trend = 0.08) and supplemental vitamin E (RR: 0.72, 95% CI: 0.47, 1.12; p-trend = 0.06) have been found to be inversely associated with RA in subjects in the Iowa Women's Health Study (Cerhan, Saag, Merlino, Mikuls, & Criswell, 2003).

Other popular dietary approaches include intake of soy products (Dijsselbloem, Vanden Berghe, De Naeyer, & Haegeman, 2004; Mohammad-Shahi et al., 2011) and avoidance of dairy, however, there are no clinical trial data. Extracts of pineapple (bromelain) (Walker, Bundy, Hicks, & Middleton, 2002), cherries (McCune, Kubota, Stendell-Hollis, & Thomson, 2011), and garlic also have anecdotal evidence. A mixed antioxidant supplement containing alpha-tocopherol (400 mg), lycopene (10 mg), palm oil carotenoids (5 mg; mainly alpha-carotene), lutein (10 mg) and supplemental vitamin C (200 mg daily) was used in an open pilot study in nonsmoking RA subjects ($N = 8$) (van Vugt, Rijken, Rietveld, van Vugt, & Dijkmans, 2008). The number of swollen and painful joints was significantly decreased, and general health significantly increased, as reflected by the disease activity score (van Vugt et al., 2008).

My own approach for dietary advice is that it should be based on a woman's preferences and habitual foods. It is important to inform a patient about known relations between foods and disease, but also to support eating favorite foods, thereby facilitating a patient's sense of well-being (Gustafsson, Ekblad, & Sidenvall, 2005).

EXERCISE AND PHYSICAL ACTIVITY

Tai chi and yoga are complementary therapies that have, during the last few decades, emerged as popular treatments for rheumatologic and musculoskeletal diseases (Uhlig, 2012). Several studies show promise for yoga with improved outcomes in RA, not just in physical function and better sleep but also in self-care (Evans et al., 2013; Middleton et al., 2013; Ward, Stebbings,

Athens, Cherkin, & Baxter, 2014; Ward, Stebbings, Cherkin, & Baxter, 2013). The concept of self-care is quantified through collecting patient-reported outcome measures related to spiritual growth, health responsibility, interpersonal relations, and stress management (Middleton et al., 2013). Even a brief, 1-week yoga intervention was found to be beneficial with decreased disability (Telles, Naveen, Gaur, & Balkrishna, 2011). It is important for patients with RA embarking on yoga to inform the instructor and adapt the postures according to joint function and ability.

Participating in shared tai chi sessions can reduce anxiety and depression and improve self-esteem, self-efficacy, and motivation (Waite-Jones, Hale, & Lee, 2013). The highly structured nature of tai chi is also felt to improve memory and offers aesthetic experiences through developing graceful, "fluid" moves (Waite-Jones et al., 2013). Tai chi for RA appears to have beneficial effects on improved joint range of motion, better muscle function, and functional status (Han et al., 2004; Uhlig, Fongen, Steen, Christie, & Odegard, 2010; Wang, 2008), though not all trials show benefit (Uhlig, Larsson, Hjorth, Odegard, & Kvien, 2005). The issue of what constitutes an optimal tai chi program for RA remains unclear. Qigong, a related technique of gentle exercise can also be used to help maintain physical strength.

There are little data on Feldenkrais or Pilates as exercise options, although personally I have recommended these techniques to select women once their arthritis was in remission to help them maintain a good range of motion and flexibility. I also recommend aquatherapy. Many fitness centers have an arthritis foundation program for water exercise in warm pool under supervision of a qualified instructor.

HOMEOPATHY

There are few controlled clinical trials investigating the efficacy of homeopathic remedies in RA. Homeopathic consultations help patients with RA cope better through enabling improved physical health, well-being and/or illness management (Brien, Leydon, & Lewith, 2012). One review summarized three RCTs (N = 266) of homeopathic treatments for RA (Jonas, Linde, & Ramirez, 2000). Two studies evaluated classical individualized homeopathy in patients with RA and did not show beneficial effects (odds ratio [OR]: 2.04, 95% CI: 0.66 to 6.34), whereas positive effects were reported in the third trial. No single homeopathic remedy emerged as more effective than the other.

Two further RCTs found no evidence that homeopathy improves symptoms of RA in patients taking NSAIDs or DMARDs (Fisher, & Scott, 2001; Brien, Lachance, Prescott, McDermott, & Lewith, 2011). High-quality research is needed to clarify which patients with RA may potentially benefit from homeopathy.

ITEMS WORN

Therapeutic devices incorporating magnets are widely available and easy to use. Studies show that static magnets are not significantly different compared with control devices (Segal et al., 2001). Magnetism, which is difficult to conceal, necessitates the use of multiple control devices, including demagnetized wrist straps and copper bracelets, and represents a concerted attempt to overcome methodological limitations associated with trials in this field (Richmond, 2008). Wearing a magnetic wrist strap or a copper bracelet did not appear to have any meaningful therapeutic effect, beyond that of a placebo, for alleviating symptoms and combating disease activity in RA (Richmond, Gunadasa, Bland, & Macpherson, 2013). There are no data in support of the widely popular copper jewelry and crystals.

MASSAGE AND MANUAL THERAPY

Massage and other practitioner-driven manual therapies have been anecdotally reported to improve health-related quality of life in people with arthritis. Although there is empirical evidence that manual therapy is beneficial for some types of arthritis, the level of effectiveness is underresearched (Cameron, 2002). Investigation of once weekly massage for upper-extremity RA involvement showed that moderate pressure massage was superior to light pressure massage. By the end of the 1-month period, the moderate pressure massage group had less pain, greater grip strength, and greater range of motion in their wrist and large upper joints (elbows and shoulders) (Field, Diego, Delgado, Garcia, & Funk, 2013).

Reiki and healing touch can be very beneficial, especially for the elderly woman with RA. There are little data on these modalities, however, in my experience, these therapies can offer a sense of well-being, relaxation, and acceptance in some patients.

MIND–BODY

Mind–body integrative therapies are varied and include guided imagery, progressive relaxation, meditation, and hypnotherapy. Most trials using hypnotherapy suggest it can be useful in pain management, and pain perception, specifically, appears to be influenced positively (Horton-Hausknecht, Mitzdorf, & Melchart, 2000; Torem, 2007). There are reports of hypnotherapy as a treatment for juvenile RA (Cioppa & Thal, 1974; Lovell & Walco, 1989). In my own experience, a few patients have taught themselves self-hypnosis, which requires patience and practice but can help in coping with symptoms of joint discomfort and pain (Yocum, Castro, & Cornett, 2000). Similarly, guided imagery and visualization can be used successfully in some women with chronic symptoms, and children particularly can become adept at this technique (Walco, Varni, & Ilowite, 1992). There are high-quality audio recordings available that can profoundly help some women cope with chronic disease.

Mindfulness meditation (Zautra et al., 2008) and the popular mindfulness-based stress reduction (MBSR) (Pradhan et al., 2007) have been studied in RA. Patients with RA who have chronic depression benefited most from mindfulness meditation across several measures, including negative and positive affect and physicians' ratings of joint tenderness (Zautra et al., 2008). Significant improvements in psychological distress and well-being ($p = .04$ and $p = .03$, respectively) were observed following an 8-week MBSR class plus a 4-month program of continued reinforcement, indicating MBSR may complement conventional disease management (Pradhan et al., 2007).

Cognitive-behavioral therapies (CBT) include the teaching of life and coping skills and the application of these skills in the patient's home and work environment (Ottonello, 2007). Studies suggest that CBT is effective in RA not only for psychological adjustment but also for physical functioning and fewer long-term doctor visits, thereby potentially reducing healthcare costs (Sharpe, Allard, & Sensky, 2008).

Other mind–body techniques include muscle relaxation and music (Pothoulaki et al., 2008; Schorr, 1993) and spa therapy, which, although not rigorously tested in clinical trials, enjoy widespread popularity. Many patients have a standing appointment or receive a reduced cost on treatments, as they go on a regular basis.

Teresa regularly listens to a guided imagery tape. She has avoided increases in medications such as steroid therapy in the short term, as she is able to manage her level of joint pain with visualization. With practice, Teresa now has a skill that allows her to go to a "safe place" immediately whenever she perceives undue stress or pain.

DIETARY SUPPLEMENTS

Fish oil supplements have been discussed earlier in this chapter. Green-lipped mussel (*Perna canaliculus*) has been shown to have anti-inflammatory effects (Halpern, 2000). however, a recent systematic review found little compelling evidence for its use in RA (Cobb & Ernst, 2006).

Probiotic supplementation with *Lactobacillus casei* may be an appropriate adjunct therapy for RA patients, helping to alleviate symptoms and improve inflammatory cytokines (Alipour et al., 2014).

Patients with RA may lack the recommended daily intake of minerals such as calcium, zinc, and selenium (Stone, Doube, Dudson, & Wallace, 1997). It is recommended therefore that patients with RA receive dietary education or supplementation. If the patient is on methotrexate, folic acid is prescribed concurrently. Selenium has been tested in an RCT and no difference in pain, swollen joint count, or morning stiffness compared with placebo were found, although both groups improved, demonstrating a placebo effect of the interventional trial (Peretz, Siderova, & Neve, 2001).

Resveratrol, a phytonutrient present in grapes, blueberries, cranberries, and other plants, has been shown to have chondroprotective and anti-inflammatory effects on the synovial expression of matrix-degrading enzymes like matrix metalloproteinases (MMPs) and bone-remodeling proteins in RA fibroblast-like synoviocytes (Glehr, Breisach, et al., 2013; Glehr, Fritsch-Breisach, et al., 2013). There are no human trials of resveratrol in RA at the time of this writing.

> Teresa had to give up her career on stage as a dancer. Instead, she began to volunteer in youth groups, became very active in her church, and learned as much as she could about her condition. She has become an empowering voice for self-care in RA and was recently invited to participate in the production of a video series in wellness solutions for arthritis. Her husband and mother also have become involved in learning about RA and are an important source of support for her.

SPIRITUAL PRACTICE AND PRAYER

Underwood and Teresi note that positive emotional experiences and expectations have been linked with favorable effects on immune functioning, independent of the negative effects of stress (Underwood & Teresi, 2002). Spirituality, defined as a psychological dimension around which individuals organize their lives, goals, values, and intentions, was an independent predictor of happiness and positive health perceptions, even after controlling for disease activity and physical functioning, for age and mood (Bartlett, Piedmont, Bilderback, Matsumoto, & Bathon, 2003; Keefe et al., 2001; McCauley, Tarpley, Haaz, & Bartlett, 2008). On the other hand, negative religious coping (such as emotional venting) in persons with RA is significantly associated with depressive symptoms (VandeCreek et al., 2004) and can pose clinical challenges for the patient as well as her doctor. Religiously trained counselors may be helpful if the patient will accept a referral. Some patients may find it helpful to start a daily journal or diary to express their positive and negative emotions on paper (Keefe et al., 2001; Smyth, Stone, Hurewitz, & Kaell, 1999).

Resources for Healthcare providers

The Arthritis Foundation maintains a very informative website (http://www.arthritis.org) that includes a guide to alternatives therapies. In addition, *Arthritis Today* magazine is published monthly by the Arthritis Foundation and prints annual supplement guides that present information on vitamins, herbs, and natural remedies.

Summary and Conclusions

An integrative approach has the potential to improve the management of symptoms and inflammation in women with RA. From the evidence presented, it would be reasonable to consider fish oil, GLA supplements, and gentle exercise such as tai chi as adjuvant therapies. Importantly, mind–body techniques and CBT offer women with RA skills to cope with and thrive with chronic illness. Effective health promotion requires a partnership between the individual, the family, and the community, as well as the health provider. Integrative healthcare and an open dialogue about all treatment options are congruent with this goal.

Table 29.1. A Comprehensive Dashboard for Rheumatoid Arthritis

Physical	Educational	Psychological	Social
Diagnostic procedures	Instruction regarding medication (dosages, adverse effects, lab monitoring)	Aid in coping with: Depression, anxiety, and anger	Finances for medical and daily living
Disease modifying treatments—DMARDs and biological therapies	Methods of compliance	Address measures for coping with fatigue	Avoidance of isolation
Joint aspiration and injections	Smoking cessation	Low self-esteem and changes in lifestyle	Employment counseling
Immunizations	Oral hygiene and avoidance of periodontitis	Suggest:	Home care
-Influenza annually	Alcohol abstinence	-Guided imagery	Sexual counseling
-Pneumovax every 5 years after age 65 years	Use of orthotics/adaptive equipment	-Daily meditation	*Manual therapies*
-Tetanus/Diphtheria every 10 years	-Contraception in women of childbearing age	-Consider mindfulness-based stress reduction program (MBSR)	-Therapeutic or healing touch
-Herpes zoster vaccination >65 years	-Advice on breastfeeding and safety with DMARDs	-Daily journal writing	-Soft tissue massage
Infectious screening	Sleep hygiene counseling	*Managing chronic fatigue consider,*	
-Hepatitis panel	Weight control—fasting in select patients	-CoQ10	
-Tuberculosis screening	*Diet and supplements,*	-Chlorophyll supplements	
-Treat periodontitis	Whole foods, limit red meat intake	*Assess for associated fibromyalgia,*	
Primary prevention	Omega-3 supplements	New diagnostic criteria	
-Coronary artery disease (blood pressure and lipid control)	Gamma-linolenic acid (GLA) supplements		
-Osteoporosis prophylaxis guided by FRAX scores	Curcumin (turmeric) with black pepper		
-Annual eye examination on hydroxychloroquine	*Exercise*		
-Consider heart rate variability (HRV) measurement	Warm water aquatherapy		
-Age-appropriate cancer screening: mammogram and colonoscopy	Tai chi, qigong, and yoga under qualified instructor		
Management of extra-articular disease (e.g., sicca symptoms)	Consider energy medicine such as acupuncture and meditation to enhance vagus (parasympathetic) nerve activity		
Splinting (e.g., wrist splints for carpal tunnel syndrome)			
Adaptive equipment			
Podiatric treatment			
Joint surgery			

REFERENCES

Ahmed, S. (2010). Green tea polyphenol epigallocatechin 3-gallate in arthritis: Progress and promise. *Arthritis Res Ther, 12,* 208.

Aho, K., & Heliovaara, M. (2004). Risk factors for rheumatoid arthritis. *Ann Med, 36,* 242–251.

Aletaha, D., Neogi, T., Silman, A. J., et al. (2010). 2010 Rheumatoid arthritis classification criteria: an American College of Rheumatology/European League Against Rheumatism collaborative initiative. *Arthritis Rheum, 62,* 2569–2581.

Aletaha, D., & Smolen, J. S. (2009). The Simplified Disease Activity Index and Clinical Disease Activity Index to monitor patients in standard clinical care. *Rheum Dis Clin North Am, 35,* 759–772, viii.

Alipour, B., Homayouni-Rad, A., Vaghef-Mehrabany, E., et al. (2014). Effects of *Lactobacillus casei* supplementation on disease activity and inflammatory cytokines in rheumatoid arthritis patients: a randomized double-blind clinical trial. *Int J Rheum Dis.*

American College of Rheumatology. (2010). Report of the American College of Rheumatology Pain Management Task Force. *Arthritis Care Res (Hoboken), 62,* 590–599.

Ansar Ahmed, S., & Penhale, W. J. (1985). Talal N. Sex hormones, immune responses, and autoimmune diseases. Mechanisms of sex hormone action. *Am J Pathol, 121,* 531–551.

Ansar Ahmed, S., & Talal, N. (1989). Sex hormones and autoimmune rheumatic disorders. *Scand J Rheumatol, 18,* 69–76.

Arbuckle, M. R., McClain, M. T., Rubertone, M. V., et al. (2003). Development of autoantibodies before the clinical onset of systemic lupus erythematosus. *N Engl J Med, 349,* 1526–1533.

Bartlett, S. J., Piedmont, R., Bilderback, A., Matsumoto, A. K., & Bathon, J. M. (2003). Spirituality, well-being, and quality of life in people with rheumatoid arthritis. *Arthritis Rheum, 49,* 778–783.

Bazzi, A., Portnoff, K., & Pischel, K. D. (2003). Is decaf a decoy? Comment on the article by Mikuls et al. *Arthritis Rheum, 48,* 862.

Belch, J. J., & Hill, A. (2000). Evening primrose oil and borage oil in rheumatologic conditions. *Am J Clin Nutr, 71*(1 Suppl), 352S–356S.

Benito-Garcia, E., Feskanich, D., Hu, F. B., Mandl, L. A., & Karlson, E. W. (2007). Protein, iron, and meat consumption and risk for rheumatoid arthritis: a prospective cohort study. *Arthritis Res Ther, 9,* R16.

Biegert, C., Wagner, I., Ludtke, R., et al. (2004). Efficacy and safety of willow bark extract in the treatment of osteoarthritis and rheumatoid arthritis: Results of 2 randomized double-blind controlled trials. *J Rheumatol, 31,* 2121–2130.

Bijlsma, J. W., Huber-Bruning, O., & Thijssen, J. H. (1987). Effect of oestrogen treatment on clinical and laboratory manifestations of rheumatoid arthritis. *Ann Rheum Dis, 46,* 777–779.

Bingham, C. O., 3rd, & Moni, M. (2013). Periodontal disease and rheumatoid arthritis: The evidence accumulates for complex pathobiologic interactions. *Curr Opin Rheumatol, 25*, 345–353.

Brien, S., Lachance, L., Prescott, P., McDermott, C., & Lewith, G. (2011). Homeopathy has clinical benefits in rheumatoid arthritis patients that are attributable to the consultation process but not the homeopathic remedy: A randomized controlled clinical trial. *Rheumatology (Oxford), 50*, 1070–1082.

Brien, S. B., Leydon, G. M., & Lewith, G. (2012). Homeopathy enables rheumatoid arthritis patients to cope with their chronic ill health: A qualitative study of patient's perceptions of the homeopathic consultation. *Patient Educ Couns, 89*, 507–516.

Calderon Artero, P., Champagne, C., Garigen, S., Mousa, S., & Block, R. (2012). Fish oil metabolites: Translating promising findings from bench to bedside to reduce cardiovascular disease. *J Glycomics Lipidomics, 2*.

Cameron, M. (2002). Is manual therapy a rational approach to improving health-related quality of life in people with arthritis? *Australas Chiropr Osteopathy, 10*, 9–15.

Cameron, M., Gagnier, J. J., & Chrubasik, S. (2011). Herbal therapy for treating rheumatoid arthritis. *Cochrane Database Syst Rev, 2*:CD002948.

Casimiro, L., Barnsley, L., Brosseau, L., et al. (2005). Acupuncture and electroacupuncture for the treatment of rheumatoid arthritis. *Cochrane Database Syst Rev, 4*:CD003788.

Cerhan, J. R., Saag, K. G., Merlino, L. A., Mikuls, T. R., & Criswell, L. A. (2003). Antioxidant micronutrients and risk of rheumatoid arthritis in a cohort of older women. *Am J Epidemiol, 157*, 345–354.

Choi, H. K. (2004). Diet and rheumatoid arthritis: Red meat and beyond. *Arthritis Rheum, 50*, 3745–3747.

Chopra, A., Saluja, M., Tillu, G., et al. (2012). Comparable efficacy of standardized Ayurveda formulation and hydroxychloroquine sulfate (HCQS) in the treatment of rheumatoid arthritis (RA): A randomized investigator-blind controlled study. *Clin Rheumatol, 31*, 259–269.

Cioppa, F. J., & Thal, A. B. (1974). Letter: Rheumatoid arthritis, spontaneous remission, and hypnotherapy. *JAMA, 230*, 1388–1389.

Clowse, M. E. (2010). The use of anti-TNFalpha medications for rheumatologic disease in pregnancy. *Int J Womens Health, 2*, 199–209.

Cobb, C. S., & Ernst, E. (2006). Systematic review of a marine nutriceutical supplement in clinical trials for arthritis: The effectiveness of the New Zealand green-lipped mussel Perna canaliculus. *Clin Rheumatol, 25*, 275–284.

Costenbader, K. H., Feskanich, D., Mandl, L. A., & Karlson, E. W. (2006). Smoking intensity, duration, and cessation, and the risk of rheumatoid arthritis in women. *Am J Med, 119*, e1–e9.

Criswell, L. A., Merlino, L. A., Cerhan, J. R., et al. (2002). Cigarette smoking and the risk of rheumatoid arthritis among postmenopausal women: Results from the Iowa Women's Health Study. *Am J Med, 112*, 465–471.

Crowson, C. S., Liang, K. P., Therneau, T. M., Kremers, H. M., & Gabriel, S. E. (2010). Could accelerated aging explain the excess mortality in patients with seropositive rheumatoid arthritis? *Arthritis Rheum, 62*, 378–382.

Crowson, C. S., Liao, K. P., Davis, J. M., 3rd, et al. (2013). Rheumatoid arthritis and cardiovascular disease. *Am Heart J, 166*, 622–628 e1.

Crowson, C. S., Matteson, E. L., Davis, J. M., 3rd, & Gabriel, S. E. (2013). Contribution of obesity to the rise in incidence of rheumatoid arthritis. *Arthritis Care Res (Hoboken), 65*, 71–77.

Crowson, C. S., Matteson, E. L., Myasoedova, E., et al. (2011). The lifetime risk of adult-onset rheumatoid arthritis and other inflammatory autoimmune rheumatic diseases. *Arthritis Rheum, 63*, 633–639.

Cutolo, M., & Lahita, R. G. (2005). Estrogens and arthritis. *Rheum Dis Clin North Am, 31*, 19–27, vii.

Das, U. N. (2011). Can vagus nerve stimulation halt or ameliorate rheumatoid arthritis and lupus? *Lipids Health Dis, 10*, 19.

Davis, J. M., 3rd, & Matteson, E. L.; American College of R, European League Against R. (2012). My treatment approach to rheumatoid arthritis. *Mayo Clin Proc, 87*, 659–673.

Davis, M. C., Okun, M. A., Kruszewski, D., Zautra, A. J., & Tennen, H. (2010). Sex differences in the relations of positive and negative daily events and fatigue in adults with rheumatoid arthritis. *J Pain, 11*, 1338–1347.

Dijsselbloem, N., Vanden Berghe, W., De Naeyer, A., & Haegeman, G. (2004). Soy isoflavone phyto-pharmaceuticals in interleukin-6 affections: Multi-purpose nutraceuticals at the crossroad of hormone replacement, anti-cancer and anti-inflammatory therapy. *Biochem Pharmacol, 68*, 1171–1185.

Efthimiou, P., Kukar, M., & Mackenzie, C. R. (2010). Complementary and alternative medicine in rheumatoid arthritis: No longer the last resort! *HSS J, 6*, 108–111.

Ernst, E. (2008). Frankincense: Systematic review. *BMJ, 337*, a2813.

Evans, S., Moieni, M., Lung, K., et al. (2013). Impact of Iyengar yoga on quality of life in young women with rheumatoid arthritis. *Clin J Pain, 29*, 988–997.

Evrengul, H., Dursunoglu, D., Cobankara, V., et al. (2004). Heart rate variability in patients with rheumatoid arthritis. *Rheumatol Int, 24*, 198–202.

Field, T., Diego, M., Delgado, J., Garcia, D., & Funk, C. G. (2013). Rheumatoid arthritis in upper limbs benefits from moderate pressure massage therapy. *Complement Ther Clin Pract, 19*, 101–103.

Fisher, P., & Scott, D. L. (2001). A randomized controlled trial of homeopathy in rheumatoid arthritis. *Rheumatology (Oxford), 40*, 1052–1055.

Fredman, G., & Serhan, C. N. (2011). Specialized proresolving mediator targets for RvE1 and RvD1 in peripheral blood and mechanisms of resolution. *Biochem J, 437*, 185–197.

Funk, J. L., Frye, J. B., Oyarzo, J. N., et al. (2006). Efficacy and mechanism of action of turmeric supplements in the treatment of experimental arthritis. *Arthritis Rheum, 54*, 3452–3464.

Funk, J. L., Frye, J. B., Oyarzo, J. N., & Timmermann, B. N. (2009). Comparative effects of two gingerol-containing *Zingiber officinale* extracts on experimental rheumatoid arthritis. *J Nat Prod, 72*, 403–407.

Gagnier, J. J., Boon, H., Rochon, P., et al. (2006). Recommendations for reporting randomized controlled trials of herbal interventions: Explanation and elaboration. *J Clin Epidemiol, 59*, 1134–1149.

Glehr, M., Breisach, M., Walzer, S., et al. (2013). The influence of resveratrol on the synovial expression of matrix metalloproteinases and receptor activator of NF-kappaB ligand in rheumatoid arthritis fibroblast-like synoviocytes. *Z Naturforsch C, 68*, 336–342.

Glehr, M., Fritsch-Breisach, M., Lohberger, B., et al. (2013). Influence of resveratrol on rheumatoid fibroblast-like synoviocytes analysed with gene chip transcription. *Phytomedicine, 20*, 310–318.

Goel, A., Jhurani, S., & Aggarwal, B. B. (2008). Multi-targeted therapy by curcumin: How spicy is it? *Mol Nutr Food Res, 52*, 1010–1030.

Goldbach-Mansky, R., Wilson, M., Fleischmann, R., et al. (2009). Comparison of Tripterygium wilfordii Hook F versus sulfasalazine in the treatment of rheumatoid arthritis: a randomized trial. *Ann Intern Med, 151*, 229–240, W49–W51.

Guimaraes, M. R., Coimbra, L. S., de Aquino, S. G., Spolidorio, L. C., Kirkwood, K. L., & Rossa, C., Jr. (2011). Potent anti-inflammatory effects of systemically administered curcumin modulate periodontal disease in vivo. *J Periodontal Res, 46*, 269–279.

Gundermann, K. J., & Muller, J. (2007). Phytodolor: Effects and efficacy of an herbal medicine. *Wien Med Wochenschr, 157*, 343–347.

Gustafsson, K., Ekblad, J., & Sidenvall, B. (2005). Older women and dietary advice: Occurrence, comprehension and compliance. *J Hum Nutr Diet, 18*, 453–460.

Hagen, K. B., Byfuglien, M. G., Falzon, L., Olsen, S. U., & Smedslund, G. (2009). Dietary interventions for rheumatoid arthritis. *Cochrane Database Syst Rev*, 1:CD006400.

Hall, G. M., Daniels, M., Huskisson, E. C., & Spector, T. D. (1994). A randomised controlled trial of the effect of hormone replacement therapy on disease activity in postmenopausal rheumatoid arthritis. *Ann Rheum Dis, 53*, 112–116.

Halpern, G. M. (2000). Anti-inflammatory effects of a stabilized lipid extract of *Perna canaliculus* (Lyprinol). *Allerg Immunol (Paris), 32*, 272–278.

Han, A., Robinson, V., Judd, M., Taixiang, W., Wells, G., & Tugwell, P. (2004). Tai chi for treating rheumatoid arthritis. *Cochrane Database Syst Rev* 3:CD004849.

He, Y., Lu, A., Zha, Y., et al. (2007). Correlations between symptoms as assessed in traditional Chinese medicine (TCM) and ACR20 efficacy response: A comparison study in 396 patients with rheumatoid arthritis treated with TCM or Western medicine. *J Clin Rheumatol, 13*, 317–321.

He, Y., Lu, A., Zha, Y., & Tsang, I. (2008). Differential effect on symptoms treated with traditional Chinese medicine and western combination therapy in RA patients. *Complement Ther Med, 16*, 206–211.

He, Y. T., Ou, A. H., Yang, X. B., et al. (2014). Traditional Chinese medicine versus western medicine as used in China in the management of rheumatoid arthritis: A randomized, single-blind, 24-week study. *Rheumatol Int*.

Holman, A. J., & Ng, E. (2008). Heart rate variability predicts anti-tumor necrosis factor therapy response for inflammatory arthritis. *Auton Neurosci, 143*, 58–67.

Holman, H. R., & Lorig, K. R. (1997). Patient education: Essential to good health care for patients with chronic arthritis. *Arthritis Rheum, 40*, 1371–1373.

Horton-Hausknecht, J. R., Mitzdorf, U., & Melchart, D. (2000). The effect of hypnosis therapy on the symptoms and disease activity in Rheumatoid Arthritis. *Psychol Health, 14*, 1089–1104.

Janssen, K. M., Vissink, A., de Smit, M. J., Westra, J., & Brouwer, E. (2013). Lessons to be learned from periodontitis. *Curr Opin Rheumatol, 25*, 241–247.

Ji, R. R., Xu, Z. Z., Strichartz, G., & Serhan, C. N. (2011). Emerging roles of resolvins in the resolution of inflammation and pain. *Trends Neurosci, 34*, 599–609.

Jonas, W. B., Linde, K., & Ramirez, G. (2000). Homeopathy and rheumatic disease. *Rheum Dis Clin North Am, 26*, 117–123, x.

Julia, A., & Marsal, S. (2013). The genetic architecture of rheumatoid arthritis: From susceptibility to clinical subphenotype associations. *Curr Top Med Chem, 13*, 720–731.

Kanis, J. A., Johnell, O., Oden, A., Johansson, H., & McCloskey, E. (2008). FRAX and the assessment of fracture probability in men and women from the UK. *Osteoporos Int, 19*, 385–397.

Kapoor, R., & Huang, Y. S. (2006). Gamma linolenic acid: an antiinflammatory omega-6 fatty acid. *Curr Pharm Biotechnol, 7*, 531–534.

Karlson, E. W., Ding, B., Keenan, B. T., et al. (2013). Association of environmental and genetic factors and gene-environment interactions with risk of developing rheumatoid arthritis. *Arthritis Care Res (Hoboken), 65*, 1147–1156.

Karlson, E. W., Mandl, L. A., Aweh, G. N., & Grodstein, F. (2003). Coffee consumption and risk of rheumatoid arthritis. *Arthritis Rheum, 48*, 3055–3060.

Kasle, S., Wilhelm, M. S., & Zautra, A. J. (2008). Rheumatoid arthritis patients' perceptions of mutuality in conversations with spouses/partners and their links with psychological and physical health. *Arthritis Rheum, 59*, 921–928.

Kay, C. R., & Wingrave, S. J. (1983). Oral contraceptives and rheumatoid arthritis. *Lancet, 1*, 1437.

Keefe, F. J., Affleck, G., Lefebvre, J., et al. (2001). Living with rheumatoid arthritis: The role of daily spirituality and daily religious and spiritual coping. *J Pain, 2*, 101–110.

Keinan, D., Leigh, N. J., Nelson, J. W., De Oleo, L., & Baker, O. J. (2013). Understanding resolvin signaling pathways to improve oral health. *Int J Mol Sci, 14*, 5501–5518.

Kemp, A. H., & Quintana, D. S. (2013). The relationship between mental and physical health: Insights from the study of heart rate variability. *Int J Psychophysiol, 89*, 288–296.

Khazai, N., Judd, S. E., & Tangpricha, V. (2008). Calcium and vitamin D: Skeletal and extraskeletal health. *Curr Rheumatol Rep, 10*, 110–117.

Klareskog, L., Ronnelid, J., Lundberg, K., Padyukov, L., & Alfredsson, L. (2008). Immunity to citrullinated proteins in rheumatoid arthritis. *Annu Rev Immunol, 26*, 651–675.

Kolasinski, S. L. (2012). Herbal medicine for rheumatic diseases: Promises kept? *Curr Rheumatol Rep, 14*, 617–623.

Kovacs, W. J., & Olsen, N. J. (2011). Sexual dimorphism of RA manifestations: Genes, hormones and behavior. *Nat Rev Rheumatol, 7*, 307–310.

Lee, Y. C., Chibnik, L. B., Lu, B., et al. (2009). The relationship between disease activity, sleep, psychiatric distress and pain sensitivity in rheumatoid arthritis: A cross-sectional study. *Arthritis Res Ther, 11*, R160.

Lee, Y. C., Frits, M. L., Iannaccone, C. K., et al. (2014). Subgrouping of rheumatoid arthritis patients based on pain, fatigue, inflammation and psychosocial factors. *Arthritis Rheumatol.*

Li, E. K., Tam, L. S., Wong, C. K., et al. (2007). Safety and efficacy of *Ganoderma lucidum* (lingzhi) and San Miao San supplementation in patients with rheumatoid arthritis: A double-blind, randomized, placebo-controlled pilot trial. *Arthritis Rheum, 57*, 1143–1150.

Linos, A., Worthington, J. W., O'Fallon, W. M., & Kurland, L. T. (1983). Case-control study of rheumatoid arthritis and prior use of oral contraceptives. *Lancet, 1*, 1299–300.

Lovell, D. J., & Walco, G. A. (1989). Pain associated with juvenile rheumatoid arthritis. *Pediatr Clin North Am, 36*, 1015–1027.

MacDonald, A. G., Murphy, E. A., Capell, H. A., Bankowska, U. Z., & Ralston, S. H. (1994). Effects of hormone replacement therapy in rheumatoid arthritis: A double blind placebo-controlled study. *Ann Rheum Dis, 53*, 54–57.

Macfarlane, G. J., Paudyal, P., Doherty, M., et al. (2012). A systematic review of evidence for the effectiveness of practitioner-based complementary and alternative therapies in the management of rheumatic diseases: Rheumatoid arthritis. *Rheumatology (Oxford), 51*, 1707–1713.

Manek, N. J., Crowson, C. S., Ottenberg, A. L., Curlin, F. A., Kaptchuk, T. J., & Tilburt, J. C. (2010). What rheumatologists in the United States think of complementary and alternative medicine: Results of a national survey. *BMC Complement Altern Med, 10*, 5.

Mao, Y. P., Tao, X. L., & Lipsky, P. E. (2000). Analysis of the stability and degradation products of triptolide. *J Pharm Pharmacol, 52*, 3–12.

Margaretten, M., Julian, L., Katz, P., & Yelin, E. (2011). Depression in patients with rheumatoid arthritis: Description, causes and mechanisms. *Int J Clin Rheumtol, 6*, 617–623.

Margaretten, M., Yelin, E., Imboden, J., et al. (2009). Predictors of depression in a multiethnic cohort of patients with rheumatoid arthritis. *Arthritis Rheum, 61*, 1586–1591.

Markle, J. G., Frank, D. N., Mortin-Toth, S., et al. (2013). Sex differences in the gut microbiome drive hormone-dependent regulation of autoimmunity. *Science, 339*, 1084–1088.

Mathur, S., Mathur, R. S., Goust, J. M., Williamson, H. O., & Fudenberg, H. H. (1979). Cyclic variations in white cell subpopulations in the human menstrual cycle: Correlations with progesterone and estradiol. *Clin Immunol Immunopathol, 13*, 246–253.

McCauley, J., Tarpley, M. J., Haaz, S., & Bartlett, S. J. (2008). Daily spiritual experiences of older adults with and without arthritis and the relationship to health outcomes. *Arthritis Rheum, 59*, 122–128.

McCloskey, E. (2013). Assessing fracture risk in patients with osteoporosis. *Practitioner*, *257*, 19–21, 2–3.

McCune, L. M., Kubota, C., Stendell-Hollis, N. R., & Thomson, C. A. (2011). Cherries and health: a review. *Crit Rev Food Sci Nutr*, *51*, 1–12.

McQueen, F. M. (2013). Imaging in early rheumatoid arthritis. *Best Pract Res Clin Rheumatol*, *27*, 499–522.

Merlino, L. A., Cerhan, J. R., Criswell, L. A., Mikuls, T. R., & Saag, K. G. (2003). Estrogen and other female reproductive risk factors are not strongly associated with the development of rheumatoid arthritis in elderly women. *Semin Arthritis Rheum*, *33*, 72–82.

Merlino, L. A., Curtis, J., Mikuls, T. R., et al. (2004). Vitamin D intake is inversely associated with rheumatoid arthritis: Results from the Iowa Women's Health Study. *Arthritis Rheum*, *50*, 72–77.

Michalsen, A. (2013). The role of complementary and alternative medicine (CAM) in rheumatology: It's time for integrative medicine. *J Rheumatol*, *40*, 547–549.

Middleton, K. R., Ward, M. M., Haaz, S., et al. (2013). A pilot study of yoga as self-care for arthritis in minority communities. *Health Qual Life Outcomes*, *11*, 55.

Mikuls, T. R., Cerhan, J. R., Criswell, L. A., et al. (2002). Coffee, tea, and caffeine consumption and risk of rheumatoid arthritis: Results from the Iowa Women's Health Study. *Arthritis Rheum*, *46*, 83–91.

Mikuls, T. R., Payne, J. B., Yu, F., et al. (2014). Periodontitis and *Porphyromonas gingivalis* in patients with rheumatoid arthritis. *Arthritis Rheum*.

Mohammad-Shahi, M., Haidari, F., Rashidi, B., Saei, A. A., Mahboob, S., Rashidi, M. R. (2011). Comparison of the effects of genistein and daidzein with dexamethasone and soy protein on rheumatoid arthritis in rats. *Bioimpacts*, *1*, 161–170.

Morris, A., Yelin, E. H., Panopalis, P., Julian, L., & Katz, P. P. (2011). Long-term patterns of depression and associations with health and function in a panel study of rheumatoid arthritis. *J Health Psychol*, *16*, 667–677.

Mravec, B. (2007). Autonomic dysfunction in autoimmune diseases: Consequence or cause? *Lupus*, *16*, 767–768.

Mur, E., Hartig, F., Eibl, G., & Schirmer, M. (2002). Randomized double blind trial of an extract from the pentacyclic alkaloid-chemotype of uncaria tomentosa for the treatment of rheumatoid arthritis. *J Rheumatol*, *29*, 678–681.

Myasoedova, E., Crowson, C. S., Kremers, H. M., Therneau, T. M., & Gabriel, S. E. (2010). Is the incidence of rheumatoid arthritis rising? Results from Olmsted County, Minnesota, 1955–2007. *Arthritis Rheum*, *62*, 1576–1582.

Naz, S. M., Farragher, T. M., Bunn, D. K., Symmons, D. P., & Bruce, I. N. (2008). The influence of age at symptom onset and length of followup on mortality in patients with recent-onset inflammatory polyarthritis. *Arthritis Rheum*, *58*, 985–989.

O'Keefe, J. H., Jr., Abuissa, H., Sastre, A., Steinhaus, D. M., & Harris, W. S. (2006). Effects of omega-3 fatty acids on resting heart rate, heart rate recovery after exercise, and heart rate variability in men with healed myocardial infarctions and depressed ejection fractions. *Am J Cardiol*, *97*, 1127–1130.

Oke, S. L., & Tracey, K. J. (2009). The inflammatory reflex and the role of complementary and alternative medical therapies. *Ann N Y Acad Sci*, 172–180.

Omachi, T. A. (2011). Measures of sleep in rheumatologic diseases: Epworth Sleepiness Scale (ESS), Functional Outcome of Sleep Questionnaire (FOSQ), Insomnia Severity Index (ISI), and Pittsburgh Sleep Quality Index (PSQI). *Arthritis Care Res (Hoboken)*, 63(Suppl 11), S287–S296.

Ottonello, M. (2007). Cognitive-behavioral interventions in rheumatic diseases. *G Ital Med Lav Ergon*, 29(1 Suppl A), A19–A23.

Park, J., & Ernst, E. (2005). Ayurvedic medicine for rheumatoid arthritis: A systematic review. *Semin Arthritis Rheum*, 34, 705–713.

Parker, J. C., Smarr, K. L., Slaughter, J. R., et al. (2003). Management of depression in rheumatoid arthritis: A combined pharmacologic and cognitive-behavioral approach. *Arthritis Rheum*, 49, 766–777.

Partlett, R., & Roussou, E. (2011). The treatment of rheumatoid arthritis during pregnancy. *Rheumatol Int*, 31, 445–449.

Pattison, D. J., Symmons, D. P., Lunt, M., et al. (2004). Dietary risk factors for the development of inflammatory polyarthritis: Evidence for a role of high level of red meat consumption. *Arthritis Rheum*, 50, 3804–3812.

Pattrick, M., Heptinstall, S., & Doherty, M. (1989). Feverfew in rheumatoid arthritis: A double blind, placebo controlled study. *Ann Rheum Dis*, 48, 547–549.

Peretz, A., Siderova, V., & Neve, J. (2001). Selenium supplementation in rheumatoid arthritis investigated in a double blind, placebo-controlled trial. *Scand J Rheumatol*, 30, 208–212.

Perry, L. M., Winthrop, K. L., Curtis, J. R. (2014). Vaccinations for rheumatoid arthritis. *Curr Rheumatol Rep*, 16, 431.

Persellin, R. H. (1976). The effect of pregnancy on rheumatoid arthritis. *Bull Rheum Dis*, 27, 922–927.

Pothoulaki, M., Macdonald, R. A., Flowers, P., et al. (2008). An investigation of the effects of music on anxiety and pain perception in patients undergoing haemodialysis treatment. *J Health Psychol*, 13, 912–920.

Pradhan, E. K., Baumgarten, M., Langenberg, P., et al. (2007). Effect of mindfulness-based stress reduction in rheumatoid arthritis patients. *Arthritis Rheum*, 57, 1134–1142.

Proudman, S. M., James, M. J., Spargo, L. D., et al. (2013). Fish oil in recent onset rheumatoid arthritis: A randomised, double-blind controlled trial within algorithm-based drug use. *Ann Rheum Dis*.

Provost, M., Eaton, J. L., & Clowse, M. E. (2014). Fertility and infertility in rheumatoid arthritis. *Curr Opin Rheumatol*, 26, 308–314.

Quandt, S. A., Chen, H., Grzywacz, J. G., Bell, R. A., Lang, W., & Arcury, T. A. (2005). Use of complementary and alternative medicine by persons with arthritis: Results of the National Health Interview Survey. *Arthritis Rheum*, 53, 748–755.

Reuter, S., Gupta, S. C., Park, B., Goel, A., & Aggarwal, B. B. (2011). Epigenetic changes induced by curcumin and other natural compounds. *Genes Nutr*, 6, 93–108.

Richmond, S. J. (2008). Magnet therapy for the relief of pain and inflammation in rheumatoid arthritis (CAMBRA): A randomised placebo-controlled crossover trial. *Trials, 9*, 53.

Richmond, S. J., Gunadasa, S., Bland, M., & Macpherson, H. (2013). Copper bracelets and magnetic wrist straps for rheumatoid arthritis—analgesic and anti-inflammatory effects: A randomised double-blind placebo controlled crossover trial. *PLoS One, 8*, e71529.

Rohleder, N., Aringer, M., & Boentert, M. (2012). Role of interleukin-6 in stress, sleep, and fatigue. *Ann N Y Acad Sci*, 88–96.

Rosen, H. R. (2011). Clinical practice. Chronic hepatitis C infection. *N Engl J Med, 364*, 2429–2438.

Rubbert-Roth, A. (2012). Assessing the safety of biologic agents in patients with rheumatoid arthritis. *Rheumatology (Oxford), 51*(Suppl 5), v38–v47.

Rutger Persson, G. (2012). Rheumatoid arthritis and periodontitis—inflammatory and infectious connections: Review of the literature. *J Oral Microbiol, 4*.

Saydah, S. H., & Eberhardt, M. S. (2006). Use of complementary and alternative medicine among adults with chronic diseases: United States 2002. *J Altern Complement Med, 12*, 805–812.

Schorr, J. A. (1993). Music and pattern change in chronic pain. *ANS Adv Nurs Sci, 15*, 27–36.

Segal, N. A., Toda, Y., Huston, J., et al. (2001). Two configurations of static magnetic fields for treating rheumatoid arthritis of the knee: A double-blind clinical trial. *Arch Phys Med Rehabil, 82*, 1453–1460.

Serhan, C. N. (2011). The resolution of inflammation: The devil in the flask and in the details. *FASEB J, 25*, 1441–1448.

Serhan, C. N., & Petasis, N. A. (2011). Resolvins and protectins in inflammation resolution. *Chem Rev, 111*, 5922–5943.

Serhan, C. N., Chiang, N., & Van Dyke, T. E. (2008). Resolving inflammation: Dual anti-inflammatory and pro-resolution lipid mediators. *Nat Rev Immunol, 8*, 349–361.

Sharpe, L., Allard, S., & Sensky, T. (2008). Five-year followup of a cognitive-behavioral intervention for patients with recently-diagnosed rheumatoid arthritis: Effects on health care utilization. *Arthritis Rheum, 59*, 311–316.

Skoldstam, L., Hagfors, L., & Johansson, G. (2003). An experimental study of a Mediterranean diet intervention for patients with rheumatoid arthritis. *Ann Rheum Dis, 62*, 208–214.

Sloan, R. P., McCreath, H., Tracey, K. J., Sidney, S., Liu, K., & Seeman, T. (2007). RR interval variability is inversely related to inflammatory markers: The CARDIA study. *Mol Med, 13*, 178–184.

Smedslund, G., Byfuglien, M. G., Olsen, S. U., & Hagen, K. B. (2010). Effectiveness and safety of dietary interventions for rheumatoid arthritis: A systematic review of randomized controlled trials. *J Am Diet Assoc, 110*, 727–735.

Smolen, J. S., Aletaha, D., Bijlsma, J. W., et al. (2010). Treating rheumatoid arthritis to target: Recommendations of an international task force. *Ann Rheum Dis, 69*, 631–637.

Smyth, J. M., Stone, A. A., Hurewitz, A., & Kaell, A. (1999). Effects of writing about stressful experiences on symptom reduction in patients with asthma or rheumatoid arthritis: A randomized trial. *JAMA, 281,* 1304–1309.

Spite, M., & Serhan, C. N. (2010). Novel lipid mediators promote resolution of acute inflammation: Impact of aspirin and statins. *Circ Res, 107,* 1170–1184.

Sterba, K. R., DeVellis, R. F., Lewis, M. A., DeVellis, B. M., Jordan, J. M., & Baucom, D. H. (2008). Effect of couple illness perception congruence on psychological adjustment in women with rheumatoid arthritis. *Health Psychol, 27,* 221–229.

Stone, J., Doube, A., Dudson, D., & Wallace, J. (1997). Inadequate calcium, folic acid, vitamin, E., zinc, and selenium intake in rheumatoid arthritis patients: Results of a dietary survey. *Semin Arthritis Rheum, 27,* 180–185.

Szekanecz, Z., Mesko, B., Poliska, S., et al. (2013). Pharmacogenetics and pharmacogenomics in rheumatology. *Immunol Res, 56,* 325–333.

Taibi, D. M., & Bourguignon, C. (2003). The role of complementary and alternative therapies in managing rheumatoid arthritis. *Fam Community Health, 26,* 41–52.

Tam, L. S., Leung, P. C., Li, T. K., Zhang, L., & Li, E. K. (2007). Acupuncture in the treatment of rheumatoid arthritis: A double-blind controlled pilot study. *BMC Complement Altern Med,* 7:35.

Tao, X., Younger, J., Fan, F. Z., Wang, B., & Lipsky, P. E. (2002). Benefit of an extract of Tripterygium Wilfordii Hook F in patients with rheumatoid arthritis: A double-blind, placebo-controlled study. *Arthritis Rheum, 46,* 1735–1743.

Task Force of the European Society of Cardiology and the North American Society of Pacing and Electrophysiology. (1996). Heart rate variability: Standards of measurement, physiological interpretation and clinical use. *Circulation, 93,* 1043–1065.

Taylor-Gjevre, R. M., Gjevre, J. A., Nair, B., Skomro, R., & Lim, H. J. (2011a). Components of sleep quality and sleep fragmentation in rheumatoid arthritis and osteoarthritis. *Musculoskeletal Care.*

Taylor-Gjevre, R. M., Gjevre, J. A., Nair, B. V., Skomro, R. P., & Lim, H. J. (2011b). Improved sleep efficiency after anti-tumor necrosis factor alpha therapy in rheumatoid arthritis patients. *Ther Adv Musculoskelet Dis, 3,* 227–233.

Telles, S., Naveen, K. V., Gaur, V., & Balkrishna, A. (2011). Effect of one week of yoga on function and severity in rheumatoid arthritis. *BMC Res Notes, 4,* 118.

Torem, M. S. (2007). Mind-body hypnotic imagery in the treatment of auto-immune disorders. *Am J Clin Hypn, 50,* 157–170.

Tracey, K. J. (2002). The inflammatory reflex. *Nature, 420,* 853–859.

Treharne, G. J., Lyons, A. C., Hale, E. D., Goodchild, C. E., Booth, D. A., & Kitas, G. D. (2008). Predictors of fatigue over 1 year among people with rheumatoid arthritis. *Psychol Health Med, 13,* 494–504.

Turesson, C., Weyand, C. M., & Matteson, E. L. (2004). Genetics of rheumatoid arthritis: Is there a pattern predicting extraarticular manifestations? *Arthritis Rheum, 51,* 853–863.

Uhlig, T. (2012). Tai chi and yoga as complementary therapies in rheumatologic conditions. *Best Pract Res Clin Rheumatol, 26,* 387–398.

Uhlig, T., Fongen, C., Steen, E., Christie, A., & Odegard, S. (2010). Exploring tai chi in rheumatoid arthritis: A quantitative and qualitative study. *BMC Musculoskelet Disord*, *11*, 43.

Uhlig, T., Larsson, C., Hjorth, A. G., Odegard, S., & Kvien, T. K. (2005). No improvement in a pilot study of tai chi exercise in rheumatoid arthritis. *Ann Rheum Dis*, *64*, 507–509.

Underwood, L. G., & Teresi, J. A. (2002). The daily spiritual experience scale: Development, theoretical description, reliability, exploratory factor analysis, and preliminary construct validity using health-related data. *Ann Behav Med*, *24*, 22–33.

VandeCreek, L., Paget, S., Horton, R., Robbins, L., Oettinger, M., & Tai, K. (2004). Religious and nonreligious coping methods among persons with rheumatoid arthritis. *Arthritis Rheum*, *51*, 49–55.

van den Broek, M., Visser, K., Allaart, C. F., & Huizinga, T. W. (2013). Personalized medicine: Predicting responses to therapy in patients with RA. *Curr Opin Pharmacol*, *13*, 463–469.

Vandenbroucke, J. P., Valkenburg, H. A., Boersma, J. W., et al. (1982). Oral contraceptives and rheumatoid arthritis: Further evidence for a preventive effect. *Lancet*, *2*, 839–842.

VanDyke, M. M., Parker, J. C., Smarr, K. L., et al. (2004). Anxiety in rheumatoid arthritis. *Arthritis Rheum*, *51*, 408–412.

van Maanen, M. A., Vervoordeldonk, M. J., & Tak, P. P. (2009). The cholinergic anti-inflammatory pathway: Towards innovative treatment of rheumatoid arthritis. *Nat Rev Rheumatol*, *5*, 229–232.

van Venrooij, W. J., van Beers, J. J., & Pruijn, G. J. (2011). Anti-CCP antibodies: The past, the present and the future. *Nat Rev Rheumatol*, *7*, 391–398.

van Vugt, R. M., Rijken, P. J., Rietveld, A. G., van Vugt, A. C., & Dijkmans, B. A. (2008). Antioxidant intervention in rheumatoid arthritis: results of an open pilot study. *Clin Rheumatol*, *27*, 771–775.

Verstappen, S. M., & Symmons, D. P. (2011). What is the outcome of RA in 2011 and can we predict it? *Best Pract Res Clin Rheumatol*, *25*, 485–496.

Virgin, H. W., Wherry, E. J., & Ahmed, R. (2009). Redefining chronic viral infection. *Cell*, *138*, 30–50.

von Kruedener, S., Schneider, W., & Elstner, E. F. (1995). A combination of Populus tremula, Solidago virgaurea and Fraxinus excelsior as an anti-inflammatory and antirheumatic drug: A short review. *Arzneimittelforschung*, *45*, 169–171.

Waite-Jones, J. M., Hale, C. A., & Lee, H. Y. (2013). Psychosocial effects of tai chi exercise on people with rheumatoid arthritis. *J Clin Nurs*, *22*, 3053–3061.

Walco, G. A., Varni, J. W., & Ilowite, N. T. (1992). Cognitive-behavioral pain management in children with juvenile rheumatoid arthritis. *Pediatrics*, *89*, 1075–1079.

Walker, A. F., Bundy, R., Hicks, S. M., & Middleton, R. W. (2002). Bromelain reduces mild acute knee pain and improves well-being in a dose-dependent fashion in an open study of otherwise healthy adults. *Phytomedicine*, *9*, 681–686.

Walsh, D. A., & McWilliams, D. F. (2014). Mechanisms, impact and management of pain in rheumatoid arthritis. *Nat Rev Rheumatol.*

Wang, C. (2008). Tai Chi improves pain and functional status in adults with rheumatoid arthritis: Results of a pilot single-blinded randomized controlled trial. *Med Sport Sci, 52,* 218–229.

Ward, L., Stebbings, S., Athens, J., Cherkin, D., & Baxter, G. D. (2014). Yoga for pain and sleep quality in rheumatoid arthritis: A pilot randomized controlled trial. *J Altern Complement Med, 20,* A87.

Ward, L., Stebbings, S., Cherkin, D., & Baxter, G. D. (2013). Yoga for functional ability, pain and psychosocial outcomes in musculoskeletal conditions: A systematic review and meta-analysis. *Musculoskeletal Care, 11,* 203–217.

Wells, G. A., Li, T., Kirwan, J. R., et al. (2009). Assessing quality of sleep in patients with rheumatoid arthritis. *J Rheumatol, 36,* 2077–2086.

Xi Bao, Y., Kwok Wong, C., Kwok Ming Li, E., et al. (2006). Immunomodulatory effects of lingzhi and san-miao-san supplementation on patients with rheumatoid arthritis. *Immunopharmacol Immunotoxicol, 28,* 197–200.

Yocum, D. E., Castro, W. L., & Cornett, M. (2000). Exercise, education, and behavioral modification as alternative therapy for pain and stress in rheumatic disease. *Rheum Dis Clin North Am, 26,* 145–159, x–xi.

Young, L. D., Bradley, L. A., & Turner, R. A. (1995). Decreases in health care resource utilization in patients with rheumatoid arthritis following a cognitive behavioral intervention. *Biofeedback Self Regul, 20,* 259–268.

Zautra, A. J., Davis, M. C., Reich, J. W., et al. (2008). Comparison of cognitive behavioral and mindfulness meditation interventions on adaptation to rheumatoid arthritis for patients with and without history of recurrent depression. *J Consult Clin Psychol, 76,* 408–421.

Zhang, J., Chen, L., Delzell, E., et al. (2014). The association between inflammatory markers, serum lipids and the risk of cardiovascular events in patients with rheumatoid arthritis. *Ann Rheum Dis.*

Zhou, H., Beevers, C. S., & Huang, S. (2011). The targets of curcumin. *Curr Drug Targets, 12,* 332–347.

Zurier, R. B., Rossetti, R. G., Jacobson, E. W., et al. (1996). Gamma-Linolenic acid treatment of rheumatoid arthritis: A randomized, placebo-controlled trial. *Arthritis Rheum, 39,* 1808–1817.

30

Eating Disorders

CAROLYN COKER ROSS

CASE STUDY

Angela was admitted for treatment of bulimia nervosa and abuse of marijuana and cocaine. Her career as an actress had been affected recently by an increase in these behaviors after she began to have flashbacks, or memories, of childhood sexual abuse.

As a child, Angela was raised in a large Midwestern city by her mother. Her parents divorced when she was 5 years old, after which time her mother's alcohol use increased. Angela is the middle child and has two sisters. Angela is the only one of her siblings who attended college. As her mother's drinking increased, Angela found herself feeling more and more alone and "lost." While inebriated, her mother often raged at her children and was physically abusive to her older sister. Angela described her childhood years as "chaotic" and violent. Despite many career opportunities, Angela had difficulty with people she worked with, which affected her access to roles she might have enjoyed playing. She reported that binging helped soothe her anxiety and made her forget her fears. After each binge, she felt like a failure, out of control, huge, fat, and ashamed. Purging helped her release some of these feelings—at least for a short while.

An integrative medicine treatment plan for this patient would include therapy to address issues associated with being an adult child of an alcoholic, which may include attendance at 12-step meetings for adult children of alcoholics (ACOA). The patient's therapy should include the use of dialectic behavior therapy to teach Angela skills of emotional regulation and distress tolerance. For her bulimia, dietary supplements would be used to address nutritional deficiencies with a multivitamin, magnesium, and zinc; digestive issues would be supported with probiotics and digestive enzymes; and the need for mood stabilization with omega-3 fatty acids and a B complex vitamin. Massage and acupuncture can be used to decrease anxiety and depression. Starting the patient on a balanced diet with three meals a day and two protein snacks will help decrease binging. In addition to the above, medication may be warranted for treatment of mood disorders.

Introduction

Eating disorders constitute a spectrum of disorders from anorexia to bulimia and binge eating disorder (BED) dating back to the fourth century AD with the first report of a high-born Roman woman, a follower of St. Jerome, who died from anorexia. Religious women were actually canonized for their fasting practices in the service of religion and were called "holy anorexics." Self-starvation reached epic levels during the Renaissance, with approximately 181 deaths reported from anorexia between 1200 and 1600 AD. Many of these women were elevated to sainthood.

Prior to that, however, Roman culture described a phenomenon similar to bulimia nervosa. "Eat, drink and be merry" included the use of "vomitoriums,"[1] where a person could vomit and then return to the feast to continue eating and drinking. Ancient Egyptians used monthly purgatives to prevent sickness.

Anorexia was identified as a medical diagnosis in 1870 and bulimia in 1903. Currently, the American Psychiatric Association recognizes anorexia nervosa, bulimia nervosa, and binge eating disorder. The category EDNOS (eating disorder not otherwise specified), which formerly included binge eating disorder, has been replaced by other specified feeding or eating disorder (OSFED), and an additional category has been added for those who do not fit any of the above called unspecified feeding and eating disorder (UFED). Between 40% and 60% of those diagnosed with one eating disorder will cross over to another

---

1. There is conflicting evidence to support the use of the term "vomitoriums" by the Romans. In some accounts, "vomitorium" is actually the architectural term for passages designed for actors/participants to enter and leave stadiums and theaters. Aldous Huxley and others used the term "vomitorium" as I have here. It seems to be accepted that Romans did vomit after feasting, and this is thought to be a standard part of the feasting experience. There are also pictures of ancient basins called "vomitoriums" that may have been used for this purpose.

eating disorder diagnosis during their lifetime (Anderluh et al., 2008). Eating disorders, therefore, might best be considered a spectrum of illnesses, rather than discrete and fixed diagnoses.

Over the past several decades, the incidence of eating disorders has increased. The lifetime prevalence in women, as reported in a large-scale national study, was 0.9% for anorexia nervosa (AN), 1.5% for bulimia nervosa (BN), and 3.5% for binge eating disorder (BED). Women are three times more likely to develop anorexia or bulimia than men (Hudson, Hiripi, Pope, & Kessler, 2007). Sixty percent of those with BED, the most common of all eating disorders, are female, and 40% male.

The average duration of bulimia and BED is approximately 8 years each (Hudson et al., 2007). Over time, approximately 50% of those with AN or BN will recover, 30% improve somewhat, and 20% will continue to be chronically ill.

There is no one known cause of eating disorders. Dieting may increase the risk of an adolescent female developing an eating disorder by sevenfold (for moderate dieting) or 18-fold (for severe dieting) (Patton et al., 1999). A study on the island of Fiji demonstrates the influence of Western culture on eating disorders. Three years after television was introduced, 80% of Fijian girls expressed a desire to lose weight, with 11% using extreme measures such as self-induced vomiting (Becker et al., 2002).

Genetics may also play a part. Relatives of an individual with anorexia are 11.3 times more likely to have anorexia and over four times more likely to develop bulimia than controls (Strober et al., 2000). Binge eating disorder also shows a familial predisposition (Bulik, 2004). Twin studies show that if an identical twin has an eating disorder (anorexia or bulimia), the other twin's risk of developing an eating disorder is higher than it would be for fraternal twins or for a nontwin sibling (Costin, 2007).

ANOREXIA NERVOSA

Anorexia nervosa (AN) is associated with one of the highest mortalities of any psychiatric diagnosis (Palmer, 2003). There is an estimated 10% mortality in anorexics that have a 10-year disease history (American Psychiatric Association, 1994). Co-occurring alcoholism or drug addiction can increase mortality in anorexics. Increasing numbers of midlife women are developing AN for the first time or having a relapse of their eating disorder (Donaldson, 1994).

The current diagnostic criteria from the DSM-5 (*Diagnostic and Statistical Manual of Mental Disorders*) for AN have changed very little. Individuals diagnosed with anorexia are unable (as opposed to "refuse" as per the previous criterion) to maintain body weight, have significantly low body weight for their developmental stage, and have severe body image distortion. The criteria no longer require the absence of three consecutive menstrual cycles as a requirement (it was not a good correlate of weight loss and it left out many people with true anorexia who were male, who were prepubertal, or who were continuing to menstruate despite significantly low weight). The DSM-5 criterion has been expanded to include not only overt fear of weight gain but also persistent behaviors that interfere with weight gain. There are two subtypes of anorexia—restricting (where food is severely cut back) or the binge-purge type (restricting alternating with binging and purging).

BULIMIA NERVOSA

Bulimia is different from anorexia in that it involves binging with compensatory behaviors to avoid weight gain. Binges are defined as eating an amount of food that is larger than most people would eat in a small period of time (usually less than 2 hours). There must also be a sense of lack of control over eating during the binge. Compensatory behaviors can include excessive exercise, self-induced vomiting, fasting, and the use of laxatives, diuretics, or diet pills. The DSM-5 criteria require binges and compensatory behaviors to occur at least once a week (instead of twice weekly in DSM-IV) for 3 months. Another criterion is that the person's self-evaluation is unduly influenced by body shape and weight.

Bulimia nervosa usually begins after age 13 and its prevalence exceeds that of anorexia by the early adult years. There is a high co-occurrence of substance use disorders in those with eating disorders. Approximately 36.8% of those with BN will also have alcohol or drug abuse or dependence (Hudson et al., 2007).

BINGE EATING DISORDER

The criteria for BED include eating large quantities of food (more than most people would eat under similar circumstances) in a small period of time, loss of control over eating, and lack of a compensatory purge. Also included in the diagnostic criteria is eating in isolation, remorse or shame after eating, eating very rapidly, and eating when not hungry and past the point of fullness. Binge eating frequency required for diagnosis is at least once weekly for at least 3 months. Binge eating disorder often goes unrecognized as up to 25% of overweight or obese individuals seeking weight loss treatment have BED and 15.7% of those seeking bariatric surgery meet the criteria for BED (Mitchell et al., 2014; Pull, 2004; Stunkard, 2004). Binge eating disorder is less common than what is sometimes referred to as compulsive overeating but is much more severe. Binge eating disorder is also associated with other co-occurring psychopathology and more subjective distress related to eating behaviors.

EXCESSIVE EXERCISE

Between 20% and 54% of individuals with eating disorders also are excessive exercisers, with purge-type anorexia having the highest prevalence. Excessive exercise interferes with normal activities. It includes distress when unable to exercise, exercise for more than 3 hours per day, and exercise performed in inappropriate places or times and despite serious injury, illness, or medical complications. Exercise can be used for affect regulation and or as a compensatory mechanism to get rid of calories. The compulsive nature of excessive exercise is a predictor of associated disordered eating or eating disorders. This can be a serious behavioral issue in those with eating disorders due to its association with a higher risk for suicide (Goodwin et al., 2014; Shroff et al., 2006; Smith, et al., 2013).

OTHER SPECIFIED FEEDING OR EATING DISORDER

There are other disorders seen clinically that did not make it into the DSM-5, and most of these are included in OSFED. To be included under OSFED, the feeding or eating behavior must be significant enough to cause impairment in functioning without meeting criteria for the aforementioned eating disorders. These include purging disorder, in which people purge to reduce weight but do not binge; night eating syndrome, BN, and BED of lower frequency or more limited duration than ascribed by the diagnostic criteria; and atypical AN, in which there are anorexic features without low weight. Individuals with night eating syndrome are distressed by a problem with their sleep-wake cycle that results in them restricting their food intake during the day and then either eating most of their calories in the evening or waking up in the middle of the night to eat. Approximately 17.7% of individuals seeking bariatric surgery may meet criteria for night eating syndrome (Mitchell et al., 2014), which if undiagnosed, could undermine potential benefits of this surgery.

UNSPECIFIED FEEDING OR EATING DISORDER

This category includes anyone who does not fit any of the other criteria for diagnosis. An example would be a person who binges and purges but does not have the weight or shape concerns required for diagnosing bulimia nervosa.

Clinicians can also use this category when there is insufficient information to make a specific diagnosis.

> I am often asked, "What is the difference between binge eating disorder and compulsive overeating (CO)?" Those with BED tend to have more severe fluctuations in their weight, higher levels of body dissatisfaction, and tend to have started binging and dieting as a child (Sorbara, 2002). Those with BED also have a higher incidence of depression and anxiety (Delgado, 2002). When placed in a laboratory setting, patients with BED given permission to eat as much as they want, will tend to eat significantly more calories than those with CO (Walsh, 2003).

MEDICAL COMPLICATIONS

The medical complications associated with eating disorders affect multiple systems of the body and many are related to nutritional deficiencies. Table 30.1 offers a summary of medical complications. For more detailed information, see Garner and Garfield (1997).

Treatment: Integrative Medicine Approach to Eating Disorders

The cornerstones of an integrative medicine approach can include:

- Medical treatment that focuses on reducing the risk of, detecting, and treating complications of the disease and on improving overall health status
- Nutritional therapies to improve nutritional status, replace nutritional deficits, help women improve their relationship with food, and improve digestion and absorption of food
- Botanical therapies to treat insomnia and depression and reduce side effects of pharmacological therapies
- Body movement to enable patients to reconnect with physical cues; learn healthy behaviors, and modify the hyperactivity of the hypothalamic-pituitary-adrenal (HPA) axis
- Psychological testing to identify co-occurring diagnoses
- Coping skills training, including cognitive-behavioral therapy and dialectical behavior therapy

Table 30.1. Eating Disorders—Medical Complications

	Anorexia	Bulimia	Binge Eating Disorder
Symptoms	Amenorrhea, constipation, headaches, fainting, cold intolerance	Bloating, fullness, lethargy, GERD, abdominal pain, sore throat, abnormal menses	Constipation, GERD, fatigue, abnormal menses, PCOS
Physical Findings	Cachexia, acrocyanosis, dry skin, hair loss, bradycardia, orthostatic hypotension, hypothermia, loss of muscle mass and subcutaneous fat, lanugo. Underweight	Knuckle calluses, dental enamel erosion, salivary gland enlargement, cardiomegaly (ipecac toxicity). Can be normal or overweight	Overweight or obese
Laboratory Findings	Hypoglycemia, leukopenia, elevated liver enzymes, euthyroid sick syndrome (low TSH, normal T3, T4), Osteopenia	Hypochloremic, hypokalemic, or metabolic acidosis (from vomiting), hypokalemia (from laxatives/diuretics, elevated amylase (from vomiting)	Hyperlipidemia, hyperglycemia, Insulin resistance, Elevated androgens
ECG Findings	Low voltage, prolonged QT interval, bradycardia	Low voltage, prolonged QT interval, bradycardia	Variable

- Complementary and alternative therapies to improve sleep and enable patients to experience deep states of relaxation, which modifies HPA axis hyperactivity and contributes to body awareness and acceptance
- Prescription medications

What keeps me from feeling hopeless about these life-threatening and difficult-to-treat diseases is the recognition that an eating disorder is a way of coping with something that the individual has difficulty tolerating—a history of trauma, abuse, neglect, or their own emotional sensitivity. At all times, I keep in mind that there is a healthy self to work with and that this self is always striving to express its soul's purpose. I concentrate my efforts on connecting with and nurturing this soul self.

Medical Treatment

The most important initial therapy for all individuals with eating disorders is nutrition. For anorexics, weight restoration should include a weight gain goal of 1 to 2 pounds per week in an inpatient setting and one-half to 1 pound per week outpatient. Individuals with BN have their highest rates of recovery between 4 and 9 years after diagnosis, with 45% showing full recovery and 27% showing considerable improvement (Steinhausen & Weber, 2009). The proportion of individuals with BED 5 years after diagnosis declines to only 10% still having BED and 18% with any eating disorder at the 5-year follow-up (Fairburn, Cooper, Doll, Norman, & O'Connor, 2000). The management of eating disorders should involve a multidisciplinary team including internists and other medical specialists, dieticians, therapists/psychologists, dentists, and psychiatrists (Chakraborty & Basu, 2010).

Medication

The American Psychiatric Association advises that decisions about the use of medication should take a back seat to weight restoration, which may, by itself, improve symptoms of depression and anxiety. Studies on antidepressants used in patients with anorexia have been hampered by high dropout rates and small numbers. In one such study on the use of olanzapine for weight gain, the drug restored weight 2 weeks faster than placebo and was more effective for obsessive symptoms, but dropout rates were too high to draw clear conclusions from the study (Bissada et al., 2008). To date there is no proven benefit in treating the acute phase of AN with medication. In contrast, antidepressants including tricyclics, selective serotonin reuptake inhibitors, and monoamine oxidase inhibitors have shown a statistically significant short-term benefit in reducing binge eating and purging in patients with BN and BED (Agras, Dorian, Kirkley, Bruce, & John, 1987; Alger, Schwalberg, Bigaouette, Michalek, & Howard, 1991; American Psychiatric Association, 2006; Leombruni et al., 2008; Walsh et al., 1988).

Nutritional Therapies

In 1950, Ancel Keys demonstrated the impact of starvation on behavior and mood (Taylor & Keys, 1950). Further research has confirmed his findings and demonstrated that nutrition affects all bodily functions including blood pressure, cholesterol, and resting heart rate (Kalm & Semba, 2005).

Several studies have consistently demonstrated deficiencies in specific nutrients that affect energy, mood, and cognition. Those with eating disorders who restrict their intake may have deficiencies in calcium, iron, riboflavin, folic acid, vitamins A, C (Beaumont, Chambers, Rouse, & Abraham, 1981), and B6; and the essential fatty acids (Langan & Farrell, 1985; Rock & Vasantharajan, 1995).

Nutritional approaches are focused on replacing missing nutrients and treating comorbid conditions.

ESSENTIAL FATTY ACIDS

In the obese patient, omega-3 fatty acid consumption has a beneficial effect on insulin sensitivity and glucose tolerance. Use of this supplement also lowers serum triglycerides (Ebbesson, Risica, Ebbesson, Kennish, & Tejero, 2005). Omega-3 fatty acids have been well studied in the treatment of major depression and bipolar disorder, which are comorbid in eating disorder patients (Adams, Lawson, Sanigorski, & Sinclair, 1996; Cott & Hibbeln, 2001; Hibbeln, 1998, 2002; Noaghiul & Hibbeln, 2003; Peet & Horrobin, 2002). A small study demonstrated decreased aggressiveness and depressive symptoms in patients with borderline personality disorder, which is more prevalent in those with bulimia and BED (Zanarini & Frankenburg, 2003).

Dosage and Side Effects

Over-the-counter preparations offer approximately 1 gram of combined DHA and EPA, which can serve as a good starting dosage. Adverse effects include a theoretical increase in bleeding time with larger doses. Side effects can include a fishy burp and stomach upset. It can be kept refrigerated or given at bedtime to avoid these side effects.

B VITAMINS

B vitamins are vital to human nutrition because they transport oxygen to the brain and offer protection from oxidative stress. B vitamins also convert glucose from our food into energy and assist in the manufacture of neurotransmitters. Deficiencies in vitamin B12 and folic acid have been found in patients with eating disorders and depression and have been implicated in poor responses to antidepressant medication (Coppen & Bolander-Gouaille, 2005; Taylor et al., 2006; Table 30.2).

Dosage and Side Effects

Supplementation of all of the B vitamins is preferable to supplementing one or two. Folic acid supplementation should not exceed 1,000 µg/day because large doses can mask B12 deficiency (Institute of Medicine, 1998). Side effects include diarrhea and itching (B12), rash (folate) and flushing (niacin).

CALCIUM

Calcium is important in patients with eating disorders for prevention of bone loss and fractures. Bone loss can be the result of amenorrhea, use of laxatives, and alcohol abuse (Hirsch & Peng, 1996; Marcus et al., 1985; US Department of Agriculture, 1994–1996). The mainstay of prevention and treatment of bone loss in anorexia is weight restoration, nutritional rehabilitation, and spontaneous resumption of menstrual cycles (Golden, 2003). Recommended dose of calcium is 1,000–1,200 mg/day from all sources. Excessive intake of calcium supplements can lead to hypercalcemia, decreased kidney function, and decreased absorption of other minerals.

VITAMIN D

Vitamin D has traditionally been recommended for bone health, but recent studies show a role for vitamin D in enhancing immunity, maintaining muscle

Table 30.2. B Vitamins for Eating Disorders

	Recommended Daily Allowance for Women Over Age 19	*Toxicity Related to High Doses*
Folate	400–1,000 µg/day	May cause seizures in those on antiseizure medications
B6	1.5 mg/day up to 100 mg/day	Neuropathy of arms and legs: reversible when supplementation is discontinued
Niacin	14 mg/day	Hyperuricemia, hyperglycemia, teratogenicity, maculopathy
B12	2.4 µg/day	None known

strength, and reducing the risk of diabetes. The obese patient (BMI > 30) may have deficient circulating vitamin D because of sequestration in fatty tissue (Wortsman, Matsuoka, Chen, Lu, & Holick, 2000). Adolescents with eating disorders also have a high prevalence of vitamin D deficiency (Modan-Moses, et al., 2014). Vitamin D levels should be checked and corrected to achieve a serum level of >30 ng/mL. (See the American Endocrine Society guidelines for more information.)

PROBIOTICS

Probiotics are beneficial microorganisms that confer a health benefit. Levels of probiotics can be decreased by the use of antibiotics, alcohol and drugs, stress, and chronic constipation. The two most common types of probiotics available in supplements are *Lactobacillus* and *Bifidobacterium*. In a study of eating disorder patients in an inpatient treatment program, the use of probiotics and digestive enzymes reduced digestive complaints from 15% to 5% (Ross, Herman, & Rojas, 2008). The inclusion of yogurt in the refeeding program for individuals with anorexia may improve immunological markers in this immunocompromised population (Nova et al., 2006). Alterations in the gut microbiome may also play a role in the development of obesity (Lin et al., 2014).

Dosage and Side Effects

The usual dose of probiotics is 5–10 billion colony forming units (CFU) of live bacteria. Adverse effects are rare and usually limited to patients with severe immune deficiency or pancreatitis.

Herbs

VALERIAN

Valeriana officinalis is effective in the treatment of anxiety due to social stress (Kohnen & Oswald, 1988), generalized anxiety (Andreatini, Sartori, Seabra, & Leite, 2002), and insomnia. When compared with placebo, valerian resulted in a decrease in slow-wave sleep onset but did not show any benefit over placebo in 14 other end points (Donath et al., 2000).

Dosage and Side Effects

The recommended starting dose of valerian for insomnia is 900–1,600 mg taken about 30 minutes before bedtime. Side effects may include headache, gastrointestinal upset, dizziness, and low body temperature.

Mind–Body Therapies

Current research suggests that reversal or attenuation of the stress response plays a significant role in the treatment and prevention of disease. The HPA axis is thought to be hyperactive in individuals with eating disorders, perhaps as a result of childhood neglect or abuse (Birketvedt et al., 2006; Zonnevylle-Bender et al., 2005). Mind–body therapies such as biofeedback, meditation, progressive muscle relaxation, and guided imagery can help address this HPA axis hyperactivity.

Biofeedback was found to reduce nervous system activation when treating anorexic and obese, binge-eating preadolescent patients (Pop-Jordanova, 2000). Guided imagery produced a 74% reduction in binging and a 75% reduction in self-induced vomiting in 50 women with bulimia (Esplen et al., 1998). A study of 55 women with bulimia showed decreases in vomiting, body dissatisfaction, and depression in those assigned to a stress management group as compared with nutritional management alone (Laessle et al., 1991).

MASSAGE THERAPY

A review of studies on massage therapy, including its use in eating disorders, shows that massage decreases levels of cortisol by an average of 31%, increases dopamine by 31%, and serotonin by 28% (Field, Hernandez-Reif, Diego, Schanberg, & Kuhn, 2005). Massage therapy may decrease stress, lower anxiety, decrease body dissatisfaction, and increase dopamine and norepinephrine in women with anorexia (Anonymous, 2001). In bulimics, massage may decrease depression and anxiety, lower cortisol, and raise dopamine levels (Field, Schanberg, & Kuhn, 1998; Ohanian, 2002). Massage and other body-centered therapies have been useful in helping those with eating disorders shift their perception and reconnect to their bodies in a more positive way.

Given the paucity of research in the use of specific complementary and alternative medicine (CAM) therapies for treating eating disorders, I have quoted several of my eating disorder patients' experiences of CAM therapies:

"The meditation class helped me get back in touch with my spiritual connection, something I'd lost after my last relapse."

"When I practiced the breathing exercises, I felt my breath moving into my belly and I experienced a difference between the 'flesh' of my belly which I'd worried about for so long (wanting to have a flat belly) and the gratitude I have for how my 'insides' all work together."

"Massage was very spiritual for me and I found it vital to my recovery."

Other Components of an Integrative Medicine Approach

The integrative medicine approach to the treatment of eating disorders also may include the use of psychometric testing, body movement therapy, and skills training.

Psychometric testing with such tools as the Eating Disorder Inventory–3 (EDI-3) is used worldwide in clinical and research studies. The EDI-3 allows the clinician to have a baseline at presentation and a means for establishing change after treatment and also supports the differences between the different eating disorder diagnoses. The EDI-3 measures drive for thinness, bulimic behaviors, body dissatisfaction, maturity fears, perfectionism, difficulties forming close relationships, and the individual's ability to differentiate between sensations and feelings and between hunger and satiety. For example, research using the EDI-3 has shown that patients with anorexia exhibit a strong drive for thinness that is mediated by the need to control their anxiety and regulate their emotions (Fiore, Ruggiero, & Sassaroli, 2014).

The use of exercise/body movement in eating disorders associated with low weight has been controversial. Compensatory exercise is strongly linked to weight and shape concerns in individuals with eating disorders and to dietary restriction (Garner, Davis-Becker, & Fischer, 2014). A recent meta-analysis on this topic highlighted the paucity of good quality studies, but did show an overall benefit to aerobic exercise, yoga, massage, and basic body awareness therapy for both anorexia and bulimia. Individuals with anorexia may actually gain weight with supervised physical therapy, and those with either anorexia or bulimia had improvements in disordered eating (Vancampfort et al., 2014). In particular, yoga has been shown to reduce eating pathology and food preoccupation, improve self-awareness, reflectiveness and the ability to self-soothe (Carei, Fyfe-Johnson, Breuner, & Brown, 2010; Douglass, 2009). There is, however, a subset of individuals with eating disorders who engage in high levels of aerobic exercise, which can prolong the time it takes for them to recover during hospitalization (Solenberger, 2001). Individuals who are on the overweight or obese end of the spectrum should be encouraged to engage in physical activity that is sustainable over the long run and which will improve their cardiometabolic profiles.

Skills training is especially important in the treatment of eating disorders across the spectrum. Individuals with eating disorders often use food in a maladaptive way to regulate their emotions or deal with negative affect. Childhood trauma is one cause of emotional dysregulation in those with eating disorders (Moulton et al., 2014). Emotional dysregulation can present as lack of emotional awareness or as impulse control difficulties in those with anorexia (Racine & Wildes, 2013). The skill set offered by dialectical behavior therapy (DBT), which combines mindfulness with cognitive behavior therapy has been shown to be effective in reducing the number of binge/purge episodes and self-harm episodes in individuals with bulimia (Fischer & Peterson, 2014; Safer, Telch, & Agras, 2001). In extremely underweight individuals with anorexia, DBT reduced eating disorder symptoms; improved quality of life and weight gain, and reduced eating disorder-related psychopathology (Lynch et al., 2013).

Dialectical behavior therapy offers a systematic way to teach individuals with eating disorders ways to tolerate emotional distress, improve interpersonal relationships, learn mindful awareness and acceptance of reality, and regulate emotions. By learning to regulate emotions, individuals with eating disorders are less likely to act impulsively from their feelings, more able to identify emotions and have other tools besides eating disorder behaviors for managing their affect and mood. (For more information on the Integrative approach to eating disorders, see Ross, 2007, 2009.)

Outcomes

In a study of anorexic patients who were weight restored in an inpatient treatment center and followed for a median of 15 months after discharge, 35% relapsed (defined as body mass index less than 17.5 for 3 months). The highest risk for relapse occurred from 6 to 17 months after discharge. The predictors of relapse included history of a suicide attempt; previous treatment for an eating disorder; severe obsessive-compulsive symptoms on admission; excessive exercise resumed immediately after discharge and ongoing weight and shape concerns at the time of discharge (Carter, Blackmore, Sutandar-Pinnock, & Woodside, 2004). Lower percent body fat after weight restoration is associated with poor clinical outcomes in the first year after treatment in individuals with anorexia (Bodell & Mayer, 2011). Relapse for individuals with anorexia who were weight restored in treatment may also be related to how able they are to change their diets. Researchers found that continued avoidance of energy-dense foods and low diet variety were associated with poor outcomes (Schebendach et al., 2008).

Relapse from BN in a study of patients completing a day treatment program who achieved symptom control was 31% over the 2-year follow-up period. The majority of relapses occurred within the first 6 months. Predictors of relapse in this study included younger age, higher frequency of purging, a higher score on the bulimia subscale of the Eating Attitudes Test before treatment, and higher scores on the interpersonal distrust subscale of the Eating Disorder Inventory at the end of treatment. Frequency of binge eating, measures of self-esteem, depression, and social adjustment were not significantly correlated to relapse (Olmsted, Kaplan, & Rockert, 1994).

In a prospective study tracking the natural course of BN and EDNOS, the probability of remission by 60 months was found to be 74% for bulimia and 83% for EDNOS. Among patients in remission, the probability of relapse was 47% for bulimia and 42% for EDNOS (Grilo et al., 2007). The degree of body image distortion has also been shown to be a predictor for relapse in bulimics and anorexics (Keel & Semba, 2005).

Studies on individuals with BED have shown some ability to predict risk of relapse on the basis of eating and shape concerns, depressive symptoms, and the overall severity of general psychopathology, including poor interpersonal skills pretreatment and at the midpoint of treatment (Dingemans, Spinhoven, & van Furth, 2007; Hilbert et al., 2007).

Conclusion

Eating disorders comprise a spectrum of disorders that are difficult to treat and have a high risk for morbidity and mortality. The integrative medicine approach offers many options to explore. While research into these therapies is still in the early stages, the benefit to risk ratio is favorable. Recovery from an eating disorder is possible, and the earlier individuals with these disorders are treated, the better the prognosis. The greatest value that physicians can offer to patients with eating disorders is the belief inherent in integrative medicine that the body, mind, and spirit all have the capacity for self-healing.

References

Adams, P. B., Lawson, S., Sanigorski, A., & Sinclair, A. J. (1996). Arachidonic acid to eicosapentaenoic acid ratio in blood correlates positively with clinical symptoms of depression. *Lipids, 31,* S157–S161.

Agras, W. S., Dorian, B., Kirkley, B. G., Bruce, A., & John, B. (1987). Imipramine in the treatment of bulimia: A double-blind controlled study. *Int J Eat Disord, 6,* 29–38.

Alger, S. A., Schwalberg, M. D., Bigaouette, J. M., Michalek, A. V., & Howard, L. J. (1991). Effect of a tricyclic antidepressant and opiate antagonist on binge-eating behavior in normoweight bulimic and obese, binge eating subjects. *Am J Clin Nutr, 53,* 865–871.

American Psychiatric Association. (1994). *Diagnostic and statistical manual of mental disorders.* 4th ed. Washington, DC: Author.

American Psychiatric Association. (2006). *Practice guideline for the treatment of patients with eating disorders* (3rd ed.). Washington, DC: Author

Anderluh, M., Tchanturia, K., Rabe-Hesketh, S., Collier, D., & Treasure, J. (2008). Lifetime course of eating disorders: Design and validity testing of a new strategy to define the eating disorders phenotype. *Psychol Med, 1,* 1–10. [Epub ahead of print]

Andreatini, R., Sartori, V. A., Seabra, M. L., & Leite, J. R. (2002). Effect of valepotriates (valerian extract) in generalized anxiety disorder: A randomized placebo-controlled pilot study. *Phytother Res, 16,* 650–654.

Anonymous. (2001). Anorexia nervosa symptoms are reduced by massage therapy. *Eat Disord, 9,* 289–299.

Beaumont, P. J., Chambers, T. L., Rouse, L., & Abraham, S. F. (1981). The diet composition and nutritional knowledge of patients with anorexia nervosa. *J Hum Nutr, 35,* 265–272.

Becker, A., Burwell, S., Gilman, D., et al. (2002). Eating behavior and attitudes following prolonged exposure to television among ethnic Fijian girls. *Br J Psychiatry, 180,* 509–514.

Birketvedt, G. S., Drivenes, E., Agledahl, I., Sundsfjord, J., Olstad, R., & Florholmen, J. R. (2006). Bulimia nervosa: A primary defect in the hypothalamic-pituitary-adrenal axis? *Appetite, 46,* 164–167.

Bissada, H., Tasca, G. A., Barber, A. M., Bradwein, J. (2008). Olanzapine in the treatment of low body weight and obsessive thinking in women with anorexia nervosa: A randomized, double-blind, placebo-controlled trial. *Am J Psychiatry, 165*(10), 1281-1288.

Bodell, L. P., & Mayer, L. E. (2011). Percent body fat is a risk factor for relapse in anorexia nervosa. *Int J Eat Disord, 44,* 118–123.

Bulik, C. M. (2004). Role of genetics in anorexia nervosa, bulimia nervosa and binge eating disorder. In T. Brewerton (Ed.), *Clinical handbook of eating disorders*. New York: Marcel Dekker.

Carei, T. R., Fyfe-Johnson, A., Breuner, C. C., & Brown, M. A. (2010). Randomized controlled clinical trial of yoga in the treatment of eating disorders. *J Adolesc Health, 46,* 346–351.

Carter, J. C., Blackmore, E., Sutandar-Pinnock, K., & Woodside, D. B. (2004). Relapse in anorexia nervosa: a survival analysis. *Psychol Med, 34,* 671–679.

Chakraborty, K., & Basu, D. (2010). Management of anorexia and bulimia nervosa: An evidence-based review. *Indian J Psychiatry, 52,* 174–186.

Coppen, A., & Bolander-Gouaille, C. (2005). Treatment of depression: Time to consider folic acid and B12. *J Psychopharmacol, 19,* 59–65.

Costin, C. (2007). *The eating disorder sourcebook* (3rd ed.). New York, NY: McGraw Hill.

Cott, J., & Hibbeln, J. R. (2001). Lack of seasonal mood change in Icelanders. *Am J Psychiatry, 158,* 328.

Delgado, C. C, Morales Gorria, M. J., Maruri Chimeno, I., et al. (2002). Eating behavior, body attitudes and psychopathology in morbid obesity. *Actas Esp Psiquitr, 30,* 376–381.

Dingemans, A. E., Spinhoven, P., & van Furth, E. F. (2007). Predictors and mediators of treatment outcome in patients with binge eating disorder. *Behav Res Ther, 45,* 2551–2562.

Donaldson, G. A. (1994). *Body image in women at midlife*. Dissertation. Boston College. AAT 9510315.

Donath, F., Quispe, S., Diefenbach, K., Maurer, A., Fietze, I., & Roots, I. (2000). Critical evaluation of the effect of valerian extract on sleep structure and sleep quality. *Pharmacopsychiatry, 33,* 47–53.

Douglass, L. (2009). Yoga as an intervention in the treatment of eating disorders: Does it help? *Eat Disord, 17,* 126–139.

Ebbesson, S. O., Risica, P. M., Ebbesson, L. O., Kennish, J. M., & Tejero, M. E. (2005). Omega-3 fatty acids improve glucose tolerance and components of the metabolic syndrome in Alaskan Eskimos: The Alaska Siberia Project. *Int J Circumpolar Health, 64,* 396–408.

Esplen, M. J., Garfinkel, P. E., Olmsted, M., et al. (1998). A randomized controlled trial of guided imagery in bulimia nervosa. *Psychol Med, 28,* 1347–1357.

Fairburn, C. G., Cooper, Z., Doll, H. A., Norman, P., & O'Connor, M. (2000). The natural course of bulimia nervosa and binge eating disorder in young women. *Arch Gen Psychiatry, 57,* 659–665.

Field, T., Hernandez-Reif, M., Diego, M., Schanberg, S., & Kuhn, C. (2005). Cortisol decreases and serotonin and dopamine increase following massage therapy. *Int J Neurosci, 115,* 1397–1413.

Field, T., Schanberg, S., & Kuhn, C. (1998). Bulimic adolescents benefit from massage therapy. *Adolescence, 33,* 555–563.

Fiore, F., Ruggiero, G. M., & Sassaroli, S. (2014). Emotional dysregulation and anxiety control in the psychopathological mechanism underlying drive for thinness. *Front Psychiatry*, 5, 43.

Fischer, S., & Peterson, C. (2014). Dialectical behavior therapy for adolescent binge eating, purging, suicidal behavior and non-suicidal self-injury: A pilot study. *Psychotherapy (Chic)*. [Epub ahead of print]

Garner, A., Davis-Becker, K., & Fischer, S. (2014). An exploration of the influence of thinness expectancies and eating pathology on compensatory exercise. *Eat Behav*, 15, 335–338.

Garner, D. M., & Garfinkel, P. E. (Eds). (1997). *Handbook of treatment for eating disorders* (2nd ed.) New York, NY. Guilford Press.

Golden, N. H. (2003). Osteopenia and osteoporosis in anorexia nervosa. *Adolesc Med*, 14, 97–108.

Goodwin, H., Haycraft, E., Meyer, C. (2014). Emotional regulation styles as longitudinal predictors of compulsive exercise: A twelve month prospective study. *J Adolesc*, 37(8), 1399–1404.

Grilo, C. M., Pagano, M. E., Skodol, A. E., et al. (2007). Natural course of bulimia nervosa and of eating disorder not otherwise specified: 5-year prospective study of remissions, relapses, and the effects of personality disorder psychopathology. *J Clin Psychiatr*, 68, 738–746.

Hibbeln, J. R. (1998). Fish consumption and major depression. *Lancet*, 351, 1213.

Hibbeln, J. R. (2002). Seafood consumption, the DHA content of mothers' milk and prevalence rates of postpartum depression: A cross-national, ecological analysis. *J Affect Disord*, 69, 15–29.

Hilbert, A., Saelens, B. E., Stein, R. I., et al. (2007). Pretreatment and process predictors of outcome in interpersonal and cognitive behavioral psychotherapy for binge eating disorder. *J Clin Psychol*, 75, 645–651.

Hirsch, P. E., & Peng, T. C. (1996). Effects of alcohol on calcium homeostasis and bone. In J. Anderson & S. Garner (Eds.), *Calcium and phosphorus in health and disease* (pp. 289–300). Boca Raton, FL: CRC Press.

Hudson, J. I., Hiripi, E., Pope, H. G., & Kessler, R. C. (2007). The prevalence and correlates of eating disorders in the national comorbidity survey replication. *Biol Psychiatry*, 61, 348–358.

Institute of Medicine. (1998). *Food and Nutrition Board. Dietary reference intakes: Thiamin, riboflavin, niacin, vitamin B6, folate, vitamin B12, pantothenic acid, biotin, and choline.* Washington, DC: National Academy Press.

Kalm, L. M., & Semba, R. D. (2005). They starved so that others could be better fed: Remembering Ancel Keys and the Minnesota Experiment. *Am Soc Nutr Sci J Nutr*, 135, 1347–1352.

Keel, P. K., Dorer, D. J., Franko, D. L., Jackson, S. C., & Herzog, D. B. (2005). Postremission predictors of relapse in women with eating disorders. *Am J Psychiatry*, 162, 2263–2268.

Kohnen, R., & Oswald, W. D. (1988). The effects of valerian, propranolol and their combination on activation, performance and mood of healthy volunteers under social stress conditions. *Pharmacopsychiatry*, *21*, 447–4488.

Laessle, R. G., Beaumont, P. J., Butow, P., et al. (1991). A comparison of nutritional management with stress management in the treatment of bulimia nervosa. *Br J Psychiatry*, *159*, 250–261.

Langan, S. M., & Farrell, P. M. (1985). Vitamin E, vitamin A and essential fatty acid status of patients hospitalized with anorexia nervosa. *Am J Clin Nutr*, *41*, 1054–1060.

Leombruni, P., Piero, A., Lavagnino, L., Brustolin, A., Campisi, S., & Fassino, S. (2008). A randomized, double-blind trial comparing sertraline and fluoxetine 6-month treatment in obese patients with Binge Eating Disorder. *Prog Neuropsychopharmacol Biol Psychiatry*. [Epub ahead of print]

Lin, C. S., Chang, C. J., Lu, C. C., et al. (2014). Impact of the gut microbiota, prebiotics and probiotics on human health and disease. *Biomed J*. [Epub ahead of print]

Lynch, T. R., Gray, K. L., Hempel, R. J., et al. (2013). Radically open-dialectical behavior therapy for adult anorexia nervosa: Feasibility and outcomes from an inpatient program. *BMC Psychiatry*, *13*, 293.

Marcus, R., Cann, C., Madvig, P., et al. (1985). Menstrual function and bone mass in elite women distance runners: Endocrine and metabolic features. *Ann Intern Med*, *102*, 158–163.

Mitchell, J. E., King, W. C., Courcoulas, A., et al. (2014). Eating behavior and eating disorders in adults before bariatric surgery. *Int J Eat Disord*. [Epub ahead of print]

Modan-Moses, D., Levy-Shraga, Y., Pinhas-Hamiel O., et al. (2014). The prevalence of vitamin D deficiency and insufficiency in adolescent inpatients diagnosed with eating disorders. *Int J Eat Disord*. [Epub ahead of print]

Moulton, S. J., Newman, E., Power, K., et al. (2014). Childhood trauma and eating psychopathology: A mediating role for dissociation and emotion dysregulation? *Child Abuse Negl*. [Epub ahead of print]

Noaghiul, S., & Hibbeln, J. R. (2003). Cross-national comparisons of seafood consumption and rates of bipolar disorders. *Am J Psychiatry*, *160*, 2222–2227.

Nova, E., Toro, O., Varela, P., et al. (2006). Effects of a nutritional intervention with yogurt on lymphocyte subsets and cytokine production capacity in anorexia nervosa patients. *Eur J Nutr*, *45*, 225–233.

Ohanian, V. (2002). Imagery rescripting within cognitive behavior therapy for bulimia nervosa: An illustrative case. *Int J Eat Disord*, *31*, 352–357.

Olmsted, M. P., Kaplan, A. S., & Rockert, W. (1994). Rate and prediction of relapse in bulimia nervosa. *Am J Psychiatry*, *151*, 738–743.

Palmer, R. L. (2003). Death in anorexia nervosa. *Lancet*, *361*, 1490.

Patton, G. C., Selzer, R., Coffey, C., et al. (1999). Onset of adolescent eating disorders: Population based cohort study over 3 years. *BMJ*, *318*, 765–768.

Peet, M., & Horrobin, D. F. (2002). A dose-ranging study of the effects of ethyl-eicosapentaenoate in patients with ongoing depression despite apparently adequate treatment with standard drugs. *Arch Gen Psychiatry*, *59*, 913–919.

Pop-Jordanova, N. (2000). Psychological characteristics and biofeedback mitigation in preadolescents with eating disorders. *Pediatr Int, 42,* 76–81.

Pull, C. P. (2004). Binge eating disorder. *Curr Opin Psychiatr, 17,* 43–48.

Racine, S. E., & Wildes, J. E. (2013). Emotion dysregulation and symptoms of anorexia nervosa: The unique roles of lack of emotional awareness and impulse control difficulties when upset. *Int J Eat Disord, 46,* 713–720.

Rock, C. L., & Vasantharajan, S. (1995). Vitamin status of eating disorder patients: Relationship to clinical indices and effect of treatment. *Int J Eat Disord, 18,* 257–262.

Ross, C. C. (2007). *Healing body, mind and spirit: An integrative medicine approach to the treatment of eating disorders.* Denver, CO: Outskirts Press.

Ross, C. C. (2009). *The binge eating and compulsive overeating workbook.* Oakland, CA: New Harbinger.

Ross, C. C., Herman, P., & Rojas, J. (2008). Integrative medicine for eating disorders. *Explore J Sci Heal, 4,* 315–320.

Safer, D. L., Telch, C. F., & Agras, W. S. (2001). Dialectical behavior therapy for bulimia nervosa. *Am J Psychiatry, 158,* 632–634.

Schebendach, J. E., Mayer, L. E., Devlin, M. J., et al. (2008). Dietary energy density and diet variety as predictors of outcome in anorexia nervosa. *J Clin Nutr, 87,* 810–816.

Shroff, H., Reba, L., Thornton, L. M., et al. (2006). Features associated with excessive exercise in women with eating disorders. *Int J Eat Disord, 39*(6), 454–461.

Solenberger, S. E. (2001). Exercise and eating disorders: A 3-year inpatient hospital record analysis. *Eat Behav, 2,* 151–168.

Smith, A. R., Fink, E. L., Anestis, M. D., et al. (2013). Exercise caution: Over-exercise is associated with suicidality among individuals with disordered eating. *Psychiatry Res, 206*(2–3), 246–255.

Steinhausen, H.-C., & Weber, S. (2009). The outcome of bulimia nervosa: Findings from one-quarter century of research. *Am J Psychiatry, 166,* 1331–1341

Sorbara, M., & Geliebter, A. (2002). Body image disturbance in obese outpatients before and after weight loss in relation to race, gender, binge eating, and age of onset of obesity. *Int J Eat Disord, 31,* 416–423.

Strober, M., Freeman, R., Lampert, C., Diamond, J., & Kaye, W. (2000). Controlled family study of anorexia nervosa and bulimia nervosa: Evidence of shared liability and transmission of partial syndromes. *Am J Psychiatry, 157,* 393–401.

Stunkard, A. J. (2004). Binge-eating disorder and the night-eating syndrome. In T. A. Wadden & A. J. Stunkard, (Eds.), *Handbook of obesity treatment.* New York: Guilford Press.

Taylor, H. L., & Keys, A. (1950). Adaptation to caloric restriction. *Science, 25,* 215–218.

Taylor, M. J., Carney, S., Geddes, J., et al. (2006). Folate for depressive disorders. *Cochrane Database of Systematic Reviews, 2.* doi: 10.1002/14651858.CD003390

U.S. Department of Agriculture. (1994–1996). *Results from the United States Department of Agriculture's 1994-1996 Continuing Survey of Food Intakes by Individuals/Diet and Health Knowledge Survey.* http://www.barc.usda.gov/bhnrc/foodsurvey/Products9496.html#foodandnutrientintakes

Vancampfort, D., Vanderlinden, J., De Hert, M., et al. (2014). A systematic review of physical therapy interventions for patients with anorexia and bulimia nervosa. *Disabil Rehabil, 36,* 628–634.

Walsh, B. T., & Boudreau, G. (2003). Laboratory studies of binge eating disorder. *Int J Eat Disord, 34*(Suppl), S30–S38.

Walsh, B. T., Gladis, M., Roose, S. P., Stewart, J. W., Stetner, F., & Glassman, A. H. (1998). Phenelzine versus placebo in 50 patients with bulimia. *Arch Gen Psychiatry, 45,* 471–475.

Wortsman, J., Matsuoka, L. Y., Chen, T. C., Lu, Z., & Holick, M. F. (2000). Decreased bioavailability of vitamin D in obesity. *Am J Clin Nutr, 72,* 690–693.

Zanarini, M. C., & Frankenburg, F. R. (2003). Omega-3 Fatty acid treatment of women with borderline personality disorder: A double-blind, placebo-controlled pilot study. *Am J Psychiatry, 160,* 167–169.

Zonnevylle-Bender, M. J., van Goozen, S. H., Cohen-Kettenis, P. T., Jansen Lucres, M. C., Annemarie, V. E., & Herman, V. E. (2005). Adolescent anorexia nervosa patients have a discrepancy between neurophysiological responses and self-reported emotional arousal to psychosocial stress. *Psychiatr Res, 15,* 45–52.

31

Cardiovascular Diseases in Women

VIVIAN A. KOMINOS

CASE STUDY

As I injected dye into the left main coronary artery, I immediately saw the critical lesion in the proximal left anterior descending. This was a typical "widow maker," the term that I had learned in medical school and training. But there was nothing typical about my patient. Beth was in her late forties and did not have the typical symptoms of chest tightness. Instead, she had noticed increasing fatigue for a year and, more recently, shortness of breath with exertion. She had seen two cardiologists before she came to me, and was told that it was all in her head. In fact, her regular exercise stress tests were normal and she was beginning to believe her doctors. Prior to her cardiac catheterization, I tried to reassure her that her nuclear stress test was probably not accurate due to breast tissue that sometimes obscures the anterior wall, but that we should just "take a look" to be certain there was no disease. In 1990, early in my practice, Beth taught me a lot and I vowed to learn all I could about women and heart disease.

Introduction

Cardiovascular disease (CVD) is the leading cause of death worldwide in both women and men (World Health Statistics [WHS], 2010). In the United States, CVD accounts for one-third of all deaths in women, but in some developing countries it accounts for half of all the deaths in women over the age of 50 (Pilote et al., 2007). Since 1984, in the United States, more women than men die of CVD (Mosca, 2007), a fact not known by many women and physicians. Cardiovascular disease kills more than 400,000 women each year in the United States (American Heart Association, 2014), more than all cancers put together, yet many women still cite breast cancer as their chief medical concern (Mosca, 2013). The good news is that cardiac death rates in women have declined to one-third of what they were in 1980 and half of this decline is secondary to risk factor prevention (Mosca, 2011). The other half is the result of treatment of acute events, such as primary coronary interventions, and therapy for primary and secondary prevention, such as statins.

Because the myth that heart disease is an old man's disease has been debunked, and because CVD can affect women differently than men, it is only fitting that CVD be examined separately for women. This chapter summarizes what is currently known about the most common forms of CVD, namely coronary heart disease (CHD) and hypertension; highlights gender-specific recommendations for CVD prevention; and discusses nutrition, supplements, pharmacotherapy, and the mind–body connection. All the recommendations that follow are obtained from data that has included women. Several studies that are repeatedly cited have been inclusive of women alone: the Nurses' Health Study (NHS), the Women's Health Study (WHS), the Women's Health Initiative (WHI), and the NIH/NHLBI-sponsored Women's Ischemia Syndrome Evaluation (WISE). This last study has been collecting data on the unique features of heart disease in women since the mid-1990s. These large prospective cohorts and trials have provided a wealth of information and have informed us that, fortunately, most CVD is preventable. I hope that this chapter will assist the reader in the prevention and treatment of CVD, the most common killer of women.

Risk Factors

Until 2013, risk stratification had been based on Framingham data, which was limited in that it did not include family history and projected only a 10-year risk of myocardial infarction (MI) and CHD. The data was also flawed when it came to assessing risk, especially among young nondiabetic women. According to Framingham, approximately 95% of women aged less than 70 years of age are at low risk (Wenger, Shaw, & Vaccarino, 2008). This does not reflect the reality that all women are at risk, as more than one-third of all women will ultimately die from CVD. In November 2013, the American College of Cardiology–American Heart Association Task Force on Practice Guidelines issued new risk assessment guidelines (Goff et al., 2013). Evidence-based guidelines specifically designed for CVD prevention in women that more accurately risk stratify women have also been published (Mosca et al., 2011) and are shown in Table 31.1.

Some risk factors are more ominous for women than for men. Women with CVD who are diabetic have a higher risk for cardiac death than men with

Table 31.1. Classification of CVD Risk in Women

Risk Status	Criteria
High risk >/= 1 of the following	Established coronary heart disease Cerebrovascular disease Peripheral arterial disease Abdominal aortic aneurysm End-stage or chronic renal disease Diabetes mellitus Ten-year predicted CVD risk of ≥ 10%
At risk	≥1 major risk factors for CVD, including: Cigarette smoking Poor diet Physical inactivity Obesity, especially central adiposity Metabolic syndrome Family history of premature CVD (CVD at <55 years of age in male relative and <65 years of age in female relative) Hypertension, whether treated or not Dyslipidemia, whether treated or not Evidence of subclinical vascular disease (e.g., coronary calcification, carotid plaque, or thickened CIMT) Systemic autoimmune disease (e.g., lupus or rheumatoid arthritis) History of preeclampsia, gestational diabetes, or pregnancy-induced hypertension Poor exercise capacity on treadmill test and/or abnormal heart rate recovery after stopping exercise.
Ideal cardiovascular health	All of the following: No risk factors Total cholesterol < 200 (untreated) Body Mass Index < 25 kg/m² Physical activity at goal for adults >20 years of age: ≥150 min/week moderate intensity, ≥75 min/week vigorous intensity, or combination Healthy diet

Table 31.2. **Diagnosis of Metabolic Syndrome Requires at Least Three of the Following**

Abdominal obesity: waist circumference >102 cm in men and >88 cm in women

Triglyceride level ≥150 mg/dL

HDL <40 mg/dL for men and <50 mg/dL for women

Systolic blood pressure ≥130 mm Hg or diastolic blood pressure ≥85 mm Hg

Fasting glucose ≥110 mg/dL

similar risks (Roche & Wang, 2013). In premenopausal women, diabetes cancels out the protective role of endogenous estrogens. In young nondiabetic women, tobacco abuse is the strongest risk factor for CVD, and yet many primary care physicians and gynecologists do not counsel their patients regarding smoking cessation. In women, 20% of CHD events occur in the absence of traditional risk factors (Khot et al., 2003). Hemoglobin A1c; high-sensitivity C-reactive protein, or hsCRP; lipoprotein (a), or Lp(a); apolipoproteins A-I and B-100; and parental history all add to the accuracy of predicting CHD events (Ridker, Buring, Rifai, & Cook, 2007). Women with polycystic ovary syndrome are much more likely to have metabolic syndrome (Moran, 2010; Table 31.2). Women more frequently than men suffer from depression, a potent risk factor that doubles the chance of a cardiac event (Nicolson et al., 2006). In women who have suffered severe childhood abuse, there is up to a 1.5-fold increase in CV events (Rich-Edwards et al., 2012). In the assessment of CV risk, our traditional classification tools are simple and sometimes incomplete. A principle of integrative medicine is that each patient's unique circumstances need to be considered.

Gender-Specific Issues Related to Heart Disease

Despite the fact that symptoms can present differently in a woman than in a man, it is disturbing that women's awareness of CVD is so lacking (Christian, Rosamond, White, & Mosca, 2007). In the last 15 years more women have become aware of heart disease as a chief health threat. Yet there is a large ethnic disparity. In 2012 only 34% of Hispanic women and 36% of African American women were aware of CVD as the leading cause of death among women as compared with 65% of white women (Mosca et al. 2013). Recent data from the WISE study have elucidated a pathophysiology of coronary artery disease (CAD) in women that differs from men. Diagnostic testing is often more difficult in women than men due to hormone-related electrocardiographic (ECG) changes and breast attenuation artifact. Treatment in women does not always yield the same results as in men. All of these factors may explain why cardiac mortality for women is not decreasing as rapidly as for men.

SYMPTOMS IN CORONARY HEART DISEASE

Most women with acute coronary syndrome present with chest pain; however, women, more often than men, also have atypical symptoms, the most common of which are nausea, vomiting, and diaphoresis (Dey et al., 2009). Women often initially present with angina instead of acute MI (Hemingway et al., 2008). Women have reported prodromal symptoms of fatigue and shortness of breath that can occur up to 1 month prior to an acute MI (McSweeney et al., 2003). Because 38% of women versus 25% of men will die within 1 year after a first heart attack, early recognition of symptoms and accurate diagnosis are paramount.

PATHOPHYSIOLOGY OF ISCHEMIC HEART DISEASE

A disproportionate number of women suffer myocardial ischemia from non-classic atherosclerotic diseases. These include microvascular dysfunction, stress-induced cardiomyopathy, inflammatory vascular conditions, and spontaneous coronary artery dissection, a rare event seen in postpartum women. In the WISE study, women with chest pain and documented myocardial ischemia were found to have a lower incidence of obstructive CAD (Merz et al., 2006). When these women had persistent symptoms, they had a significant increased risk of MI or death even if coronary angiography revealed no, or nonobstructive, CAD (Gulati et al., 2009). In these women coronary microvascular dysfunction is likely the source of ischemia. Instead of the traditional plaque that protrudes into the lumen and is easy to visualize on coronary angiography, women may have intramural atherosclerosis as evidenced by intravascular ultrasound. In fatal acute coronary syndrome, women are more likely to have plaque erosion than plaque rupture (Merz et al., 2006). Women with coronary artery calcifications had greater mortality rates than men with the same coronary artery calcium score (Raggi, Shaw, Berman, & Callister, 2004). Stress-induced "takotsubo" cardiomyopathy occurs following acute emotional stress or life-threatening illness and is more common in postmenopausal women (Akashi, Goldstein& Ueyama, 2008). Excessive stress-induced catecholamines, microvascular dysfunction, and multivessel epicardial spasm have been proposed as mechanisms, yet there is no known reason why women are disproportionately affected when compared with men. Traditional pharmacotherapy has been unsuccessful in the prevention and treatment of microvascular dysfunction, and research is underway to determine whether acupuncture, lifestyle modification, and mind–body medicine will reduce cardiovascular events.

NONINVASIVE DIAGNOSTIC TESTING

Because symptoms may be less reliable in women than in men, the threshold for diagnostic testing should be lower in women. However, there is lower use of stress testing in women than in men in all age groups (Mieres et al., 2005). The diagnostic accuracy of exercise ECG is lower in women due to multiple factors including Bayesian factors (i.e., lower pretest probability), hormonal factors (estrogen has a "digoxin"-like effect of ST segments), and anatomy (e.g., mitral valve prolapse). Exercise duration and the ability to exercise to maximal stress are the strongest prognostic indicators for both men and women (Mieres et al., 2005). The inability to achieve five METS, the equivalent of the physical work that is required to perform activities of daily living signifies poor prognosis.

Clinical Tip

In general, if a nondiabetic patient has a normal resting ECG, and is able to exercise, refer her for an exercise treadmill test. If she has diabetes, is at high risk, has an abnormal resting ECG, or has poor exercise capacity, refer her for a stress test with cardiac imaging or a stress echocardiogram.

OUTCOME DIFFERENCES AND TREATMENT

Women less than 65 years old who present with an acute MI have higher morbidity and mortality rates than age-matched men (Vaccarino et al., 2013). The higher incidence of comorbid risk factors such as diabetes, renal failure, and heart failure explain only part of the mortality difference between women and men. No major mortality difference is seen in older women presenting with an acute MI when compared with age-matched men (Vaccarino et al., 2013). Approximately one-third of all coronary artery bypass surgery (CABG) is performed on women. After CABG, women fair worse than men, even after adjusting for comorbid factors (Vaccarino et al., 2003). Women had twice the incidence of depression, almost twice the rate of hospital readmission, more physical symptoms and side effects, and lower physical function when compared with men. The majority of the studies reveal higher mortality rates in women than in men after CABG (Wenger, Lewis, Welty, Herrington, & Bitner, 2008). Approximately one-third of all percutaneous coronary interventions (PCI) procedures are on women. For acute ST-segment elevation MI, PCI is superior to thrombolytics in both men and women (Lansky et al., 2005). In acute coronary syndrome, women had a reduction in death or MI with PCI if they were high risk (elevated CPK-MB or troponin, higher TIMI (thrombolysis in myocardial infarction) risk score, hsCRP, and brain natriuretic protein). For those women not at high risk, the results are mixed. There has been overall improvement in outcomes in women undergoing PCI (Singh et al., 2008). With newer drug-coated and biodegradable stents, women have a lower death and complication rate than men (Zhang et al., 2013).

Aspirin Use in Women

PRIMARY PREVENTION

The WHS randomized 39,876 women at low risk for CVD to receive 100 mg of aspirin every other day versus placebo (Ridker et al., 2005). In a 10-year follow-up there was a 17% reduction in ischemic strokes. In a subgroup analysis, women ≥ 65 years of age had a 26% reduction in CVD events and 34% reduction in MI. In the NHS, a prospective observational study of 79,439 low-risk women followed for 24 years, the group that self-selected to take aspirin had a significant relative risk reduction of 25% in all-cause mortality and 38% in cardiovascular death (Chan et al., 2007). The benefit of aspirin in high-risk women has been well established in a meta-analysis of 287 studies (Antithrombotic Trialists' Collaboration [ATC], 2002).

Clinical Tip

The United States Preventive Services Task Force (USPSTF) recommends aspirin for men age 45 to 79 to prevent MI, but offers no such recommendation for women despite the data from WHS and NHS indicating effectiveness of aspirin for primary prevention! However, it does recommend aspirin to prevent ischemic stroke in women age 55 to 79 (Wolff, Miller, & Ko 2009). Based on WHS data, aspirin should be given to women for prevention of MI who are over age 65 or at high risk. Use low-dose, 81 mg, non-enteric-coated aspirin. Enteric coating may prevent absorption and has been the cause of what was thought to be "aspirin resistance" (Grosser et al., 2013).

SECONDARY PREVENTION

A reduction of mortality from the administration of low-dose aspirin was seen regardless of gender: 33 events were prevented for every 1,000 women treated (ATC, 1994). Based on evidence, low-dose, 81 mg, aspirin should be recommended to women with no contraindications who have known CHD. Currently it is estimated that low-dose aspirin is used by only 50% of women who are aspirin eligible (Berger et al., 2006).

DUAL ANTIPLATELET THERAPY

In acute coronary syndrome, there is treatment benefit when adding clopidogrel to aspirin in both men and women (Yusef, Zhao, Mehta, Chrolavicius, & Tognoni, 2001). Dual antiplatelet therapy post stent implantation is also as effective in women as in men (Zhang et al., 2013).

Nutritional Recommendations

Few topics are debated more emotionally than diet for the prevention of heart disease. Data from diet studies has been confusing, and the charged atmosphere surrounding the high-fat versus low-fat controversy is fitting for sensational tabloids rather than academic discourse. Keep in mind that one diet does not fit all and that food has emotional, cultural, geographic, and traditional attachments that go beyond lab values and statistics. Epidemiologic data has shown that the Mediterranean, anti-inflammatory, and Indo-Mediterranean diets have a favorable effect on CVD. In general, a heart-healthy diet incorporates whole grains, high fiber foods, and oily fish a few times a week, limits the consumption of saturated fats and sodium, and recommends avoidance of trans fats. Specific nutritional recommendations follow.

OMEGA-3 FATTY ACIDS

In the NHS, there was a 38%–40% decreased risk of sudden myocardial death in the women that had the highest intake of omega-3 fatty acids, but there was no decrease in nonfatal CVD events after controlling for other risk factors (Albert et al., 2005; Hu et al., 2002). In Japan, where fish intake exceeds that of the United States, there was a strong inverse relationship seen between high dietary intake of fish (up to eight servings a week) and risk of nonfatal

MI and coronary events but no relationship was seen with fatal cardiac events (Iso et al., 2006). The inconsistent results have not been explained. Although the mechanisms by which omega-3 fatty acids may reduce sudden death are not fully understood, a cohort study found increased heart rate variability (HRV) in those adults with the highest intake (Mozaffarian, Stein, Prineas, & Siscovick, 2008). Omega-3 fatty acids are also indicated for treatment of hypertriglyceridemia, and the prescription Lovaza has FDA approval for triglyceride (TG) levels ≥ 500 mg/dL. In view of the proinflammatory state caused by our modern diets with high ratios of omega-6 to omega-3 fatty acids intake, an increase in omega-3-rich foods such as fish, flaxseed, canola, pumpkin seed, walnut, and soybeans may be beneficial both for primary and secondary prevention. An ongoing large primary prevention randomized, double-blind, placebo-controlled trial of 1 g/day of omega-3 fatty acid with 2,000 IU of vitamin D3 will hopefully answer whether these supplements will decrease CVD (Manson et al., 2012).

FIBER

Soluble fiber has been associated with lowering of total and LDL cholesterol, lowering of blood pressure, weight control, and improvement in insulin resistance and in clotting factors (Anderson & Hanna, 1999). The NHS revealed that a 10-g/day increase in total fiber intake was associated with a significant decrease in risk of CHD events (Wolk et al., 1999). Another large prospective cohort study of women found that intake of dietary fiber was inversely associated with risk of MI and CVD, but when adjusting for other CVD risk factors the association was not statistically significant (Liu et al., 2002). Nonetheless, due to the overwhelming evidence that high-fiber diets prevent many of the risks associated with CVD, the Adult Treatment Panel III recommends a diet that includes 5–10 g of soluble fiber per day (Grundy et al., 2004). Good sources of soluble fiber include flaxseed, oat bran, psyllium, guar, and pectin.

SOY

Epidemiologic data has shown that postmenopausal women who consume diets rich in phytoestrogens, especially in the form of isoflavones, have a lower incidence of CVD (Kokubo et al., 2007). In addition, high intake of phytoestrogens has been associated with lower waist to hip ratios and lower TGs (de Kleijn, van der Schouw, Wilson, Grobbee, & Jacques, 2002), and reduced fasting glucose levels, insulin levels, and inflammatory markers when compared with placebo (Atteritano et al., 2007). When soy nuts were added to a thera-peutic lifestyle changes (TLC) diet in postmenopausal women, blood pressure and LDL cholesterol improved in hypertensive women and BP was reduced in normotensive women (Welty, Lee, Lew, & Zhou, 2007). Although there is no conclusive evidence that soy has a beneficial or negative effect on CVD, based on epidemiologic data from Japan, it may be advisable to recommend that women obtain one serving of protein a day from natural soy foods such as tofu, tempeh, and soybeans.

TEA

Green tea has been used for medicinal purposes in China for thousands of years. Recent studies have shown that the polyphenolic compounds in teas have anticancer, neuroprotective, and antioxidant properties (Yang, Chen, & Wu, 2014). The Rotterdam study revealed that fatal and nonfatal MI was lower in tea drinkers with a daily intake greater than 375 mL (Geleijnse et al., 2002). A prospective cohort revealed an inverse relationship between green tea consumption and cardiovascular mortality (Kuriyama et al., 2006). This association was stronger in women than in men, with the max-imum benefit obtained with 3 to 4 cups of green tea a day. Concentrated catechins from green tea (500 mg or the equivalent of 6 to 7 cups of green tea) resulted in a significant decrease in plasma oxidized LDL (Inami et al., 2007). The consumption of at least 3 cups of tea per day was associated with less carotid plaque in women but not in men (Debette et al., 2008). The addition of milk counteracted the flow-mediated vasodilation that was seen with plain black tea (Lorenz et al., 2007). In a meta-analysis study of over 190,000 people there was no association with black tea and CVD; however, drinking 3 or more cups of green tea a day was associated with a 21% lower stroke risk than those people who drank 1 cup or less (Arab & Elashoff, 2009).

GARLIC

Garlic (*Allium sativum*) is the herbal supplement that has the most evidence for prevention or treatment of CVD, mainly through its effects on lipids (Knox & Gaster, 2007). The German Commission E has approved garlic for hyperlip-idemia. A meta-analysis of 13 randomized, double-blind, placebo-controlled trials found garlic was superior to placebo in reducing cholesterol but that the decrease was small and of questionable clinical benefit (Stevinson, Pittler, &

Ernst, 2000). In a review of the more recent data, however, there is evidence that garlic has plasma lipid-lowering abilities and anticoagulant and antioxidant properties in vitro (Gorinstein et al., 2007). Herbalists have used garlic for hypertension and there is a meta-analysis that has shown its effectiveness (Silagy & Neil, 1994). Recommended dosages are one to two cloves of raw garlic a day, 300 mg dried garlic powder tablet (standardized to 1.3% allicin or 0.6% allicin yield) two to three times per day, or 7.2 g of aged garlic extract per day. Precaution: garlic can increase risk of bleeding; use with caution in those taking warfarin or heparin.

NUTS

Three large prospective cohort studies that have included women have found an inverse relationship between nut consumption and CVD events (Albert, Gaziano, Willett, & Manson, 2002; Fraser, Sabate, Beeson, & Strahan, 1992; Hu et al., 1998). In the NHS, women who consumed more than 5 ounces of nuts a week had a significantly reduced risk of fatal and nonfatal CHD than women who consumed less than 1 ounce a month (Hu et al., 1998). Although nut consumption improves serum lipids, the 35% CHD risk reduction (Kris-Etherton, Hu, Ros, & Sabate, 2007) that is found in the epidemiologic data cannot be explained by this factor alone. Other beneficial nutrients in nuts such as arginine, magnesium, folate, plant sterols, and soluble fiber along with omega-3 fatty acids and vitamin E also play a beneficial role (Vogel et al., 2005). Nuts are often avoided as a high-calorie food, however, studies reveal eating 5 servings a week is associated with weight loss (Mozaffarian, Hao, Rimm, Willett, & Hu, 2011).

ALCOHOL

Moderate alcohol intake of one to two drinks a day has been shown to be related to decreased incidence of MI, ischemic stroke, peripheral vascular disease, and death after an MI and CHF (Vogel et al., 2005). In patients who have survived an MI, binge drinking (more than two drinks in 1 to 2 hours) was associated with twice the risk of cardiac and overall mortality (Mukamal, Maclure, Muller, & Mittleman, 2005). Although moderate alcohol does not result in increased morbidity, heavier intake poses significant hazards and can result in cardiomyopathy, hypertension, hemorrhagic stroke, arrhythmias, and sudden death. The risks and benefits must therefore be discussed with the patient.

SPECIFIC DIETS

The anti-inflammatory and Mediterranean diets are covered elsewhere.

Ornish Diet

The Dr. Dean Ornish Program for Heart Disease Reversal uses a vegetarian, low-fat diet. Fats are limited to no more than 10% of total calories: those that occur naturally in fruits, beans, legumes, soy, grains, and vegetables. Avocados, nuts, oils, coconuts, and seeds are excluded. Nonfat dairy products are allowed. This diet is used in conjunction a lifestyle program that includes 3 hours of aerobic exercise weekly, group support, and daily meditation. This program resulted in angiographic reversal of heart disease and decreased CV events and mortality in patients with established coronary artery disease (Ornish et al., 1998).

Atkins Diet

The Atkins diet is a multiphasic plan that includes fats from all sources, is high in protein, and limits carbohydrates. During the 2-week induction phase only proteins and fats are consumed. Carbohydrates are allowed over the next few phases. Emphasis is placed on weight loss. There is evidence that the Atkins diet improves cardiovascular risk markers: HDL cholesterol increases, LDL particle size increases (small particle size is associated with increase atherogenesis) and triglycerides decrease (Paoli et al., 2013). Evidence regarding actual CV events, however, is lacking.

Supplement Use in Cardiovascular Disease

Trials of supplement use have often yielded mixed or negative results. These are summarized in Table 31.3.

Herbal Preparations

Several drugs used for cardiovascular treatment have their origins in plants. These include aspirin, digoxin, atropine, reserpine, and amiodarone. Few herbal products available in the United States have undergone adequate testing

Table 31.3. Supplement Use in Cardiovascular Disease

Supplements with Evidence for Cardiovascular Benefit and No Deleterious Effects

Vitamin E: May be beneficial for older women and women with known CVD; recommended dose is 400 IU/day.	WHS (2005): Women 65 years and older treated with 600 IU of natural source Vitamin E taken every other day had a significant reduction (26%) in major cardiovascular events ($p = .009$), but in younger women supplementation had no effect. The Heart Outcomes Prevention Evaluation (HOPE) Study Investigators. (2000): No detriment or benefit in 4.5-year follow up. Cook et al. (2007): Mild reduction in subgroup of women with prior CVD.
Magnesium: Magnesium relaxes smooth muscle, stabilizes cardiac conductivity, and decreases neural excitability. More than 60% of Americans have inadequate intake, especially the elderly and Caucasian and African American women (Ford & Mokdah, 2003). Deficiency is also present in patients on diuretics. Dosage is usually 400 mg/day.	Appel et al. (1997): Prevention of hypertension in normotensives and lowering of BP in hypertensives with the DASH diet (see also: "Hypertension" section) Bashir et al. (1993): reduction in sustained ventricular tachycardia with supplement. Ma et al. (1995): Carotid artery thickness was inversely related to intake.
Vitamin D Deficiency is associated with higher risk for multiple diseases including CVD, CHF, some cancers, diabetes, and autoimmune diseases (Holick, 2007). Supplementation is encouraged for those who are deficient. Deficiency is more common in women than in men. Dosage is based on degree of deficiency; 1,000 IU/day are recommended for the general population.	Autier and Gangini (2007): Meta-analysis of 18 randomized trials: decrease in all-cause mortality.

(continued)

Table 31.3. Continued

Supplements with Evidence for Cardiovascular Benefit and No Deleterious Effects

Coenzyme Q10: Depletion is seen in patients on statins. Usual dosage is 200 mg/day.	Morisco, Trim Arco, and Condor Elli (1993): 38%–61% decrease in hospitalizations and pulmonary edema in patients with NYHA class II or IV CHF. Watson et al. (1999): No improvement in advanced CHF. Marcoff (2007): 200 mg of coenzyme Q10 are recommended for statin myopathy
L-Carnitine: Usual dosage is 3–6 g/day but it can potentiate the effect of warfarin.	Colonna and Iliceto (2000): Patients with an acute MI who received L-carnitine within 24 hours had improvements in LV volumes at 3, 6, and 12 months. There are no outcomes data regarding CVD events. Hiatt et al. (2001); Brevetti, Diehm, and Lambert (1999): In patients with peripheral vascular disease, there was improvement in maximum walking capacity and symptoms of claudication. Witte, Clark, and Cleland (2001): Patients with CHF did not improve in terms of exercise capacity.

Supplements That May Be Harmful or Have No Proven Benefit in Cardiovascular Disease

Beta-carotene	Rapola et al. (1996), Rapola et al. (1998): Increased angina pectoris. Osganian et al. (2003): Increase in all-cause mortality and cardiovascular health.
Folic acid, vitamin B6, and vitamin B12: Prevention trials aimed at lowering homocysteine levels have not shown reduced CVD risk.	Bonaa et al. (2006): Increased cardiovascular events in folic acid plus B12 group. HOPE 2 Investigators (2006): Fewer patients had strokes; more were hospitalized with unstable angina; no CVD risk reduction in treatment groups. Lange et al. (2004): Increase in stent-restenosis.
Vitamin C	Kushi et al. (1996): Small, but nonsignificant increase in CHD mortality and stroke. Osganian et al. (2003): 28% reduction in fatal and nonfatal CHD event in those who took supplements versus diet alone. Knekt et al. (2004): 700 mg/day correlated to a 25% reduction in cardiovascular risk. In General: trials of vitamin C alone or combined with other vitamins have found no effect on CVD events or all cause mortality and no harm.

(continued)

Table 31.3. Continued

Supplements That May Be Harmful or Have No Proven Benefit in Cardiovascular Disease

L-ARGININE	Blum et al. (2000): No increase in nitric oxide levels or decrease in inflammatory markers. Schulman, Becker, and Kass (2006): Study was stopped prematurely due to increased death rate in patients with acute MI in the treatment group. Long term L-Arginine exposure can accelerate endothelial cell senescence (Xiong, 2014).
Calcium	Bolland et al. (2008): Higher incidence of MI, TIA, stroke and sudden death in postmenopausal women treated with 1 g of elemental calcium. Hsia et al. (2007): No increase or decrease in cardiovascular risk. In the WHI, there was no difference in coronary artery calcium scores in women who were randomized to receive 1000 mg of elemental calcium/ 400 IU vitamin D supplementation, as compared to controls (Manson, 2010).

Abbreviations: CHD, coronary heart disease; CHF, congestive heart failure; CVD, cardiovascular disease; LV, left ventricle; MI, myocardial infarction; NYHA, New York Heart Association; TIA, transient ischemic attack.

for CVD. Table 31.4 summarizes the more common herbs. Red yeast rice is described under the "Hyperlipidemia" section and garlic under the "Nutrition" section of this chapter. Guggulipid and policosanol are widely advertised as having lipid-lowering abilities, yet do not have good efficacy data; they will not be reviewed here.

Treatment of Dyslipidemia

In November 2013, the American College of Cardiology–American Heart Association Task Force on Practice Guidelines issued their new cholesterol guideline (Stone et al., 2014). This is the first major update since 2002, when the National Cholesterol Education Program released the Adult Treatment Panel III report. The old guidelines concentrated treatment to specific target LDL levels: lower than 160 for people at low risk, lower than 130 for those at moderate risk, lower than 100 for those at high risk, and lower than 70

Table 31.4. Herbal Preparations Used for the Treatment of Cardiovascular Disease

Herb	Disease	Method of Action	Dosing	Contraindication
Hawthorn (*Cratagus spp.*)	CHF Reviewed in meta-analysis of randomized trials	Increases stroke volume Reduces afterload Peripheral vasodilator	Minimum effective dose 300 mg of leaf extract (160–1800 mg of standardized extract used in trials)	Safer than digoxin: can be used with renal impairment, less arrhythmogenic potential. Clinician should always be alert to drug interactions, but the large multicenter SPICE trial failed to note any AER between hawthorn and digoxin, beta-blockers, and class III antiarrhythmics
Ginkgo biloba	Peripheral artery disease In a meta-analysis of eight RPCDB trials pain-free walking increased by 34 min	Mechanism of action not known	120–160 mg/day or extract standardized to provide 24% ginkgoflavones and 6% terpenes	Can increase risk of bleeding; use with caution in those taking aspirin, or NSAIDS. Do not use with warfarin or heparin
Horse chestnut (*Aesculus hippocastanum*)	Chronic venous insufficiency: 14 RPC trials effective in decreasing lower leg volume and leg pain	Hydroxicoumarin derivative, glycosides aescin, and aesculin	300 mg extract containing 50 mg aescin per day	Generally well tolerated

Abbreviations: CHF, congestive heart failure; NSAIDS, nonsteroidal anti-inflammatory drug; RPC, randomized, placebo-controlled; RPCDB, randomized, placebo-controlled, double-blind

Source: Adapted from Vogel et al. (2005)

for those with established CVD. There is little evidence from randomized controlled trials to support these target levels. Instead, the new guidelines rely heavily on trials that use fixed doses of statins for groups at risk. An emphasis is placed on lifestyle and aim to treat the *person* rather than a cholesterol level.

Using the latest randomized controlled trials, the expert panel found that four groups had decreased atherosclerotic cardiovascular disease (ASCVD) events from cholesterol lowering with statin therapy. The guidelines are the same for women as for men.

1. Individuals with clinical ASCVD
2. Individuals with primary elevations of LDL–C ≥190 mg/dL.
3. Individuals 40 to 75 years of age with diabetes and LDL–C 70 to 189 mg/dL without clinical ASCVD
4. Individuals without clinical ASCVD or diabetes who are 40 to 75 years of age with LDL–C 70 to 189 mg/dL and have an estimated 10-year ASCVD risk of 7.5% or higher.

In these groups high-intensity statin therapy is recommended to reduce LDL levels by at least 50%. Moderate intensity statin therapy is used for those who cannot tolerate high-intensity therapy or for those with diabetes and a 10-year risk of less than 7.5%.

Statin therapy is not recommended for the following groups:

1. An age of more than 75 years, unless clinical ASCVD is present;
2. A need for hemodialysis; or
3. New York Heart Association class II, III, or IV heart failure.

The expert panel also found no evidence to support the use of nonstatin therapies either alone or in combination with statins.

The advances of the new guidelines are summarized here:

1. Move away from treating a lab value;
2. Recommend the use of proven medications; focus on the medications that work: statins;
3. Treat only those patients that have the most to gain from therapy;
4. Involve the patient in the decision process.

> ### Clinical Tip
>
> Remember, these are guidelines, not dictates. And no risk calculator or guideline is perfect. I believe, when compared with previous guidelines, these are definitely a step in the right direction. There are ongoing discussions and controversies surrounding the new guidelines and risk calculator. There will likely be refinements in the future based on evidence.

HORMONAL INFLUENCES

Hormonal influences on lipoproteins are complex and help explain, at least partially, the increase of CVD after menopause. Prepubertal boys and girls are similar in terms of lipid levels (Bittner, 2005). During puberty, women's HDL-C rises and is maintained at roughly 10 mg/dL higher than men's HDL-C throughout their lifetime. However, many women with MI have HDL-C ≥ 60 mg/dL (Bittner et al., 2000), a level that is considered protective against CHD. During the premenopause years, lipoprotein levels vary and are affected by the menstrual cycle, pregnancy, and use of oral contraceptives. With oral contraceptives, TGs can increase by 13%–75% (Godsland et al., 1990), and LDL-C particle size can decrease (Foulon et al., 2001). In the postmenopausal years, total cholesterol increases, LDL-C particle size decreases, and there is a greater increase in postprandial lipoproteins (Bittner, 2005). Oral hormone replacement therapy decreases LDL-C and Lp(a) and increases HDL-C and triglycerides. Selective estrogen receptor modulators slightly affect lipoproteins, causing up to an 8% increase in triglycerides and up to 10% decrease in LDL-C (Barrett-Connor et al., 2002). Fertility therapy does not appear to increase the risk of CVD later in life (Udell, Lu, & Redelmeier, 2013). In fact those women who received fertility therapy had fewer cardiovascular events, all-cause mortality, thromboembolic events, depression, and alcoholism.

STATINS FOR SECONDARY PREVENTION

Statin therapy in women with established CHD significantly reduces CHD mortality, nonfatal MI, and revascularization. The effects of statins are similar in men and women, and recent trials have provided evidence that women achieve the same clinical end points with statins as men (Bittner, 2005). In the treating to new targets (TNT) study, in which 19% of the participants were women, there was a similar reduction in cardiovascular events with intensive lipid lowering in men and women (Wenger, Lewis, et al., 2008).

Clinical Tip

Supplementation with Coenzyme Q10 (see Table 31.3) is recommended for statin and red yeast rice users.

STATINS FOR PRIMARY PREVENTION

There has been debate about statins for primary prevention in women partly because women had been underrepresented in early statin trials and partly because low-risk women were being given statins. The MEGA Study was the first trial to show a statistically significant reduction of CVD events in women (Mizuno et al., 2008). Women constituted over 68% of the 7,832 participants in this prospective randomized, open label trial with a 10-year follow-up. Among women randomized to receive pravastatin, there was a 26%–27% decrease in CVD events, with the most benefit seen in women who were 60 years of age or older. The randomized, placebo-controlled JUPITER trial gave 20 mg of rosuvastatin to healthy women and men, without hyper-lipidemia, with elevated hsCRP of ≥ 2 mg/L (Ridker et al., 2008). The women in the trial had a 46% decrease in CVD events and death in the rosuvastatin group. This trial highlights the effectiveness of statins in women and the importance of screening for CVD risk with hsCRP and raises the question of whether the indications for statin use should be expanded. However, the trial has several limitations, which should prevent an immediate rush to use statins in everyone with elevated hsCRP: it did not look at the effects of statins on normal levels of hsCRP; the long-term safety of decreasing LDL cholesterol to 55 mg/dL in a healthy population is not known; levels of gly-cated hemoglobin and diabetes were higher in the rosuvastatin group; and CVD is affected by multiple factors in the participants other than hsCRP (Hlatky, 2008).

Clinical Tip

Statin use should be individualized to each woman's unique set of risk factors and preferences. I measure hsCRP in each of my patients and use it to help guide me for the prescription of statins along with aspirin use and lifestyle modification.

OTHER PHARMACOTHERAPY

Trials of clofibrate and colestipol have not included women. Trials on ezetimibe (Zetia) have shown similar success of lipid lowering in women and men, but clinical outcome data is lacking.

RED YEAST RICE

Red yeast rice (RYR) contains monacolin K (lovastatin) and eight other monacolins, along with sterols, isoflavones, and monounsaturated fatty acids. This family of substances probably explains why RYR is more effective at reducing cholesterol than what would be expected with the small amount of lovastatin that it contains. Based on a meta-analysis of randomized controlled trials of RYR, HDL-C can be raised by 15%–22%, LDL-C can be lowered by 27%–32%, and TGs lowered by 27%–38% (Liu et al., 2006). The recommended dosage is 1,200 mg twice a day with meals. Side effects include headaches and gastrointestinal discomfort. Lipid profiles and liver enzymes should be monitored 8 weeks after the initiation of RYR both to determine its effectiveness and to rule out any significant liver abnormalities. Red yeast rice is often well tolerated when statins are not. Outcome data with RYR is not available as it is for statins.

PHYTOSTEROLS

A dose of 1.8 to 2 g/day, divided over two meals, can result in a decrease of LDL-C by 9%–20% (Katan et al., 2003; Woodgate, Chan, & Conquer, 2006). HDL-C and TGs are not affected. Plant stanols/sterols can be effectively combined with statins, niacin, or RYR and are relatively safe with the exception of the rare person with familial sitosterolemia. There is no outcome data regarding phytosterol use and CVD.

NIACIN

Prior to the advent of statins, niacin was widely used to manage dyslipidemia. Doses of up to 3,000 mg/day can increase HDL-C by 30%, decrease LDL-C by 21%, decrease TGs by 44%, and decrease Lp(a) by 26% (Goldberg et al., 2000). But "improving the numbers" does not translate into efficacy. Two secondary prevention trials with niacin did not find reduced cardiovascular events. In the AIM-HIGH trial the addition of niacin to 40 mg of simvastatin was compared with placebo and simvastatin (Boden & Probstfield, 2011). This trial was stopped early due to futility and a trend toward a higher risk of ischemic stroke in the niacin group. The HPS2-THRIVE study evaluated the effect of extended-release niacin in combination with laropipract (a prostraglandin receptor antagonist) versus placebo in more than 24,000 patients treated with statin (The HPS2-THRIVE Collaborative Group, 2014). In this trial, niacin did not reduce cardiovascular events but the niacin group had increased side effects including infection, bleeding, and myalgias.

Niacin can still be considered, and is included in the current treatment guidelines for those statin-intolerant patients at high risk for cardiovascular events. Niaspan is a prescription preparation that is long acting and can be used once a day. The "No Flush" over-the-counter preparations should not be used, because they may not contain any free nicotinic acid, which is responsible for the cholesterol-lowering effects. In addition to flushing, side effects include GI disturbances, asthma exacerbation, acanthosis nigricans, and elevations in serum transaminases. Patients should be told about the side effect of flushing and of its usual improvement over the course of several weeks. Niacin should be taken in the evening, with dinner or a snack, up to 1 hour after taking an enteric-coated low-dose aspirin in order to decrease flushing. Start dosing at 375–500 mg/day, increasing in increments of 250–500 mg every 2 weeks with careful monitoring of serum transaminases and lipid profiles. Niacin can be combined with statins or RYR and phytosterols.

FISH OIL

Omega-3 fatty acids are diverse in their effects on CVD risk reduction and are covered in greater detail in the "Nutrition" section of this chapter. They are effective in reduction of TGs, and the prescription Lovaza has been approved for use in patients with TG levels of at least 500 mg/dL. Omega-3 fatty acids reduce the synthesis and secretion of VLDL particles, and increase the removal of TG from VLDL and chylomicrons through up-regulation of enzymes such as lipoprotein lipase (Bays, Tighe, Sadovsky, & Davidson, 2008). Omega-3 fatty acids can be safely added to statin therapy. An RDBPC trial comparing fish oil

4 g/day combined with simvastatin versus simvastatin alone showed a significant increase in HDL-C levels of 3.4%, and a decrease in non-HDL-C (defined as total cholesterol minus HDL-C; or the sum of LDL-C and VLDL-C) levels of 9.0% (Davidson et al., 2007). Dosages of 1–4 g/day are recommended.

Hypertension

One of three adults in America has hypertension (Ong, Cheung, Man, Lau, & Lam, 2007). Although hypertension affects men at younger ages than women, the rise in hypertension is steeper in women as they age. The overall prevalence of hypertension in men is slightly higher than in women (30.7 vs. 28.2); women are more aware then men when they are affected (67.6% vs. 66.7%); and more women are treated than men (58.0% vs. 52.1%). Yet fewer women than men have control of their hypertension (Ong et al., 2007). Women who had gestational hypertension have higher risk for stroke and CVD later in life. Women who take oral contraceptives are two to three times more likely to have hypertension than women who are not on oral contraceptives, especially if they are older or obese (Chobanian et al., 2003).

Hypertension carries a significant decrease in life expectancy (Franco et al., 2005b) and contributes to the incidence of stroke, renal disease, CHD, and heart failure. Until the age of 50, diastolic and systolic blood pressures rise in tandem, whereas after the age of 50, systolic blood pressure (SBP) continues to rise while diastolic blood pressure (DBP) falls or remains the same. Above the age of 60, elevated SBP has a higher relative risk for CHD than DBP, whereas prior to the age of 50, DBP is a more potent risk predictor (Franklin et al., 2001). According to a meta-analysis, each 20 mm Hg increase in SBP over 115, and each 10 mm Hg in DBP over 75 doubles the risk of a fatal cardiovascular event with the absolute risk also rising with age (Lewington, Clarke, Qizilbash, Peto, & Collins, 2002). The risk of cardiovascular events increases 2.5-fold in women and 1.6-fold in men with prehypertension. As such, aggressive approaches for prevention and treatment must be employed. Decreases in BP bring about rapid decreases in CVD morbidity and mortality, with a 50%–60% decrease in stroke death and a 40%–50% decrease in CAD death for every 10 mm Hg decrease in SBP and 5 mm Hg decrease in DBP (Lewington et al., 2002).

PREVENTION AND GUIDELINES FOR TREATMENT

Hypertension is a multifactorial illness that is affected by lifestyle, mental-emotional health, genetics, illness, drugs, and supplements. The successful prevention and treatment of hypertension should address all these aspects, but unfortunately pharmacotherapy has been the mainstay of treatment to the exclusion of proper nutrition, adequate exercise, supplements and botanicals, and relaxation techniques. New guidelines for pharmacotherapy released by the Eighth Joint National Committee (JNC 8) in December of 2013 take race into account and include comorbidies of diabetes and chronic renal disease.

DIET

Excess caloric intake and supraphysiologic intake of sodium contribute to hypertension. The fiber rich DASH diet, which emphasizes whole grains, low-fat dairy, and nuts, and which is low in sodium and high in magnesium and potassium, has been shown to be very effective in lowering BP to goal in 71% of patients with Stage 1 hypertension (Svetkey et al., 2004). When the DASH diet was used with lower sodium intake, SBP was reduced by up to 7.1 mm Hg in nonhypertensive individuals and 11.5 mm Hg in hypertensive participants (Sacks et al., 2001). Twenty-four-year follow-up data from over 80,000 women enrolled in the NHS revealed that there was a significant reduction of CHD and stroke in those women who followed a DASH-style diet (Fung et al., 2008).

In epidemiologic studies, the Mediterranean diet is associated with a lower incidence of hypertension even after adjusting for other risk factors (Nunez-Cordoba et al., 2009).

MIND–BODY TECHNIQUES

Breathing exercises with device-guided breathing can lower SBP by approximately 10 mm Hg and DBP by approximately 5 mm Hg (Meles et al, 2004; Schein et al, 2001). "Resperate" is such a device that has FDA approval. Biofeedback-assisted relaxation methods can be effective in select individuals who have high anxiety, rapid pulse, high urinary cortisol levels, and cool hand temperatures (McGrady, Nadsady, & Schumann-Brzezinski, 1991; Yonker, Tan, Fine, & Woerner,1981).

Transcendental meditation has been shown to reduce SBP by 4.7 mm Hg and DBP by 3.2 mm Hg (Anderson, Liu, & Kryscio, 2008). Yoga regulates the sympathetic nervous system and is a useful adjunct in the treatment of hypertension (Cramer et al., 2014). Studies on tai chi and qigong have shown improvement in SBP and DBP with no adverse effects (Yeh, Wang, Wayne, & Phillips, 2008).

PHYSICAL ACTIVITY

Physical activity reduces BP in hypertensive individuals even in the absence of weight loss. Aerobic activity causes a decrease in BP that can last an entire day. As little as 30 minutes of aerobic activity three times a week has an antihypertensive effect (Elley & Arroll, 2005). The American College of Sports Medicine recommends that at least 30 minutes of continuous aerobic exercise be performed on all or most days of the week. Acutely, BP reductions of up to 5 to 7 mm Hg are seen with effects lasting up to 22 hours post exercise. With regular exercise training, decreases in catecholamines, improvement in peripheral artery resistance, and insulin resistance are seen.

DIETARY SUPPLEMENTS

Several supplements can prevent and treat hypertension: magnesium, vitamin D, omega-3 fatty acids, and L-arginine. Magnesium deficiencies are associated with an increased risk for hypertension and are common in the typical American diet. A comprehensive analytical review of 44 human studies found that oral magnesium supplementation (230–460 mg per day) enhanced the BP-lowering effects of antihypertensive medications in patients with stage 1 hypertension (Rosanoff, 2010).

Vitamin D deficiency activates the renin angiotensin system and increases parathyroid hormone, which increases the risk for hypertension, left ventricular hypertrophy, and diabetes. Epidemiological studies have shown that vitamin D deficiency is prevalent in 30%–50% of the population and is associated with cardiovascular disease risk factors and events. In a meta-analysis of 18 randomized, controlled trials, vitamin D supplementation has been linked to a decrease in all-cause mortality (Autier & Gandini, 2007). Outcomes data on vitamin D supplementation and the reduction of hypertension are not available, although the evidence is mounting that vitamin D deficiency must be corrected in order to decrease the risk of all CVD.

Omega-3 fatty acid supplementation causes a small but significant decrease in BP that may account, in part, for the cardiovascular benefit seen with polyunsaturated fatty acids. Omega-3 fatty acids decrease the production of vasoconstrictor eicosanoids, reduce ACE activity and angiotensin II formation, enhance endothelial nitric oxide production, and activate the parasympathetic nervous system (Cicero, Erick, & Borghi, 2009).

A meta-analysis of 11 randomized trials evaluating the effect of L-arginine, an amino acid and substrate of nitric oxide synthase, on blood pressure concluded that compared with placebo, L-arginine significantly lowered SBP by 5.39 mm Hg and DBP by 2.66 mm Hg (Dong et al., 2011).

There are a number of botanicals that have been shown to lower blood pressure in randomized controlled trials including hibiscus, grape seed, olive leaf, and beetroot. Hibiscus (*Hibiscus sabdariffa*) tea and extract made from the calyces or sepals, the leaf-like spikes that surround the base of a flower, have been shown to significantly lower SBP and DBP in adults with prehypertension to moderate essential hypertension and type 2 diabetes (Hopkins, Lamm, Funk, & Ritenbaugh, 2013). Dose is typically 1,000 mg of hibiscus taken two to three times per day.

A meta-analysis of studies of grape seed extract (*Vitis vinifera*), which is high in catechin, epicatechin, and oligomeric proanthocyanidins, found that it significantly reduces SBP and heart rate, with no effect on blood lipids or C-reactive protein (Feringa, Laskey, Dickson, & Coleman, 2011). Doses used in the studies were 150–300 mg per day of the extract.

Olive leaf has been shown to act as a calcium channel blocker, and one 8-week randomized double-blinded comparative trial found olive leaf extract (500 mg twice daily) was similarly effective to captopril (12.5–25 mg twice daily) for lowering blood pressure in patients with stage 1 hypertension (Susalit et al., 2011).

In a meta-analysis of randomized trials, consumption of beetroot juice (*Beta vulgaris*) was associated with a significant reduction in SBP (-4.4 mm Hg) (Siervo, Lara, Ogbonmwan, & Mathers, 2013). Doses vary but are typically 4 ounces one to two times daily. While herbal diuretics, such as parsley leaf and seed (*Petroselinum sativum*), dandelion leaf (*Taraxacum officinale*), and fennel seed (*Foeniculum vulgare*), are widely used in the management of hypertension by integrative practitioners, there are no randomized controlled trials to evaluate their efficacy.

PHARMACOTHERAPY

In December 2013, JNC 8 released new guidelines for pharmacotherapy of hypertension (James et al., 2014), which is the same for men and women. The SBP and DBP goals are based on age and comorbidities of diabetes mellitus (DM) or chronic kidney disease (CKD). The major differences from JNC 7 include a higher pharmacotherapy threshold of SBP of 150 mm Hg for those 60 years of age or older and blood pressure goals of less than 140/90 for those younger than 60 and for all ages if DM or CKD is present. Beta-blockers were removed as first-line antihypertensive therapy: initiation of therapy with angiotensin receptor blockers (ARB), angiotensin converting enzyme inhibitors

(ACE), calcium-channel blockers, and thiazide diuretics are appropriate for the nonblack population, while thiazide diuretics or calcium-channel blockers are indicated for the black population, regardless of whether DM or CKD is present. A full discussion of recommendations for drug therapy is found in James et al. (2014).

Exercise and the Heart

Both women and men achieve cardiovascular benefit from exercise, with women possibly gaining more benefit than men (Shiroma & Lee, 2010). Data from the NHS and the WHI Obesity Study reveal that women in the highest quintiles of physical activity gain the most benefit when compared with sedentary women (Manson et al., 1999; Manson et al., 2002). Women who were sedentary had three times the risk of CVD or death when compared with women in the highest quintile of physical activity (Stevens, Cal, Evenson, & Thomas, 2002). These studies revealed a strong dose-response gradient. Further, the benefit of exercise carried through every weight category (Stevens et al., 2002), and sedentary lifestyle remains an independent risk factor for CVD after multivariate analysis (Franco, de Laet, et al., 2005).

The American College of Sports Medicine recommends at least 150 minutes per week of moderate intensity cardiorespiratory exercise (defined as walking at a brisk pace of 3 miles per hour) or 75 minutes per week of vigorous intensity exercise (Garber et al., 2011). Resistance exercises for each of the major muscle groups along with neuromotor exercise for balance, flexibility, and coordination should be performed 2 to 3 days a week. If patients cannot walk at a brisk pace, they should be encouraged to walk at a 2–2.9 mile/hr pace, which reduces the risk of cardiovascular events by approximately 25% (Manson et al., 1999). Vigorous activity, examples of which include running, bicycling, swimming, tennis, and calisthenics, has added cardiovascular benefit. Because epidemiologic evidence has proven that the prescribed physical activity can prevent at least 30%–40% of the cardiovascular events that occur in women, it is of utmost importance that we give our patients a "prescription" for exercise.

Emotions and the Heart

Socioeconomic stress such as marital stress, caregiver strain, social isolation, lack of a sense of purpose, and financial hardship; and psychoaffective disorders such as depression, anxiety, anger, and hostility have all been associated with an increased risk of CVD (Rozanski, 2014). The INTERHEART case-control study, which included 12,461 men and women with acute MI in 52 countries and 14,637 matched controls, revealed that psychosocial stress was an independent risk factor for MI, regardless of geographic or ethnic background (Rosengren et al., 2004). Although there has been increasing data on the impact of stress on the heart, and although most physicians easily grasp this notion, they often fail to recognize depression in patients with CVD. In depressed patients hospitalized with acute coronary syndrome, only 24.5% were accurately diagnosed by their physicians with depression (Amin, Jones, Nugent, Rumsfeld, & Spertus, 2006). The current AHA guidelines recommend screening women with CVD for depression, but no guidelines are given regarding treatment.

DEPRESSION

Epidemiologic studies support both major depression and depressive symptoms as a significant risk for CHD. Eleven cohort studies have shown that patients with depression have 2.5 times the risk of having an acute MI as nondepressed patients (Rugulies, 2002). The presence of depression with a recent MI doubles the risk of death in both men and women, but the prevalence of depression in women is twice that of men (Naqvi, Naqvi, & Merz, 2005). Diabetic women are more depressed than diabetic men, and depressed diabetic women have a more aggressive form of CVD than nondepressed diabetic women. Younger women with CHD have the highest prevalence of depression (Mallik et al., 2006) and have the highest risk of death after an acute MI.

Antidepressants

Tricyclic antidepressants (TCAs) can slow intraventricular conduction, thereby causing heart block or ventricular reentry arrhythmias (Glassman & Preud'homme, 1993) and cause severe orthostatic hypotension (Glassman & Bigger, 1981). Because TCAs may cause a decrease in left ventricular (LV) function, they are contraindicated in patients with impaired LV function or CHD. In the SADHART trial, sertraline, a selective serotonin reuptake inhibitor (SSRI) was shown to be safe in patients with CVD who have a major depressive disorder. In a double-blind, placebo-controlled trial that randomized 369 eligible patients to sertraline or placebo, sertaline did not reduce LV ejection fraction, increase ventricular arrhythmias or heart block (Glassman et al., 2002). Sertraline was superior to placebo in the treatment of depression, and there was a trend toward decreased cardiovascular events. However, the trial was a safety study and was not powered to determine whether sertaline was effective for the reduction of cardiovascular events. It is the only prospective randomized control published to date. One review found that SSRI use was associated with decreased CVD morbidity and mortality in six studies, increased CHD events in two studies, and had no significant effect in four studies (Von Ruden, Adson, & Kotlyar, 2008).

Psychological Intervention

A meta-analysis by the Cochrane Collaboration of psychological intervention trials found only a small benefit in the reduction of total mortality, revascularization, or nonfatal MI by such interventions (Cochrane Heart Group, 2011). In some trials, psychosocial stress was not reduced and therefore CV events were not reduced. For example, women who were randomized to therapy in the randomized trial follow-up to the Ischemic Heart Disease Study had higher mortality than those receiving usual care, but the therapy was not successful in reducing their stress (Cossette, Frasure-Smith, & Lesperance, 2001; Frasure-Smith et al., 1997). In others trials, such as the ENRICHD study, both intervention and control groups received treatment that almost equally reduced stress (The ENRICHD Investigators, 2003). As such, CV events were reduced in both groups and the "intervention" did not appear effective. In contrast, the Stockholm Women's Intervention Trial for Coronary Heart Disease that randomized 237 women to either psychosocial intervention or usual care after an acute cardiac event showed positive effects (Orth-Gomer et al., 2009). The intervention group met in 20 small-group sessions led by an RN over 1 year. Therapy was aimed at women's unique stressors and was successful in reducing stress. At the end of 7 years, there was a 67% reduction in death in the intervention group compared with controls, and this difference could not be explained by other risk factors. These results suggest a powerful protective effect of targeted successful psychological intervention.

Exercise and Cardiac Rehabilitation

Lower depression scores have been seen in both ill and healthy people who are physically active (Lawlor & Hopker, 2001). In a randomized, controlled study of 156 men and women with major depressive disorder followed for 16 weeks, exercise was as effective as sertraline in the treatment of depression (Blumenthal et al., 1999). In another randomized controlled trial in patients with CHD, exercise and stress management decreased depression, improved HRV, and improved flow-mediated dilation (Blumenthal et al., 2005).

Cardiac rehabilitation (CR) trials have shown a decrease in cardiovascular mortality when CR was successful in reducing psychosocial stress (Dusseldorp, van Elderen, Maes, Meulman, & Kraaij, 1999; Linden, Stossel, & Maurice, 1996). Depressed patients who entered CR had a 63% decrease in depression and a 73% decrease in cardiovascular morbidity and mortality over a 5-year period (Milani & Lavie, 2007). Persistence of depression following CR, however, was associated with over a fourfold higher risk of cardiac mortality when compared with nondepressed patients. Women report more psychosocial symptoms prior to CR than men. Although depression, anxiety, and panic improve in both men and women after CR, anger and relationship dissatisfaction improved only in men (Hazelton et al., 2014). Only half of patients who are eligible participate in CR, and women, especially minority and older women, are 55% less likely to attend CR than men (Witt et al., 2004). This lack of participation is partly due to lack of physician support or referral. It is imperative to offer this life-saving modality to heart disease patients.

ACUTE EMOTIONAL STRESS AND CARDIOMYOPATHY

The "broken heart" syndrome, or takotsubo cardiomyopathy, occurs in the absence of obstructive coronary atherosclerosis and disproportionately affects postmenopausal women (Virani, Khan, Mendoza, Ferreira, & de Marchena, 2007). There are no chronic symptoms, but an acute emotional or physical stressor initiates symptoms that can be clinically identical to an acute MI. Rapid and complete recovery of left ventricular dysfunction is a hallmark of this syndrome and if systolic function has not recovered in 4 to 6 weeks, a different diagnosis should be considered (Wittstein, 2007). Treatment includes usual care and medications, but there is no consensus on how long to continue medications once LV function has recovered. The recurrence rate is approximately 3.5% (Gianni et al., 2006), but there are no data on prevention. Many questions remain regarding why it affects mostly women and whether this syndrome represents an exaggeration of the normal stress response, or a pathologic defect.

PSYCHOLOGICAL STRESS AND VENTRICULAR ARRHYTHMIAS

Ventricular arrhythmias (VAs) occur because vagal efferents richly innervate atrial muscle and the sinoatrial (SA) and atrioventricular (AV) nodes and only sparsely innervate ventricular tissue. Sympathetic efferents are widespread throughout the heart. Therefore, the ventricles are vulnerable to sympathetic discharge. It is estimated that 20% of VAs are precipitated by emotional stress. In patients with implantable cardiac defibrillators (ICD), anger was significantly more likely to be identified by patients prior to a shock, and the VA was faster and more difficult to terminate (Lampert et al., 2002). There was a 37% increased incidence of sudden cardiac death (SCD) in patients with mild depression and a 77% increased risk of SCD in patients with severe depression when compared with controls (Empana et al., 2006).

PSYCHOLOGICAL STRESS AND ATRIAL ARRHYTHMIAS

Patients with atrial fibrillation (AF) and palpitations from atrial ectopy commonly report emotional stress. The Framingham Offspring Study revealed that anxiety predicted AF in men and correlated with increased overall mortality in men and women (Eaker, Sullican, Kelly-Hayes, D'Agostino, & Benjamin, 2005). Examinations of HRV from holter monitors revealed that there was higher sympathetic to parasympathetic activity until 10 minutes prior to the start of the AF (Ziegelstein, 2007).

Acupuncture

Acupuncture is used to treat stable angina arrhythmias (Lomuscio, A et al., 2011) (Richter, Herlitz, & Hjalmarson, 1991), Raynaud's syndrome (Vogel et al., 2005), and hypertension (Chiu, Chi, & Reid, 1997). The ability of acupuncture to inhibit sympathetic outflow may account for its effectiveness. The specific acupuncture points used for the treatment of CVD are the *Neiguan* or *Zusanli* acupoints, which overlie the median and deep peroneal nerves (Guo, Jai, Cao, Guo, & Li, 1981). A placebo effect has been suggested. Because both acupuncture and the placebo effect involve the endogenous opioid system, there is a narrow window between a placebo effect and a true response (Vogel et al., 2005). But a study using sham acupuncture as a control indicates that acupuncture is effective. When compared with amiodarone, acupuncture was as effective in preventing the recurrence of AF post cardioversion, while sham acupuncture was ineffective (Lomuscio et al., 2011).

Studies are underway to determine effective meridian points for chronic stable angina (Li et al., 2014). Many cardiac patients benefit from acupuncture, and it has therefore entered mainstream cardiology, even while its effectiveness is still being investigated.

Chelation

Chelation therapy with ethylenediamine tetra-acetic acid (EDTA) for the treatment of CAD has been controversial since its inception in the 1950s. The Trial to Assess Chelation Therapy (TACT) was the first large-scale double-blind randomized control study to show the benefit of intravenous chelation with oral high-dose vitamins in post-MI patients (Lamas et al., 2014). Over 1,700 patients (only 18% were female and 97% were Caucasian) were randomized to one of four groups: chelation with vitamins, chelation with placebo pills, IV placebo infusions with vitamins, and IV placebo with placebo pills. At the end of 5 years, the chelation plus vitamin group had statistically significant fewer end points (CV death, MI, need for revascularization, angina, or stroke) when compared with the placebo plus placebo group (26% versus 30%). The groups with one active therapy had no statistically significant difference in end points compared with the nontreatment group. The maximum benefit of chelation with vitamins was seen in diabetic patients. As the first and only well-designed trial showing modest benefit of IV chelation with vitamin therapy in a stable post MI population, TACT has not changed cardiology practice, and the routine use of chelation therapy is still not advised. However, TACT does offer options, especially for the post-MI diabetic patient, and opens up research for many unanswered questions. Does oral chelation, which is used frequently in alternative practices, work? Does chelation depend on the appropriate use of high-dose vitamins? Does chelation benefit those with subclinical atherosclerosis?

Summary

This chapter has outlined the unique nature of women's cardiovascular health, and I hope that you will find the following brief summary for risk assessment and disease prevention helpful.

1. Listen to the woman. She is blessed with incredible intuitive powers after years of hormonal cycling and after being a caretaker for her family or friends. Be aware that typical symptoms of chest discomfort may or may not be present and that she may describe fatigue or dyspnea as her anginal equivalent.
2. Determine her cardiovascular risk from her unique life experiences, as well as from the factors on Table 31.1
3. Order appropriate diagnostic testing and/or refer to a cardiologist you trust. All diabetic and high-risk women can benefit from seeing a good preventive cardiologist.

4. Recommend appropriate preventive measures in ALL women:
    a. Nutritional counseling for weight reduction/maintenance, hypertension, or hyperlipidemia;
    b. Exercise recommendations to improve physical conditioning, strength, flexibility, balance, and mental health;
    c. Psychosocial intervention when appropriate;
    d. Aspirin as outlined in this chapter;
    e. Supplement use as outlined in this chapter, especially omega-3 fatty acids and magnesium;
    f. Mind–body techniques for relaxation and stress management; and
    g. Pharmacotherapy to achieve goal levels of BP and lipids and to control diabetes.
5. Lastly, find joy in your practice so that you can be a better healer and improve your own cardiovascular health.

REFERENCES

Akashi, Y. J., Goldstein, D. S., & Ueyama, T. (2008). Takotsubo cardiomyopathy: A new form of acute, reversible heart failure. *Circulation, 7*, 1171–1176.

Albert, C. M., Gaziano, J. M., Willett, W. C., & Manson, J. E. (2002). Nut consumption and decreased risk of sudden cardiac death in the Physicians' Health Study. *Arch Intern Med, 162*, 1482–1387.

Albert, C. M., Oh, K., Whang, W., et al. (2005). Dietary alpha-linolenic acid intake and risk of sudden cardiac death and coronary heart disease. *Circulation, 112*, 3232–3238.

American Heart Association. (2014). *Heart disease and stroke statistics—2014 update.* Dallas, TX: American Heart Association.

Amin, A. A., Jones, A. M., Nugent, K., Rumsfeld, J. S., & Spertus, J. A. (2006). The prevalence of unrecognized depression in patients with acute coronary syndrome. *Am Heart J, 152*, 928–934.

Anderson, J. W., & Hanna, T. J. (1999). Impact of nondigestible carbohydrates on serum lipoproteins and risk for cardiovascular disease. *J Nutr, 129*, 1457S–1466S.

Anderson, J. W., Liu, C., & Kryscio, R. J. (2008). Blood pressure response to transcendental meditation: A meta-analysis. *Am J Hypertens, 21*, 310–316.

Antithrombotic Trialists' Collaboration (ATC). (1994). Collaborative overview of randomized trials of antiplatelet therapy: Prevention of death, myocardial infarction, and stroke by prolonged antiplatelet therapy in various categories of patients. *BMJ, 308*, 81–106.

Antithrombotic Trialists' Collaboration (ATC). (2002). Collaborative meta-analysis of randomised trails of antiplatelet therapy for prevention of death, myocardial infarction, and stroke in high risk patients. *BMJ, 324*, 71–86.

Appel, L. J., Moore, T. J., Obarzanek, E., et al. (1997). A clinical trial of the effects of dietary patterns on blood pressure. DASH Collaborative Research Group. *N Engl J Med, 336*, 1117–1124.

Arab, L., & Elashoff, D. (2009). Green and black tea consumption and the risk of stroke: A meta-analysis. *Stroke, 40*, 1786–1792.

Arslanian-Engoren, C., Patel, A., Fang, J., et al. (2006). Symptoms of men and women presenting with acute coronary syndromes. *Am J Cardiol, 98*, 1177–1181.

Atteritano, M., Marini, H., Minutoli, L., et al. (2007). Effects of the phytoestrogen genistein on some predictors of cardiovascular risk in osteopenic, postmenopausal women: A 2-years randomized, double-blind, placebo-controlled study. *J Clin Endocrinol Metab, 92*, 3068–3075.

Autier, P., & Gandini, S. (2007). Vitamin D supplementation and total mortality: A meta-analysis of randomized controlled trials. *Arch Intern Med, 167*, 1730–1737.

Barrett-Connor, E., Grady, D., Sashegyi, A., et al. (2002). Raloxifene and cardiovascular events in osteoporotic postmenopausal women. *JAMA, 287*, 847–857.

Bashir, Y., Sneddon, J. F., Staunton, H. A., et al. (1993). Effects of long-term oral magnesium chloride replacement in congestive heart failure secondary to coronary artery disease. *Am J Cardiol, 72*, 1156–1162.

Bays, H. E., Tighe, A. P., Sadovsky, R., & Davidson, M. H. (2008). Prescription omega-3 fatty acids and their lipid effects: Physiologic mechanisms of action and clinical implications. *Expert Re Cardiovasc Ther, 6*, 391–409.

Berger, J. S., Roncaglioni, M. C., Avanzini, F., Pangrazzi, I., Tognoni, G., & Brown, D. L. (2006). Aspirin for the primary prevention of cardiovascular events in women and men: A sex-specific meta-analysis of randomized controlled trails. *JAMA, 295*, 306–313.

Bittner, V. (2005). Perspectives on dyslipidemia and coronary heart disease in women. *J Am Coll Cardiol, 46*, 1628–1635.

Bittner, V., Simon, J. A., Fong, J., Blumenthal, R. S., Newby, K., & Stefanick, M. L. (2000). Correlates of high HDL cholesterol among women with coronary heart disease. *Am Heart J, 139*, 288–296.

Blum, A., Hathaway, L., Mincemoyer, R., et al. (2000). Effects of oral l-arginine on endothelium-dependent vasodilation and markers of inflammation in healthy postmenopausal women. *J Am Coll Cardiol, 35*, 271–276.

Blumenthal, J. A., Babyak, M. A., Moore, K. A., et al. (1999). Effects of exercise training on older patients with major depression. *Arch Intern Med, 159*, 2349–2356.

Blumenthal, J. A., Sherwood, A., Babyak, M. A., et al. (2005). Effects of exercise and stress management training on markers of cardiovascular risk in patients with ischemic heart disease. *JAMA, 293*, 1626–1634.

Boden, W. E., & Probstfield, J. L. (2011). Niacin in patients with low HDL cholesterol levels receiving intensive statin therapy. *NEJM, 67*, 2255–2267.

Bolland, M. J., Barber, P. A., Doughty, R. N., et al. (2008). Vascular events in healthy older women receiving calcium supplementation: Randomised controlled trial. *BMJ, 336*, 262–266.

Bonaa, K. H., Njolstad, I., Ueland, P. M., et al. (2006). Homocysteine lowering and cardiovascular events after acute myocardial infarction. *N Engl J Med, 354*, 1578–1588.

Brevetti, G., Diehm, C., & Lambert, D. (1999). European multicenter study on propionyl-l-carnitine in intermittent claudication. *J Am Coll Cardiol, 34*, 1618–1624.

Canto, J. G., Goldberg, R. J., Hand, M. M., et al. (2007). Symptom presentation of women with acute coronary syndromes: Myth vs. reality. *Arch Intern Med, 167*, 2405–2413.

Chan, A. T., Manson, J. E., Feskanich, D., Stampfer, M. J., Colditz, G. A., & Fuchs, C. S. (2007). Long-term aspirin use and mortality in women. *Arch Intern Med, 167*, 562–572.

Chiu, Y. J., Chi, A., & Reid, I. A. (1997). Cardiovascular and endocrine effects of acupuncture in hypertensive patients. *Clin Exp Hypertens, 19*, 1047–1063.

Chobanian, A. V., Bakris, G. L., Clack, H. R., et al. (2003). The seventh report of the joint national committee on prevention, detection, evaluation, and treatment of high blood pressure: The JNC 7 report. *JAMA, 289*, 2560–2572.

Christian, A. H., Rosamond, W., White, A. R., & Mosca, L. (2007). Nine-year trends and racial and ethnic disparities in women's awareness of heart disease and stroke: AN American Heart Association national study. *J Womens Health (Larchmt), 16*(1), 68–81.

Cicero, A. F., Erick, S., & Borghi, C. (2009). Omega-3 polyunsaturated fatty acids: Their potential role in blood pressure prevention and management. *Curr Vasc Pharmacol, 7*, 330–337.

Cochrane Heart Group. (2011). *Psychological interventions for coronary heart disease.* Published online. Retrieved August 8, 2014. doi: 10.1002/14651858.CD002902.pub3

Colonna, P., & Iliceto, S. (2000). Myocardial infarction and left ventricular remodeling: Results of the CEDIM trial. L-carnitine Ecocardiografia Digitalizzata Infarto Miocardico. *Am Heart J, 139*(2 Pt 3), S124–S130.

Cook, N. R., Albert, C. M., Gaziano, J. M., et al. (2007). A randomized factorial trial of vitamins C and E and beta carotene in the secondary prevention of cardiovascular events in women: Results from the Women's Antioxidant Cardiovascular Study. *Arch Intern Med, 167*, 1610–1618.

Cossette, S., Frasure-Smith, N., & Lesperance, F. (2001). Clinical implications of a reduction in psychological distress on cardiac prognosis in patients participating in a psychosocial intervention program. *Psychosom Med, 63*, 257–266.

Cramer, H., Haller, H., et al. (2014). A systematic review and meta-analysis of yoga for hypertension. *Am J Hypertension.*[Epub ahead of print]

Davidson, M. H., Stein, E. A., Bays, H. E., et al. (2007). Efficacy and tolerability of adding prescription omega-3 fatty acids 4 g/d to simvastatin 40 mg/d in hypertriglyceridemic patients: An 8-week, randomized, double-blind, placebo-controlled study. *Clin Ther, 29*, 1354–1367.

de Kleijn, M. J., van der Schouw, Y. T., Wilson, P. W., Grobbee, D. E., & Jacques, P. R. (2002). Dietary intake of phytoestrogens is associated with a favorable metabolic cardiovascular risk profile in postmenopausal U.S. women: The Framingham study. *J Nutr, 132*, 276–282.

Debette, S., Courbon, D., Leone, N., et al. (2008). Tea consumption is inversely associated with carotid plaques in women. *Arterioscler Thromb Vasc Biol, 28,* 353–359.

Department of Health and Human Services. (1996). *Physical activity and health, a report of the Surgeon General.* Atlanta: Department of Health and Human Services, Centers for Disease Control and Prevention, National Center for Chronic Disease Prevention and Health Promotion.

Dey, S., Flather, M. D., et al. (2009). Sex related differences in the presentation, treatment and outcomes among patient with acute coronary syndromes: The Global Registry of Acute Coronary Events. *Heart, 95,* 20–26.

Dong, J. Y., Qin, L. Q., Zhang, Z., et al. (2011). Effect of oral L-arginine supplementation on blood pressure: A meta-analysis of randomized, double-blind, placebo-controlled trials. *Am Heart J, 162,* 959–965.

Dusseldorp, E., van Elderen, T., Maes, S., Meulman, J., & Kraaij, V. (1999). A meta-analysis of psychoeducational programs for coronary heart disease patients. *Health Psychol, 18,* 506–519.

Eaker, E. D., Sullican, L. M., Kelly-Hayes, M., D'Agostino, R. B., & Benjamin, E. J. (2005). Tension and anxiety and the prediction of the 10-year incidence of coronary heart disease, atrial fibrillation, and total mortality: The Framingham offspring study. *Psychosom Med, 67,* 692–696.

Empana, J. P., Jouven, X., Lemaitre, R. N., et al. (2006). Clinical depression and risk of out-of-hospital cardiac arrest. *Arch Intern Med, 166,* 195–200.

Elley, C. R., & Arroll, B. (2005). Refining the exercise prescription for hypertension. *Lancet, 366,* 1248–1249.

Feringa, H. H., Laskey, D. A., Dickson, J. E., & Coleman, C. (2011). The effect of grape seed extract on cardiovascular risk markers: A meta-analysis of randomized controlled trials. *J Am Diet Assoc, 111,* 1173–1181.

Ford, E. S., & Mokdad, A. H. (2003). Dietary magnesium intake in a national sample of US adults. *J Nutr, 133,* 2879–2882.

Foulon, T., Payen, N., Laporte, F., et al. (2001). Effects of two low-dose oral contraceptives containing ethinylestradiol and either desogestrel or levonorgestrel on serum lipids and lipoproteins with particular regard to LDL size. *Contraception, 64,* 11–16.

Franco, O. H., de Laet, C., Peeters, A., Jonker, J., Mackenbach, J., & Nusselder, W. (2005). Effects of physical activity on life expectancy with cardiovascular disease. *Arch Intern Meda, 165,* 2355–2360.

Franco, O. H., Peeters, A., Conneux, L., & de Laet, C. (2005). Blood pressure in adulthood and life expectancy with cardiovascular disease in men and women: Life course analysis. *Hypertension, 46,* 280–286.

Franklin, S. S., Larson, M. G., Khan, S. A., et al. (2001). Does the relation of blood pressure to coronary heart disease risk change with aging? *Circulation, 103,* 1245–1249.

Fraser, G. E., Sabate, J., Beeson, W. L., & Strahan, T. M. (1992). A possible protective effect of nut consumption on risk of coronary heart disease. *Arch Intern Med, 152,* 1416–1426.

Frasure-Smith, N., Lesperance, F., Prince, R. H., et al. (1997). Randomised trial of home-based psychosocial nursing intervention for patients recovering from myocardial infarction. *Lancet, 350,* 473–479.

Fung, T. T., Chiuve, S. E., McCullough, M. L., Rexrode, K. M., Logroscino, G., Hu, F. B. (2008). Adherence to a DASH-Style diet and risk of coronary heart disease and stroke in women. *Arch Intern Med, 168,* 713–720.

Fung, T. T., van Dam, R., et al. (2010). Low-carbohydrate diets and all-cause-specific mortality: Two cohort studies. *Ann Intern Med, 153,* 289–298.

Garber, C. E., Blissmer B., Deschenes, M. R., et al. (2011). American College of Sports Medicine position stand: Quantity and quality of exercise for developing and maintaining cardiorespiratory, musculoskeletal, and neuromotor fitness in apparently healthy adults: Guidance for prescribing exercise. *Med Sci Sports Exerc, 43,* 1334–1359.

Geleijnse, J. M., Launer, L. J., Van de Kuip, D. A., Hofman, A., & Witteman, J. C. (2002). Inverse association of tea and flavenoid intakes with incident myocardial infarction: The Rotterdam Study. *Am J Clin Nutr, 75,* 880–886.

Gianni, M., Dentali, F., Grandi, A. M., Summer, G., Hiralal, R., & Lonn, E. (2006). Apical ballooning syndrome or takotsubo cardiomyopathy: A systematic review. *Eur Heart J, 27,* 1523–1529.

Glassman, A. H., & Bigger, J. T. (1981). Cardiovascular effects of therapeutic doses of tricyclic antidepressants. *Arch Gen Psychiatry, 38,* 815–820.

Glassman, A. H., & Preud'homme, X. A. (1993). Review of the cardiovascular effects of heterocyclic antidepressants. *J Clin Psychiatry, 54,* 16–22.

Glassman, A. H., O'Connor, C. M., Califf, R. M., et al. (2002). Sertraline treatment of major depression in patients with acute MI or unstable angina. *JAMA, 288,* 701–709.

Goff, D. C., Lloyd-Jones, D. M., et al. (2014). 2013 ACC/AHA Guidelines on the Assessment of Cardiovascular Risk: A Report of the American College of Cardiology/American Heart Association Task Force on Practice Guidelines. *Circulation, 129,* 549–573.

Godsland, I. F., Crook, D., Simpson, R., et al. (1990). The effects of different formulations of oral contraceptive agents on lipid and carbohydrate metabolism. *N Engl J Med, 323,* 1375–1381.

Goldberg, A., Alagona, P., Jr., Capuzzi, D. M., et al. (2000). Multiple-dose efficacy and safety of an extended-release form of niacin in the management of hyperlipidemia. *Am J Cardiol, 85,* 1100–1105.

Gorinstein, S., Jastrzebski, Z., Namiesnik, J., Leontowicz, H., Leontowicz, M., & Trakhtenberg, S. (2007). The atherosclerotic heart disease and protecting properties of garlic: Contemporary data. *Mol Nutr Food Res, 51,* 1365–1381.

Grosser, T., Fries, S., et al. (2013). Drug resistance and pseudoresistance: An unintended consequence of enteric coated aspirin. *Circulation, 127,* 377–385.

Grundy, S. M., Cleeman, J. I., Merz, N. B., et al., for the Coordinating Committee of the National Cholesterol Education Program. (2004). Implications of recent clinical trials for the National Cholesterol Education Program Adult Treatment Panel III Guidelines. *Circulation, 110,* 227–239.

Gulati, M., Cooper-DeHoff, R. M., et al. (2009). Adverse cardiovascular outcomes in women with nonobstructive coronary artery disease. *Arch Intern Med*, *169*, 843–850.

Guo, X. Q., Jai, R. J., Cao, Q. Y., Guo, Zd, & Li, P. (1981). Inhibitory effect of somatic nerve afferent impulses on the extrasystole induced by hypothalamic stimulation. *Acta Physiolo Sin*, *33*, 334–350.

Hazelton, G., Williams, J., et al. (2014). Psychosocial benefits of cardiac rehabilitation among women compared to men. *J Cardiopulm Rehab Prev*, *34*, 21–28.

Hemingway, H., Langenberg, C., Damant, J., Frost, C., Pyörälä, K., & Carrett-Connor, E. (2008). Prevalence of angina in women versus men. *Circulation*, *117*, 1526–1536.

Hiatt, W. R., Regensteiner, J. G., Creager, M. A., et al. (2001). Propionyl-L-carnitine improves exercise performance and functional status in patients with claudication. *Am J Med*, *110*, 616–622.

Hlatky, M. A. (2008). Expanding the orbit of primary prevention—Moving beyond JUPITER. *NEJM*, *359*, 2280–2282.

Holick, M. F. (2007). Vitamin D deficiency. *N Engl J Med*, *357*, 266–281.

Hopkins, A. L., Lamm, M. G., Funk, J. L., & Ritenbaugh, C. (2013). Hibiscus sabdariffa L. in the treatment of hypertension and hyperlipidemia: A comprehensive review of animal and human studies. *Fitoterapia*, *85*, 84–94.

Hsia, J., Heiss, G., Ren, H., et al. (2007). Calcium/vitamin D supplementation and cardiovascular events. *Circulation*, *115*, 846–854.

Hu, F. B., Bronner, L., Willett, W. C., et al. (2002). Fish and omega-3 fatty acid intake and risk of coronary heart disease in women. *JAMA*, *287*, 1815–1821.

Hu, F. B., Stampfer, M. J., Manson, J. E., et al. (1998). Frequent nut consumption and risk of coronary heart disease in women: Prospective cohort study. *BMJ*, *317*, 1341–1345.

Inami, S., Takano, M., Yamamoto, M., et al. (2007). Tea catechin consumption reduces circulation oxidized low-density lipoprotein. *Int Heart J*, *48*, 725–732.

Iso, H., Kobayashi, M., Ishihara, J., et al. (2006). Intake of fish and n3 fatty acids and risk of coronary heart disease among Japanese: The Japan Public Health Center-Based (JPHC) Study Cohort I. *Circulation*, *113*, 195–202.

James, P. A., Oparil, S., et al. (2014). 2013 evidence-based guideline for the management of high blood pressure in adults: A report from the panel members appointed to the Eight Joint National Committee (JNC8). *JAMA*, *311*, 507–520.

Jones, D. A., & West, R. R. (1996). Psychological rehabilitation after myocardial infarction: Multicentre randomized controlled trial. *BMJ*, *313*, 1517–1521.

Katan, M. B., Grundy, S. M., Jones, P., Law, M., Miettinen, T., Paoletti, R., & Stresa Workshop Participants. (2003). Efficacy and safety of plant stanols and sterols in the management of blood cholesterol levels. *Mayo Clin Proc*, *78*, 965–978.

Khot, U. N., Khot, M. B., Bajzer, C. T., et al. (2003). Prevalence of conventional risk factors in patients with coronary heart disease. *JAMA*, *290*, 898–904.

Knekt, P., Ritz, J., Pereira, M. A., et al. (2004). Antioxidant vitamins and coronary heart disease risk: A pooled analysis of 9 cohorts. *Am J Clin Nutr*, *80*, 1508–1520.

Knox, J., & Gaster, B. (2007). Dietary supplements for the prevention and treatment of coronary artery disease. *J Altern Complement Med*, *13*, 83–95.

Kokubo, Y., Iso, H., Ishihara, J., Okada, K., Inoue, M., & Tsugane, S. (2007). Association of dietary intake of soy, beans, and isoflavones with risk of cerebral and myocardial infarctions in Japanese populations: The Japan Public Health Center-Based (JPHC) Study Cohort I. *Circulation, 116,* 2553–2562.

Kris-Etherton, P. M., Hu, F. B., Ros,E., & Sabate, J. (2007). The Role of Tree Nuts and Peanuts in the Prevention of Coronary Heart Disease: Multiple Potential Mechanisms. *The Journal of Nutrition, 2007 Nuts and Health Symposium.*

Kuriyama, S., Shimazu, T., Ohmori, K., et al. (2006). Green tea consumption and mortality due to cardiovascular disease, cancer, and all causes in Japan: The Ohsaki study. *JAMA, 296,* 1255–1265.

Kushi, L. H., Folsom, A. R., Prineas, R. J., Mink, P. J., Wu, Y., & Bostick, R. M. (1996). Dietary antioxidant vitamins and death from coronary heart disease in postmenopausal women. *N Engl J Med, 334,* 1156–1162.

Lamas, G. A., Boineau, R., et al. (2014). EDTA chelations therapy along and in combination with oral high-dose multivitamins and minerals for coronary disease: The factorial group results of the Trial to Assess Chelation Therapy. *Am Health J, 168,* 37–44.

Lampert, R., Joska, T., Burg, M. M., Batsford, W. P., McPherson, C. A., & Jain, D. (2002). Emotional and psychical precipitants of ventricular arrhythmia. *Circulation, 106,* 1800–1805.

Lange, H., Suryapranato, H., DeLuca, G., et al. (2004). Folate therapy and in-stent restenosis after coronary stenting. *N Engl J Med, 350,* 2673–2681.

Lansky, A. J., Hochman, J. S., Ward, P. A., et al. (2005). Percutaneous coronary intervention and adjunctive pharmacotherapy in women: A statement for healthcare professionals from the American Heart Association. *Circulation, 111,* 940–953.

Lawlor, D. A., & Hopker, S. W. (2001). The effectiveness of exercise as an intervention in the management of depression: Systematic review and meta-regression analysis of randomised controlled trials. *BMJ, 322,* 763–767.

Lee, I. M., Cook, N. R., Gaziano, J. M., et al. (2005). Vitamin E in the primary prevention of cardiovascular disease and cancer: The Women's Health Study: A randomized controlled trial. *JAMA, 294,* 56–65.

Lewington, S., Clarke, R., Qizilbash, N., Peto, R., & Collins, R. (2002). Age-specific relevance of usual blood pressure to vascular mortality: A meta-analysis of individual data for one million adults in 61 prospective studies. *Lancet, 360,* 1903–1913.

Li, D., Yang, M., et al. (2014). Acupuncture for chronic, stable angina pectoris and an investigation of the characteristics of acupoint specificity: Study protocol for a multicenter randomized controlled trial. *Trials, 15,* 50.

Linden, W., Stossel, C., & Maurice, J. (1996). Psychosocial interventions for patients with coronary artery disease: A meta-analysis. *Arch Intern Med, 156,* 745–752.

Liu, J., Zhang, J., Shi, Y., Grimsgaard, S., Alraek, T., & Fonnebo, V. (2006). Chinese red yeast rice (Monascus purpureus) for primary hyperlipidemia: A meta-analysis of randomized controlled trials. *Chin Med, 23,* 1–4.

Liu, S., Burin, J. E., Sesso, H. D., Rimm, E. B., Willett, W. C., & Manson, J. E. (2002). A prospective study of dietary fiber intake and risk of cardiovascular disease among women. *J Am Coll Cardiol, 39,* 49–56.

Lomuscio, A., Belletti, S., et al. (2011). Efficacy of acupuncture in preventing atrial fibrillation recurrences after electrical cardioversion. *J Cardiovasc Eletrophysiol, 22,* 241–247.

Lorenz, M., Jochmann, N., von Krosigk, A., et al. (2007). Addition of milk prevents vascular protective effects of tea. *Eu Heart J, 28,* 219–223.

Ma, J., Folso, A. R., Melnick, S. L., et al. (1995). Associations of serum and dietary magnesium with cardiovascular disease, hypertension, diabetes, insulin, and carotid arterial wall thickness: The ARIC study. Atherosclerosis Risk in Communities Study. *J Clin Epidemiol, 48,* 927–940.

Mallik, S., Spertus, J. A., Reid, K. J., et al. (2006). Depressive symptoms after acute myocardial infarction: Evidence for highest rates in younger women. *Arch Intern Med, 166,* 876–883.

Manson, J. E., Bassuk, S. S., et al. (2012). The vitamin D and Omega-3 trial (VITAL): Rationale and design of a large randomized controlled trial of vitamin D and marine omega-3 fatty acid supplements for the primary prevention of cancer and cardiovascular disease. *Contemp Clin Trials, 33,* 159–171.

Manson, J. E., Greenland, P., LaCroix, A. Z., et al. (2002). Walking compared with vigorous exercise for the prevention of cardiovascular events in women. *N Engl J Med, 347,* 716–725.

Manson, J. W., Hu, F. B., Rich-Edwards, J. W., et al. (1999). A prospective study of walking as compared with vigorous exercise in the prevention of coronary heart disease in women. *N Engl J Med, 341,* 650–658.

Marcoff, L., & Thompson, P. D. (2007). The role of coenzyme Q10 in statin-associated myopathy *J Am Coll Cardiol, 49,* 2231–2237.

McGrady, A., Nadsady, P. A., & Schumann-Brzezinski, C. (1991). Sustained effects of biofeedback-assisted relaxation therapy in essential hypertension. *Biofeedback Self Regul, 16,* 399–411.

McGrady, A. V., Yonker, R., Tan, S. Y., Fine, T. H., & Woerner, M. (1981). The effect of biofeedback-assisted relaxation training on blood pressure and selected biochemical parameters in patients with essential hypertension. *Biofeedback Self Regul, 6,* 343–353.

McSweeney, J. C., Cody, M., O'Sullivan, P., Elberson, K., Moser, D. K., & Garvin, B. J. (2003). Women's early warning symptoms of acute myocardial infarction. *Circulation, 108,* 2619–2623.

Meles, E., Giannattasio, C., Failla, M., Gentile, G., Capra, A., & Mancia, G. (2004). Nonpharmacologic treatment of hypertension by respiratory exercise in the home setting. *Am J Hypertens, 17,* 370–374.

Merz, C. N. B., Shaw, L. J., Reis, S. E., et al. (2006). Insights from the NHLBI-sponsored women's ischemia syndrome evaluation (WISE) study. *J Am Coll Cardiol, 47,* 21S–29S.

Mieres, J. H., Shaw, L. J., Arai, A., et al. (2005). Role of noninvasive testing in the clinical evaluation of women with suspected coronary artery disease. *Circulation, 111,* 682–696.

Milani, R. V., & Lavie, C. J. (2007). Impact of cardiac rehabilitation on depression and its associated mortality. *Am J Med, 120*, 799–806.

Milner, K. A., Funk, M., Richards, S., Wilmes, R. M., Vaccarino, V., & Krumholz, H. M. (1999). Gender differences in symptom presentation associated with coronary heart disease. *Am J Cardiol, 84*, 396–399.

Mizuno, K., Nakaya, N., Ohashi, Y., et al. (2008). Usefulness of Pravastatin in primary prevention of cardiovascular events in women: Analysis of the management of elevated cholesterol in the primary prevention group of adult Japanese. *Circulation, 117*, 494–502.

Moran, L. J., Misso, M. L., et al. (2010). Impaired glucose tolerance, type 2 diabetes and metabolic syndrome in polycystic ovary syndrome: A systematic review and meta-analysis. *Hum Reprod Update, 16*, 347–363.

Morisco, C., Trim Arco, B., & Condor Elli, M. (1993). Effect of coenzyme Q10 therapy in patients with congestive heart failure: A long-term multicenter randomized study *Clin Investig, 71*(Suppl), S134–S136.

Mosca, L., et al. (2011). Effectiveness based guidelines for the prevention of cardiovascular disease in women-2011 update. *Circulation, 123*, 1243–1262.

Mosca, L., Banka, C. L., Benjamin, E. J., et al. (2007). Evidence-based guidelines for cardiovascular disease prevention in women: 2007 update. *Circulation, 115*, 1481–1501.

Mosca, L., Hammond, G., Mochari-Greenberger, H., Towfighi, A., & Albert MA; American Heart Association Cardiovascular Disease and Stroke in Women and Special Populations Committee of the Council on Clinical Cardiology, Council on Epidemiology and Prevention, Council on Cardiovascular Nursing, Council on High Blood Pressure Research, and Council on Nutrition, Physical Activity and Metabolism. (2013). Fifteen-year trends in awareness of heart disease in women: Results of a 2012 American Heart Association national survey. *Circulation, 19, 127*, 1254–1263.

Mosca, L., Mochari, H., Christian, A., et al. (2006). National study of women's awareness, preventative action, and barriers to cardiovascular health. *Circulation, 113*, 525–534.

Mozaffarian, D., Hao, T., Rimm, E. B., Willett, W. C., & Hu, F. B. (2011). Changes in diet and lifestyle and long-term weight gain in women and men. *N Engl J Med, 364*, 2392–2404.

Mozaffarian, D., Stein, P. K., Prineas, R. J., & Siscovick, D. S. (2008). Dietary fish and omega-3 fatty acid consumption and heart rate variability in US adults. *Circulation, 117*, 1130–1137.

Mukamal, K. J., Maclure, M., Muller, J. E., & Mittleman, M. A. (2005). Binge drinking and mortality after acute myocardial infarction. *Circulation, 112*(25), 3839–3845.

Naqvi, T. Z., Naqvi, S. S., & Merz, C. N. (2005). Gender differences in the link between depression and cardiovascular disease. *Psychosom Med, 67*, S15–S18.

Nicolson, A., Kuper, H., et al. (2006). Depression as an aetiologic and prognostic factor in coronary heart disease: A meta-analysis of 6362 events among 146,538 participants in 54 observational studies. *European Heart Journal, 27*, 2763–2774.

Nunez-Cordoba, J. M., Valencia-Serrano, F., et al. (2009). The Mediterranean diet and incidence of hypertension: The Segulmiento Universidad de Navarra (SUN) Study. *Am J Epidemiol, 169*, 339–346.

Ong, K. L., Cheung, B. M. Y., Man, Y. B., Lau, C. P., & Lam, K. S. L. (2007). Prevalence, awareness, treatment, and control of hypertension among United States adults 1999–2004. *Hypertension, 49*, 69.

Ornish, D., Scherwitz, L. W., et al. (1998). Intensive lifestyle changes for reversal of heart disease. *JAMA, 280*, 2001–2007.

Orth-Gomer, K., Schneiderman, N., et al. (2009). Stress reduction prolongs life in women with coronary disease: The Stockholm Women's Intervention Trial for Coronary Heart Disease (SWITCHD). *Circ Cardiovasc Qual Outcomes, 2*, 25–32.

Osganian, S. K., Stampfer, M. J., Rimm, E., et al. (2003). Vitamin C and risk of coronary heart disease in women. *J Am Coll Cardiol, 42*, 246–252.

Paoli, A., Rubini, A., et al. (2013). Beyond weight loss: A review of the therapeutic uses of very-low-carbohydrate (ketogenic) diets. *Eur J Clin Nutr, 67*, 789–796.

Pate, R. R., Pratt, M., Blair, S. N., et al. (1995). Physical activity and public health. A recommendation from the Centers for Disease Control and Prevention and the American College of Sports Medicine. *JAMA, 273*, 402–407.

Patel, H., Rosengren, A., & Ekman, I. (2004). Symptoms in acute coronary syndromes: Does sex make a difference? *Am Heart J, 148*, 27–33.

Pilote, L., Dasgupta, K., Guru, V.,et al. (2007). A comprehensive view of sex-specific issues related to cardiovascular disease. *CMAJ, 176*(6), S1–44.

Raggi, P., Shaw, L. J., Berman, D. S., & Callister, T. Q. (2004). Gender-based differences in the prognostic value of coronary calcification. *J Women Health (Larchmt), 13*, 273–283.

Rapola, J. M., Virtamo, J., Haukka, J. K., et al. (1996). Effect of vitamin E and beta carotene on the incidence of angina pectoris: A randomized, double-blind, controlled study. *JAMA, 275*, 693–698.

Rapola, J. M., Virtamo, J., Ripatti, S., et al. (1998). Effects of alpha tocopherol and beta carotene supplements on symptoms, progression, and prognosis of angina pectoris. *Heart, 79*, 454–458.

Rich-Edwards, J. W., Mason, S., et al. (2012). Physical and sexual abuse in childhood as predictors of early-onset cardiovascular events in women. *Circulation, 126*, 920–927.

Ridker, P. M., Buring, J. E., Rifai, N., & Cook, N. R. (2007). Development and validation of improved algorithms for the assessment of global cardiovascular risk in women. *JAMA, 297*, 611–619.

Ridker, P. M., Cook, N. R., Lee, I., et al. (2005). A randomized trial of low-dose aspirin in the primary prevention of cardiovascular disease in women. *N Engl J Med, 352*, 1293–1304.

Ridker, P. M., Danielson, E., Fonseca, F., et al., for the JUPITER Study Group. (2008). Rosuvastatin to Prevent Vascular Events in Men and Women with Elevated C-Reactive Protein. *NEJM, 359*, 2195–2207.

Richter, A., Herlitz, J., & Hjalmarson, A. (1991). Effect of acupuncture in patients with angina pectoris. *Eur Heart J, 12*, 175–178.

Roche, M. M., & Wang, P. P. (2013). Sex differences in all cause and cardiovascular mortality, hospitalization for individuals with and without diabetes and patients with diabetes diagnosed early and late. *Diabetes Care, 36*, 2582–2590.

Rosanoff, A. (2010). Magnesium supplements may enhance the effect of antihypertensive medications in stage 1 hypertensive subjects. *Magnes Res, 23*, 27–40.

Rosendorff, C., Black, H. R., Cannon, C. P., et al. (2007). Treatment of hypertension in the prevention and management of ischemic heart disease. *Circulation, 115*, 2761–2788.

Rosengren, A., Hawken, S., Ounpuu, S., et al. (2004). Association of psychosocial risk factors with risk of acute myocardial infarction in11 119 cases and 13 648 controls from 52 countries (the INTERHEART study): Case-control study. *Lancet, 364*, 953–962.

Rozanski, A. (2014). Behavioral cardiology. *J Am Coll Cardiol, 64*, 100–110.

Rugulies, R. (2002). Depression as a predictor for coronary heart disease: A review and meta-analysis. *Am J Prev Med, 23*, 51–61.

Sacks, F. M., Svetsky, L. P. O., Vollmer, W. M., et al. (2001). Effects on blood pressure of reduced dietary sodium and the dietary approaches to stop hypertension (DASH) diet. *N Engl J Med, 344*, 3–10.

Shiroma, E. J., & Lee, I.-M. (2010). Exercise in cardiovascular disease: Physical activity and cardiovascular health: Lessons learned from epidemiological studies across age, gender, and race/ethnicity. *Circulation, 122*, 743–752.

Siervo, M., Lara, J., Ogbonmwan, I., & Mathers, J. C. (2013). Inorganic nitrate and beetroot juice supplementation reduces blood pressure in adults: A systematic review and meta-analysis. *J Nutr Jun, 143*, 818–826.

Schein, M. H., Gavish, B., Herz, M., et al. (2001). Treating hypertension with a device that slows and regularises breathing: A randomised double-blind controlled study *J Hum Hypertens, 15*, 271–278.

Schulman, S. P., Becker, L. C., & Kass, D. A. (2006). L-arginine therapy in acute myocardial infarction: The vascular interaction with age in myocardial infarction (VINTAGE MI) randomized clinical trial. *JAMA, 295*, 58–64.

Silagy, C. A., & Neil, H. A. (1994). A meta-analysis of the effect of garlic on blood pressure. *J Hypertens, 12*, 463–468.

Singh, M., Charanjit, S. R., Gersh, B. J., et al. (2008). Mortality differences between men and women after percutaneous coronary Interventions. *JACC, 51*, 2313–2322.

Stevens, J., Cal, J., Evenson, K. R., & Thomas, R. (2002). Fitness and fatness as predictors of mortality from all causes and from cardiovascular disease in men and women in the lipid research clinics study. *Am J Epidemiol, 156*, 832–841.

Stevinson, C., Pittler, M. H., & Ernst, E. (2000). Garlic for treating hypercholesterolemia. *Ann Intern Med, 133*, 420–429.

Stone, N. J., Robinson, J. G., et al. (2014). ACC/AHA Guideline on the treatment of blood cholesterol to reduce atherosclerotic cardiovascular risk in adults: A report of the American College of Cardiology/American Heart Association Task Force on Practice Guidelines. *J Am Coll Cardiol, 63*(25 Pt B), 2889–2934.

Susalit, E., Agus, N., Effendi, I., et al. (2011). Olive (Olea europaea) leaf extract effective in patients with stage-1 hypertension: Comparison with Captopril. *Phytomedicine, 18*, 251–258.

Svetkey, L. P., Simons-Morton, D. G., Proschan, M. A., et al. (2004). Effect of the dietary approaches to stop hypertension diet and reduced sodium intake on blood pressure control. *J Clin Hypertension (Greenwich), 6*, 373–381.

The ATBC Cancer Prevention Study Group. (1994). The alpha-tocopherol, beta-carotene lung cancer prevention study: Design, methods, participant characteristics, and compliance. *Ann Epidemiol, 4*, 1–10.

The ENRICHD Investigators. (2003). Effects of treating depression and low perceived social support on clinical events after myocardial infarction: The enhancing recovery in coronary heart disease patients (ENRICHD) randomized trial. *JAMA, 289*, 3106–3116.

The Heart Outcomes Prevention Evaluation (HOPE) 2 Investigators. (2006). Homocysteine lowering with folic acid and B vitamins in vascular disease. *N Engl J Med, 354*, 1567–1577.

The Heart Outcomes Prevention Evaluation (HOPE) Study Investigators. (2000). Vitamin E supplementation and cardiovascular events in high-risk patients. *N Engl J Med, 342*, 154–160.

The HPS2-THRIVE Collaborative Group. (2014). Effects of extended-release niacin with laropiprant in high-risk patients. *N Engl J Med, 371*, 203–212.

Udell, J. A., Lu, H., & Redelmeier, D. A. (2013). Long-term cardiovascular risk in women prescribed fertility therapy. *J Am Coll Cardiol, 62*, 1704–1712.

Vaccarino, V., Lin, Z. Q., Kasl, S. V., et al. (2003). Gender differences in recovery after coronary artery bypass surgery *J Am Coll Cardiol, 41*, 307–314.

Vaccarino, V., Badimon, L., et al. (2013). Presentation, management and outcomes of ischaemic heart disease in women. *Nat Rev Cardiol, 10*, 508–518.

Virani, S. S., Khan, A. N., Mendoza, C. E., Ferreira, A. C., & de Marchena, E. (2007). Takotsubo cardiomyopathy, or broken-heart syndrome. *Tex Heart Inst J, 34*, 76–79.

Von Ruden, A. E., Adson, D. E., & Kotlyar, M. (2008). Effect of selective serotonin reuptake inhibitors on cardiovascular morbidity and mortality. *J Card Pharm Ther, 13*, 32–40.

Vogel, J. H. K., Bolling, S. F., Costello, R. B., et al. (2005). Integrating complementary medicine into cardiovascular medicine *J Am Coll Cardiol, 46*, 184–221.

Watson, P. S., Scalia, G. M., Galbraith, A., Burstow, D. J., Bett, N., & Aroney, C. N. (1999). Lack of effect of coenzyme Q on left ventricular function in patients with congestive heart failure *J Am Coll Cardiol, 33*, 1549–1552.

Welty, R. K., Lee, K. S., Lew, N. S., & Zhou, J. R. (2007). Effect of soy nuts on blood pressure and lipid levels in hypertensive, prehypertensive, and normotensive postmenopausal women. *Arch Intern Med, 167*, 1060–1067.

Wenger, N. K. (2008). Drugs for cardiovascular disease prevention in women. *Drugs, 68*, 339–358.

Wenger, N. K., Lewis, S. J., Welty, F. K., Herrington, D. M., & Bitner, V. (2008a). Beneficial effects of aggressive low-density lipoprotein cholesterol lowering in women with stable coronary heart disease in the Treating to New Targets (TNT) study. *Heart, 94,* 434–439.

Wenger, N. K., Shaw, L. J., & Vaccarino, V. (2008). Coronary heart disease in women: Update 2008. *Clin Pharmacol Therb, 83,* 37–51.

Witt, B. J., Jacobsen, S. J., Weston, S. A., et al. (2004). Cardiac rehabilitation after myocardial infarction in the community *J Am Coll Cardiol, 44,* 988–996.

Witte, K. K. A., Clark, A. L., & Cleland, J. G. F. (2001). Chronic heart failure and micronutrients. *J Am Coll Cardiol, 37,* 1765–1774.

Wittstein, I. S. (2007). The broken heart syndrome. *Cleveland Clin J Med, 74*(Suppl 1), S17–S22.

Wolff, T., Miller, T., & Ko, S. (2009). Aspirin for the primary prevention of cardiovascular events: An update of the evidence for the US Preventive Services Task Force. *Ann Intern Med, 150,* 405–410.

Wolk, A., Manson, J. E., Stampfer, M. J., et al. (1999). Long-term intake of dietary fiber and decreased risk of coronary heart disease among women. *JAMA, 281,* 1998–2004.

Woodgate, D., Chan, C. H., & Conquer, J. A. (2006). Cholesterol-lowering ability of a phytostanol softgel supplement in adults with mild to moderate hypercholesterolemia. *Lipids, 41,* 127–132.

World Health Statistics (WHS). (2010). Geneva: World Health Organization.

Yang, C. S., Chen, G., Wu, Q. Recent scientific studies of a traditional chinese medicine, tea, on prevention of chronic diseases. *J Tradit Complement Med, 4*(1), 17–23.

Yeh, G. Y., Wang, C., Wayne, P. M., & Phillips, R. S. (2008). The effect of tai chi exercise on blood pressure: A systematic review. *Prev Cardiol, 11,* 82–89.

Yusef, S., Zhao, F., Mehta, S. R., Chrolavicius, S., & Tognoni, G. (2001). Clopidogrel in unstable angina to prevent recurrent events trial investigators: Effects of clopidogrel in addition to aspirin in patients with acute coronary syndromes without ST-segment elevation. *N Engl J Med, 345,* 494–502.

Zhang, L., Qiao, B., et al. (2013). Gender difference on five-year outcomes of EXCEL biodegradable polymer-coated sirolimus-eluting stents implantation results from the CREATE study. *Chin Med J (Engl), 126,* 1039–1045.

Ziegelstein, R. C. (2007). Acute emotional stress and cardiac arrhythmias. *JAMA, 298,* 324–329.

32

Osteoporosis

LOUISE GAGNÉ

CASE STUDY

At age 52, Margot was diagnosed as having osteopenia. Her T scores were -1.7 at the lumbar spine and -1.2 at the femoral neck. Margot had struggled with low-grade depression and anxiety for a number of years, but was otherwise in good health. She expressed concern that her bones were "already weak" at her age. Her goal was to avoid becoming disabled by osteoporosis.

Margot had experienced a sudden transition into menopause at age 48, after having a hysterectomy and bilateral oophorectomy for uterine fibroids. She used a multivitamin and a calcium supplement irregularly and was on no medications. She described her level of exercise as "close to zero." Routine blood work was unremarkable, other than her 25-hydroxy vitamin D (25-OHD), which was in the deficient range at 13 ng/mL (32 nmol/L).

An integrative bone health program was planned with Margot, and over the following year she made a number of changes to her lifestyle. She began eating more fruits, vegetables, and fish. She started taking supplements regularly and corrected her vitamin D deficiency. She began walking to work and purchased a self-hypnosis CD to help her unwind at the end of the day. A follow-up dual X-ray absorptiometry (DXA) scan showed her bone density had remained essentially the same, with only a slight improvement in the T score for her lumbar spine. Margot was relieved that she had managed to halt further bone loss, but hoped to improve her bone density if possible. She also expressed delight at how good she was feeling generally, stating that she had "so much more energy." She had started to enjoy cooking and inviting friends over instead of "having popcorn for supper." Her mood had improved markedly. It was suggested to Margot that she step up her exercise regime to include weight lifting 2–3 times per week. She was referred to a physiotherapist to review correct technique and to set up a structured exercise program.

I love the "side benefits" that often happen for patients who embark on an integrative health program. A plan that was designed to support Margot's bone health also enhanced her mood and increased her sense of overall well-being.

Introduction

I ntegrative medicine aims to support the health of the whole person and in doing so, to promote health and healing in all body systems. Fragile bones do not exist in isolation. Thus, an integrative approach to osteoporosis includes a bone nourishing, anti-inflammatory diet; appropriate supplements; exercise and mind–body practices; and pharmaceutical medicines when indicated.

EPIDEMIOLOGY

Osteoporosis is a significant cause of pain, disability, and death in aging populations throughout the world. The incidence of osteoporotic fractures varies widely among populations, with relatively low rates in Africa and Latin America and comparatively high rates in northern Europe and North America (Dhanwal, Dennison, Harvey, & Cooper, 2011). More than 10 million Americans have osteoporosis, and there are over 2 million osteoporosis-related fractures per year (Siris et al., 2001). Women are at higher risk and account for approximately 75% of all cases. Using the World Health Organization (WHO) criteria, approximately 16% of postmenopausal women aged ≥50 years have osteoporosis and 61% have osteopenia (Looker, Borrud, Dawson-Hughes, Shepherd, & Wright, 2012). The costs to the US healthcare system are significant, totaling over $18 billion annually (Cauley, 2013). As the population ages, the costs related to osteoporosis prevention and treatment are expected to continue to climb (Burge et al., 2007).

PATHOPHYSIOLOGY

Osteoporosis is a skeletal disorder characterized by low bone mass, increased bone fragility, and an increased risk of fracture. It is a multifactorial disease arising from genetic, hormonal, metabolic, mechanical, and immunological factors.

Bone provides a critical support structure for the body, protects vital organs, and plays a central role in mineral and acid/base balance. Bone mass reaches its peak around age 30 and begins to decline after age 40 to 50. However, repair and renewal of bone continues throughout adult life, with approximately 15% of bone mass turning over each year.

There are two major types of bone cells. Osteoblasts synthesize the organic bone matrix and its calcification. The organic matrix is composed mainly of type 1 collagen, as well as a number of noncollagenous proteins such as osteocalcin, osteonectin, and sialoproteins. The inorganic component is composed mainly of hydroxyapatite crystals. Osteoclasts reabsorb bone in order to allow for metabolic requirements and for repair and remodeling of bone to take place. Together, these cell types carry out a finely tuned metabolic dance. Bone begins to deteriorate when bone resorption outpaces bone formation.

SCREENING AND DIAGNOSIS

Assessing Bone Strength

Bone strength is determined by bone quality as well as bone mass. Bone quality is influenced by bone microarchitecture and the composition of the bone matrix and mineral (Compston, 2006). There is no established way to assess bone quality in a clinical practice setting. Bone mass or bone mineral density (BMD) is most commonly assessed using a DXA scan.

Osteoporosis is defined as a BMD more than 2.5 standard deviations (SD) below the mean for young adults. Osteopenia is defined as a BMD 1–2.5 SD below the young adult mean. Established osteoporosis is diagnosed when the BMD falls more than 2.5 SD below the mean for young adults and there are one or more fragility fractures. However, it is recognized that an isolated BMD measurement may or may not accurately reflect fracture risk (Cummings et al., 1993; Guyatt et al., 2002; Wainwright et al., 2005). A wide overlap exists between the bone densities of women who will eventually suffer a fracture and those who will not (Marshall, Johnell, & Wedel, 1996).

The Fracture Risk Algorithm (FRAX) developed by the World Health Organization (WHO) includes a number of risk factors to more

accurately predict 10-year fracture risk (http://www.shef.ac.uk/FRAX/tool.
aspx?country=9). These include a history of prior fracture, thinness, smoking,
rheumatoid arthritis, excessive alcohol intake, and history of hip fracture in
a parent. FRAX can be a valuable tool to identify women at high risk of fracture, even without the inclusion of BMD (see Figure 32.1) (Kanis, McCloskey,
Johansson, Oden, & Leslie, 2012). The North American Menopause Society
(NAMS) recommends that BMD be measured in all women ≥ 65 years and
in all postmenopausal women with medical causes of bone loss. The NAMS
also recommends consideration of BMD in postmenopausal women age 50
or over who have one or more of the risk factors listed in the FRAX algorithm
([Anonymous], 2010).

Measuring biochemical markers of bone turnover, such as C- and
N-telopeptides and bone alkaline phosphatase, combined with BMD may also
provide a more precise prediction of future fracture risk. However a recent
systematic review found insufficient evidence to inform the choice of which
bone turnover marker to use in routine clinical practice to monitor osteoporosis treatment response (Burch et al., 2014). International reference standards
have not yet been developed (Vasikaran et al., 2011).

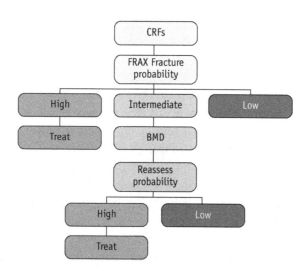

FIGURE 32.1. Management algorithm for the assessment of individuals at risk of frac-
ture. CRFs = clinical risk factors.
Source: From Kanis et al. (2008). Image used with permission of the WHO Collaborating
Centre for Metabolic Bone Diseases, University of Sheffield. FRAX® is registered to
Professor JA Kanis, University of Sheffield.

Risk Factors for Osteoporotic Fracture

The focus of osteoporosis screening programs should be to ultimately reduce the risk of fracture. Osteoporosis prevention strategies should aim to ameliorate all modifiable risk factors (see Box 32.1).

Box 32.1 Factors That Increase Fracture Risk

Factors leading to poor bone strength and/or an increased risk of falls:

- nutritional deficiencies
- smoking
- high alcohol intake
- excessive caffeine
- premature menopause
- malabsorption disorders
- autoimmune/inflammatory disease
- low body weight
- small body frame
- family history of osteoporosis
- female gender
- Caucasian or Asian descent
- impaired vision
- dizziness or balance problems
- fainting or loss of consciousness
- physical frailty
- medication-related side effects
- vitamin D deficiency

Medications:

- glucocorticoids
- anticonvulsants
- sedatives
- anticholinergics
- antihypertensives
- heparin
- cyclosporin
- proton pump inhibitors
- intramuscular medroxyprogesterone acetate

THE ROLE OF INFLAMMATION

Chronic inflammation is implicated in the process of aging (Bruunsgaard & Pedersen, 2003; Chung, Sung, Jung, Zou, & Yu., 2006) and plays a role in the development of a wide range of chronic diseases, including cardiovascular disease, Alzheimer's disease, diabetes, and cancer (Pradhan, Manson, Rifai, Buring, & Ridker, 2001; Ridker, Rifai, Stampfer, & Hennekens, 2000). There is growing evidence that osteoporosis is also, in part, a result of chronic low-grade inflammation (Clowes, Riggs, & Khosla, 2005; Ginaldi, Di Benedetto, & De Martinis, 2005; J. Koh et al., 2005; Sampaio Lacativa, & Fleiuss de Farias, 2010). Women with chronic inflammatory diseases such as rheumatoid arthritis and inflammatory bowel disease are known to be at increased risk of developing osteoporosis (Sampaio Lacativa, & Fleiuss de Farias, 2010). Elevated levels of high sensitivity C-reactive protein (hsCRP) are associated with lower BMD in healthy women as well as in women with inflammatory conditions (Goldring, 2003). Pro-inflammatory cytokines such as interleukin-6 (IL-6), interleukin-1 (IL-1), and tumor necrosis factor-alpha (TNF-alpha) promote accelerated bone loss via activation of osteoclasts, inhibition of collagen production in osteoblasts, and enhanced breakdown of the extracellular matrix (Ginaldi, Di Benedetto, & De Martinis, 2005; Ding, Parameswaran, Udayan, Burgess, & Jones, 2008).

Foods rich in anti-inflammatory compounds, such as fruits, vegetables (New et al., 2000), and omega-3 fatty acids (Das, 2000) have been found to decrease the risk of developing osteoporosis. Fruit and vegetable consumption is associated with both increased peak bone mass and with improved bone health in older populations (Lanham-New, 2008; Prynne et al., 2006; Tucker et al., 1999). The bone building effects of fruits and vegetables may be due to a number of factors: anti-inflammatory and antioxidant phytonutrients, alkalinizing effects; the nutrients, such as flavonoids, potassium, vitamin K, and vitamin C, that they provide; and the presence of other unknown compounds and synergistic effects. For all the above reasons, an anti-inflammatory diet is recommended as the foundation of an integrative bone health plan (see Box 32.2).

Nutrition for Bone Health

CALCIUM

Calcium is an essential nutrient for building and maintaining healthy bones. And yet, high calcium intakes do not ensure strong bones and lower calcium intakes do not necessarily lead to weaker bones (Bischoff-Ferrari et al., 2007;

Box 32.2 Anti-Inflammatory Diet

- Enjoy 8–10 servings per day from a variety of deeply colored fruits and vegetables
- Choose healthy fats: extra virgin olive oil, avocados, nuts, and fatty, cold-water ocean fish such as wild salmon, black cod, sardines, and halibut
- Use anti-inflammatory spices/herbs/teas such as turmeric, ginger, rosemary, green tea
- Choose whole grain, low glycemic load carbohydrates
- Reduce consumption of partially hydrogenated oils, vegetables oils (safflower, sunflower, corn, soy), and saturated animal fats
- Avoid foods that provoke allergy or intolerance
- Cultivate healthy bowel flora

Feskanich, Willett, & Colditz, 2003; Nordin, 2000). Calcium requirement is determined by absorptive efficiency versus the rate that calcium is lost via the bowels, kidneys, skin, hair, and nails (World Health Organization, Food and Agriculture Organization, 2004). To improve calcium absorption and/ or decrease calcium excretion, maintain an optimum intake of vitamin D (Heaney, Dowell, Hale, & Bendich, 2003) and vitamin K1 and K2 (Vermeer, & Theuwissen, 2011); increase fruits and vegetables (Barzel, & Massey, 1998); obtain a healthy balance of essential fatty acids (Kruger, & Horrobin, 1997); consume adequate but not excessive protein (Barzel, & Massey, 1998); lower dietary sodium to less than 2,400 mg/day (Harrington, & Cashman, 2003; Heaney, 2006); avoid excess caffeine (Hallstrom, Wolk, Glynn, & Michaelsson, 2006); and eat fewer highly refined carbohydrates (Thom, Bishop, Blacklock, & Morris, 1978). It has been estimated that adequate calcium intake may range from ~450 mg to ~1,150 mg per day depending on the influence of these types of factors. For instance, it has been estimated that a low animal protein intake of 20 g/day, coupled with a low sodium intake of 1.15 g/day could lower calcium requirements by 390 mg/day. Maximum calcium absorption from optimal vitamin D intake could lower the calcium requirement even further (World Health Organization, Food and Agriculture Organization, 2004). The combined influence of a wide range of dietary and lifestyle factors may explain the "calcium paradox" whereby hip fracture rates are less common in developing countries where calcium intakes are lower (World Health Organization, Food and Agriculture Organization, 2004).

In the United States, the current calcium dietary reference intakes (DRIs) for women are: 1,300 mg/day for ages 9–18, 1,000 mg/day for ages 19–50, and 1,200 mg/day for ages 50 and up. The need for calcium supplementation should be based on a careful assessment of all existing dietary sources, including baseline intake (~250 mg/day), dairy products, fortified beverages, and calcium that may be present in multivitamins or other supplements. The difference between this total and the DRI can then be used to estimate the amount of supplement needed. A meta-analysis by Tang et al. found that for people over the age of 50, 1,200 mg of calcium alone or in combination with vitamin D reduced fracture risk by 12% as well as bone loss rates (Tang, Eslick, Nowson, Smith, & Bensoussan, 2007). Some studies have linked the use of calcium supplements with an increased risk of kidney stones and cardiovascular disease (Bolland, 2010), though the validity of these findings has been challenged (Heaney et al., 2012); Rautiainen, Wang, Manson, & Sesso, 2013; Xiao, & Park, 2013). A study by Langsetmo et al. found that increased calcium intake from diet and supplements may actually lower mortality in women (Langsetmo et al., 2013). When dietary intake is insufficient, calcium supplementation is recommended, but should always be part of a broader strategy that includes adequate vitamin D, vitamin K2, and other bone-building foods and nutrients (see Box 32.3).

Box 32.3 Advising Patients About Calcium Supplementation

Large, compressed calcium tablets may be difficult to swallow and may not fully disintegrate in the stomach particularly in the presence of low stomach acid. Calcium supplements in the form of powders, capsules, and liquids may be better tolerated.

Recommended Calcium Supplements

Calcium carbonate: It is best taken with meals and is less expensive than calcium citrate. However those with low stomach acid may have diminished dissolution and absorption. Calcium carbonate provides 40% elemental calcium.

Calcium citrate: This form of calcium is well absorbed with or without meals and is often recommended for patients on proton pump inhibitors and those over 50 (Sakhaee, Bhuket, Adams-Huet, & Rao, 999). Calcium citrate provides 21% elemental calcium.

Calcium from dolomite, oyster shell, or coral is not recommended.

Avoid taking calcium supplements along with psyllium or with foods high in oxalic acid (e.g. spinach) or phytic acid (e.g. wheat bran). Calcium supplementation of 500 mg or more should be taken in divided doses to maximize absorption.

ACID/BASE ISSUES

In bone, minute downward shifts in the local pH can stimulate osteoclast activity, while also impairing the activity of osteoblasts (Arnett, 2003). A diet high in animal protein and low in fruits and vegetables may produce a chronic low-grade metabolic acidosis that could prove harmful to the skeleton (Cordain et al., 2005; Lanham-New, 2008; Marangella et al., 2004; Maurer, Riesen, Muser, Hulter, & Krapf, 2003; Sebastian, Frassetto, Sellmeyer, Merriam, & Morris, 2002). Fruits and vegetables generate bicarbonate that can buffer the acidifying effects of animal protein, alkalinize the urine and significantly lower urinary calcium excretion (Barzel & Massey, 1998). In a study by Buclin et al., acid-forming diets increased calcium excretion by 74% as compared with base-forming diets (Buclin et al., 2001). Balanced diets with adequate protein along with abundant fruits and vegetables are therefore recommended (Alexy, Remer, Manz, Neu, & Schoenau, 2005; Sebastian, 2005).

VITAMIN D

Vitamin D is essential for calcium absorption and for bone health. The hormonally active form of vitamin D, 1,25-OHD, induces active transport of calcium across the intestinal mucosa. Vitamin D also stimulates the absorption of phosphate and magnesium ions and acts synergistically with vitamin K to stimulate bone mineralization.

Vitamin D deficiency and insufficiency is common throughout North America (Holick, 2006; Jacobs et al., 2008). Breastfed infants, women, the elderly, the obese, and people with darker skin tones are at higher risk of deficiency. An international epidemiological study found that 64% of postmenopausal women with osteoporosis had inadequate vitamin D concentrations (<30 ng/mL) (Lips et al., 2006). Supplementation with 700–800 IU/day of vitamin D has been shown to reduce fracture risk in older adults (Bischoff-Ferrari, Willett, et al., 2005; Trivedi, Doll, & Khaw, 2003). A positive dose response has been shown for higher doses of vitamin D3 (>400 IU/day) and higher serum levels of 25-OHD and nonvertebral and hip fractures (Bischoff-Ferrari, Willett, et al., 2009). Vitamin D also reduces the risk of falls (Bischoff-Ferrari, Dawson-Hughes, et al., 2009) and improves lower-extremity function (Bischoff-Ferrari, Dietrich, Orav, Dawson-Hughes, 2004) in older adults.

All women should be screened at least once for vitamin D deficiency. A serum vitamin D (25-OHD) of at least 34 ng/mL (85 nmol/L) is necessary for optimum calcium absorption (Heaney et al., 2003), and optimum fracture prevention is reached at 40 ng/mL (100 nmol/L) (Bischoff-Ferrari, Willett, et al., 2005). Each incremental increase in 25-OHD is associated with an increase in BMD (Bischoff-Ferrari, Dietrich, et al., 2004; Fradinger, & Zanchetta, 2001; Mezquita-Raya et al., 2001).

Vitamin D can be obtained through sunlight exposure, from a limited number of foods, or from supplements. Sunlight exposures of 10–15 minutes, without sunblock, at the appropriate latitude and season, can be a good source of endogenously produced vitamin D. A few foods are naturally rich in vitamin D: fatty ocean fish such as salmon, sardines, and black cod, and sun-exposed mushrooms. Fortified foods include some brands of orange juice, milk, fortified milk substitutes, and some yogurts. Vitamin D supplementation is an inexpensive and reliable way to ensure an optimum serum concentration of 40 ng/mL (100 nmol/L). For most adults, a supplement of at least 1,000 IU/day will be needed to achieve this serum concentration (Bischoff-Ferrari, 2007; Cannell, Hollis, Zasloff, & Heaney, 2008). Vitamin D3 (cholecalciferol) is the preferred form to use (Armas, Hollis, & Heaney, 2004) and should be taken with meals.

ESSENTIAL FATTY ACIDS

Both omega-6 (n-6) and omega-3 (n-3) polyunsaturated fatty acids are essential nutrients (Simopoulos, 2000). They are incorporated into cell membranes, where they influence membrane characteristics and become precursors for eicosanoids such as prostaglandins, leukotrienes, and thromboxanes. These fats perform opposing roles in the body, and the balance between them plays a significant role in regulating the inflammatory response (Simopoulos, 2008). Western diets tend to be relatively high in omega-6 fats and low in omega-3s. While there have been suggestions of an "ideal" ratio of omega-6 to omega-3, there is no consensus other than most Americans need to significantly increase their intake of the latter.

Omega-3 fatty acids suppress production of interleukin 1-beta (IL-beta), TNF-alpha, and IL-6, and are known to have anti-inflammatory effects (Simopoulos, 2011). Certain omega-6 fatty acids, such as gamma-linolenic acid (GLA) also have anti-inflammatory effects. On the other hand, the omega-6 fatty acid linoleic acid (LA) has pro-inflammatory effects and leads to increased production of IL-beta, TNF-alpha, and IL-6 cytokines.

The intake and ratio of essential fatty acids in the diet appears to play an important role in bone health. In animal studies, fish oils rich in omega-3s have been found to attenuate bone loss associated with estrogen withdrawal (Fernandes, Lawrence, & Sun, 2003). Animal studies have also shown that the omega-3 fatty acid eicosapentaenoic acid (EPA) enhances calcium absorption, reduces calcium excretion, and increases calcium deposition in bone (Kruger, Coetzer, de Winter, Gericke, & van Papendorp, 1998).

In human studies, supplementation with calcium, EPA, and GLA resulted in a decrease in bone turnover and an increase in lumbar and femoral bone density in elderly women (Kruger et al., 1998). In the Rancho Bernardo study, higher ratios of omega-6 to omega-3 fatty acids were associated with lower BMD in the hip for all women studied (Weiss, Barrett-Connor, & von Muhlen, 2005). A study of postmenopausal Chinese women found that higher intake of sea fish, as opposed to fresh water fish, was associated with greater bone mass and a lower risk of osteoporosis (Y. Chen, Ho, & Lam, 2010). While the systematic review by Orchard et al. found the data mixed in outcomes and strength, it does appear that omega-3 fatty acids tend to have positive effects on bone if ingested for 18 months or more and if given with a mixture of fatty acids along with calcium. An increased intake of alpha-linolenic acid (ALA) as opposed to EPA and docosahexaenoic acid (DHA) appeared to be particularly beneficial (Orchard, Pan, Cheek, Ing, & Jackson, 2012).

Although more study is needed, omega-3 fatty acids appear to enhance calcium absorption, reduce calcium excretion, and improve mineralization of bone matrix and bone strength (Knopp, Diner, Blitz, Lyritis, & Rowe, 2005; Kruger, & Horrobin, 1997). There are also many known health benefits of reducing omega-6 fatty acids and increasing omega-3 fatty acid intake in the diet (Simopoulos, 2008).

PROTEIN

Adequate protein is essential for the growth and maintenance of healthy bones (Cooper et al., 1996). Protein tends to have anabolic effects on bone: it provides the structural matrix of bone, increases insulin-like growth factor (IGF-1) levels, and increases intestinal absorption of calcium (Heaney & Layman, 2008). Protein also increases urinary calcium excretion; however, other constituents in foods, such as phosphorus in meat and potassium in legumes appear to partially offset this effect (Massey, 2003).

Studies on the effect on bone of animal versus plant proteins and high versus low protein intakes have shown mixed results. A number of studies have found that high levels of animal protein in the diet are associated with increased fracture rates and accelerated bone mineral loss (Abelow, Holford, & Insogna, 1992; Feskanich, Willett, Stampfer, & Colditz, 1996; Marsh, Sanchez, Mickelsen, Keiser, & Mayor, 1980). In the Nurses' Health Study, protein intakes higher than 95 g/day were associated with significantly higher forearm fracture rates compared with protein intakes less than 68 g/day (Feskanich,

Willett, et al., 1996). In another study, lowering protein intakes to current recommended daily allowance guidelines (0.8 g/kg) resulted in significant reductions in urinary calcium excretion and in markers of bone resorption (Ince, Anderson, & Neer, 2004). Several studies have also shown that an increased ratio of vegetable to animal protein is protective against fractures (Frassetto, Todd, Morris, & Sebastian, 2000; Sellmeyer, Stone, Sebastian, & Cummings, 2001; Weikert et al., 2005). On the other hand, the Framingham Osteoporosis Study found that higher protein intakes (60–83 g/d in quartiles 2–4 versus 46 g/d in the lowest quartile) in elderly men and women (mean age 75 years) were associated with a 37% decreased risk of hip fracture (D. Misra et al., 2011). Data from the Women's Health Initiative found that a 20% increase in protein intake (from 15% to 18% of energy intake) improved BMD maintenance and marginally lowered forearm fracture risk (Beasley et al., 2014). A systematic review by Calvez et al. concluded, "no clinical data support the hypothesis of a detrimental effect of HP (high protein) diet on bone health, except in the context of inadequate calcium supply" (Calvez, Poupin, Chesneau, Lassale, & Tome, 2012). Other studies support the idea that, in the presence of adequate dietary calcium and vitamin D, increasing protein intake may have a favorable effect on bone health (Dawson-Hughes & Harris, 2002; Heaney & Layman, 2008). It should be noted that most studies looking at "higher" protein diets have looked at modest increases in protein intake, not the effects on bone of protein intakes in the range of 30% or more of energy intake.

In summary, an adequate but not excessive intake of protein is recommended alongside a balanced diet that includes abundant fruits and vegetables and adequate calcium. Choosing some vegetarian sources of protein, such as quinoa and soy foods is also highly recommended for bone and overall health.

VITAMIN K

There are two naturally occurring forms of vitamin K: phylloquinone (K1), synthesized by plants, and menaquinone (K2), which either is the result of bacterial action in the gastrointestinal tract converting K1 to K2 or is directly obtained from food sources such as meat, egg yolks, fermented dairy, and fermented soy (e.g., miso, natto). As previously mentioned, vitamin K and vitamin D act synergistically to stimulate bone mineralization. Menaquinone appears to play a particularly important role in the prevention and therapy of osteoporosis (Bolton-Smith et al., 2007; Kanellakis et al., 2012; Ushiroyama, Ikeda, & Ueki, 2002). Vitamin K2 is essential for the gamma carboxylation of osteocalcin; it stimulates the synthesis of osteoblastic markers and inhibits bone resorption by inhibiting the formation and activity of osteoclasts (Adams

& Pepping, 2005; Prabhoo & Prabhoo, 2010). Epidemiological studies consistently show a link between higher vitamin K status and reduction of fracture risk. Booth et al. found that elderly men and women in the highest quartile of dietary vitamin K had a relative risk for hip fracture of 0.35 (Booth et al., 2000). Women who consume one or more servings of lettuce per day (a source of K1) have been found to have a relative risk of 0.55 for hip fracture (Feskanich et al., 1999). Patients with osteoporotic fractures of the spine and femoral neck have been found to be markedly deficient in K1 and the MK-7 and MK-8 forms of K2 (Hodges, Akesson, Vergnaud, Obrant, & Delmas, 1993; Hodges et al., 1991). A systematic review by Cockayne et al. found that the majority of vitamin K intervention studies showed a reduction in BMD loss and improved bone biomarkers (Cockayne et al., 2006). A 3-year trial of K2 (mk-7 180 mcg/day) supplementation in postmenopausal women showed preservation of BMD in the lumbar spine and slowing of the rate of bone loss in the femoral neck (Knapen, Drummen, Smit, Vermeer, & Theuwissen, 2013).

Subclinical vitamin K deficiency is common, and typical dietary intakes are below the levels associated with decreased fracture risk (Kaneki, 2006). The current vitamin K DRI for adult women is 90 mcg, but amounts of 254 mcg/day or higher may be needed for optimum bone health (Pearson, 2007). A number of researchers have called for separate DRIs for each type of vitamin K, as K2 appears to have an important role in the prevention of vascular calcification and cancer (Vermeer & Theuwissen, 2011). The best food sources of K1 are green leafy vegetables such as lettuce, collards, spinach, and kale, as well as other vegetables rich in chlorophyll, such as broccoli. Vitamin K2 is found in animal foods such as cheese, egg yolks, butter, goose liver, chicken liver, chicken, and beef. Natto, a fermented soybean food, is also a very rich source of K2 (Schurgers & Vermeer, 2000). When used as a supplement, the mk-7 form of vitamin K2 is recommended, because it results in significantly higher, more stable vitamin K serum levels when compared with K1 or the mk-4 form of K2 (Sato, Schurgers, & Uenishi, 2012; Schurgers et al., 2007).

Note: Vitamin K supplementation should be avoided by patients on anticoagulants (Beulens et al., 2013).

MAGNESIUM

Magnesium is essential for bone health. Low magnesium intakes can reduce the number and function of osteoblasts, increase the number and activity of osteoclasts, and promote inflammation and oxidative stress (Castiglioni, Cazzaniga, Albisetti, & Maier, 2013). Magnesium is also required for the conversion of vitamin D to 1,25-dihydroxycholecalciferol (calcitriol) (Castiglioni et al., 2013). Epidemiological studies have linked higher magnesium intakes with increased BMD (Ryder et al., 2005; Tucker et al., 1999). Some intervention trials of magnesium supplementation have also shown an increase in BMD as well as reduced fracture rates (Sojka, & Weaver, 1995; Stendig-Lindberg, Tepper, & Leichter, 1993). Approximately 50% of women in the United States do not obtain the daily requirement of 320 mg of magnesium. Low magnesium intakes are also associated with a number of other chronic health conditions such as type 2 diabetes and hypertension (Rosanoff, Weaver, & Rude, 2012). Good sources of magnesium include dark green leafy vegetables, nuts and seeds, legumes, and whole grains.

TRACE MINERALS

A number of trace minerals including zinc, copper, and manganese act as cofactors for specific enzymes important for bone metabolism. Serum concentrations of zinc and copper have been found to be lower in osteoporotic women than in controls (Gur et al., 2002). A varied, whole food diet plus a good quality multivitamin/mineral supplement should ensure an adequate supply of these nutrients.

VITAMIN C

Vitamin C (ascorbic acid) is an essential cofactor for collagen formation. It also plays a key antioxidant role in the body. Plasma levels of vitamin C and other antioxidants have been found to be significantly lower in postmenopausal women with osteoporosis compared with age-matched controls (Maggio et al., 2003). The Framingham Osteoporosis Study found that elderly men and women in the highest tertile of total and supplemental vitamin C intake had significantly fewer hip and nonvertebral fractures. A total intake of ~200 mg/day was associated with the lowest prevalence of fracture (Sahni et al., 2009). The best dietary sources of vitamin C are fruits and vegetables such as papaya, pineapple, oranges, broccoli, and bell peppers.

SOY

Soybeans are good sources of high-quality plant protein, phytoestrogens, minerals, vitamins, essential fatty acids, and fiber. Studies of soy foods and soy isoflavones (SI) in relation to bone health have been mixed. A 3-year trial of SIs in postmenopausal women showed nil effects, other than a modest bone sparing effect at the femoral neck (Alekel et al., 2010). On the other hand, a systematic review of SI supplements by Wei et al. found that isoflavones increased BMD by 54% and decreased deoxypyridinoline (DPD), a bone resorption marker, by 23%. The effects were greatest for postmenopausal women using an SI dose greater than 75mg/day (Wei, Liu, Chen, & Chen, 2012). Several large population-based studies of soy food intake have also shown beneficial effects. The Shanghai Women's Health Study found a relative risk of fracture of 0.63 in the highest quintile of soy protein intake (≥13 g/day) (Zhang et al., 2005). The Singapore Chinese Health Study found a significant reduction in hip fracture risk for women with higher soy intakes (W. Koh et al., 2009).

There is reason to believe that a dietary pattern that includes whole soy foods, as they have been traditionally eaten, is more beneficial to bone health than isolated constituents of soy (Lanou, 2011; Reinwald & Weaver, 2010). Based on the available evidence, 1–2 servings/day of whole soy foods, such as tofu, tempeh, and edamame are recommended.

Substances That May Be Harmful to Bone Health

SODIUM

Average sodium intake in the United States (3,500 mg/day) exceeds the recommended intake of <2,400 mg/day, and high-salt diets are known to increase urinary calcium excretion (Harrington & Cashman, 2003). The DASH II diet (Dietary Approaches to Stop Hypertension and Sodium Reduction), which included 9.5 servings of fruits and vegetables per day, low-fat dairy products, whole grains, and reduced meat and sodium intake, resulted in decreased calcium losses and reduced bone turnover (Lin et al., 2003). The bone benefits of the DASH II diet appear to be related to its overall effects rather than to the reduction in sodium per se. Increasing calcium and potassium intakes can substantially offset the urinary losses of calcium caused by high sodium intakes (Heaney, 2006). However, a high sodium intake along with a low calcium intake may lead to detrimental effects on bone health (Bedford & Barr, 2011). Patients should be advised to stay within the recommended sodium intake of <2,400 mg/day.

CAFFEINE

Excessive caffeine intake is associated with a modest increase in the risk of osteoporotic fracture (Hallstrom et al., 2006). The increased risk appears to occur in women who consume >300 mg of caffeine/day or approximately 4 cups of coffee, and who also have a low calcium intake. While excessive caffeine intake should be avoided, women with optimal calcium intakes should not experience any negative effects on bone health from moderate intake of caffeinated beverages (Heaney, 2002).

VITAMIN A

Preformed vitamin A (retinol) intakes of >5,000 mcg/day have been associated with an increased risk of hip fracture (Melhus et al., 1998), however, more recent data has failed to confirm this effect. An intervention study found no increase in fracture risk among 2,322 adults who took a controlled, high-dose retinol supplement (25,000 IU retinyl palmitate/day) for as long as 16 years (Ambrosini et al., 2013).

CIGARETTE SMOKING

Cigarette smoking is an independent risk factor for low BMD, and the negative effect increases with amount and duration of smoking (Yoon, Maalouf, & Sakhaee, 2012). Smoking also has negative effects on bone health unrelated to BMD (Dimai & Chandran, 2011). In the Nurses' Health Study, smokers had a relative risk of 1.2 for hip fracture, and this figure rose to 1.4 for those who smoked 25 or more cigarettes/day (Cornuz, Feskanich, Willett, & Colditz, 1999). A meta-analysis involving more than 59,000 men and women found that smokers have a relative risk of 1.13 for any fracture and a relative risk of 1.6 for hip fractures (Kanis et al., 2005). Clearly, for many reasons, women should be encouraged not to begin smoking. Current smokers who quit will obtain benefits to their bone health after a period of 10 years (Cornuz et al., 1999).

ALCOHOL

In animal studies, chronic heavy alcohol consumption, especially during adolescence and young adulthood, can significantly damage bone health (Sampson, 2002). On the other hand, low or moderate consumption of alcohol in adulthood appears to have protective effects on bone (Berg et al., 2008; Sommer et al., 2013). Moderate alcohol consumption has recognized cardiovascular benefits (Vogel, 2002) but can also increase the risk of breast cancer in women (Mezzetti et al., 1998) and has other potentially detrimental effects on health (Anonymous, 2006). All things considered, adult women should be advised to limit their alcoholic drinks to fewer than seven per week.

Botanical Medicines

Numerous in vitro and animal studies and a smaller number of human trials have examined the potential of herbal medicines to enhance bone health (Putnam, Scutt, Bicknell, Priestley, & Williamson, 2007). A study of Shen Gu (traditional Chinese medicine mixture for nourishing kidney and strengthening bone: *Fructus psoraleae* 16 g, *Radix codonopsis* 16 g, *Rhizoma drynariae* 16 g, *Cortex eucommiae* 16 g, *Radix Rehmanniae preparata* 20 g, *Radix astragali* 20 g, *Radix glycyrrhizae* 6 g; the treatment group was given 25 mL of the formula twice a day for 6 months) in 96 osteoporotic patients found significant beneficial effects on bone (Mingyue et al., 2005). The Ayurvedic preparation Reosto, which contains a mixture of botanicals and organic calcium (Ingredients per tablet: *Terminalia arjuna* 45 mg, *Withania somnifera* 45 mg, *Commiphora wightii* 235 mg, *Sida cordifolia* 45 mg, *Vanda roxburghi* 50 mg, *Godanti bhasma* 120 mg, *Kukkutandatvak bhasma* 35 mg; the treatment group received two tablets twice a day for 12 months) was found to significantly increase BMD (Shah & Kolhapure, 2004). Deng et al. published the first study of a Fufang (herbal formula: *Herba epimedii, Rehmannia glutinosa, Dioscorea batatas, Cornus officinalis, Cinnamomum cassia, Drynaria fortunei, Morinda officinalis*; the treatment group received a dose of 10 g/day of dried granules; the doses of each herb are not available) using fracture as one of the primary end points. Postmenopausal women improved their BMD and had an impressive 43% reduction in fragility fractures over a 5-year period (Deng et al., 2012). *Dioscorea spongiosa* (Yin, Kouda, et al., 2004; Yin, Tezuka, et al., 2004), *Astragalus membranaceus* (Kim et al., 2003), walnut extract (*Juglans regia*; Papoutsi et al., 2008), and curcumin, a compound found in turmeric root (*Curcuma longa*; Bharti, Takada, & Aggarwal, 2004), have shown osteoprotective effects in laboratory and animal studies. Further studies are needed to assess the role of botanical medicines in the prevention and treatment of osteoporosis.

Tea (*Camellia sinensis*)

Tea has anti-inflammatory effects, cardiovascular benefits, and cancer protective properties (De Bacquer, Clays, Delanghe, & De Backer, 2006; Gardner, Ruxton, & Leeds, 2007). Tea drinking appears to have beneficial effects on bone, and several studies have linked tea consumption to modest increases in BMD (Z. Chen et al., 2003; De Bacquer, Clays, Delanghe, & De Backer, 2006).

The Mind–Body Connection

Chronic stress, through activation of the sympathetic nervous system (SNS), tends to exert catabolic effects on the body, resulting in the breakdown of energy stores and body tissues. In animal studies, both chronic stressors and the administration of glucocorticoids have been shown to stimulate bone resorption (Jia, O'Brien, Stewart, Manolagas, & Weinstein, 2006; Patterson-Buckendahl, Pohorecky, & Kvetnansky, 2007). Major depression (Cizza, Ravn, Chrousos, & Gold, 2001) and anorexia nervosa (D. Misra et al., 2008) are associated with elevation of serum cortisol levels and with increased bone loss. Increased SNS activity stimulates resorption of bone by osteoclasts and inhibits bone formation by osteoblasts (Togari, Arai, & Kondo, 2005).

Stress reduction, using mind–body practices such as meditation, self-hypnosis, guided imagery, breath work, or biofeedback games is highly recommended as part of an integrative plan to support bone health and overall well-being (see the side bar text).

> Many of my patients enjoy listening to hypnosis or guided imagery CDs. There is nothing they need to do, other than to get comfortable. Busy women are delighted to hear that it's something they can do even while sleeping!

Exercise

Exercise is key to building and maintaining strong bones. Both general physical activity and mechanical loading contribute to building peak bone mass, beginning in the prepubertal years (Anderson, 2000; Heinonen et al., 2000). Bone density at all skeletal sites is strongly correlated with muscle mass, and muscle mass is strongly linked to physical activity (Proctor et al., 2000). Muscle mass generally increases until around age 30 and begins to decline after age 50. Muscle strength losses tend to be most striking after age 70. However, regular exercise at any age, even in the very elderly, can result in increased muscle strength, balance, and functional capacity (Evans, 1997; Fiatarone et al., 1994).

Exercise programs for women have been shown to consistently prevent or reverse bone loss in the lumbar spine and the femoral neck (Wolff, van Croonenborg, Kemper, Kostense, & Twisk, 1999). The Bone Estrogen Strength

Training (BEST) Study found that postmenopausal women who received 800 mg/day of calcium citrate, along with a structured exercise program, increased their muscle mass by 11%–21% and increased their BMD by ~2% (Cussler et al., 2005). Even women with established osteoporosis can improve their bone mass with a low-impact exercise program (Todd & Robinson, 2003). Walking for at least 4 hours per week has been found to decrease hip fracture risk by 41% (Feskanich, Willett, & Colditz, 2002). A 2-year program of back-strengthening exercises was found to reduce vertebral fractures in post-menopausal women (Sinaki et al., 2002).

Recommended physical activities include walking, aerobic exercise, jumping, running, weight training, and racquet sports. Women should aim for 30 to 45 minutes of exercise, 5 or more times per week. Weight training exercise is best done on alternate days. Tai chi may have a number of beneficial effects including reducing fall frequency, improving balance and strength, and maintaining BMD (Voukelatos, Cumming, Lord, & Rissel, 2007; Wayne et al., 2007).

Considerations in Younger Women

Ideally, every woman should reach her peak bone mass by age 30–35. Peak bone mass is influenced by genetic factors and also by diet and physical activity during childhood, adolescence, and young adulthood. It is of concern that in the United States only 15% of girls ages 9–13 and 13% of young women ages 14–18 meet their daily calcium requirement (Bailey et al., 2010). Young women should be counseled about the importance of a healthy diet, maintaining an ideal body weight, and regular exercise (Lloyd, Petit, Lin, & Beck, 2004).

Young women who use depot medroxyprogesterone acetate (DMPA) for contraception are at risk for bone loss (Walsh, Eastell, & Peel, 2008), though BMD tends to recover after discontinuation of DMPA (Kaunitz, Arias, & McClung, 2008). Smoking, heavy alcohol consumption, anorexia nervosa (M. Misra et al., 2008), late-onset menarche, amenorrhea (Gordon & Nelson, 2003), primary ovarian failure, and autoimmune diseases (Lloyd et al., 2002) are other risk factors that may prevent young women from achieving their peak bone mass.

Some bone loss normally accompanies pregnancy and lactation and is then usually recovered after infants are weaned (Kalkwarf & Specker, 2002). Epidemiologic studies show that multiple pregnancies and periods of lactation are not associated with lower bone mass or increased fracture risk (Melton et al., 1993).

Pharmaceuticals

Osteoporosis is best approached with a lifelong, comprehensive prevention program. Women of all ages should be aware of the diet and lifestyle choices that will support their bone health. Ongoing strategies should include optimum diet, appropriate supplementation, regular physical activity, and fall prevention. Secondary causes of osteoporosis should be corrected where possible.

In addition, pharmacologic therapy for prevention and/or treatment of osteoporosis may be recommended. The National Osteoporosis Foundation (NOF) has issued guidelines for osteoporosis treatment which incorporate the FRAX algorithm. The NOF recommends pharmacologic intervention for postmenopausal women who have a history of hip or vertebral fracture; a T score of 2.5 or higher (DXA) at the femoral neck or spine; a T score between −1 and −2.5 at the femoral neck or spine; and a 10-year probability of hip fracture of 3% or higher or a 10-year probability of any major osteoporosis-related fracture of 20% or higher (National Osteoporosis Foundation, 2010). Some women may wish to begin an extensive bone-building program and continue to monitor their bone density before making a decision to begin medication.

THE ROLE OF ESTROGEN

Bone loss is known to rapidly accelerate in the years following menopause, as estrogen levels naturally fall. The primary action of estrogen on bone is to inhibit the osteoclast by increasing the amount of osteoprotegerin (OPG) produced by osteoblasts (Fitzpatrick, 2006). Estrogen also has anti-inflammatory effects and acts to suppress the production of bone-resorbing cytokines (Bilezikian, 1998; Manolagas, Bellido, & Jilka, 1995; Pacifici, 1996). Consequently, at the time of menopause, the concentration of inflammatory cytokines that can induce osteoclastogenesis rises (Cenci et al., 2000; Horowitz, 1993).

Postmenopausal hormone therapy (HT) has beneficial effects on bone, reduces the risk of colon cancer, and can alleviate hot flashes and vaginal dryness. On the other hand, women who use estrogen-progestin HT have an increased risk of cardiovascular disease, stroke, thromboembolic events, and breast cancer (Nelson, Humphrey, Nygren, Teutsch, & Allan, 2002). In the Women's Health Initiative (WHI) trial, women receiving HT had increased BMD and lower fracture rates. However, the study authors concluded, "When considering the effects of hormone therapy on other important disease outcomes in a global model, there was no net benefit, even in women considered to be at high risk of fracture" (Cauley et al., 2003). What remains unclear is whether a very low dose transdermal estrogen would prevent osteoporosis without significantly increasing the risks of cardiovascular disease, stroke, thromboembolic events, and breast cancer. A randomized controlled study of 417 postmenopausal women explored a transdermal dose of .014 mg estradiol and found improved lumbar spine and hip bone density and reduced bone turnover as compared with controls (Ettinger et al., 2004). In 2012, the US Preventive Services Task Force continued to recommend against the use of HT for the prevention of chronic disease (Moyer, 2013). Thus, treatment with HT should be individualized, based on a careful exploration of the risks and benefits for each woman.

BISPHOSPHONATES

Bisphosphonates are indicated for both prevention and treatment of post-menopausal osteoporosis and are the usual choice of first-line therapy. Anti-resorptive therapies reduce fracture risk by inhibiting the activity of osteoclasts and reducing bone turnover, thus increasing bone mass. High bone turnover is particularly relevant in the pathogenesis of vertebral fractures (Compston, 2006). The most common side effects are dyspepsia, esophagitis, nausea, and abdominal pain. Osteonecrosis of the jaw is a serious, rare event associated with bisphosphonate use. There is also concern that bisphosphonates may impair microdamage repair and thus increase the brittleness of bone (Mashiba et al., 2000; Turner, 2002).

Alendronate has been shown to increase BMD and to reduce the incidence of fractures of the spine and hip in women with osteoporosis (Bauer et al., 2004). The usual dose range is 35–70 mg weekly. Risendronate also increases BMD and reduces vertebral and some nonvertebral fracture rates (Harris et al., 1999). The usual dose is 35 mg weekly. Ibandronate has similar indications and side effects as the two bisphosphonates mentioned previously. It is usually given as monthly oral dose of 150 mg (McCarus, 2006). Zoledronic acid is normally administered intravenously, in a 5 mg dose once a year. It has been found to decrease spine and hip fractures in postmenopausal women and may be useful for women who cannot tolerate oral bisphosphonates (Black et al., 2007).

DENOSUMAB

Receptor activator for nuclear factor kappa-B ligand (RANKL) is critical for the production and function of osteoclasts. Denosumab is a fully human monoclonal antibody that inhibits osteoclastogenesis by blocking the action of RANKL on the osteoclast. This leads to a decrease in bone resorption, an increase in BMD, and a decreased risk of vertebral, nonvertebral, and hip fractures. Side effects include musculoskeletal pain, hypercholesterolemia, cystitis, and eczema. Denosumab is contraindicated in patients with hypocalcemia. The usual dose is 60 mg given subcutaneously every 6 months (Silva-Fernandez, Rosario, Martinez-Lopez, Carmona, & Loza, 2013).

SELECTIVE ESTROGEN RECEPTOR MODULATORS

Selective estrogen receptor modulators (SERMS) act as estrogen agonists on bone and lipid metabolism while also having antagonist actions on breast and endometrial tissue. Raloxifene is effective at reducing postmenopausal bone loss and the risk of vertebral fractures (Ettinger et al., 1999). Raloxifene also significantly reduces the risk of breast cancer and improves lipid profiles (Barrett-Connor et al., 2004). The usual dose is 60 mg/day. Side effects include deep vein thrombosis (DVT) and pulmonary embolism.

CALCITONIN

Calcitonin is produced by thyroid C cells and acts to inhibit bone resorption by inhibiting osteoclast activity. Calcitonin from salmon has been used to treat osteoporosis in women who are 5 or more years post menopause. It is effective in reducing the pain associated with acute compression fractures of the vertebrae (Knopp et al., 2005). It is normally given as a daily intranasal spray of 200 IU. Calcitonin is not considered a first-line drug for osteoporosis, because other more effective medications are available. Side effects include flushing, nausea, and diarrhea. Calcitonin may also be associated with an increased risk of malignancy (Overman, Borse, & Gourlay, 2013).

RECOMBINANT PARATHYROID HORMONE

Recombinant parathyroid hormone (PTH), either full length (1–84) or fragment (1–34), has been found to have anabolic effects on bone, stimulating osteoblast cell proliferation and bone formation. These medications may be useful in reducing the incidence of new vertebral and nonvertebral fractures in postmenopausal women (Bilezikian, Rubin, & Finkelstein, 2005; McCarus,

2006; Reginster & Sarlet, 2006). They are normally given as a once-daily sub-cutaneous injection for a period of up to 2 years. The length of treatment is limited due to concerns of a possible increased risk of osteosarcoma (Tashjian & Chabner, 2002). Recombinant PTH therapy may be followed by an antiresorptive agent. Side effects include nausea and headaches.

Summary

Osteoporosis is a costly and potentially disabling condition affecting millions of women. An integrative approach encompassing diet, exercise, supplements, and mind–body therapies, as well as pharmaceutical medications when indicated, is recommended to prevent and treat this disorder. The good news for women is that essentially the same strategies that help them to build healthy bones will also protect them against heart disease, diabetes, depression, and a host of other chronic conditions.

RECOMMENDATIONS TO BUILD AND MAINTAIN HEALTHY BONES

1. An anti-inflammatory diet that includes an abundance of fruits and vegetables, healthy fats, whole grains, and anti-inflammatory herbs, teas, and spices.
2. Total calcium intake for postmenopausal women (from diet plus supplements) of 1,200 mg per day.
3. A serum 25-OH D concentration in the range of 40 ng/mL (100 nmol/L).
4. Adequate intake of vitamin K1 and K2.
5. Increased intake of omega-3 fatty acids.
6. Adequate but not excessive protein (0.8 g/kg), including some vegetarian sources.
7. 1–2 servings per day of whole soy foods.
8. A good quality multivitamin/mineral supplement.
9. Physical activity for 30–45 minutes most days of the week. Include weight bearing, aerobic, and weight lifting exercise.
10. A daily mind–body practice.
11. Avoid: cigarette smoking and excessive intake of alcohol and caffeine.
12. Reduce the risk of falls and, if possible, avoid medications that harm bone or increase the risk of falls.
13. Pharmaceutical therapies should be individualized and risk and benefits explored with each woman.

Acknowledgment

I thank my sister MaryLynn Gagné for her patient and dedicated technical help in the preparation of this chapter.

REFERENCES

[Anonymous]. (2006). Alcohol over time: Still under control? For women, there's not much leeway between healthful and harmful drinking, especially as we get older. *Harv Womens Health Watch, 13*, 1–3

[Anonymous]. (2010). Management of osteoporosis in postmenopausal women: 2010 position statement of The North American Menopause Society. *Menopause, 17*, 25–54; quiz 55–56. doi: 10.1097/gme.0b013e3181c617e6

Abelow, B. J., Holford, T. R., & Insogna, K. L. (1992). Cross-cultural association between dietary animal protein and hip fracture: A hypothesis. *Calcif Tissue Int, 50*, 14–18. doi: 10.1007/BF00297291

Adams, J., & Pepping, J. (2005). Vitamin K in the treatment and prevention of osteoporosis and arterial calcification. *American Journal of Health-System Pharmacy, 62*, 1574–1581. doi: 10.2146/ajhp040357

Alekel, D. L., Van Loan, M. D., Koehler, K. J., et al. (2010). The Soy Isoflavones for Reducing Bone Loss (SIRBL) Study: A 3-y randomized controlled trial in postmenopausal women. *Am J Clin Nutr, 91*, 218–230. doi: 10.3945/ajcn.2009.28306

Alexy, U., Remer, T., Manz, F., Neu, C. M., & Schoenau, E. (2005). Long-term protein intake and dietary potential renal acid load are associated with bone modeling and remodeling at the proximal radius in healthy children. *Am J Clin Nutr, 82*, 1107–1114.

Ambrosini, G. L., Bremner, A. P., Reid, A., et al. (2013). No dose-dependent increase in fracture risk after long-term exposure to high doses of retinol or beta-carotene. *Osteoporosis Intl*, 1285–1293.

Anderson, J. J. B. (2000). The important role of physical activity in skeletal development: How exercise may counter low calcium intake. *Am J Clin Nutr, 71*, 1384–1386.

Armas, L. A. G., Hollis, B. W., & Heaney, R. P. (2004). Vitamin D(2) is much less effective than vitamin D(3) in humans. *J Clin Endocrinol Metab, 89*, 5387–5391. doi: 10.1210/jc.2004-0360

Arnett, T. (2003). Regulation of bone cell function by acid-base balance. *Proc Nutr Soc, 62*, 511–520. doi: 10.1079/PNS2003268

Bailey, R. L., Dodd, K. W., Goldman, J. A., et al. (2010). Estimation of total usual calcium and vitamin D Intakes in the United States. *J Nutr, 140*, 817–822. doi: 10.3945/jn.109.118539

Barrett-Connor, E., Cauley, J. A., Kulkarni, P. M., Sashegyi, A., Cox, D. A., & Geiger, M. J. (2004). Risk-benefit profile for raloxifene: 4-year data from the Multiple Outcomes of Raloxifene Evaluation (MORE) randomized trial. *J Bone Miner Res, 19*, 1270–1275. doi: 10.1359/JBMR.040406

Barzel, U. S., & Massey, L. K. (1998). Excess dietary protein can adversely affect bone. *J Nutr, 128*, 1051–1053.

Bauer, D. C., Black, D. M., Garnero, P., et al. (2004). Change in bone turnover and hip, non-spine, and vertebral fracture in alendronate-treated women: The Fracture Intervention Trial. *J Bone Miner Res, 19*, 1250–1258. doi: 10.1359/JBMR.040512

Beasley, J. M., LaCroix, A. Z., Larson, J. C., et al. (2014). Biomarker-calibrated protein intake and bone health in the Women's Health Initiative clinical trials and observational study (1–3). *Am J Clin Nutr, 99*, 934–940. doi: 10.3945/ajcn.113.076786

Bedford, J. L., & Barr, S. I. (2011). Higher urinary sodium, a proxy for intake, is associated with increased calcium excretion and lower hip bone density in healthy young women with lower calcium intakes. *Nutrients, 3*, 951–961. doi: 10.3390/nu3110951

Berg, K. M., Kunins, H. V., Jackson, J. L., et al. (2008). Association between alcohol consumption and both osteoporotic fracture and bone density. *Am J Med, 121*, 406–418. doi: 10.1016/j.amjmed.2007.12.012

Beulens, J. W. J., Booth, S. L., van den Heuvel, E. G. H. M., Stoecklin, E., Baka, A., & Vermeer, C. (2013). The role of menaquinones (vitamin K-2) in human health. *Br J Nutr, 110*, 1357–1368. doi: 10.1017/S0007114513001013

Bharti, A. C., Takada, Y., & Aggarwal, B. B. (2004). Curcumin (diferuloylmethane) inhibits receptor activator of NF-kB ligand-induced NF-kB activation in osteoclast precursors and suppresses osteoclastogenesis. *J Immunol, 172*, 5940–5947.

Bilezikian, J. P. (1998). Estrogens and postmenopausal osteoporosis: Was Albright right after all? *J Bone Miner Res, 13*, 774–776. doi: 10.1359/jbmr.1998.13.5.774

Bilezikian, J. P., Rubin, M. R., & Finkelstein, J. S. (2005). Parathyroid hormone as an anabolic therapy for women and men. *J Endocrinol Invest, 28*(8 Suppl), 41–49.

Bischoff-Ferrari, H. A. (2007). How to select the doses of vitamin D in the management of osteoporosis. *Osteoporosis Int, 18*, 401–407. doi: 10.1007/s00198-006-0293-9

Bischoff-Ferrari, H. A., Dawson-Hughes, B., Baron, J. A., et al. (2007). Calcium intake and hip fracture risk in men and women: A meta-analysis of prospective cohort studies and randomized controlled trials. *Am J Clin Nutr, 86*, 1780–1790.

Bischoff-Ferrari, H. A., Dawson-Hughes, B., Staehelin, H. B., et al. (2009). Fall prevention with supplemental and active forms of vitamin D: A meta-analysis of randomised controlled trials. *Br Med J, 339*, b3692-b3692. doi: 10.1136/bmj.b3692

Bischoff-Ferrari, H. A., Dietrich, T., Orav, E. J., Dawson-Hughes, B. (2004). Positive association between 25-hydroxy, vitamin D levels and bone mineral density: A population-based study of younger and older adults. *Am J Med, 116*, 634–639. doi: 10.1016/j.amjmed.2003.12.029

Bischoff-Ferrari, H. A., Willett, W. C., Wong, J. B., et al. (2009). Prevention of nonvertebral fractures with oral vitamin d and dose dependency: A meta-analysis of randomized controlled trials. *Arch Intern Med, 169*, 551–561.

Bischoff-Ferrari, H. A., Willett, W. C., Wong, J. B., Giovannucci, E., Dietrich, T., & Dawson-Hughes, B. (2005). Fracture prevention with vitamin D supplementation: A meta-analysis of randomized controlled trials. *JAMA, 293*, 2257–2264. doi: 10.1001/jama.293.18.2257

Black, D. M., Delmas, P. D., Eastell, R., et al. (2007). Once-yearly zoledronic acid for treatment of postmenopausal osteoporosis. *N Engl J Med, 356,* 1809–1822. doi: 10.1056/NEJMoa067312

Bolland, M. J. (2010). Effect of calcium supplements on risk of myocardial infarction and cardiovascular events: Meta-analysis. *Br Med J, 341,* c6923–c6923. doi: 10.1136/bmj.c6923

Bolton-Smith, C., McMurdo, M. E. T., Paterson, C. R., et al. (2007). Two-year randomized controlled trial of vitamin K-1 (phylloquinone) and vitamin D-3 plus calcium on the bone health of older women. *Journal of Bone and Mineral Research, 22,* 509–519. doi: 10.1359/JBMR.070116

Booth, S. L., Tucker, K. L., Chen, H. L., et al. (2000). Dietary vitamin K intakes are associated with hip fracture but not with bone mineral density in elderly men and women. *Am J Clin Nutr, 71,* 1201–1208.

Bruunsgaard, H., & Pedersen, B. K. (2003). Age-related inflammatory cytokines and disease. *Immunol Allergy Clin North Am, 23,* 15–39. doi: 10.1016/S0889-8561(02)00056-5

Buclin, T., Cosma, M., Appenzeller, M., et al. (2001). Diet acids and alkalis influence calcium retention in bone. *Osteoporosis Int, 12,* 493–499. doi: 10.1007/s001980170095

Burch, J., Rice, S., Yang, H., et al. (2014). Systematic review of the use of bone turnover markers for monitoring the response to osteoporosis treatment: The secondary prevention of fractures, and primary prevention of fractures in high-risk groups. *Health Technol Assess, 18,* 1–180.

Burge, R., Dawson-Hughes, B., Solomon, D. H., Wong, J. B., King, A., & Tosteson, A. (2007). Incidence and economic burden of osteoporosis-related fractures in the United States, 2005–2025. *J Bone Miner Res, 22,* 465–475. doi: 10.1359/JBMR.061113

Calvez, J., Poupin, N., Chesneau, C., Lassale, C., & Tome, D. (2012). Protein intake, calcium balance and health consequences. *Eur J Clin Nutr, 66,* 281–295. doi: 10.1038/ejcn.2011.196

Cannell, J. J., Hollis, B. W., Zasloff, M., & Heaney, R. P. (2008). Diagnosis and treatment of vitamin D deficiency. *Expert Opin Pharmacother, 9,* 107–118. doi: 10.1517/14656566.9.1.107

Castiglioni, S., Cazzaniga, A., Albisetti, W., & Maier, J. A. M. (2013). Magnesium and osteoporosis: Current state of knowledge and future research directions. *Nutrients, 5,* 3022–3033. doi: 10.3390/nu5083022

Cauley, J. A. (2013). Public health impact of osteoporosis. *J Gerontol A Biol Sci Med Sci, 68,* 1243–1251. doi: 10.1093/gerona/glt093

Cauley, J. A., Robbins, J., Chen, Z., et al. (2003). Effects of estrogen plus progestin on risk of fracture and bone mineral density: The Women's Health Initiative randomized trial. *JAMA, 290,* 1729–1738. doi: 10.1001/jama.290.13.1729

Cenci, S., Weitzmann, M. N., Roggia, C., et al. (2000). Estrogen deficiency induces bone loss by enhancing T-cell production of T NF-alpha. *J Clin Invest, 106,* 1229–1237. doi: 10.1172/JCI11066

Chen, Y. M., Ho, S. C., & Lam, S. S. (2010). Higher sea fish intake is associated with greater bone mass and lower osteoporosis risk in postmenopausal Chinese women. *Osteoporosis Int, 21,* 939–946. doi: 10.1007/s00198-009-1029-4

Chen, Z., Pettinger, M. B., Ritenbaugh, C., et al. (2003). Habitual tea consumption and risk of osteoporosis: A prospective study in the women's health initiative observational cohort. *Am J Epidemiol, 158,* 772–781. doi: 10.1098/aje/kwg214

Chung, H. Y., Sung, B., Jung, K. J., Zou, Y., & Yu., B. P. (2006). The molecular inflammatory process in aging. *Antioxid Redox Signal, 8,* 572–581. doi: 10.1089/ars.2006.8.572

Cizza, G., Ravn, P., Chrousos, G. P., & Gold, P. W. (2001). Depression: A major, unrecognized risk factor for osteoporosis? *Trends Endocrinol Metab, 12,* 198–203. doi: 10.1016/S1043-2760(01)00407-6

Clowes, J. A., Riggs, B. L., & Khosla, S. (2005). The role of the immune system in the pathophysiology of osteoporosis. *Immunol Rev, 208,* 207–227. doi: 10.1111/j.0105-28 96.2005.00334.x

Cockayne, S., Adamson, J., Lanham-New, S., Shearer, M. J., Gilbody, S., & Torgerson, D. J. (2006). Vitamin K and the prevention of fractures: Systematic review and meta-analysis of randomized controlled trials. *Arch Intern Med, 166,* 1256–1261. doi: 10.1001/archinte.166.12.1256

Compston J. (2006). Bone quality: What is it and how is it measured? *Arq Bras Endocrinol Metabol, 50,* 579–585.

Cooper, C., Atkinson, E. J., Hensrud, D. D., et al. (1996). Dietary protein intake and bone mass in women. *Calcif Tissue Int, 58,* 320–325. doi: 10.1007/BF02509379

Cordain, L., Eaton, S. B., Sebastian, A., et al. (2005). Origins and evolution of the western diet: Health implications for the 21st century. *Am J Clin Nutr, 81,* 341–354

Cornuz, J., Feskanich, D., Willett, W. C., & Colditz, G. A. (1999). Smoking, smoking cessation, and risk of hip fracture in women. *Am J Med, 106,* 311–314. doi: 10.1016/S0002-9343(99)00022-4

Cummings, S. R., Black, D. M., Nevitt, M. C., et al. (1993). Bone-density at various sites for prediction of hip-fractures. *Lancet, 341,* 72–75. doi: 10.1016/0140-6736(93)92555-8

Cussler, E. C., Going, S. B., Houtkooper, L. B., et al. (2005). Exercise frequency and calcium intake predict 4-year bone changes in postmenopausal women. *Osteoporosis Int, 16,* 2129–2141. doi: 10.1007/s00198-005-2014-1

Das, U. N. (2000). Essential fatty acids and osteoporosis. *Nutrition, 16,* 386–390. doi: 10.1016/S0899-9007(00)00262-8

Dawson-Hughes, B., & Harris, S. S. (2002). Calcium intake influences the association of protein intake with rates of bone loss in elderly men and women. *Am J Clin Nutr, 75,* 773–779.

De Bacquer, D., Clays, E., Delanghe, J., & De Backer, G. (2006). Epidemiological evidence for an association between habitual tea consumption and markers of chronic inflammation. *Atherosclerosis, 189,* 428–435. doi: 10.1016/j.atherosclerosis.2005.12.028

Deng, W., Zhang, P., Huang, H., et al. (2012). Five-year follow-up study of a kidney-tonifying herbal Fufang for prevention of postmenopausal osteoporosis and fragility fractures. *J Bone Miner Metab, 30,* 517–524. doi: 10.1007/s00774-012-0351-7

Dhanwal, D. K., Dennison, E. M., Harvey, N. C., & Cooper, C. (2011). Epidemiology of hip fracture: Worldwide geographic variation. *Indian J Orthop, 45,* 15–22. doi: 10.4103/0019-5413.73656

Dimai, H. P., & Chandran, M.; FRAX Position Dev Conf Members. (2011). Official positions for FRAX (R) clinical regarding smoking. *Journal of Clinical Densitometry, 14,* 190–193. doi: 10.1016/j.jocd.2011.05.011

Ding, C., Parameswaran, V., Udayan, R., Burgess, J., & Jones, G. (2008). Circulating levels of inflammatory markers predict change in bone mineral density and resorption in older adults: A longitudinal study. *J Clin Endocrinol Metab, 93,* 1952–1958. doi: 10.1210/jc.2007-2325

Ettinger, B., Black, D. M., Mitlak, B. H., et al. (1999). Reduction of vertebral fracture risk in postmenopausal women with osteoporosis treated with raloxifene: Results from a 3-year randomized clinical trial. *JAMA, 282,* 637–645. doi: 10.1001/jama.282.7.637

Ettinger, B., Ensrud, K., Wallace, R., et al. (2004). Effects of ultralow-dose transdermal estradiol on bone mineral density: A randomized clinical trial. *Obstet Gynecol, 104,* 443–451.

Evans, W. (1997). Functional and metabolic consequences of sarcopenia. *J Nutr, 127,* S998–S1003.

Fernandes, G., Lawrence, R., & Sun, D. (2003). Protective role of n-3 lipids and soy protein in osteoporosis. *Prostaglandins Leukot Essent Fatty Acids, 68,* 361–372. doi: 10.1016/S0952-3278(03)00060-7

Feskanich, D., Weber, P., Willett, W. C., Rockett, H., Booth, S. L., & Colditz, G. A. (1999). Vitamin K intake and hip fractures in women: a prospective study. *Am J Clin Nutr, 69,* 74–79.

Feskanich, D., Willett, W. C., & Colditz, G. A. (2003). Calcium, vitamin D, milk consumption, and hip fractures: a prospective study among postmenopausal women. *Am J Clin Nutr, 77,* 504–511.

Feskanich, D., Willett, W. C., Stampfer, M. J., & Colditz, G. A. (1996). Protein consumption and bone fractures in women. *Am J Epidemiol, 143,* 472–479.

Feskanich, D., Willett, W., & Colditz, G. (2002). Walking and leisure-time activity and risk of hip fracture in postmenopausal women. *JAMA, 288,* 2300–2306. doi: 10.1001/jama.288.18.2300

Fiatarone, M. A., Oneill, E. F., Ryan, N. D., et al. (1994). Exercise training and nutritional supplementation for physical frailty in very elderly people. *N Engl J Med, 330,* 1769–1775. doi: 10.1056/NEJM199406233302501

Fitzpatrick, L. A. (2006). Estrogen therapy for postmenopausal osteoporosis. *Arq Bras Endocrinol Metabol, 50,* 705–19. doi: 10.1590/S0004-27302006000400016

Fradinger, E. E., & Zanchetta, J. R. (2001). Vitamin D and bone mineral density in ambulatory women living in Buenos Aires, Argentina. *Osteoporosis Int, 12,* 24–27. doi: 10.1007/s001980170153

Frassetto, L. A., Todd, K. M., Morris, R. C., & Sebastian, A. (2000). Worldwide incidence of hip fracture in elderly women: Relation to consumption of animal and vegetable foods. *J Gerontol A Biol Sci Med Sci, 55,* M585–M592.

Gardner, E. J., Ruxton, C. H. S., & Leeds, A. R. (2007). Black tea—helpful or harmful? A review of the evidence. *Eur J Clin Nutr, 61,* 3–18. doi: 10.1038/sj.ejcn.1602489

Ginaldi, L., Di Benedetto, M. C., & De Martinis, M. (2005). Osteoporosis, inflammation and ageing. *Immun Ageing, 2,* 14–14. doi: 10.1186/1742-4933-2-14

Goldring, S. R. (2003). Inflammatory mediators as essential elements in bone remodeling. *Calcif Tissue Int, 73*, 97–100. doi: 10.1007/s00223-002-1049-y

Gordon, C. M., & Nelson, L. M. (2003). Amenorrhea and bone health in adolescents and young women. *Curr Opin Obstet Gynecol, 15*, 377–384. doi: 10.1097/01.gco.0000094698.87578.21

Gur, A., Colpan, L., Nas, K., et al. (2002). The role of trace minerals in the pathogenesis of postmenopausal osteoporosis and a new effect of calcitonin. *J Bone Miner Metab, 20*, 39–43. doi: 10.1007/s774-002-8445-y

Guyatt, G. H., Cranney, A., Griffith, L., et al. (2002). Summary of meta-analyses of therapies for postmenopausal osteoporosis and the relationship between bone density and fractures. *Endocrinol Metab Clin North Am, 31*, 659+. doi: 10.1016/S0889-8529(02)00024-5

Hallstrom, H., Wolk, A., Glynn, A., & Michaelsson, K. (2006). Coffee, tea and caffeine consumption in relation to osteoporotic fracture risk in a cohort of Swedish women. *Osteoporosis Int, 17*, 1055–1064. doi: 10.1007/s00198-006-0109-y

Harrington, M., & Cashman, K. D. (2003). High salt intake appears to increase bone resorption in postmenopausal women but high potassium intake ameliorates this adverse effect. *Nutr Rev, 61*, 179–183. doi: 10.1301/nr.2003.may.179–183

Harris, S. T., Watts, N. B., Genant, H. K., et al. (1999). Effects of risedronate treatment on vertebral and nonvertebral fractures in women with postmenopausal osteoporosis: A randomized controlled trial. *JAMA, 282*, 1344–1352. doi: 10.1001/jama.282.14.1344

Heaney, R. P. (2002). Effects of caffeine on bone and the calcium economy. *Food and Chemical Toxicology, 40*, 1263–1270. doi: 10.1016/S0278-6915(02)00094-7

Heaney, R. P. (2006). Role of dietary sodium in osteoporosis. *J Am Coll Nutr, 25*, 271S–276S.

Heaney, R. P., & Layman, D. K. (2008). Amount and type of protein influences bone health. *Am J Clin Nutr, 87*, 1567S–1570S.

Heaney, R. P., Dowell, M. S., Hale, C. A., & Bendich, A. (2003). Calcium absorption varies within the reference range for serum 25-hydroxyvitamin D. *J Am Coll Nutr, 22*, 142–146.

Heaney, R. P., Kopecky, S., Maki, K. C., Hathcock, J., MacKay, D., & Wallace, T. C. (2012). A review of calcium supplements and cardiovascular disease risk. *Adv Nutr, 3*, 763–771. doi: 10.3945/an.112.002899

Heinonen, A., Sievanen, H., Kannus, P., Oja, P., Pasanen, M., & Vuori, I. (2000). High-impact exercise and bones of growing girls: A 9-month controlled trial. *Osteoporosis Int, 11*, 1010–1017.

Hodges, S. J., Akesson, K., Vergnaud, P., Obrant, K., & Delmas, P. D. (1993). Circulating levels of vitamin-K1 and vitamin-K(2) decreased in elderly women with hip fracture. *Journal of Bone and Mineral Research, 8*, 1241–1245.

Hodges, S. J., Pilkington, M. J., Stamp, T. C. B., et al. (1991). Depressed levels of circulating menaquinones in patients with osteoporotic fractures of the spine and femoral-neck. *Bone, 12*, 387–389. doi: 10.1016/8756-3282(91)90027-G

Holick, M. F. (2006). High prevalence of vitamin D inadequacy and implications for health. *Mayo Clin Proc, 81*, 353–373.

Horowitz, M. C. (1993). Cytokines and estrogen in bone: Anti-osteoporotic effects. *Science, 260,* 626–627. doi: 10.1126/science.8480174

Ince, B. A., Anderson, E. J., & Neer, R. M. (2004). Lowering dietary protein to US recommended dietary allowance levels reduces urinary calcium excretion and bone resorption in young women. *J Clin Endocrinol Metab, 89,* 3801–3807. doi: 10.1210/jc.2003-032016

Jacobs, E. T., Alberts, D. S., Foote, J. A., et al. (2008). Vitamin D insufficiency in southern Arizona. *Am J Clin Nutr, 87,* 608–613.

Jia, D., O'Brien, C. A., Stewart, S. A., Manolagas, S. C., & Weinstein, R. S. (2006). Glucocorticoids act directly on osteoclasts to increase their life span and reduce bone density. *Endocrinology, 147,* 5592–5599. doi: 10.1210/en.2006-0459

Kalkwarf, H. J., & Specker, B. L. (2002). Bone mineral changes during pregnancy and lactation. *Endocrine, 17,* 49–53. doi: 10.1385/ENDO:17:1:49

Kaneki, M. (2006). [Protective effects of vitamin K against osteoporosis and its pleiotropic actions]. *Clin Calcium, 16,* 1526–1534.

Kanellakis, S., Moschonis, G., Tenta, R., et al. (2012). Changes in parameters of bone metabolism in postmenopausal women following a 12-month intervention period using dairy products enriched with calcium, vitamin, D., and phylloquinone (vitamin K-1) or menaquinone-7 (vitamin K-2): The Postmenopausal Health Study II. *Calcif Tissue Int, 90,* 251–262. doi: 10.1007/s00223-012-9571-z

Kanis, J. A., Johnell, O., Oden, A., et al. (2005). Smoking and fracture risk: A meta-analysis. *Osteoporosis Int, 16,* 155–162. doi: 10.1007/s00198-004-1640-3

Kanis, J. A., McCloskey, E., Johansson, H., Oden, A., & Leslie, W. D. (2012). FRAX(A(R)) with and without bone mineral density. *Calcif Tissue Int, 90,* 1–13. doi: 10.1007/s00223-011-9544-7

Kaunitz, A. M., Arias, R., & McClung, M. (2008). Bone density recovery after depot medroxyprogesterone acetate injectable contraception use. *Contraception, 77,* 67–76. doi: 10.1016/j.contraception.2007.10.005

Kim, C., Ha, H., Lee, J. H., Kim, J. S., Song, K., & Park, S. W. (2003). Herbal extract prevents bone loss in ovariectomized rats. *Arch Pharm Res, 26,* 917–924. doi: 10.1007/BF02980200

Knapen, M. H. J., Drummen, N. E., Smit, E., Vermeer, C., & Theuwissen, E. (2013). Three-year low-dose menaquinone-7 supplementation helps decrease bone loss in healthy postmenopausal women. *Osteoporosis Int, 24,* 2499–2507. doi: 10.1007/s00198-013-2325-6

Knopp, J. A., Diner, B. M., Blitz, M., Lyritis, G. P., & Rowe, B. H. (2005). Calcitonin for treating acute pain of osteoporotic vertebral compression fractures: A systematic review of randomized, controlled trials. *Osteoporosis Int, 16,* 1281–1290. doi: 10.1007/s00198-004-1798-8

Koh, J. M., Khang, Y. H., Jung, C. H., et al. (2005). Higher circulating hsCRP levels are associated with lower bone mineral density in healthy pre- and postmenopausal women: Evidence for a link between systemic inflammation and osteoporosis. *Osteoporosis Int, 16,* 1263–1271. doi: 10.1007/s00198-005-1840-5

Koh, W. P., Wu, A. H., Wang R., et al. (2009). Gender-specific associations between soy and risk of hip fracture in the Singapore Chinese Health Study. *Am J Epidemiol*, *170*, 901–909. doi: 10.1093/aje/kwp220

Kruger, M. C., Coetzer, H., de Winter, R., Gericke, G., & van Papendorp, D. H. (1998). Calcium, gamma-linolenic acid and eicosapentaenoic acid supplementation in senile osteoporosis. *Aging-Clin Exp Res*, *10*, 385–394.

Kruger, M. C., & Horrobin, D. F. (1997). Calcium metabolism, osteoporosis and essential fatty acids: A review. *Prog Lipid Res*, *36*, 131–151. doi: 10.1016/S0163-7827(97)00007-6

Langsetmo, L., Berger, C., Kreiger, N., et al. (2013). Calcium and vitamin D intake and mortality: Results from the Canadian Multicentre Osteoporosis Study (CaMos). *J Clin Endocrinol Metab*, *98*, 3010–3018. doi: 10.1210/jc.2013-1516

Lanham-New, S. A. (2008). The balance bone health: Tipping the scales on favor of potassium-rich, bicarbonate-rich foods. *J Nutr*, *138*, 172S–177S.

Lanou, A. J. (2011). Soy foods: Are they useful for optimal bone health? *Ther Adv Musculoskelet Dis*, *3*, 293–300. doi: 10.1177/1759720X11417749

Lin, P. H., Ginty, F., Appel, L. J., et al. (2003). The DASH diet and sodium reduction improve markers of bone turnover and calcium metabolism in adults. *J Nutr*, *133*, 3130–3136.

Lips, P., Hosking, D., Lippuner, K., et al. (2006). The prevalence of vitamin D inadequacy amongst women with osteoporosis: An international epidemiological investigation. *J Intern Med*, *260*, 245–254. doi: 10.1111/j.1365-2796.2006.01685.x

Lloyd, T., Beck, T. J., Lin, H. M., et al. (2002). Modifiable determinants of bone status in young women. *Bone*, *30*, 416–421. doi: 10.1016/S8756-3282(01)00675-5

Lloyd, T., Petit, M. A., Lin, H. M., & Beck, T. J. (2004). Lifestyle factors and the development of bone mass and bone strength in young women. *J Pediatr*, *144*, 776–782. doi: 10.1016/j.jpeds.2004.02.047

Looker, A. C., Borrud, L. G., Dawson-Hughes, B., Shepherd, J. A., & Wright, N. C. (2012). *NCHS Data Brief: Osteoporosis or low bone mass at the femur neck or lumbar spine in older adults: United States, 2005–2008*. Retrieved June 22, 2014, from http://www.cdc.gov/nchs/data/databriefs/db93.htm.

Maggio, D., Barabani, M., Pierandrei, M., et al. (2003). Marked decrease in plasma antioxidants in aged osteoporotic women: Results of a cross-sectional study. *J Clin Endocrinol Metab*, *88*, 1523–1527. doi: 10.1210/jc.2002-021496

Manolagas, S. C., Bellido, T., & Jilka, R. L. (1995). New insights into the cellular, biochemical, and molecular-basis of postmenopausal and senile osteoporosis—roles of Il-6 and Gp130. *Int J Immunopharmacol*, *17*, 109–116. doi: 10.1016/0192-0561(94)00089-7

Marangella, M., Di Stefano, M., Casalis, S., Berutti, S., D'Amelio, P., & Isaia, G. C. (2004). Effects of potassium citrate supplementation on bone metabolism. *Calcif Tissue Int*, *74*, 330–335. doi: 10.1007/s00223-003-0091-8

Marsh, A. G., Sanchez, T. V., Mickelsen, O., Keiser, J., & Mayor G. (1980). Cortical bone-density of adult lacto-ovo-vegetarian and omnivorous women. *J Am Diet Assoc*, *76*, 148–151.

Marshall, D., Johnell, O., & Wedel, H. (1996). Meta-analysis of how well measures of bone mineral density predict occurrence of osteoporotic fractures. *Br Med J, 312*, 1254–1259.

Mashiba, T., Hirano, T., Turner, C. H., Forwood, M. R., Johnston, C. C., & Burr, D. B. (2000). Suppressed bone turnover by bisphosphonates increases microdamage accumulation and reduces some biomechanical properties in dog rib. *J Bone Miner Res, 15*, 613–620. doi: 10.1359/jbmr.2000.15.4.613

Massey, L. K. (2003). Dietary animal and plant protein and human bone health: A whole foods approach. *J Nutr, 133*, 862S–865S.

Maurer, M., Riesen, W., Muser, J., Hulter, H. N., & Krapf, R. (2003). Neutralization of Western diet inhibits bone resorption independently of K intake and reduces cortisol secretion in humans. *Am J Physiol Renal Physiol, 284*, F32–F40. doi: 10.1152/ajprenal.00212.2002

McCarus, D. C. (2006). Fracture prevention in postmenopausal osteoporosis: A review of treatment options. *Obstet Gynecol Surv, 61*, 39–50. doi: 10.1097/01.ogx.0000197807.08697.06

Melhus, H., Michaelsson, K., Kindmark, A., et al. (1998). Excessive dietary intake of vitamin A is associated with reduced bone mineral density and increased risk for hip fracture. *Ann Intern Med, 129*, 770+.

Melton, L. J., Bryant, S. C., Wahner, H. W., et al. (1993). Influence of breast-feeding and other reproductive factors on bone mass later in life. *Osteoporosis Int, 3*, 76–83. doi: 10.1007/BF01623377

Mezquita-Raya, P., Munoz-Torres, M., Luna, J. D., et al. (2001). Relation between vitamin D insufficiency, bone density, and bone metabolism in healthy postmenopausal women. *J Bone Miner Res, 16*, 1408–1415. doi: 10.1359/jbmr.2001.16.8.1408

Mezzetti, M., La Vecchia, C., Decarli, A., Boyle, P., Talanmini, R., & Franceschi, S. (1998). Population attributable risk for breast cancer: Diet, nutrition, and physical exercise. *J Natl Cancer Inst, 90*, 389–394. doi: 10.1093/jnci/90.5.389

Mingyue, W., Ling, G., Bei, X., Junqing, C., Peiqing, Z., & Jie, H. (2005). Clinical observation on 96 cases of primary osteoporosis treated with kidney-tonifying and bone-strengthening mixture. *J Tradit Chin Med, 25*, 132–136.

Misra, D., Berry, S. D., Broe, K. E., et al. (2011). Does dietary protein reduce hip fracture risk in elders? The Framingham osteoporosis study. *Osteoporosis Int, 22*, 345–349. doi: 10.1007/s00198-010-1179-4

Misra, M., Prabhakaran, R., Miller, K. K., et al. (2008). Weight gain and restoration of menses as predictors of bone mineral density change in adolescent girls with anorexia nervosa-1. *J Clin Endocrinol Metab, 93*, 1231–1237. doi: 10.1210/jc.2007-1434

Moyer, V. (2013). Menopausal hormone therapy for the primary prevention of chronic conditions: US Preventive Services Task Force recommendation statement. *Ann Intern Med, 158*, 47–54 doi: 10.7326/0003-4819-158-1-201301010-0053

National Osteoporosis Foundation. (2010). *Clinician's guide to prevention and treatment of osteoporosis*. Retrieved June 22, 2014, from http://nof.org/files/nof/public/content/file/344/upload/159.pdf

Nelson, H. D., Humphrey, L. L., Nygren, P., Teutsch, S. M., & Allan, J. D. (2002). Postmenopausal hormone replacement therapy: Scientific review. *JAMA*, *288*, 872–881. doi: 10.1001/jama.288.7.872

New, S. A., Robins, S. P., Campbell, M. K., et al. (2000). Dietary influences on bone mass and bone metabolism: Further evidence of a positive link between fruit and vegetable consumption and bone health? *Am J Clin Nutr*, *71*, 142–151.

Nordin, B. E. C. (2000). Calcium requirement is a sliding scale. *Am J Clin Nutr*, *71*, 1381–1383.

Orchard, T. S., Pan, X., Cheek, F., Ing, S. W., & Jackson, R. D. (2012). A systematic review of omega-3 fatty acids and osteoporosis. *Br J Nutr*, *107*, S253–S260. doi: 10.1017/S0007114512001638

Overman, R. A., Borse, M., & Gourlay, M. L. (2013). Salmon calcitonin use and associated cancer risk. *Ann Pharmacother*, *47*, 1675–1684. doi: 10.1177/1060028013509233

Pacifici, R. (1996). Estrogen, cytokines, and pathogenesis of postmenopausal osteoporosis. *J Bone Miner Res*, *11*, 1043–1051

Papoutsi, Z., Kassi, E., Chinou, I., Halabalaki, M., Skaltsounis, L. A., & Moutsatsou, P. (2008). Walnut extract (*Juglans regia*, L.) and its component ellagic acid exhibit anti-inflammatory activity in human aorta endothelial cells and osteoblastic activity in the cell line KS483. *Br J Nutr*, *99*, 715–722. doi: 10.1017/S0007114507837421

Patterson-Buckendahl, P., Pohorecky, L. A., & Kvetnansky, R. (2007). Differing effects of acute and chronic stressors on plasma osteocalcin and leptin in rats. *Stress*, *10*, 163–172. doi: 10.1080/10253890701317601

Pearson, D. A. (2007). Bone health and osteoporosis: the role of vitamin K and potential antagonism by anticoagulants. *Nutr Clin Pract*, *22*, 517–544. doi: 10.1177/011542 6507022005517

Prabhoo, R., & Prabhoo, T. R. (2010). Vitamin K2: A novel therapy for osteoporosis. *J Indian Med Assoc*, *108*, 253–254, 256–258.

Pradhan, A. D., Manson, J. E., Rifai, N., Buring, J. E., & Ridker, P. M. (2001). C-reactive protein, interleukin 6, and risk of developing type 2 diabetes mellitus. *JAMA*, *286*, 327–334. doi: 10.1001/jama.286.3.327

Proctor, D. N., Melton, L. J., Kosla, S., Crowson, C. S., O'Connor, M. K., & Riggs, B. L. (2000). Relative influence of physical activity, muscle mass and strength on bone density. *Osteoporosis Int*, *11*, 944–952. doi: 10.1007/s001980070033

Prynne, C. J., D Mishra, G., O'Connell, M. A., et al. (2006). Fruit and vegetable intakes and bone mineral status: a cross-sectional study in 5 age and sex cohorts. *Am J Clin Nutr*, *83*, 1420–1428.

Putnam, S. E., Scutt, A. M., Bicknell, K., Priestley, C. M., & Williamson, E. M. (2007). Natural products as alternative treatments for metabolic bone disorders and for maintenance of bone health. *Phytother Res*, *21*, 99–112. doi: 10.1002/ptr.2030

Rautiainen, S., Wang, L., Manson, J. E., & Sesso, H. D. (2013). The role of calcium in the prevention of cardiovascular disease: A review of observational studies and randomized clinical trials. *Curr Atheroscler Rep*, *15*, 362–362. doi: 10.1007/s11883-013-0362-4

Reginster, J., & Sarlet, N. (2006). The treatment of severe postmenopausal osteoporosis: A review of current and emerging therapeutic options. *Treat Endocrinol, 5,* 15–23. doi: 10.2165/00024677-200605010-00003

Reinwald, S., & Weaver, C. M. (2010). Soy components vs. whole soy: Are we betting our bones on a long shot? *J Nutr, 140,* 2312S–2317S. doi: 10.3945/jn.110.124008

Ridker, P. M., Rifai, N., Stampfer, M. J., & Hennekens, C. H. (2000). Plasma concentration of interleukin-6 and the risk of future myocardial infarction among apparently healthy men. *Circulation, 101,* 1767–1772.

Rosanoff, A., Weaver, C. M., & Rude, R. K. (2012). Suboptimal magnesium status in the United States: Are the health consequences underestimated? *Nutr Rev, 70,* 153–164. doi: 10.1111/j.1753-4887.2011.00465.x

Ryder, K. M., Shorr, R. I., Bush, A. J., et al. (2005). Magnesium intake from food and supplements is associated with bone mineral density in healthy older white subjects. *J Am Geriatr Soc, 53,* 1875–1880. doi: 10.1111/j.1532-5415.2005.53561.x

Sahni, S., Hannan, M. T., Gagnon, D., et al. (2009). Protective effect of total and supplemental vitamin C intake on the risk of hip fracture: A 17-year follow-up from the Framingham Osteoporosis Study. *Osteoporosis Int, 20,* 1853–1861. doi: 10.1007/s00198-009-0897-y

Sakhaee, K., Bhuket, T., Adams-Huet, B., & Rao, D. S. (1999). Meta-analysis of calcium bioavailability: A comparison of calcium citrate with calcium carbonate. *Am J Ther, 6,* 313–21. doi: 10.1097/00045391-199911000-00005

Sampaio Lacativa, P. G., & Fleiuss de Farias, M. L. (2010). Osteoporosis and inflammation. *Arq Bras Endocrinol Metabol, 54,* 123–132.

Sampson, H. W. (2002). Alcohol and other factors affecting osteoporosis risk in women. *Alcoh Res Health, 26,* 292–298.

Sato, T., Schurgers, L. J., & Uenishi, K. (2012). Comparison of menaquinone-4 and menaquinone-7 bioavailability in healthy women. *Nutr J, 11,* 93.

Schurgers, L. J., Teunissen, K. J. F., Hamulyak, K., Knapen, M. H. J., Vik, H., & Vermeer, C. (2007). Vitamin K-containing dietary supplements: Comparison of synthetic vitamin K-1 and natto-derived menaquinone-7. *Blood, 109,* 3279–3283. doi: 10.1182/blood-2006-08-040709

Schurgers, L. J., & Vermeer, C. (2000). Determination of phylloquinone and menaquinones in food: Effect of food matrix on circulating vitamin K concentrations. *Haemostasis, 30,* 298–307.

Sebastian, A. (2005). Dietary protein content and the diet's net acid load: Opposing effects on bone health. *Am J Clin Nutr, 82,* 921–922.

Sebastian, A., Frassetto, L. A., Sellmeyer, D. E., Merriam, R. L., & Morris, R. C. (2002). Estimation of the net acid load of the diet of ancestral preagricultural Homo sapiens and their hominid ancestors. *Am J Clin Nutr, 76,* 1308–1316.

Sellmeyer, D. E., Stone, K. L., Sebastian, A., & Cummings, S. R. (2001). A high ratio of dietary animal to vegetable protein increases the rate of bone loss and the risk of fracture in postmenopausal women. *Am J Clin Nutr, 73,* 118–122.

Shah, A., & Kolhapure, S. (2004). Evaluation of efficacy and safety of Reosto in senile osteoporosis: a randomized, double-blind placebo-controlled clinical trial. *Indian J Clin Pract, 15,* 25–36.

Silva-Fernandez, L., Rosario, M. P., Martinez-Lopez, J. A., Carmona, L., & Loza, E. (2013). Denosumab for the treatment of osteoporosis: A systematic literature review. *Reumatol Clin, 9,* 42–52. doi: 10.1016/j.reuma.2012.06.007

Simopoulos, A. P. (2000). Human requirement for n-3 polyunsaturated fatty acids. *Poult Sci, 79,* 961–970.

Simopoulos, A. P. (2008). The importance of the omega-6/omega-3 fatty acid ratio in cardiovascular disease and other chronic diseases. *Exp Biol Med, 233,* 674–688. doi: 10.3181/0711-MR-311

Simopoulos, A. P. (2011). Evolutionary aspects of diet: The omega-6/omega-3 ratio and the brain. *Mol Neurobiol, 44,* 203–215. doi: 10.1007/s12035-010-8162-0

Sinaki, M., Itoi, E., Wahner, H. W., et al. (2002). Stronger back muscles reduce the incidence of vertebral fractures: A prospective 10 year follow-up of postmenopausal women. *Bone, 30,* 836–841. doi: 10.1016/S8756-3282(02)00739-1

Siris, E. S., Miller, P. D., Barrett-Connor, E., et al. (2001). Identification and fracture outcomes of undiagnosed low bone mineral density in postmenopausal women—results from the National Osteoporosis Risk Assessment. *JAMA, 286,* 2815–2822. doi: 10.1001/jama.286.22.2815

Sojka, J. E., & Weaver, C. M. (1995). Magnesium supplementation and osteoporosis. *Nutr Rev, 53,* 71–74.

Sommer, I., Erkkila, A. T., Jarvinen, R., et al. (2013). Alcohol consumption and bone mineral density in elderly women. *Public Health Nutr, 16,* 704–712. doi: 10.1017/S136898001200331X

Stendig-Lindberg, G., Tepper, R., & Leichter, I. (1993). Trabecular bone density in a two year controlled trial of peroral magnesium in osteoporosis. *Magnesium Res, 6,* 155–163.

Tang, B. M. P., Eslick, G. D., Nowson, C., Smith, C., & Bensoussan, A. (2007). Use of calcium or calcium in combination with vitamin D supplementation to prevent fractures and bone loss in people aged 50 years and older: a meta-analysis. *Lancet, 370,* 657–666. doi: 10.1016/S0140-6736(07)61342-7

Tashjian, A. H., & Chabner, B. A. (2002). Commentary on clinical safety of recombinant human parathyroid hormone 1–34 in the treatment of osteoporosis in men and postmenopausal women. *J Bone Miner Res, 17,* 1151–1161. doi: 10.1359/jbmr.2002.17.7.1151

Thom, J. A., Bishop, A., Blacklock, N. J., & Morris, J. E. (1978). Influence of refined carbohydrate on urinary calcium excretion. *Br J Urol, 50,* 459–464. doi: 10.1111/j.1464-410X.1978.tb06191.x

Todd, J. A., & Robinson, R. J. (2003). Osteoporosis and exercise. *Postgrad Med J, 79,* 320–323. doi: 10.1136/pmj.79.932.320

Togari, A., Arai, M., & Kondo, A. (2005). The role of the sympathetic nervous system in controlling bone metabolism. *Expert Opin Ther Targets, 9,* 931–940. doi: 10.1517/14728222.9.5.931

Trivedi, D. P., Doll, R., & Khaw, K. T. (2003). Effect of four monthly oral vitamin D-3 (cholecalciferol) supplementation on fractures and mortality in men and women living in the community: Randomised double blind controlled trial. *Br Med J, 326,* 469–472. doi: 10.1136/bmj.326.7387.469

Tucker, K. L., Hannan, M. T., Chen, H. L., Cupples, L. A., Wilson, P. W. F., & Kiel, D. P. (1999). Potassium, magnesium, and fruit and vegetable intakes are associated with greater bone mineral density in elderly men and women. *Am J Clin Nutr, 69*, 727–736.

Turner, C. H. (2002). Biomechanics of bone: Determinants of skeletal fragility and bone quality. *Osteoporosis Int, 13*, 97–104. doi: 10.1007/s001980200000

Ushiroyama, T., Ikeda, A., & Ueki, M. (2002). Effect of continuous combined therapy with vitamin K-2 and vitamin D-3 on bone mineral density and coagulofibrinolysis function in postmenopausal women. *Maturitas, 41*, 211–221. doi: 10.1016/S0378-5122(01)00275-4

Vasikaran, S., Eastell, R., Bruyere, O., et al. (2011). Markers of bone turnover for the prediction of fracture risk and monitoring of osteoporosis treatment: A need for international reference standards. *Osteoporosis Int, 22*, 391–420. doi: 10.1007/s00198-010-1501-1

Vermeer, C., & Theuwissen, E. (2011). Vitamin K, osteoporosis and degenerative diseases of ageing. *Menopause Int, 17*, 19–23. doi: 10.1258/mi.2011.011006

Vogel, R. A. (2002). Alcohol, heart disease, and mortality: A review. *Rev Cardiovasc Med, 3*, 7–13.

Voukelatos, A., Cumming, R. G., Lord, S. R., & Rissel, C. (2007). A randomized, controlled trial of tai chi for the prevention of falls: The Central Sydney Tai Chi Trial. *J Am Geriatr Soc, 55*, 1185–1191. doi: 10.1111/j.1532-5415.2007.01244.x

Wainwright, S. A., Marshall, L. M., Ensrud, K. E., et al. (2005). Hip fracture in women without osteoporosis. *J Clin Endocrinol Metab, 90*, 2787–2793. doi: 10.1210/jc.2004-1568

Walsh, J. S., Eastell, R., & Peel, N. F. A. (2008). Effects of depot medroxyprogesterone acetate on bone density and bone metabolism before and after peak bone mass: A case-control study. *J Clin Endocrinol Metab, 93*, 1317–1323. doi: 10.1210/jc.2007-2201

Wayne, P. M., Kiel, D. P., Krebs, D. E., et al. (2007). The effects of tai chi on bone mineral density in postmenopausal women: A systematic review. *Arch Phys Med Rehabil, 88*, 673–680. doi: 10.1016/j.apmr.2007.02.012

Wei, P., Liu, M., Chen, Y., & Chen, D. C. (2012). Systematic review of soy isoflavone supplements on osteoporosis in women. *Asian Pac J Trop Med, 5*, 243–248. doi: 10.1016/S1995-7645(12)60033-9

Weikert, C., Walter, D., Hoffmann, K., Kroke, A., Bergmann, M. M., & Boeing, H. (2005). The relation between dietary protein, calcium and bone health in women: Results from the EPIC-Potsdam cohort. *Ann Nutr Metab, 49*, 312–318. doi: 10.1159/000087335

Weiss, L. A., Barrett-Connor, E., & von Muhlen, D. (2005). Ratio of n-6 to n-3 fatty acids and bone mineral density in older adults: The Rancho Bernardo study. *Am J Clin Nutr, 81*, 934–938.

Wolff, I., van Croonenborg, J. J., Kemper, H. C. G., Kostense, P. J., & Twisk, J. W. R. (1999). The effect of exercise training programs on bone mass: A meta-analysis of published controlled trials in pre- and postmenopausal women. *Osteoporosis Int, 9*, 1–12. doi: 10.1007/s001980050109

World Health Organization, Food and Agriculture Organization. (2004). *Vitamin and mineral requirements in human nutrition.* Report of a joint FAO/WHO expert consultation, Bangkok, Thailand, 21–30 September 1998.

Xiao, Q., & Park, Y. (2013). Dietary and supplemental calcium intake and mortality reply. *JAMA Intern Med, 173,* 1841–1842. doi: 10.1001/jamainternmed.2013.9232

Yin, J., Kouda, K., Tezuka, Y., et al. (2004). New diarylheptanoids from the rhizomes of *Dioscorea spongiosa* and their antiosteoporotic activity. *Planta Med, 70,* 54–58. doi: 10.1055/s-2004-815456

Yin, J., Tezuka, Y., Kouda, K., et al. (2004). Antiosteoporotic activity of the water extract of Dioscorea spongiosa. *Biol Pharm Bull, 27,* 583–586. doi: 10.1248/bpb.27.583

Yoon, V., Maalouf, N. M., & Sakhaee, K. (2012). The effects of smoking on bone metabolism. *Osteoporosis Int, 23,* 2081–2092. doi: 10.1007/s00198-012-1940-y

Zhang, X. L., Shu, X. O., Li, H. L., et al. (2005). Prospective cohort study of soy food consumption and risk of bone fracture among postmenopausal women. *Arch Intern Med, 165,* 1890–1895. doi: 10.1001/archinte.165.16.1890

PART V

Special Topics in Women's Health

33

Sexuality

KAREN KOFFLER

If sexuality is one dimension of our ability to live passionately in the world, then in cutting off our sexual feelings, we diminish our overall power to feel, know, and value deeply.

—Judith Plaskow, *Standing Again at Sinai: Judaism from a Feminist Perspective*

CASE STUDY

JL is a 48-year-old perimenopausal woman who has three teenagers and a full-time job. In the course of our initial conversation, she shared her complete disinterest in sex, saying, "I would rather sleep than have sex." Her husband of 18 years was understanding, but his libido remained strong and his attraction to his wife unwavering. We addressed her digestive disorder, which was her primary complaint, through an elimination diet, probiotics, and digestive enzymes, and in follow-up, I asked whether she wanted to explore the possibility of improving her libido. JL was interested, so we explored other possibilities, beyond exhaustion, as to why her once satisfactory libido was absent. There were no significant traumas, no physical limitations or pain, no significant marital issues. Biochemically, her adrenal reserve was low as were her progesterone levels; her free testosterone levels were particularly low. We discussed the importance of self-care, especially given her multiple roles. She committed to her desire to carve out time for a weekly yoga session and evening walks after dinner. I recommended acupuncture treatments and placed her on supplements that supported her adrenals. Her diet required minor changes and included abstaining from coffee after noon and incorporating a protein-rich snack at about 4 pm. She began feeling better, noting more restorative sleep and better energy. We added gyrotonics weekly (a system of rhythmic circular movements that correlate with the breath), and she began to describe that she felt more connected to her body. Because of her nearly absent free testosterone, her risk for osteoporosis, and a demanding job that required strong mental acumen, I discussed adding low-dose topical testosterone. She was interested and began using it 6 days/week. After several weeks, I received an e-mail from JL describing her experience of having occasional spontaneous sexual thoughts come to her mind at unusual times. She even planned an intimate adventure with her husband, something she hadn't done since her children were born. From my perspective, every change she made toward greater self-care created the possibility for her to reconnect with herself and reclaim a lighter, more playful and sensual side that had gotten left behind in the demanding world she had unintentionally created.

One hundred years ago, a woman who loved sex was considered mentally disturbed. Today, a woman who does not love sex is thought to be suffering from dysfunction. This radical change in female sexuality illustrates the ephemeral nature of this particular topic in women's health. In reality, women may vacillate between extremes throughout their lives. It would seem, then, what is "normal" is for a woman to have a varying definition of her sexual experience from one moment to the next. Whether or not a woman is being fed and fueled by her sexuality is dependent on a whole host of factors, some of which may be obvious, such as pain. But "dysfunction" is a broad term used today, which may mean diminished sexual desire, arousal, or orgasm in addition to pain. These "dysfunctions" may cause some women great distress; others feel perfectly satisfied to never engage in sexual activity again. Understanding women's sexuality means understanding the individual in a nonjudgmental way because, clearly, what constitutes "normal" is variable.

Why should a practitioner get involved in such murky waters? A basic tenet of integrative medicine is an appreciation of the whole person and the various lifestyle behaviors that contribute to their wellness. Sexual satisfaction makes an important contribution to well-being (Dean et al., 2013), and dysfunction in this area of a woman's life is associated with decreased quality of life (Davison, Bell, LaChina, Holden, & Davis, 2009).

It turns out that sexual dysfunction in women is very common, up to 76% experience it at some point in their lives, and yet is rarely discussed in the primary care setting (Munarriz, Kim, Goldstein, & Traish, 2003). Understanding that sexuality contributes significantly to a woman's well-being in a variety of ways provides us an opportunity to help her realize a better state of health. It is also reasonable to suggest that improving a woman's sexual health may contribute to a more satisfying relationship with her partner.

But getting to the root of the issues of sexual dissatisfaction can be challenging given that anything from hormonal imbalance, to prior trauma or abuse, stress and exhaustion, to unresolved resentment can interfere with a woman's ability to express and derive pleasure from her sexuality. Furthermore, we have only a rudimentary understanding of female sexuality, and the scientific community is in its infancy in providing insight. Fortunately, there is a growing list of practitioners that are experienced in this arena: sex therapists, pelvic floor physical therapists, and tantra practitioners in addition to gynecologists and integrative practitioners.

In understanding female sexuality, it is valuable to gain perspective by looking into the past. Through archeological findings, we have learned that our ancestors experienced a variety of sexual activities including having more than one partner, same-sex partners, and even group sex. In many cultures over time, varied male desires, including homosexuality and multiple partners, were culturally acceptable. There is little evidence that these same practices were widely acceptable for women.

Marriage, as construed today in the West, with the expectation that all needs of an individual are met within the context of the relationship, is a very new concept. What used to require a village is now is the responsibility of one's partner. The concept of romantic love coupled with committed relationship is an early 20th-century creation. There are still cultures today that have not embraced the confining notion that security, sexuality, coparenting, and more are all to be manifested in a single union. Family therapist and author Esther Perel, in her book *Mating in Captivity* (2006), asks the important question, Does intimacy make for great sex?

Another example of our sexual evolution is what is considered physically attractive in a woman. Throughout time, a round, voluptuous female body was considered desirable, however, by today's standards these full-figured women would be considered overweight. Whole industries have developed in response to the demand to be thin and yet voluptuous. This cultural norm has had a dramatic effect on women at every age in our society. Tremendous resources go into creating the "perfect body," but far less attention is given to the psyche and spirit of sexuality. Furthermore, overweight women are often judged and judge themselves harshly and withdraw from their sexual selves, as if they are somehow less deserving of a satisfying experience.

Understanding the sexual response is a relatively new area of study. While it is true that one of the earliest works on sexual behavior was the Kama Sutra, composed between 400 BCE and 200 CE (in a culture where historically women have been repressed), it was the controversial figure Alfred Kinsey who in 1953 offered insight into the female sexual experience in the West. His work is considered to be a driving force behind the 1960s sexual revolution in the United States. Soon after, Masters and Johnson authored *The Human Sexual Response*, in which they proposed four stages of sexual response: excitement (arousal), plateau, orgasm, and resolution. This theory has recently been questioned by Gina Ogden, PhD, who created the ISIS survey (Integrating Spirituality in Sexuality), which revealed that not everyone moves through the sexual experience in the same way. Ogden's survey of 3,800 men and women revealed that intercourse and orgasm were not necessary for a satisfying sexual experience as Masters and Johnson had suggested (Ogden, 2008). In addition, Dr. Rosemary Basson has shown that rather than the linear progression of the sexual response described by Masters and Johnson, many women move in a more circular pattern (Basson, 2005).

What we can appreciate in this brief review of women's sexuality over time is that it is not stagnant, but is rather an experience shaped by culture, religious beliefs, economics, and individual experiences.

The Biology of Sexual Dysfunction

Libido thrives best in a healthy body, and sexuality is often the first domain of a woman's life that is impacted by a health issue. Pain causing physical distress is enormously distracting and is a common cause of sexual dissatisfaction.

Common issues, such as low back pain, may make intercourse difficult. Physical therapists have insight into appropriate positions that will prevent further aggravation of back pain. There are many kinds of props to help get around this issue and physical therapists can make appropriate recommendations.

Pain with intercourse due to menopausal changes in vaginal tissue can dampen sexual interest for both the woman and her partner, who does not want to cause harm. Enormous benefit can be derived from intravaginal estrogen (especially for mucosal atrophy) or topical dehydroepiandrosterone (DHEA) or testosterone applied in the area of the vulva (these tissues are denser in androgen receptors, whereas vaginal tissues have a greater density of estrogen receptors). Furthermore, intravaginal DHEA improved several parameters of vaginal health including pH and the architecture of both superficial and deeper cell layers and may be a superior choice to intravaginal estrogen when exposure to the latter is of concern (Basson, Brotto, Petkau, & Labrie, 2010). Women can work with a gynecologist or primary care doctor who is comfortable using these hormones.

Over-the-counter lubricants can also be effective and can be water-, oil-, or silicone-based. Of the three, silicone seems to be preferred by many women because it does not cause vaginal irritation with prolonged intercourse as much as oil- and water-based lubricants do. In addition, there is a higher incidence of candida overgrowth in women using oil-based products.

Vaginismus is painful spasmodic contractions of the vagina in response to physical contact or pressure; sexual intercourse can be a significant trigger. Manual therapy can be very effective in decreasing these muscle contractions. In addition to these conditions, there can be several other causes of pain with intercourse, and patients should be assessed by a pelvic floor physical therapist. Women who have received pelvic radiation for cancer treatment may suffer from vaginal stenosis. Dilators can be an effective treatment; it takes time and motivation to use them effectively. Diabetes can result in neuronal damage creating pain or dulled sensation and diminished lubrication. This is a difficult issue to overcome. Pelvic floor physical therapy is a possible treatment, but thus far has little outcomes data.

Hysterectomy can be associated with several adverse consequences from a sexual standpoint. Surgery can affect neuronal inputs to the vagina and clitoris dampening sensation. Scar tissue can cause adhesions that contribute to pain. Hormone levels in the premenopausal woman drop abruptly with surgical menopause. Even when the ovaries are spared, blood flow disturbances postoperatively often lead to a cessation of hormone production within 2 years. Oophorectomy can significantly lessen desire due to the cessation of testosterone production, which normally continues to be manufactured in the ovarian stroma even after menopause. Judicious replacement of hormones can make a significant impact on many of these issues. A variety of forms of hormones and routes of administration are readily available today (see the chapter "Menopause") and is best managed by a physician well versed in hormonal therapy. Generally speaking, topical administration is safest for both estrogen and testosterone, and screening tests before initiation of treatment as well as careful follow-up to avoid supraphysiologic dosing is essential. Contraindications may include women with hormonally driven cancers.

Being obese can both contribute to other health issues and erase a woman's sense of sexiness. In fact, 30% of women in heterosexual relationships say that their body image negatively impacts their sexual function. Obesity reduces circulating testosterone, which contributes to female libido, lessening desire from a biochemical standpoint. Weight loss can improve this. Other readily correctable metabolic issues that can sometimes contribute to diminished libido include hypothyroidism, high prolactin, low magnesium, B6, and B12 (Bartlik, 2010).

Sleep deprivation, a pervasive condition in today's society, throws the body into fight-or flight mode, which in my clinical experience robs a woman of her interest in sex. In order to maintain the higher levels of cortisol needed to respond to chronic stress, other steroidogenic hormones are reduced, which can inhibit libido. Exhaustion itself can abolish sexual interest. Treatment plans geared toward addressing sexuality should take stress-modifying strategies into account. I have found that doing so can significantly impact a woman's sense of sexuality.

Diseases like cancer can alter a woman's view of her body and virtually eliminate her sexual energy even in the setting of successful treatment. Many factors contribute to this, including chemically induced menopause, negative body image, and a lost sense of femininity. Research suggests that one important factor that assists women in recovering her sexuality in this context is the quality of her primary relationship (Gilbert, Ussher, & Perz, 2010).

In addition to the physical impact associated with hormonal changes, hormonal imbalance will often show up as a loss of libido. Simply stated, it is generally thought that estrogen and testosterone turn on a sex drive and progesterone turns it off. In the perimenopausal period, a time of significant hormonal fluxes, a common symptom women describe is a lack of sexual interest. It is likely there are several contributors to this, and lower estrogen levels and diminished testosterone may play a significant role. For many women, hormone replacement, particularly testosterone, can improve desire.

As mentioned above, several studies support the use of hormones alone (i.e., testosterone) or in combination with estradiol (Davis & Braunstein, 2012; Davis et al., 2008; Nappi et al., 2010). The combination of testosterone and the erectile dysfunction drug sildenafil has been shown to be a promising treatment for hypoactive sexual desire (Poels et al., 2013), but sildenifil alone has not been shown to be of benefit (Basson & Brotto, 2003). In addition, there are herbal products and supplements that can be of use. Maca (*Lepidium meyenii*) at 3.5 g/day has been shown to lower measures of sexual dysfunction (Brooks et al., 2006). Zestra, a novel blend of topical herbal extracts including borage oil, evening primrose oil, angelica root, and coleus has been shown to improve desire and arousal (Ferguson, Hosmane, & Heiman, 2010). Another commercially available product, Arginmax for women, has been shown to increase desire, satisfaction, and vaginal dryness in both pre- and post-menopausal women (Ito, Polan, Whipple, & Trant, 2006). This product contains arginine, damiana, ginseng, ginkgo, vitamins, and minerals, and its effect does not appear to be mediated via estrogen receptors, making it a reasonable consideration for women who have had or are at risk for estrogen-related cancers (Polan, Hochberg, Trant, & Wuh, 2004). There have been other studies examining ginkgo alone and yohimbine as potentially having an impact on sexual arousal, but the results have been mixed (Meston & Worcel, 2002).

A surprising paradox is that not all women with waning hormones experience a loss of libido. Some women find improved libido at menopause, perhaps from being free from the possibility of getting pregnant as well as having reduced caretaking responsibilities of children. In fact, in studies evaluating vaginal responsiveness to erotica, there was no difference seen between pre- and postmenopausal women (Van Lunsen & Laan, 2004). Another important point to remember is that women on birth control pills often experience a significant reduction in libido. A possible mechanism is that these exogenous hormones increase sex hormone–binding globulin, thereby lowering testosterone levels. The hormonal contribution has to be understood in relation to many other factors in a woman's life: her relationships, her life's circumstances, her emotional connectedness to herself, and so forth. The neurobiology of sexuality is complex, and there does not appear to be a direct corollary between hormonal levels and libido in all women.

Both anxiety and depression will typically create a lack of sexual desire. Dopamine and serotonin, neurotransmitters impacting mood, contribute to sexual interest. Oddly enough, medications used to treat depression frequently have a profound negative effect on libido and the ability to achieve orgasm. Recent data shows this medication side effect can be offset by acupuncture and exercise (Khamba et al., 2013, Lorenz & Meston, 2014). Bupropion has also been shown to improve sexual desire and lubrication when used adjunctively in the setting of SSRI use (Safarinejad, 2010). One study of premenopausal women with SSRI-related sexual dysfunction, especially difficulty with orgasm, found Viagra to be of help. A randomized double-blind, placebo-controlled trial found that 3 g/day of maca root significantly improved libido in men and women with SSRI-induced sexual dysfunction (Dording et al., 2008).

There are many other medications that can have a negative impact on sexual function. In addition to antidepressants, several classes of antihypertensives and medications used to treat breast cancer (selective estrogen-receptor modulators and aromatase inhibitors) are the most common. Ideally, the goal would be to minimize these medications by addressing lifestyle and using less problematic therapies (i.e., diet, exercise, supplements, therapy, and acupuncture, to name a few).

It is important to appreciate the role that aging and childbirth have on the pelvic floor including muscle tone, sensitivity, and its relationship with sexual satisfaction. Studies have shown that microtears following vaginal delivery weaken the levator musculature. In many countries, it is routine for postpartum women to undergo a series of pelvic floor physical therapy treatments to help them regain strength (Citak et al., 2010). These exercises include biofeedback to learn to control pelvic floor and core musculature, Kegel exercises, the use of weights to strengthen vaginal walls and pelvic floor, and pelvic tilts and bridges alone and with a Bosu ball.

A prevalent and challenging contributor to sexual dysfunction is previous sexual abuse. An estimated 20% of women have had a history of childhood sexual abuse, making this a common source of diminished sexual satisfaction in adulthood (www.victimsofcrime.org). Cognitive-behavioral therapy has been shown to be of benefit, as can mindfulness-based interventions that emphasize present-moment, nonjudgmental awareness (Brotto, Basson, & Luria, 2008). Both approaches are common tools used by sex therapists, and local providers can be found through the International Society for the Study of Women's Sexual Health.

Crisis of Desire

In my clinic, when I ask my patients about their libido, the most common response is, "What libido?" I find this is independent of age. On occasion, I have a female patient who has a strong libido, is confident in her body and sexual prowess and views sex as a practice that invigorates her life. Her sexual appetite may outpace her partner's. More often, though, women seem to be dissociated from their bodies and from their sexuality and so the ability to give and receive pleasure is compromised. These women may find themselves acquiescing to sex in order to keep their partners "happy." They may have given up on the concept that sexual activity can also make them happy.

This dissociation between mind and body has many root causes: cultural values that cast shame, early traumas, lack of trust, chronic multitasking that distracts, exhaustion, boredom, anger, and, very importantly, the devoted practice of parenting, to name a few. It is ironic that one of the biggest selling pharmaceuticals today is medication for men to optimize erectile function and yet these same men may have partners that are disinterested in sex!

My patients experiencing a lack of sexual interest are not unique. It is estimated that low libido affects up to 70% of women at various times and while they may be concerned about it, they are not likely to raise the issue themselves in a clinical setting. As I engage with my patient, I often find that her lack of libido is tied to a general lack of pleasure, joyfulness, and spontaneity in her life, the nectar that gives our lives dimension. She may have forgotten to engage in activities that are not immediately purposeful or practical. Pleasure has seemingly become frivolous. She may well have disconnected from the sensations of her body. But sexual energy is a primary driving force in our lives. It is intertwined with self-esteem, power, optimism, sensuality, and playfulness. A lack of libido can undermine her principle relationship with her partner. Understanding a woman's desire and what drives it is a challenge. So as clinicians, can we inspire desire?

The sex therapist, Esther Perel, in her book *Mating in Captivity* (2006), describes the fate of many married couples today: that of "dwindling desire and a long list of sexual alibis" resulting in the death of Eros. Part of the challenge with desire, according to Perel, is that it does not necessarily mesh well with love, especially committed love that creates a sense of security, and especially over the long haul. In fact, parenthood and the chronic selflessness that comes with it, in her clinical experience as well as mine, creates a withdrawal from eroticism for individuals, and often it is the woman who is affected more. Adventure and excitement become rare in the setting of running a household, and desire may become a distant memory. Lust in the setting of predictability is a hard sell.

Many of us want the security, stability, and reliability that a committed relationship brings. And at the same time, we have a yearning for novelty, risk, and the unknown. But all is not lost. Perel suggests that we have the opportunity to create desire even in the midst of familiarity. Instead of the illusion of certainty in which we think we know our partner (let alone ourselves), we can regain our curiosity by opening to the mystery of our partners and the separateness of them, because it is that tension that ignites passion. This takes a willingness to "see with new eyes" the aspects of our partners we really do not know. That sense of discovering additional dimensions of our partners (and ourselves) can be intoxicating. Of course, "getting there" is the bridge many people have the toughest time crossing. It begins with a sincere and persistent willingness to experience the relationship differently. Tapping into what may have become a dormant imagination is another key ingredient. These are not quick fixes, but according to Perel, they are effective. There are many resources today to help women and couples redefine this area of their lives (see references).

One popular strategy to address female sexuality is to remake ourselves physically. In our culture, sexiness is a hot medical commodity. We have available all kinds of means to *appear* sexier: breast augmentation, buttocks augmentation, lip augmentation and the ability to shave off fat to create specific contours. As women, we seem to be willing to undergo surgical procedures and their attendant risks in order to convey something different. And yet, in my practice, these efforts do not necessarily seem to be paying off. In addition to looking sexy, women want to feel sexier. They want to experience *desire*.

"Oh darling! The only good sex is illicit sex!"

(Response of my 72-year-old patient when I asked her about sexual activity with her husband of 43 years. Her answer was a resounding no.)

But the question of what creates desire for women looms. It is a question being studied by a small group of scientists with some fascinating findings worth reviewing.

An article in *Psychology Today* offers us new insight (Castleman, 2009). Societal lore is that desire precedes arousal. This is true for men who experience sexual desire like a hunger or thirst. They become aroused when they feel desire. However, this is not necessarily the path for women, according to University of British Columbia psychiatrist Rosemary Basson. She discovered, through interviews with hundreds of women, that contrary to the conventional model, for many women, desire is not the *cause* of lovemaking, but rather, it is the *result*. "Women," Basson explains, "often begin sexual experiences feeling sexually neutral." But as things heat up, so do they, and they eventually experience desire (Castleman, 2009). Understanding this can help us with strategies to inspire women. I often hear my patients' comment that once they "get going" they are able to enjoy their sexual experience. Perhaps if couples understood this as normal, they would be more likely to engage, rather than roll over and resist their partner.

Arousal in men is accompanied by an obvious event: an erection. Chivers and colleagues have shown that women's sexual arousal is tied to an emotional state, not a physical one. In fact, women may show signs of physical arousal (engorgement of vulva and vaginal tissues) in response to stimuli, but not be aware of it. In other words, a woman may not perceive arousal despite the fact that her genitals are receptive to sexual activity (Chivers, Seto, Lalumière, Laan, & Grimbos, 2010).

This discrepancy has been explored further. Meredith Chivers's work using a plethysmograph placed within the walls of the vagina to record engorgement, was coupled with her subjects simultaneously reporting their *feelings* of arousal all while watching various kinds of erotica (Chivers et al., 2010). As with Meston, the two recordings hardly matched: that is, objective measurements of arousal (blood flow within the vagina) and subjective scores of arousal were very likely to be different, meaning that a woman may become aroused without realizing it. This disconnection between a physical sense and a felt sense for women is something we do not see in men.

Chivers's work has elucidated something else. In her studies, which included watching 90-second segments of a variety of sexual encounters: women with men, women with women, men with men, and sexual encounters between Bonobo apes (Bonobos are a matriarchal society, and they use sexual activity freely including to dissipate stress within a tribe and when they encounter differing tribes) some surprising discoveries were made. It turns out that women are far more likely to respond to a broad variety of sexual stimuli than men, either heterosexual or homosexual. Every sexual scenario brought about a physical response in women (with the exception of viewing a flaccid penis) including witnessing the sexual activity of Bonobo apes. However, men responded consistently to the sexual activity that corresponded with their sexual orientation only, and not at all to apes. What we can learn from this is that women's sexual responsiveness is broader than they, or society perceives, especially when compared with men; yet women are often emotionally cut off from that physical response. One explanation for this difference is in the structures that get aroused: penises extend and men are acutely aware of that change. In women, there is no overt physical difference.

Teri Fisher's group at Ohio State University designed a brilliant study to investigate another aspect of female sexuality (Alexander & Fisher, 2003). She had co-ed college students answer questionnaires inquiring about sexual practices, masturbation, and porn use. Prior to answering the questions, she informed the participants that they were going to (1) hand their completed survey to a fellow student, (2) have their responses kept anonymous, or (3) be hooked up to a polygraph machine while filling out the questionnaire.

The men involved in the study had the same replies regardless of how it was reviewed; their answers were not influenced by who would see them. The women, on the other hand, tailored their responses depending on the viewer. The women who handed their responses to another student never checked anything X-rated. If they were in the group promised to have answers kept anonymous, they answered a significantly greater number of questions positively. And if they thought they were being recorded by a polygraph, they answered with the greatest number of affirmatives. In fact, with similar frequency and often more than the men. Dr. Fisher interpreted this study to show that women feel judged about their sexual interests in a way that men do not. Without coercion, they distance themselves from their sexual interests in a way that men do not.

This does not hold true for all women or even younger generations of women. According to Nielsen, the consumer tracking company, one in three online porn viewers are female and 13 million American women are logging on to porn sites at least once a month. Clearly, there is an anonymity associated with logging on and viewing. But the important point is that this goes squarely against societal assumptions that female sexuality thrives in the setting of an emotional connection. Today, there is a phenomenon of younger women "hooking up" for casual sex with no implicit interest in commitment. Indeed, pop fiction/erotica like *50 Shades of Gray* and television shows like *Girls* are highlighting a diverse sexual appetite in women that has not been entertained publicly before.

This behavior has also been examined in the lab. In a study involving listening to audiotapes of sexual encounters, women physically responded more to scenarios involving strangers (with both men and women) than with people they knew. As previously described, there was a disconnection in the subjects between their physical response of arousal and their awareness of what *seemed* arousing (Chivers & Timmers, 2012).

It is becoming clear that women respond to erotic rawness, yet consciously acknowledging this arousal is not permissible. Why is this? Is it physical? Cultural? And are we at the dawn of seeing women free themselves of those limitations? And will this awareness impact societal expectations of women?

What We Can Do as Clinicians

Female sexuality is an ever-changing alchemy of internal and external stimuli; of cultural norms and personal experience; of modern-day demands and the goal of personal fulfillment; and of the time of life and conditions a woman finds herself in. For many women, duty and obligation seek to find a balance with passion and spontaneity. Emerging literature and social media confirm that women often have robust fantasy lives when they allow it to register. Manifesting sexual satisfaction may well contribute to her overall health.

As clinicians, our role is to facilitate well-being at every level of a woman's life. Sexual expression is an important part of most women's lives. We can help by considering these approaches:

1. Become comfortable inquiring about sexual health. Rarely does a woman have a chance to discuss this domain of her life with a

professional. I begin simply by asking, "How is your libido? Are you satisfied with the sexual aspect of your life?" Most patients appreciate the inquiry. Be sure to emphasize safety in appropriate patients. Allow space to have the patient reflect on their satisfaction with their partner.

2. Identify the general root of a dysfunction. If the matter can be traced to psychological distress, referring to a sex therapist can begin the process of reframing the woman's experience. If the matter seems to be more physical, an integrative gynecologist and pelvic floor physical therapist can be of great benefit. Bear in mind the enormous impact that stress-modifying strategies have on well being including sexual well-being. A basic workup once dysfunction is identified includes:

   • Inquiry into self-care practices, stress-hardiness, and sleep. This can give an indication as to the degree of sympathetic overdrive a woman may be experiencing, and mind–body practices can be immediately instituted. In particular, mindfulness meditation has been studied in this setting and found to be of great benefit (Brotto, 2014).

   • Physical exam with an emphasis on signs of inflammation, palpation of the thyroid gland, and a pelvic exam.

   • Hormone levels including 4 point salivary cortisol, DHEAs to help identify the role of stress, free and total testosterone, midcycle (if menstruating) estradiol and progesterone, full thyroid panel, evaluation for anemia and nutritional deficiencies (B12 and RBC magnesium in particular). Address any imbalances.

   • Referral to integrative providers who can reacquaint a woman with the sensual nature of her body. I have found the sweeping circular movement of gyrotonics to be of great benefit, as well as more subtle energy practices such as acupuncture and healing energy.

3. Encourage the concept of sexuality as an open-ended personal project. Frame the conversation such that regardless of past experience, a different and more satisfying sex life is possible. Exploration beyond an individual woman's conventions may bring added depth to her sexual life.

REFERENCES

Adeniyi, A. F., Adeleye, J. O., & Adeniyi, C. Y. (2010). Diabetes, sexual dysfunction and therapeutic exercise: A 20 year review. *Curr Diabetes Rev, 6*, 201–206.

Alexander, M. G., & Fisher, T. D. (2003). Truth and consequences: Using the bogus pipeline to examine sex differences in self-reported sexuality, *J Sex Res, 40*, 27–35.

Bartlik, B. (2010). Ask the expert: Sexual dysfunction medication, hormones, and nutrition. *Focus, 8,* 547–549.

Basson, R. (2005). Women's sexual dysfunction: Revised and expanded definitions *CMAJ, 172,* 1327–1333.

Basson, R. (2010). Testosterone therapy for reduced libido in women. *Ther Adv Endocrinol Metab, 1,* 155–164.

Basson, R., & Brotto, L. A. (2003). Sexual psychophysiology and effects of sildenafil citrate in oestrogenised women with acquired genital arousal disorder and impaired orgasm: A randomized control trial. *BJOG, 110,* 1014–1024.

Basson, R., Brotto, L. A, Petkau, A. J., & Labrie, F. (2010). Role of androgens in women's sexual dysfunction. *Menopause, 17,* 962–971.

Bergner, D. (2013). *What do women want?* New York, NY: HarperCollins.

Bloemers, J., van Rooij, K., Poels, S., et al. (2013). Toward personalized sexual medicine: Part 1. Integrating the "dual control model" into differential drug treatments for hypoactive sexual desire disorder and female sexual arousal disorder. *J Sex Med, 10,* 791–809.

Brooks, N. A., Wilcox, G., Walker, K. Z., Ashton, J. F., Cox, M. B., & Stojanovska L. (2008). Beneficial effects of *Lepedium meyenii* (Maca) on psychological symptoms and measures of sexual dysfunction in postmenopausal women are not related to estrogen or androgen content. *Menopause, 15,* 1157–1162.

Brotto, L. A., & Basson R. (2014). Group mindfulness-based therapy significantly improves sexual desire in women. *Behav Res Ther, 57,* 43–54.

Brotto, L. A., Basson, R., & Luria, M. (2008). A mindfulness-based group psychoeducational intervention targeting sexual arousal disorder in women. *J Sex Med, 5,* 1646–1659.

Castleman, M. (2009). Desire in women: Does it lead to sex? Or result from it? *Psychology Today,* July 15.

Cattanach, J. (1985). Oestrogen deficiency after tubal ligation. *Lancet, 1,* 847–849.

Chivers, M. L., Seto, M. C., Lalumière, M. L., Laan, E., & Grimbos, T. (2010). Agreement of self-reported and genital measures of sexual arousal in men and women: A meta-analysis. *Arch Sex Behav, 39,* 5–56.

Chivers, M. L., & Timmers, A. D. (2012). The effects of gender and relationship context clues in audio narratives in heterosexual women's and men's genital and subjective sexual response. *Archives of Sexual Behavior, 41,* 185–197.

Citak, N., Cam, C., Arslan, H., Karateke, A., Tug, N., Ayaz, R., & Celik, C. (2010). Postpartum sexual function of women and the effects of early pelvic floor muscle exercises. *Acta Obstet Gynecol Scand, 89,* 817–822.

Davis, S. R., & Braunstein, G. D. (2012). Efficacy and safety of testosterone in the management of hypoactive sexual desire disorder in postmenopausal women. *J Sex Med, 9,* 1134–1148.

Davis, S. R., Moreau, M., Kroll, R., et al.; APHRODITE Study Team. (2008). Testosterone for low libido in postmenopausal women not taking estrogen. *N Engl J Med, 359,* 2005–2017.

Davison, S. L., Bell, R. J., LaChina, M., Holden, S. L., & Davis, S. R. (2009). The relationship between self-reported sexual satisfaction and general well-being in women. *J Sex Med, 6,* 2690–2697.

Dean, A., Shechter, A., Vertkin, A., Weiss, P., Yaman, O., Hodik, M., & Ginovker, A. (2013). Sexual Health and Overall Wellness (SHOW) survey in men and women in selected European and Middle Eastern countries. *Int Med Res*, *14*, 482–492.

Dording, C. M., et al. (2008). A double-blind, randomized, pilot dose-finding study of maca root (*L. meyenii*) for the management of SSRI-induced sexual dysfunction. *CNS Neurosci Ther*, *14*, 182–191.

Ferguson, D., Hosmane, B., & Heiman, J. (2010). Randomized, placebo-controlled double-blind, parallel design trial of the efficacy and safety of Zestra in women with mixed desire/interest/arousal/orgasm disorders. *J of Sex and Marital Therapy*, *36*, 66–86.

Field, N., Mercer, C. H., Sonnenberg, P., et al. (2013). Associations between health and sexual lifestyles in Britain: Findings from the third National Survey of Sexual Attitudes and Lifestyles. *Lancet*, *382*, 1830–1844.

Gilbert, E., Ussher, J. M., & Perz, J. (2010). Sexuality after breast cancer: A review. *Maturitas*, *66*, 397–407.

Goldstein, A., & Brandon, M. (2004). *Reclaiming desire*. New York, NY: Rodale Press.

Hartmann, U., Philippsohn, S., Heiser, K., & Rüffer-Hesse C. (2004). Low sexual desire in midlife and older women: Personality factors, psychosocial development, present sexuality *J Menopause*, *11*(6 Pt 2), 726–740.

Holstein, L. L., & Taylor, D. J. (2001). *How to have magnificent sex: The dimensions of vital sexual connection*. New York, NY: Harmony Books.

Ito, T. Y., Polan, M. L., Whipple, B., & Trant, A. S. (2006). The enhancement of female sexual function with ArginMax, a nutritional supplement, among women differing in menopausal status. *J Sex and Marital Therapy*, *32*, 369–378.

Kennedy, S. H., Eisfeld, B. S., Dickens, S. E., Bacchiochi, J. R., & Bagby, R. M. (2000). Antidepressant-induced sexual dysfunction during treatment with moclobemide, paroxetine, sertraline, and venlafaxine. *J Clin Psychiatry*, *61*, 276–281.

Khamba, B., Aucoin, M., Lytle, M., et al. (2013). Efficacy of acupuncture treatment of sexual dysfunction secondary to antidepressants. *J Altern Complement Med*, *19*, 862–869.

Landa, J, & Hopkins, V. (2012). *The sex drive solution for women*. Ocala, FL: Atlantic.

Lorenz, T. A., & Meston, C. M. (2014). Exercise improves sexual function in women taking antidepressants: Results from a randomized crossover trial. *Depress Anxiety*, *31*, 188–195.

Martinez, C. S., Ferreira, F. V., Castro, A. A., & Gomide, L. B. (2014). Women with greater pelvic floor muscle strength have better sexual function. *Acta Obstet Gynecol Scand*, *93*, 497–502.

Meston, C. M., & Worcel, M. (2002). The effects of yohimbine plus L-arginine glutamate on sexual arousal in postmenopausal women with sexual arousal disorder. *Arch Sex Behav*, *31*, 323–332.

Moorman, P. G., Myers, E. R., Schildkraut, J. M., Iversen, E. S., Wang, F., & Warren, N. (2011). Effect of hysterectomy with ovarian preservation on ovarian function. *Obstet Gynecol*, *118*, 1271–1279.

Munarriz, R., Kim, N., Goldstein, I., & Traish, A. (2003). *Biology of female sexual function*. http://www.bumc.bu.edu/sexualmedicine/physicianinformation/biology-of-female-sexual-function

Nappi, R. E., Albani, F., Santamaria, V., et al. (2010). Menopause and sexual desire: The role of testosterone. *Menopause Int, 16*, 162–168.

North American Menopause Society. (2013). Position Statement: Management of symptomatic vulvovaginal atrophy: 2013 position. *Menopause, 20*, 888–902.

Nurnberg, H. G., Hensley, P. L., Heiman, J. R., Croft, H. A., Debattista, C., & Paine, S. (2008). Sildenafil treatment of women with antidepressant-associated sexual dysfunction. *JAMA, 300*, 395–404.

Ogden, G. (2008). *The return of desire: A guide to rediscovering your sexual passion.* Boston, MA: Shambala.

Perel, E. (2006). *Mating in captivity.* New York, NY: HarperCollins.

Poels, S., Bloemers, J., van Rooij, K., et al. (2013). Toward personalized sexual medicine: Part 2. Testosterone combined with a PDE5 inhibitor increases sexual satisfaction in women with HSDD and FSAD, and a low sensitive system for sexual cues. *J Sex Med, 10*, 810–823.

Polan, M. L., Hochberg, R. B., Trant, A. S., & Wuh, H. C. (2004). Estrogen bioassay of ginseng extract and ArginMax, a nutritional supplement for the enhancement of female sexual function. *J Women's Health, 13*, 427–430.

Rosen, R. C., Connor, M. K., Miyasato, G., et al. (2012). Sexual desire problems in women seeking healthcare: A novel study design for ascertaining prevalence of hypoactive sexual desire disorder in clinic-based samples of U.S. women. *J Womens Health (Larchmt), 21*, 505–515.

Safarinejad, M. R. (2011). Reversal of SSRI-induced female sexual dysfunction by adjunctive buproprion in menstruating women: A double-blind, placebo-controlled and randomized study. *J Psychopharmacol, 25*, 370–378.

Serati, M., Braga, A., di Dedda, M. C., et al. (2014). Benefit of pelvic floor muscle therapy in improving sexual function in women with stress urinary incontinence: A pretest-posttest intervention study. *J Sex Marital Ther.*

Stephenson, K. R., & Meston CM. (2013). The conditional importance of sex: Exploring the association between sexual well-being and life satisfaction. *J Sex Marital Ther.* [Epub ahead of print, October 10]

Suschinsky, K. D., Lalumière, M. L., & Chivers, M. L. (2009). Sex differences in patterns of genital sexual arousal: Measurement artifacts or true phenomena? *Arch Sex Behav, 38*, 559–573.

Van Lunsen, R. H., & Laan, E. (2004). Genital vascular responsiveness and sexual feelings in midlife women: Psychophysiologic, brain, and genital imaging studies. *Menopause, 11*(6 Pt 2), 741–748.

34

Lesbian, Bisexual, and Transgender Health

MARNIE LAMM AND BARBARA ECKSTEIN

CASE STUDY

Elaine was a 23-year-old pregnant woman who came into our clinic, as a new patient, accompanied by her friend. Elaine had been up all night nauseated and vomiting; she was unable to get a timely appointment with her regular provider. During the visit, Elaine and her friend revealed that they were partners, and the three of us discussed a treatment and follow-up plan. After the visit, a nurse came to tell me that Elaine's friend had requested a work excuse for her time in the clinic that morning. The nurse, who later realized she might have made a mistake, told the woman that only patients and their direct family members were able to get work excuses.

Introduction

Lesbian and bisexual women represent a diverse group of individuals of all ages, ethnicities, religions, and cultural and socioeconomic backgrounds whose lifestyles, identities, mannerisms, appearance, family structures, health needs, sexual practices, and identities may be fluid over time. While many lesbians identify a primary attraction to women from childhood, the adoption of the identity as a lesbian may not come until later in life, sometimes not until after marriage and childbearing. Some women may have intimate physical relationships with other women yet not identify as lesbian or bisexual (Kerker, Mostashari, & Thorpe, 2006). Healthcare considerations are, in many ways, the same for lesbians and bisexuals as for they are heterosexual women, yet there are important differences to be aware of in order to provide appropriate and sensitive care.

Approximately 1%–4% of women in the United States identify as lesbian or bisexual (Chandra, Mosher, Copen, & Sionean, 2011). Population data on lesbian and bisexual health is limited due to an omission of sexual orientation in most state and federal health surveillance programs. In 2011, the Institute of Medicine (IOM) recommended inclusion of sexual orientation in the electronic health record and Health and Human Services announced that by 2013 it would begin collecting data on sexual orientation in its nationwide population health surveys. Currently available data comes from states that are more accepting of sexual minorities and where greater support services are already in place (Box 34.1).

Barriers to Healthcare

Lesbian and bisexual women have lower rates of preventative care than their heterosexual counterparts due to a lack of routine care (Aaron et al., 2001; Austin & Irwin, 2013; Diamant, 2001; Harrison & Silenzio, 1996; Hutchinson, Thompson, & Cedarbaum, 2006; McNair et al., 2011; Valanis et al., 2000) and lack of provider knowledge regarding appropriate screening (American College of Obstetricians and Gynecologists [ACOG], 2012; Bonvincini & Perlin, 2003; Marques, 2014; White & Dull, 1998). Lesbian and bisexual women interface less with the healthcare system for numerous reasons, including fear of discrimination, real (lack of a need for birth control or prenatal care) versus perceived (belief of low or no risk of sexually transmitted infections) need for routine health services, and lack of insurance coverage (in part due to insurance plans not covering same-sex partners; Blosnich & Silenzio, 2013). The Affordable Care Act, signed into law in March 2010, prohibits insurance companies from discriminating against people based on sexual orientation and gender identity, allowing for coverage of same-sex spouses and their children. Self-esteem, social support, community support, and degree of being "out" are all associated with a greater likelihood of using healthcare services (Austin, 2013).

Issues Relating to Disclosure of Sexual Orientation and Sexual Practices

A large proportion of lesbians do not to disclose their orientation to their healthcare providers (Austin & Irwin, 2013; Barbara, Quant, & Anderson,

Box 34.1 Terminology

Ally—Someone who has a concern for the well-being of lesbian, gay, bisexual, trans, and intersex people and a belief that heterosexism, homophobia, biphobia, and transphobia are social justice issues.

Bisexual: A person who is emotionally, physically, and/or sexually attracted to more than one gender. Also called "bi."

Disorders of sex development (DSD)—also referred to as **intersex**, DSD refers to a variety of congenital conditions in which chromosomal, gonadal, or anatomic sex development is not typically male or female.

Gender identity—an individual's sense of their gender; this may be male, female, or other.

Gender dysphoria—official DSM-5 diagnosis for the condition in which someone's gender identity does not match their biological sex and in which this mismatch causes significant personal distress or impairment in social, occupational, or other areas of functioning. This term replaces "Gender Identity Disorder" in DSM-IV. (APA gender dysphoria fact sheet)

Female-to-male (FtM)—adjective used to describe an individual whose biological sex at birth was female and who is transitioning/has transitioned to living as a man. An FtM individual is sometimes also referred to as a **transman.**

LGBTQA—Lesbian, Gay, Bisexual, Transgender, and Queer or Questioning, Ally

Lesbian—A lesbian is a woman whose sexual and affectional preferences are directed toward other women. Behavior may range from exclusively homosexual, to bisexual, to situationally heterosexual, prompted by economic status, cultural factors, or sexual desire. Not all women who partner with women consider themselves lesbian. (Rankow, 1995)

Male-to-female (MtF)—adjective used to describe an individual whose biological sex at birth was male and who is transitioning/has transitioned to living as a woman. An MtF individual is sometimes also referred to as a **transwoman.**

Transgender—umbrella term/adjective used to describe a community of individuals whose gender identities vary to differing degrees from their biological sex.

Transsexual—term, used mostly in medical setting, to describe someone who has transitioned from their biological gender to their self-identified gender.

Queer—a term used by some LGBT people to describe themselves. This has traditionally been a pejorative term and should not be used to describe someone unless they themselves use the term.

2001), and bisexual women are even less likely to do so (McNair et al., 2013). Women often fear that the importance of disclosure will not be fully appreciated and that doing so may lead to discrimination, breaches of confidentiality, judgment, and even compromised care. Women may choose not to discuss their sexual orientation because they want to get to know their physician better or they are waiting to be asked. In one study, both women and their physicians believed that it was easier if the other initiated the process, and both sides felt that sexual orientation was not relevant to the clinical context (McNair et al., 2012). Women who are able to disclose their orientation report better health-care experiences (Mosach, Brouwer, & Petroll, 2013) and receive appropriate screening tests more often than those who do not (Kerker et al., 2006; Rankow & Tessaro, 1998). Barriers that healthcare providers cite to discussing sexual orientation and practices include lack of knowledge of relevant issues, fear of offending heterosexual patients, lack of time, assuming patients do not want to disclose, and not wanting to be intrusive (McNair et al., 2012; Box 34.2).

Health Maintenance and Screening

Lesbian and bisexual women should receive the same routine screening and preventative services that heterosexual women receive based on individual and family history plus risk factor assessment. Since routine screening is often tied to reproductive health services that lesbian and bisexual women may be less likely to engage in, it is important to consider any office visit an opportunity to review and create a healthcare maintenance plan.

Cancer

The number of lesbians with breast, cervical, endometrial, and other cancers is unknown at this time, because major surveys such as the National Cancer Institute (NCI) Surveillance, Epidemiology, and End Results (SEER) and state cancer registries do not currently collect information regarding sexual orientation. Studies have suggested that lesbians have greater risk factors for breast and endometrial cancer such as nulliparity, higher body mass index (BMI), and higher rates of alcohol use (Case et al., 2004; Davis et al., 2000; Zaritsky & Dibble, 2010). Although small early studies suggested that lesbian and bisexual women have a two to three times greater risk of breast cancer, later studies have shown that the disparity may not be as great (Dibble, Roberts, & Nussey, 2004). Ecological studies have shown that in geographic areas with greater female sexual minority density, there is a greater incidence of lung and breast cancer after controlling for race/ethnicity and poverty (Boehmer, Miao, Maxwell, & Ozonoff, 2014). Population-level data is needed to gain a more accurate picture of cancer incidence and prevalence in general.

There is an erroneous assumption among some women and their providers that women who have sex exclusively with women do not need Pap smears.

Box 34.2 Questions for Providers

How effectively do you identify and cultivate community resources for your LGBTQ patients?

Consider developing a resource list for appropriate referrals for special LGBT health concerns.

Is the environment welcoming of LGBTQ patients and their families?

Consider having visual cues in the waiting room such as rainbow colored items, Safe Zone (see resources section) signs and magazines geared to LGBTQ audiences to acknowledge you are inclusive.

Consider having unisex restrooms, realizing that sex-segregated services may cause dilemmas for some patients.

Are health forms appropriate for LGBTQ patients?

Consider having more inclusive options on intake forms such as single, married to man/woman, living with partner, and so forth. For gender, in addition to M and F, add a third category for other with space for explanation.

Questions regarding families should provide alternatives for children with more than two parents.

How are the privacy rights of LGBTQ patients protected?

Consider having a written policy stating: "We do not discriminate on the basis of age, race, sex, sexual orientation, gender identity, religion, language, or disability" posted in a conspicuous place and appropriately conveyed to persons with disabilities and to those for whom English is not their primary language.

Consider including a section on all forms explaining how confidentiality will be protected. Offer the patient the right to refuse to answer a question on the form knowing that further discussion will be possible during the visit.

Do LGBTQ patient's significant others participate in care decisions?

Be sure to acknowledge and include any companion that a person brings to a visit as appropriate.

Do LGBTQ patients feel that they are understood and are getting appropriate care?

Consider explaining why you are asking about personal details: "It is helpful for me to understand patient's lifestyle and habits so I can fully assess your health needs and make appropriate recommendations."

Ask about current and past sexual practices in an open, nonjudgmental way: "Over your lifetime, have your partners been men, women or both?" "Do you follow safe sex practices or have any questions regarding safe sex practices?" "I understand that your primary sexual relations are with women, do you feel you have any need for contraception?"

Don't be afraid to acknowledge your own lack of understanding: "I am not sure what you mean by that term, can you help me understand?"

Is there a way to improve and monitor quality of services for LGBTQ patients?

Consider providing an evaluation form to assess patient satisfaction and to solicit feedback.

Consider providing regular training to all staff members regarding diversity, harassment, antidiscrimination resources, and LGBTQ related issues.

A population-based study of over 18,000 women ages 18 to64 in New York City showed that, compared with heterosexual women, lesbians and bisexual women were 10 times more likely not to have received appropriate Pap testing and four times more likely not to have received mammograms, regardless of access to healthcare, sexual identity, and other confounding factors (Kerker et al., 2006). Another study showed that lesbian and bisexual women were 3 times less likely than heterosexual women to have had appropriate Pap testing and also that subsets of lesbian and bisexual women have increased risk factors for cervical dysplasia including number of male partners, unprotected intercourse, younger age at first coitus, and higher HIV seroprevalence (Diamant, Schuster, McGuigan, & Lever, 1999). Approximately 80% of women who identify as lesbian report having had sex with men (Koh et al., 2005; Marazzo et al., 2001; Rankow & Tessaro, 1998). Studies have shown that human papillomavirus (HPV) infections do occur in women who report sex only with other women (Marazzo et al., 1998).

Sexually Transmitted Infections

Women who identify as lesbian or bisexual should be asked about all sexual contacts, because infection risk is tied to actual behavior and not sexual orientation. Providers should offer sexually transmitted infection (STI) screening to all women, regardless of hetero- or homosexual behaviors, including HIV, syphilis, and chlamydia/gonorrhea screening (Marazzo, 2004; Workowski & Berman, 2010).

A majority of lesbian and bisexual women who have had sex with men report engaging in vaginal intercourse without condom use (Diamante, Schuster, & Lever, 1999; Marrazzo et al., 2001), putting them at equal risk for STIs as heterosexual women who have unprotected intercourse. In certain subpopulations, particularly adolescent and bisexual women, risk behaviors associated with STIs and HIV transmission are actually increased (Eisenberg, 2001; Koh et al., 2005; Matthews, Brandenburg, Johnson, & Hughes, 2004). There have been reports of sexual transmission of bacterial vaginosis (Berger et al., 1995), trichomoniasis (Kellock & O'Mahony, 1996), syphilis (Campos-Outcalt & Hurwitz, 2002), human papilloma virus (Marrazzo, et al., 1998) and genotype-concordant HIV between women (Kwakwa & Ghobiral, 2003). Many lesbians believe that they cannot contract HIV by having sex with women, even if their partners engage in high-risk behaviors such as IV drug use (Stevens & Hall, 2001). Another potential route of HIV transmission is through donor sperm if women are using samples other than those obtained from regulated sperm banks. Lesbian and bisexual women should be counseled that while lower, there is still a significant risk of STI transmission during female homosexual contact and that safe sex practices are an important consideration.

Psychosocial Issues

ASSAULT AND INTIMATE PARTNER VIOLENCE

Screening for violence and domestic abuse should be as routinely done with lesbian and bisexual women as it is with heterosexual women. A study of university students showed lesbians are 1.6 and bisexual women are 3.1 times more likely to be sexually assaulted than heterosexual women (Martin, Fisher, Warner, Krebs, & Linquist, 2011). Approximately 40% lesbian and bisexual women reported a lifetime history of sexual assault, as compared with 11%–17% of heterosexual women (Rothman, Exner, & Baughman, 2011). In the National Intimate Partner and Sexual Violence Survey, 61.1% of bisexual women, 42.8% of lesbians, and 35% of heterosexual women reported being victims of rape, physical violence, or stalking by an intimate partner (National Institute of Intimate Partner Violence, 2010). The process of disclosing intimate partner violence can be doubly difficult for a woman who has yet to disclose her sexual orientation to her provider. Both the process of concealing a lesbian identity or revealing it can cause significant stress and withdrawal from traditional support systems in the home, school, and community. Discussion of an individual's support system can provide a fuller picture of ability to deal with stress, victimization, and relationship difficulties.

CHILDREN AND FAMILY

While many lesbian and bisexual women are raising families, they often lack the social and legal support structures available to heterosexual women. Over 27% of female couples are raising children (Krivikas & Lofquist, 2011), and this number is growing, particularly as more same-sex couples are exploring different fertility options. Additionally, same-sex couples are four times more likely to be raising adopted children and six times more likely to be raising foster children than heterosexual couples (Gates, 2013). In general, same-sex married or domestic partners do not have legal protections such as joint adoption rights, family medical leave benefits, and shared social security, insurance, and retirement benefits. Hospital visitation rights for same-sex partners were not guaranteed until 2011, when the revised standards of the Joint Commission specified a hospitalized patient's right to designate the support person of their choice regardless of whether that person is a family member, spouse, or same-sex domestic partner.

ADOLESCENT ISSUES

The consensus from both the American Academy of Pediatrics and the Society for Adolescent Health and Medicine is that lesbian, gay, bisexual, transgender, and queer (LGBTQ) youth are generally healthy, well-adjusted, resilient teenagers and young adults who go on to become healthy adults. Providers are encouraged to be a resource for sexual minority youth and their families, providing information in the context that being LGBTQ is "normal, just different."

High-risk behavior and higher rates of depression and suicide in this group reflects reactions to nonacceptance and lack of family, community, and societal acceptance (Kann et al., 2011). Gay and lesbian youths are two to three times more likely to attempt suicide than their heterosexual counterparts and have higher rates of tobacco, alcohol, and illegal drug use (King et al., 2008). Lesbian- and bisexual-identified youth are more likely to report intercourse before the age of 13, to report intercourse with multiple partners, and to be less likely to use contraceptives than their exclusively heterosexual peers (Goodenow, Sazalacha, Robin, & Westheimer, 2008; Herrick, Matthews, & Garofalo, 2010).

The Society for Adolescent Health and Medicine recommends that providers ask youth how they self-identify and be guided by the individual's language and self-concept keeping in mind that many youths have yet to "come out" to their family and friends and that disclosure of their sexual orientation may have serious repercussions. The American Academy of Pediatrics recommends that sexually active adolescents who have not engaged in high-risk sex be tested for STIs once yearly and that high-risk individuals with multiple or anonymous partners, having unprotected intercourse or with substance abuse history, be tested at shorter intervals (American Academy of Pediatrics, Committee on Adolescence, 2013). Additional guidelines include offering HPV vaccine at ages 11–12 and catch-up through age 26, routine cervical cancer screening, and discussion of condoms for sex toys, use of dental dams, and routine and emergency birth control methods.

AGING

Older lesbian and bisexual women may be a particularly vulnerable and isolated population. Although there has been extensive research regarding the growing elderly population in general, little is known about the issues aging lesbian and bisexual women face. What we do know from qualitative data is that older lesbian and bisexual women report a significant history of discrimination including embarrassment, rejection, hostility, and breach of confidentiality that often leads to avoidance of routine healthcare and less use of elderly housing and other social support services (Addis, Davies, Greene, MacBride-Stewart, & Shepard, 2001; Brotman, Ryan, & Cormier, 2003; Harrison & Silenzio, 1996).

Transgender Health

CASE STUDY

Harold was a 57-year-old male with uncontrolled diabetes, hypertension, hypercholesterolemia, and obesity who was referred to me from a colleague because he had told the provider that he believed he was transgender. I told Harold I would gladly work with him on his transgender health needs as well as his other medical needs, but disclosed to him that he was my first transgender patient and that I would be learning as we went along.

Transgender individuals are people whose intrinsic gender identity does not match their biological sex. Many transgender people experience gender dysphoria—distress that results from the discordance of biological sex and experienced gender (American Psychiatric Association, 2013). Treatment for gender dysphoria, considered to be highly effective, includes physical, medical, and/or surgical treatments to more closely align an individual's physical appearance with their self-identified gender (World Professional Association for Transgender Health, 2011). (See Box 34.3 for various treatment strategies). It is important to note that each transgender person will have their own vision of how much they need or want to transition physically, and that some may not choose to transition at all. One male-to-female transgender person may choose to undergo laser facial hair removal and take feminizing hormones while another may proceed with breast implants, sexual reassignment, and facial feminization surgeries.

Research on transgender individuals is sparse and usually consists of small convenience samples; however there are several risk factors that consistently emerge among studies and are worth mentioning. Transgender patients are at high risk of stigmatization, discrimination (including housing and employment), harassment, physical and sexual violence (hate crimes as well as intimate partner violence), tobacco and other substance abuse, depression,

Box 34.3 Transgender Treatment Options

Voice and Communication Therapy (verbal [pitch, intonation] and nonverbal [gestures, posture])

Physical modifications (e.g., laser hair removal, breast binding or padding, genital tucking, or penile prosthesis)

Hormone Replacement Therapy (HRT): Male to Female

Estrogen (IM or TD preferred, PO)
Spironolactone PO
Finasteride PO
Progesterone (IM preferred)—use is controversial
GnRH Agonists—used in adolescents

Hormone Replacement (HRT): Female to Male

Testosterone (IM or TD)

Surgery: Male to Female (MtF)

Breast augmentation
Genital surgery (SRS): penectomy, orchiectomy, vaginoplasty
Facial feminization surgery
Reduction thyroidchondroplasty
Voice Surgery
Buttock augmentation

Surgery: Female to Male (FtM)

Bilateral mastectomy/chest reconstruction
Genital surgery (SRS): hysterectomy, oophorectomy, metoidoplasty, phalloplasty, scrotoplasty

SRS—sexual reassignment surgery

suicide, HIV/STIs, and childhood abuse (Institute of Medicine, 2011; Xavier, Honnold, & Bradford, 2007).

Caring for transgender adults is well within the scope of primary care and does not require specialist referral to an endocrinologist for general care (ACOG, 2011; Gardner & Safer, 2013; Unger, 2014, UCSF Center of Excellence for Transgender Health, n.d.). Box 34.4 lists useful resources for clinicians treating transgender patients, including guidelines and straightforward protocols for initiating and maintaining hormone replacement therapy.

Box 34.4 Useful Resources

General Information and Guidelines

Gay and Lesbian Medical Association—Information regarding resources creating comprehensive systems of care for LGBT people. Includes ability to register your practice as LGBT friendly and also has free educational webinars for providers and staff. http://www.glma.org/

Lesbian Health and Resource Center—comprehensive, user-friendly website that provides clinically useful tools, tips, and further resources. http://www.lesbian-healthinfo.org/
http://www.cdc.gov/lgbthealth/links.htm

Improving the Health Care of Lesbian, Gay, Bisexual, and Transgender (LGBT) People: Understanding and Eliminating Health Disparities—Comprehensive overview of major health issues, demographics, terminology, and recommended steps for improvement of patient-centered care. http://www.lgbthealtheducation.org/publications/top/

National LGBT Tobacco Control Network—Guide for substance abuse treatment—although geared toward substance abuse treatment, this guide provides a comprehensive overview of issues and consideration for working with LGBT individuals. Has good templates for sexual orientation intake form and feedback forms. http://www.lgbttobacco.org/files/Provider%20Introduction%20to%20 Substance%20Abuse%20Treatment.pdf

Transgender Health and Clinical Guidelines

World Professional Association for Transgender Health (formerly the Harry Benjamin International Gender Dysphoria Association) **Standards of Care v7**—comprehensive document addressing scope of TG care; includes useful tables on effects and expected time course of specific HRT medications, as well as risks associated with HRT. http://www.wpath.org/uploaded_files/140/files/Standards%20of%20Care,%20V7%20 Full%20Book.pdf

Tom Waddell Protocol—excellent, concise reference document with specific HRT doses and formulations, relative and absolute contraindications, and monitoring parameters; also nicely outlines some general social, health, and mental health concerns in trans population. https://www.sfdph.org/dph/comupg/oservices/medSvs/hlthCtrs/TransGendprotocols122006.pdf

UCSF Center of Excellence for Transgender Health Primary Care, Protocol for Transgender Patient Care—comprehensive, well-organized site that helps practitioner address full scope of transgender health needs including general preventive care and screening, fertility, and aging issues. http://www.transhealth.ucsf.edu/trans?page=protocol-00-00

Transsexual Road Map—excellent resource for patients navigating their transition; as such, serves as a rich source of nonmedical information for providers to better

(continued)

Box 34.4 Continued

understand what their transgender patients face and go through in transitioning.
http://www.tsroadmap.com/index.html

Intersex Association of America (ISNA) and **Accord Alliance**—resources for intersex individuals, their families, advocates, and practitioners.
http://www.isna.org and http://www.accordalliance.org

Patient Handouts and Posters

GLBT Health—Online resource for professional LGBT friendly posters, handouts, and brochures for use in healthcare settings.
http://www.glbthealth.org/HAPMaterials.htm

Training Resources

The Gay Alliance Safe Zone—Information regarding short training program that aims to increase the awareness, knowledge, and skills for staff to create a safe, welcoming environment for LGBTQ individuals. Provides materials to signify that your facility is a safe zone. (Often colleges and universities offer this training locally.)
http://www.gayalliance.org/safezonet.html

Straight for Equality (A PFLAG project)—offers local training programs for health-care staff to identify and change barriers to providing culturally competent care.
http://www.straightforequality.org/

Gay, Lesbian, Bisexual, and Transgender Health Access Project—foster the development and implementation of comprehensive, culturally appropriate, quality health promotion policies and healthcare services. Organization also offers free onsite trainings in Massachusetts.
http://www.glbthealth.org/CommunityStandardsofPractice.htm

Gender and Health Collaborative Curriculum Project—online interactive sexual diversity learning module for healthcare providers. http://www.genderandhealth.ca/en/modules/

LGBT Elders

Services and Advocacy for Lesbian, Gay, Bisexual, and Transgender Elders—provides resources regarding healthcare and social service issues including information on end-of-life planning, healthcare proxy, and living wills.
http://www.sageusa.org

LGBT Youth

The Trevor Project—suicide hotline and web resources including issues related to psychosocial and health issues for LGBTQ youth.
http://www.thetrevorproject.org/

Phone and Online Support for Patients

Mautner Project—offers ongoing phone and online peer support for LBT women nationwide with professionally trained staff to answer health-related questions. This

(continued)

Box 34.4 Continued

site also has online support groups for lesbian, bisexual, and transgender women dealing with serious illness, bereavement, or caregiving issues.
http://www.whitman-walker.org/mautnerproject

Fenway Health: Lesbian, Gay, Bisexual and Transgender Helpline and Peer Listening Line—provides trained telephone support and information on local resources for LGBTQ adults and youth.
http://www.fenwayhealth.org/site/PageServer?pagename=FCHC_srv_services_tollfree

Note: While female-to-male transgender persons do not identify as women, they are being included in this chapter on women's health because some female health considerations do apply to them. Intersex, or disorders of sex development, is not the same as transgender and is a separate and complex topic. Please see Box 34.4 for resources on issues related to intersex individuals.

Over the course of 6 years, Harold transitioned to living full-time as a woman. Based on Harold's preference, I began using the female pronoun once she started presenting to the clinic as Susanna. Her HRT regimen included estrogen, finasteride, and spironolactone. She brought her diabetes, hypertension, and cholesterol under control within months of starting HRT, though she continued to struggle with her weight. Susanna came out to her ex-wife and children, and while conversations where difficult, they were ultimately supportive. Based on samples Susanna provided me, I wrote supporting letters requesting her gender be changed to female on both her driver's license and birth certificate, requests that were both granted.

I was very lucky that Susanna was my first transgender patient, as she was willing to work with me as I learned how to help her. Given the discrimination that transgender patients have had within the healthcare field and the paucity of trained providers, you will find that if you are accepting and supportive of a transgender patient, he or she will be more than happy to work with you as you learn about how to meet his or her healthcare needs.

Summary and Recommendations

The practice of integrative medicine includes an emphasis on the patient–practitioner interaction as a healing modality *in and of itself* and an effort toward understanding the whole person by taking into account the biopsychosocial factors that affect health and well-being. Lesbian, bisexual, and transgender individuals have unique life and health issues that are often poorly understood. Cultural humility, nonjudgmental interest and efforts to create an inclusive environment can help foster mutual trust and understanding that can be instructive and healing on many levels.

REFERENCES

Aaron, D. J., Markovic, N., Danielson, M. E., Honnold, J. A., Janosky, J. E., & Schmidt, N. J. (2001). Behavioral risk factors for disease and preventive health practices among lesbians. *Am J Public Health, 91*, 972–975.

Addis, S., Davies, M., Greene, G., MacBride-Stewart, S., & Shepard, M. (2009). The health, social care and housing needs of lesbian, gay, bisexual and transgender older people: A review of the literature. *Health Soc Care Comm, 17*, 647–658.

American Academy of Pediatrics, Committee on Adolescence. (2013). Office-based care for the lesbian, gay, bisexual, transgender, and questioning youth. *Pediatrics, 132*, 198–203.

American College of Obstetricians and Gynecologists (ACOG). (2011). Committee on Health Care for Underserved Women, Opinion No. 512. Health care for transgender individuals. *Obstet Gynecol, 118*, 1454–1458.

American College of Obstetricians and Gynecologists (ACOG). (2012). Committee on Health Care for Underserved Women, Opinion 525. Health care for lesbian and bisexual women. *Obstet Gynecol, 119*, 1077–1080.

American Psychiatric Association. (2013). *Diagnostic and statistical manual of mental disorders* (5th ed.). Arlington, VA: Author.

American Psychiatric Association. (2013). Gender dysphoria. Retrieved April 30, 2014, from http: www.dsm5.org/Documents/Gender%20Dysphoria%20Fact%20Sheet.pdf.

Austin, E. L. (2013). Sexual orientation disclosure in to health care providers among urban and non-urban southern lesbians. *Women Health, 53*, 41–55.

Austin, E. L., & Irwin, J. A. (2012). Health behaviors and health care utilization of southern lesbians. *Women Health Iss, 20*, 178–184.

Barbara, A., Quant, S., & Anderson, R. (2001). Experiences of lesbians in the health care environment. *Women Health, 34*, 45–62.

Berger, B. J., Kolton, S., Zenilman, J. M., Cummings, M. C., Felldman, J., & McCormack, W. M. (1995). Bacterial vaginosis in lesbians: A sexually transmitted disease. *Clin Infect Dis 21*, 1402–1405.

Blosnich, J. R., & Silenzio, V. M. B. (2013). Physical health indicators among lesbian, gay, and bisexual U.S. veterans. *Ann Epidemiol, 23*, 448–451.

Boehmer, U., Miao, X., Maxwell, N. I., & Ozonoff, A. (2014). Sexual minority population density and increase of lung, colorectal and female breast cancer in California. *BMJ Open, 4*, e004461.

Brotman, S., Ryan, B., & Cormier, R. (2003). The health and social service needs of gay and lesbian elders and their families in Canada. *Gerontologist, 43*,192–202.

Campos-Outcalt, D., & Hurwitz, S. (2002). Female-to-female transmission of syphilis: A case report. *Sex Trans Dis, 29*, 119–120.

Case, P., Austin, B., Hunter, D. J., Manson, J. E., Malspeis, S., Willett, W. C., & Spiegelman, D. (2004). Sexual orientation, health risk factors, and physical functioning in the Nurses' Health Study II. *J Womens Health, 13*, 1033–1047.

Chandra, A., Mosher, W. D., Copen, C., & Sionean, C. (2011). Sexual behavior, sexual attraction, and sexual identity in the United States: Data from the 2006–28 National Survey of Family Growth. *Natl Health Stat Report, 36*, 1–36.

Davis, V., Chrislaw, E., Edwards, C., et al. (2000). Lesbian health guidelines. *J Soc Obstet Gynaecol Can, 22*, 202–205.

Diamant, A. L., Schuster, M. A., McGuigan, K., & Lever, J. (1999). Lesbians' sexual history with men: Implications for taking a sexual history. *Arch Intern Med, 159*, 2730–2736.

Diamant, A. L., Schuster, M. A., & Lever, J. (2000). Receipt of preventive health care services by lesbians. *Am J Prev Med, 19*, 141–148.

Dibble, S. L., Roberts, S. A., & Nussey, B. (2004). Comparing breast cancer risk between lesbians and their heterosexual sisters. *Womens Health Iss, 14*, 60–68.

Eisenberg, M. (2001). Differences in sexual risk behaviors between college students with same-sex and opposite-sex experience: Results from a national survey. *Arch Sex Behav, 30*, 575–589.

Gardner, I. H., & Safer, J. D. (2013). Progress on the road to better medical care for transgender patients. *Curr Opin Endocrinol Obes, 20*, 553–558.

Gates, G. (2013). LGBT parenting in the United States. The Williams Institute. Retrieved April 15, 2014, from http: williamsinstitute.law.ucla.edu/research/census-lgbt-demographics-studies/family-formation-and-raising-children-among-same-sex-couples/

Goodenow, C., Sazalacha, L., Robin, L. E., & Westheimer, K. (2008). Dimensions of sexual orientation and HIV-related risk among adolescent females: Evidence from a statewide survey. *Am J Public Health, 98*, 1051–1058.

Harrison, A. E., & Silenzio, V. M. B. (1996). Comprehensive care of lesbian and gay patients and families. *Prim Care, 23*, 31–47.

Herrick, A. L., Matthews, A. K., & Garofalo, R. (2010). Health risk behaviors in a urban sample of young women who have sex with women. *J Lesbian Stud, 14*, 80–92.

Hutchinson, M. K., Thompson, A., & Cedarbaum, J. (2006). Multisystem factors contributing to disparities in preventive health care among lesbian women. *JOGNN, 35*, 393–402.

Institute of Medicine. (2011). The health of lesbian, gay, bisexual, and transgender people: Building a foundation for better understanding. Washington, DC: Institute of Medicine.

Kann, L., Olsen, E. O., McManus, T., et al. Centers for Disease Control and Prevention. (2011). Sexual identity, sex of sexual contacts, and health risk behaviors among students in grade 9–12—Youth risk behavior surveillance, selected sites, United States, 2001–2009. *MMWR Surveill Summ*, *60*, 1–133.

Kellock, D., & O'Mahony, C. P. (1996). Sexually acquired metronidazole-resistant trichomoniasis in a lesbian couple. *Genitourin Med*, *72*, 60–61.

Kerker, B. D., Mostashari, F., & Thorpe, L. (2006). Health care access and utilization among women who have sex with women: Sexual behavior and identity. *J Urban Health*, *83*, 970–979.

King, M., Semlyeni J. Tae, S. S., Killaspy, H., Osborn, D., Popelyuki, D., & Nazareth, I. (2008). A systematic review of mental disorder, suicide and deliberate self harm in lesbian, gay and bisexual people. *BMC Psychiatry*, *8*, 70.

Koh, A. S., Gomez, C. A., Shade, S., et al. (2005). Sexual risk factors among self-identified lesbians, bisexual women, and heterosexual women accessing primary care settings. *Sex Transm Dis*, *32*, 563–569.

Krivickas, K. M., & Lofquist, D. (2011). *Demographics of same-sex couples households with children*. US Census Bureau, Fertility and Family Statistics Branch. SEHSD Working Paper Number 2011–11. Retrieved April 29, 2014, from https://www.census.gov/hhes/samesex/files/Krivickas-Lofquist%20PAA%202011.pdf

Kwakwa, H. A., & Ghobiral, M. W. (2003). Female-to-female transmission of human immunodeficiency virus. *Clin Infect Dis*, *36*, e40–e41.

Marrazzo, J. M. (2004). Barriers to infectious disease care among lesbians. *Emerg Infect Dis*, *10*, 1974–1978.

Marrazzo, J. M., Koutsky, L. A., Kiviat, N. B., et al. (2001). Papanicolaou test screening and prevalence of genital human papillomavirus among women who have sex with women. *Am J Public Health*, *91*, 947–952.

Marrazzo, J. M., Koutsky, L. A., Stine, K. L., et al. (1998). Genital human papillomavirus infection in women who have sex with women. *J Infect Dis*, *178*, 1604–1609.

Martin, S. L., Fisher, B. S., Warner, T. D., Krebs, C. P., & Linquist, C. H. (2011). Women's sexual orientation and their experiences of sexual assault before and during university. *Womens Health Issues*, *3*, 199–205.

Marques, A. M., Noquierra, C., & de Olivera, J. M. (2014). Lesbians on medical encounters: Tales of heteronormativity, deception and expectations. *Health Care Women Int*, *60*, e1–19.

Matthews, A. K., Brandenburg, D. L., Johnson, T. P., & Hughes, T. L. (2004). Correlates of underutilization of gynecological cancer screening among lesbian and heterosexual women. *Prev Med*, *38*, 105–113.

McNair, R. P., Szalacha, L. A., & Hughes, T. L. (2011). Health status, health service use and satisfaction according to sexual identity of young Australian women. *Womens Health Iss*, *21*, 40–47.

McNair, R. P., Hegarty, K., & Taft, A. (2012). From silence to sensitivity: A new identity disclosure model to facilitate disclosure for same-sex attracted women in general practice consultations. *Soc Sci Med*, *75*, 208–216.

Mosack, K. E., Brouwer, A. M., & Petroll, A. E. (2013). Sexual identity, identity disclosure, and health care experiences: Is there evidence for differential homophobia in primary care practice? *Womens Health Iss*, *23*, e341–e346.

National Institute of Intimate Partner Violence. (2010). *Findings on victimization by sexual orientation*. Retrieved April 15, 2014, from http: www.cdc.gov/violenceprevention/nisvs

Rankow, E. J. (1995). Lesbian health issues for the primary care provider. *J Fam Practice, 40*, 486–496.

Rankow, E. J., & Tessaro, I. (1998). Cervical cancer risk and Papanicolaou screening in a sample of lesbian and bisexual women. *J Fam Practice, 47*, 139–143.

Rothman, E. F., Exner, D., & Baughman, A. L. (2011). The prevalence of sexual assault against people who identify as gay, lesbian or bisexual in the United States: A systematic review. *Trauma Violence Abuse, 12*, 55–66.

Stevens, P. E., & Hall, J. M. (2001). Sexuality and safer sex: The issues for lesbians and bisexual women. *JOGNN, 4*, 439–447.

UCSF Center of Excellence for Transgender Health. (n.d.). *Primary care protocol for transgender patient care*. Retrieved April 30, 2014, from http://www.transhealth.ucsf.edu/trans?page=protocol-00-00

Unger, C. A. (2014). Care of the transgender patient: The role of the gynecologist. *American Journal of Obstetrics and Gynecology, 210*, 16–26.

Valanis, B. G., Bowen, D. J., Bassford, T., Whitlock, E., Charney, P., & Cater, R. A. (2000). Sexual orientation and health: Comparison in the Women's Health Initiative Sample. *Arch Fam Med, 9*, 843–853.

White, J. C., & Dull, V. T. (1998). Health risk factors and health seeking behavior in lesbians. *J Womens Health, 6*, 103–112.

Workowski, K. A., & Berman, S. M. (2010). Centers for Disease Control and Prevention. Sexually transmitted diseases guidelines. *MMWR 2010, 59*(RR-12), 1–110.

World Professional Association for Transgender Health (WPATH). (2011). *Standards of care for the health of transsexual, transgender, and gender nonconforming people* (7th ed.). Retrieved April 30, 2014, from http://www.wpath.org/uploaded_files/140/files/Standards%20of%20Care,%20V7%20Full%20Book.pdf

Xavier, J., Honnold, J., & Bradford, J. (2007). *The health, health-related needs, and life course experiences of transgender Virginians*. Virginia HIV Community Planning Committee and Virginia Department of Health. Richmond, VA: Virginia Department of Health. Retrieved April 30, 2014, from http://www.vdh.virginia.gov/epidemiology/diseaseprevention/documents/pdf/THISFINALREPORTVol1.pdf

Zaritsky, E., & Dibble, S. L. (2010). Risk factors for reproductive and breast cancers among older lesbians. *J Womens Health, 19*, 125–131.

35

Environmental Exposures and Women's Health

MANIJEH BERENJI AND JOANNE L. PERRON

CASE STUDY

A pregnant woman participating in a research study conducted by the University of California at San Francisco on exposures to chemicals and toxicants was found to have serum mercury almost three times greater than the Centers for Disease Control (CDC) reporting threshold (5.8 µg/L). The cord blood level was also elevated (7.43 µg/L). Investigation of the home environment found face creams obtained in Mexico with mercury levels up to 30,000 parts per million (ppm), a level markedly higher than the FDA standard for face creams (<1 ppm). After removal of these products, the pregnant woman was lost to follow-up. Chelation therapy is usually not recommended in pregnant women, but given the high mercury exposures in this case, the benefit of chelation would have to be considered. The infant could not be assessed for sequelae of in utero mercury exposure (Dickenson, Woodruff, Stotland, Dobraca, & Das, 2012).

Introduction

Environmental health is concerned with all of the external factors (physical, chemical, and biological) that have an impact on human health, behavior, and disease. Reproductive environmental health is focused on exposures from environmental chemicals during the life course and especially during vulnerable developmental periods (preconception, pregnancy, and early childhood) that adversely impact human health.

Occupational health seeks to mitigate workplace hazards, including chemical exposures. The number of women in the workplace has more than doubled over the past 40 years, from 30 million in 1970 to 67 million in 2007 (American College of Occupational and Environmental Medicine, 2011). In 2004, more than 28 million women ages 18–44 were employed full-time (McDiarmid & Gehle, 2006). Despite the increasing number of women employed in industries using heavy metals, organic solvents, and pesticides, many of these industrial agents have not been vigorously tested for reproductive toxicity (Till, Koren, & Rovet, 2008).

The emerging evidence from historical events, animal toxicology research, and epidemiological studies of exposed populations demonstrates robust associations between exposure to environmental toxicants and adverse health outcomes. According to a recent American College of Obstetricians and Gynecologists Committee Opinion, the increases in adverse health outcomes since World War II cannot be explained by genetic changes alone (American College of Obstetricians and Gynecologists, 2013). The President's Cancer Panel declared in 2010 that abundant and robust evidence exists linking cancer to environmental and occupational chemical exposures (President's Cancer Panel, 2010).

Environmental toxicants are industrial or naturally occurring, organic and inorganic chemicals that harm human health across the life span, more so during critical developmental windows. Examples include pesticides, components of air pollution, flame retardants, solvents, heavy metals, and numerous other chemicals found in everyday household products and consumer goods. Over 80,000 chemicals are registered for use in the United States with an estimated 2,000 new ones introduced every year (National Toxicology Program, n.d.). Contrary to the extensive testing of pharmaceutical chemicals before introduction to the marketplace, environmental toxicants *do not* undergo premarket human safety testing. The regulatory hurdles that the United States Environmental Protection Agency (US EPA) must satisfy to ban harmful substances are significant, so that even asbestos, a known carcinogen, is not outlawed.

The Evidence for Health Effects and Mechanisms of Action

The evidence stream linking toxic chemical exposure to adverse developmental effects includes human observational studies as well as *in vitro* and *in vivo* toxicological testing. For ethical reasons, there are no direct experimental human data in the form of randomized control trials (RCTs) to assess the relationship between exposure to environmental chemicals and adverse developmental health outcomes. Reliance on cell lines and animal studies to determine human harm is supported by the National Academy of Science, which concluded that there is conservation of function across species, concordance of developmental and reproductive effects, and that humans are as, or more, sensitive, than the most sensitive animal species (National Research Council, 2000).

Many of these chemicals act as endocrine disruptors, which are "chemicals that may interfere with the body's endocrine system and produce adverse developmental reproductive, neurological, and immune effects in both humans and wildlife" (National Institute for Environmental Health Sciences [NIEHS], n.d.). Endocrine disruptors can act through traditional nuclear hormone receptor pathways (estrogen, progesterone, androgen, thyroid, and retinoid) and more diverse avenues such as nonnuclear, neurotransmitter, or orphan receptors and enzymatic pathway interference (Diamanti-Kandarakis et al., 2009). The dose-response curves of EDCs do not follow the traditional paradigm of Paracelsus (with increasing concentrations of a compound there will be increasing toxic effects on the organism). Paradoxically, exposure to miniscule amounts during vulnerable windows of development may be more damaging than higher exposures at other times (Diamanti-Kandarakis et al., 2009).

Endocrine disruptors can directly interfere with ovarian steroid hormone production or alter the control and action of ovarian hormones at the level of the hypothalamic-pituitary-gonadal axis (Mendola & Louis, 2010). Furthermore, endocrine disruptors can have multiple hormonal effects. For example, the pesticide dichlorodiphenyltrichloroethane (DDT) is an estrogen disruptor, while its metabolite dichlorodiphenyldichloroethylene (DDE) is an androgen antagonist (Diamanti-Kandarakis et al., 2009). Endocrine-disrupting chemicals do not cause genetic mutations or change the DNA sequence. Rather, EDCs can alter gene expression via the epigenome and effects may be transmitted transgenerationally (Skinner, Manikkam, & Guerrero-Bosagna, 2010).

Endocrine disruptors can be naturally occurring or man-made. Examples include phytoestrogens, diethylstilbestrol (DES; see Box 35.1), certain pesticides, plasticizers (such as bisphenol A [BPA] and phthalates), or halogenated hydrocarbons (such as dioxins, polychlorinated biphenyls [PCBs], and polybrominated diphenyl ethers [PBDEs]) (NIEHS, n.d.). The molecular structure of an endocrine disruptor often includes a central ring, which mimics that found in steroid hormones, with added halogen side groups (chlorine, bromine, fluorine) that confer various properties such as molecular stability (Diamanti-Kandarakis et al., 2009).

Neuroendocrine disruptors are defined as pollutants in the environment that are capable of acting as agonists/antagonists or modulators of the synthesis and/or metabolism of neuropeptides, neurotransmitters, or neurohormones. These agents can alter diverse physiological, behavioral, or hormonal processes, affecting an animal's capacity to reproduce, develop, and grow, or deal with stress and other challenges (Trudeau, Kah, & Bourguignon, 2011).

Exposures to Environmental Chemicals

The most common routes of exposure to chemicals occur through ingestion, inhalation, or dermal contact. For children, the ingestion route is the most prevalent route of exposure, as they tend to explore their surroundings and may inadvertently touch and eat a compound with significant concentrations of a toxic substance. For adults, exposures can occur in the home (i.e., hobbies involving use of chemicals, such as woodworking or painting) or at the workplace (by means of specific industrial processes and the resulting air emissions). The Fourth National Report on Human Exposure to Environmental Chemicals by the CDC evaluated and assessed the presence of over 200 chemicals in a representative sample of civilian and noninstitutionalized Americans (CDC, 2009).

Chemical exposures that occur during fetal development are associated with adverse birth outcomes such as low birth weight, preterm delivery, decreased fetal growth, birth defects, pregnancy loss, and developmental delays (Stillerman, Mattison, Giudice, & Woodruff, 2008). Many chemicals are ubiquitous in these CDC biomonitoring results. While lead levels have markedly decreased due to widespread public health measures, chemicals banned in the 1970s, such as DDT and PCBs are still present in a significant portion of the population, even pregnant women (Woodruff, Zota, & Schwartz, 2011).

Maternal nutritional deficits and environmental stressors can perturb fetal development, as demonstrated by epidemiological studies from the Dutch famine. These studies had shown that adult health outcomes were dependent on the timing of gestational exposure. Those exposed to famine early in gestation had the most significant adverse health outcomes (including coronary heart disease, abnormal lipid profiles, and obesity); midgestation famine exposure was associated with greater obstructive airway disease; and those with late gestation were more likely to develop glucose intolerance as adults (Painter, Roseboom, & Bleker, 2005).

Historical incidents of fetal exposures to methyl mercury, thalidomide, and DES, as well as common exposures to alcohol, tobacco, and drugs of abuse have demonstrated that the placenta is not a stalwart barrier to toxicants. Chemicals measured in maternal serum and urine have been found in amniotic fluid, cord blood, and meconium (Barr, 2007).

The heavy metals mercury, lead, and selenium exhibit a substantial maternal–fetal transfer. Results from an inner-city African American cohort found mercury cord red blood cell (RBC) levels that were 1.5 times greater than maternal RBC levels. Furthermore, higher mercury levels in both the mother and fetus were associated with preterm births and low birth weight (Chen et al., 2014).

Although breast milk is considered the healthiest way to feed babies and infants, exposure to harmful chemicals through breastfeeding has been documented since 1951, beginning with DDT. Since then, additional chemicals have been identified worldwide in breast milk (Mead, 2008). The most worrisome are persistent organic pollutants (POPs), lipophilic halogenated compounds, which according to the US EPA are associated with myriad adverse human health effects (US EPA, 2014a). The immense benefits of breastfeeding on infant and adult health are well-established. Studies linking ingestion of contaminated breast milk with adverse health outcomes are limited due to the ubiquitous nature of toxicant exposures and the length of time required to determine the effects on health.

A fetus and young child are more sensitive to harmful chemicals because of a higher metabolic rate, under-developed liver detoxifying mechanisms as well as immune system, and subfunctioning blood-brain barrier (Newbold & Heindal, 2010). Disruptions can occur in the fetus or child at exposure levels that may have no lasting effects on adults (Schettler, 2001). Thus, developmental exposure to toxicants can cause myriad outcomes ranging from fetal death and congenital malformations to neurodevelopmental problems and adverse health outcomes diagnosed decades later (Newbold & Heindal, 2010).

In utero and early life exposures to industrial chemicals and contaminants such as methyl mercury (Box 35.2), lead (Box 35.3), PCBs, arsenic, and toluene are well-known to contribute to neurodevelopmental disorders at doses lower than those affecting adult brain function (Grandjean & Landrigan, 2006). Emerging evidence is now linking exposures to manganese, high fluoride

Box 35.2 Mercury Case Study

Mercury is a developmental neurotoxicant that was first documented on a large-scale after widespread aquatic contamination in the fishing village of Minimata, Japan, during the 1950s (World Health Organization, 2007). Mothers were unaffected while their babies suffered severe neurologic sequelae (Rusyniak, Furbee, & Pascuzzi, 2005).

levels, tetrachloroethylene, certain pesticides, and flame retardants with adverse neurodevelopmental outcomes (Grandjean & Landrigan, 2014).

Fetal neurodevelopment is an exquisite biological orchestration that is vulnerable to perturbation during neuronal proliferation, migration, connectivity, and myelination, as well as during neurotransmitter formation and receptor development (Rodier, 2004). Normal neurodevelopment depends on these processes occurring during a tightly-controlled time frame and in a specific sequence. Adverse effects depend on the developmental stage when exposure occurs, on cumulative interactions between contaminants, and on a mosaic of additional environmental and genetic factors.

Pesticides

Pesticides are distinguished by the category of pest they target. Pesticides target pests, insecticides target insects, herbicides target weeds, fungicides target fungi or fungal spores, and rodenticides target rodents. Chemical pesticides

Box 35.3 Lead Case Study

In 2012, the *Morbidity and Mortality Weekly Report* (MMWR) described six cases of elevated lead levels in foreign-born pregnant women from ingestion of Ayurvedic medications produced in India. Blood lead levels (BLL) ranged from 16 to 64 µg/dL (CDC, 2012). Two of six women miscarried in the late first trimester. Newborn BLL measured in two of the babies were 7 and 23 µg/dL. Neurodevelopmental effects such as diminished intelligence, low birth weight, and behavioral problems can occur at any BLL, therefore, there are no safe lead levels in pregnancy (CDC, 2010). During pregnancy, stored lead is released from the maternal bones, exposing the developing fetus (Gulson Jameson Mahaffey Mizon & Korsch, 1997). Additionally, an elevated BLL in pregnancy is associated with gestational hypertension and spontaneous miscarriage (CDC, 2010).

(synthetically-derived), consist of four main classes: organophosphates (which irreversibly interfere with an enzyme that regulates the neurotransmitter acetylcholine), organochlorines (which act by targeting the sodium channel in nerve cells; most are banned, though some countries use them for malaria control), carbamates (which reversibly interfere with an enzyme that regulates the neurotransmitter acetylcholine), and pyrethroids (synthetic version of the naturally occurring pesticide pyrethrin found in chrysanthemums). These pesticides are also used as insecticides and rodenticides. There are over 20 chemical classes of herbicides, insecticides, and rodenticides. There are also biological pesticides, which include microbial pesticides, plant-incorporated protectants (PIPs), and naturally occurring biochemical pesticides.

Pesticides often combine an active ingredient and inert substances designed to facilitate the effectiveness of the active ingredient. Inert chemicals are proprietary to the manufacturer. Inert, however, does not imply safe, as some have harmful effects.

Agricultural workers are the most common occupational cohort to have persistent chronic pesticide exposures. Besides those who apply the pesticides and work in the fields, others are exposed to pesticides by virtue of pesticide usage in homes, schools, and recreational areas. Exposure can also be related to pesticide drift and proximity to agricultural areas depending on pesticide volatility, persistence in the environment, and weather conditions.

Pesticides can be unintentionally absorbed through the skin or mucous membranes, inhaled into the lungs, or ingested. The National Institute for Occupational Safety and Health (NIOSH) established the Sentinel Event Notification System for Occupational Risks—Pesticides Program (SENSOR-Pesticides) in 1987 to reduce the number of injuries and illnesses associated with occupational pesticide exposures (Department of Health and Human Services, NIOSH, 2011). The US EPA is currently proposing changes to the agricultural Worker Protection Standard (WPS) to protect agricultural workers and their families from pesticide exposure (US EPA, 2011).

US EPA Safety Assessment for Pesticides

In conducting health risk assessments for pesticides, the US EPA first identifies the hazard in question, performs a dose-response assessment to see how much of the specific pesticide is required to cause an effect, delineates the exposure route, and lastly does a risk characterization.

According to the US EPA, there are currently 1,234 active pesticide ingredients and 19,881 pesticides products (including restricted use) registered in the United States (Sutton, Perron, Giudice, & Woodruff, 2011). The total pesticide amount used in the United States (agricultural and nonagricultural) was approximately 1.1 billion pounds of pesticides in both 2006 and 2007 (US EPA, 2013a). It should be noted that there are also many pesticides that are not registered with the US EPA. These "illegal" pesticides have been notably found in tick repellants for pets and mothballs, among other household items (US EPA, 2012b). For healthcare professionals trying to identify causative agents in cases of environmental exposures, pinpointing the active ingredients on the product label is key to doing a thorough investigation. The US EPA's Pesticide Product Label System allows individuals to determine the status of a particular pesticide, using the US EPA Registration Number (which appears on all registered pesticides sold in the United States).

Many pesticides target the nervous system of the insect or pest. Because of the similarity in brain chemistry, neurotoxicity also occurs in mammals. While the acute neurological effects of pesticide exposure are well-known, the neurodevelopmental effects are still being elucidated. Approximately 100 pesticides have been listed as human neurotoxicants based on acute exposures. It is likely, due to lack of complete information on developmental neurotoxicity, that this list underrepresents the actual number of pesticides that are neurotoxic to humans (Grandjean & Landrigan, 2014).

Experimental studies suggest that these compounds can cause developmental neurotoxicity by varied mechanisms. Familiar mechanisms include oxidative stress and perturbation of membrane ion channels. A more novel characterization is neuroendocrine disruption.

In addition to occupational exposure, the most vulnerable populations are pregnant women and developing children in agricultural and poverty-stricken inner-city areas (Sutton et al., 2011). A white paper on the reproductive harm of pesticides by the Program on Reproductive Health and the Environment (PRHE) has summarized the science of adverse human health outcomes. Pesticides exposures, either in utero or during childhood, are associated with childhood leukemia and other childhood cancers, diminished semen quality, male sterility, prostate cancer, early female puberty, irregularities in menstrual and ovarian function, diminished female fertility/fecundity, early menopause, and breast cancer (Sutton et al., 2011).

The American Cancer Society published a review of the scientific literature from occupational studies describing the greater cancer risk due to pesticide exposure (Alavanja, Ross & Bonner, 2013). The authors of this paper discuss specific cancers that have the most scientific evidence of having a link to pesticide exposure: non-Hodgkin lymphoma (NHL), leukemia, multiple myeloma (MM), and breast and prostate cancer. Many of the carcinogenic pesticides (such as DDT) have been restricted because of definitive evidence of

Table 35.1. Cancer-Causing Pesticides

Cancer	Pesticides
Non-Hodgkin Lymphoma	2,4-D, MCPA, Glyphosate, and Atrazine
Adult Leukemia	Diazinon, Metribuzin, Alachlor, and EPTC
Multiple Myeloma	Permethrin, Captan, and Carbaryl

Source: Alavanja, Ross, & Bonner (2013)

carcinogenicity, yet others in the marketplace are not restricted because policymakers do not believe the body of evidence is strong enough.

The following registered pesticides have population-based evidence (mostly occupational, and in some cases animal toxicology) of associations with NHL: 2,4-dichlorophenoxyacetic acid (2,4-D), 2-methyl-4-chlorophenoxyacetic acid (MCPA), glyphosate, and atrazine. Adult leukemia is associated with occupational exposure to diazinon, metribuzin, alachlor, and S-ethyl dipropylcarbamothioate (EPTC). Finally, MM has associations with occupational exposure to permethrin, captan, and carbaryl. The authors did not find any specific pesticide exposure to be strongly linked with breast cancer (Alavanja et al., 2013; Table 35.1).

Perfluorooctanoic Acid/Perfluorooctane Compounds (PFCs)

Perfluorooctanoic acid (PFOA) is a synthetic chemical used in the production of non-stick cooking vessels or water-resistant materials. Perfluorooctane sulfonate (PFOS) is found in stain-resistant textiles or carpets, and is also found as a by-product of other fluoridated compounds that are used to line microwave popcorn bags and pizza boxes. For the average person, consumption of contaminated food, ingestion of dust, and inhalation of air are the major exposure pathways for PFCs. The pathways are product- and age-dependent. For example, infants, toddlers, and children have exposure from carpets and rugs due to hand-mouth contact, while food packaging is a more important exposure route for teenagers and adults (Trudeau et al., 2011).

Flame Retardants

Polybrominated diethyl ethers are flame retardants that have been used in foam in most household furniture and carpet padding as well as in consumer

---

Box 35.4 PFOA—Example of an Accidental Community Exposure

Also called C8, PFOA was released into the air and the Ohio River from the 1950s to 2000 from DuPont's Washington, West Virginia, facility. In 2002, contaminated groundwater was found to have affected local water districts in the surrounding area of Parkersburg, West Virginia (C8 Science Panel, 2013b). An epidemiological study looked at more than 25,000 residents residing in the area of water contaminated by C8 and found an increased risk of kidney and testicular cancers (Barry, Winquist, & Steenland, 2013). Furthermore, the C8 science panel states that there is a probable link between C8 exposure and elevated cholesterol, ulcerative colitis, thyroid disease, and pregnancy-induced hypertension (C8 Science Panel, 2013a). However, a recent systematic review found no causal relationship between exposure to PFOA/PFOS and the risk of cancer, even occupationally. These authors believe that the Parkersburg findings were unreliable due to chance, confounding, and bias (Chang Hans-Olov, & Boffetta, 2014).

---

electronics for the past 30 years. Since these PBDEs are not bound to the products that contain them, they can leach out and accumulate in the environment, in household dust and in the water supply. Humans can either inhale contaminated air where these products are used or ingest the PBDEs (through eating seafood). Given the increasing use of PBDEs in consumer products, PBDEs are increasingly being found in humans.

According to a review of PBDE wildlife neurotoxicology (which documents the vast effects on fish, birds, and terrestrial and aquatic animals) these compounds have been detected worldwide (from the Baltic Sea to the Pacific and the Arctic Oceans) at exponentially-increasing levels exceeding PCBs by several-fold (Basu & Head, 2010). Consequently, the food system contains PBDEs and other brominated flame retardants (BFRs). A 2008 market survey found that fish had the highest levels of BFRs at 616 ppb followed by meat 190, dairy 32, and vegetables at 12 ppb (Schecter et al., 2008).

Flame retardants have been called the "asbestos of our time" by prominent environmental health scientists and advocates (Blum, 2014). More than 175 flame-retardants are currently in the marketplace. Touted by industry for their ability to inhibit flame ignition and spread, prominent scientists are increasingly concerned that any benefit derived from them is negated by the emerging science demonstrating adverse environmental and human health outcomes (Birnbaum & Bergman, 2010; Shaw, Blum, & Weber, 2010).

Those that contain halogen components (chlorine or bromine) are similar in structure and nature to PCBs, which were banned in 1977. Due to chemical stability, halogenated compounds resist breakdown, remain in the environment for decades, and bioaccumulate as they move up the food chain. Their lipophilic nature allows accumulation and storage in mammalian fatty tissue (Janssen, 2005). These halogen-containing flame-retardants are worrisome because of their potential to act as carcinogens, mutagens, reproductive toxicants, immune-toxicants, and endocrine disruptors (Birnbaum & Bergman, 2010). In addition, there are concerns that flame-retardants, behaving like PCBs, may also be significant and pervasive neurodevelopmental toxicants (Janssen, 2005).

A flame retardant called polybrominated biphenyl (PBB), with a similar structure to PCBs, was involved in a large-scale accidental contamination of Michigan livestock, which resulted in the exposure of nine million people, and prompted the stoppage of PPBs production in 1979 (Janssen, 2005). According to the Michigan PBB registry, exposed women were more likely to have menstrual irregularities (as did their breastfed daughters) and exposed men had more thyroid disease. Additionally, daughters of exposed women were more likely to have miscarriages and sons to have genital or urinary disorders (Emory, Rollins School of Public Health, Department of Epidemiology, 2014).

After restriction of PBBs in the United States, the use of PBDEs in consumer products dramatically increased over the ensuing decades. Structurally similar to both PCBs and PBBs, flame retardants have the potential for similar behavior (Birnbaum & Bergman, 2010). All PBDEs (with their two halogenated phenyl rings), are more similar to thyroid hormone than PCBs (which are known thyroid disruptors) (Zoeller, 2010). Several reviews have summarized the current body of knowledge delineating the reproductive and neurodevelopmental toxicological outcomes and mechanisms of action that BFRs/PBDEs demonstrate in animal studies (Costa & Giordano, 2007; Darnerud, 2008; Dingemans, van den Berg, & Westerink, 2011; Fonnum & Mariussen, 2009; Janssen, 2005; Legler, 2008; Zoeller, 2010). In addition to promoting oxidative stress, mitochondrial damage, apoptosis, altering calcium homeostasis and signaling, and disrupting gene expression, PBDEs and other flame retardants are considered endocrine disruptors of estrogen, androgen, and thyroid hormone. Depending on the specific PBDE congener, the chemicals serve as antagonists or agonists at androgen, progesterone, and estrogen receptors, and increase adverse reproductive outcomes (Costa & Giordano, 2007; Darnerud, 2008; Legler, 2008).

Children are most vulnerable to the effects of PDBEs. Levels of PBDE in California children aged 2 to 5 years are 10- to 1,000-times higher than European children, five times higher than other US children, and two to 10 times higher than US adults. Additionally, the levels in these children approach and often exceed levels measured in occupationally exposed US polyurethane foam recyclers and carpet installers (Rose, Bennett, Bergman, Fangstrom, & Hertz-Picciotto, 2010).

Data from NHANES demonstrate that specific PBDEs are present in high concentrations in the bloodstreams of most Americans, as compared with Europeans (CDC, 2009). The CHAMACOS (Center for the Health Assessment of Mothers and Children of Salinas) study (a longitudinal birth cohort study started in 1998 and continuing to this day) has examined environmental chemicals and their impact on children's health. Data generated from this study have found that higher PBDE exposures during pregnancy were associated with decreased female fertility, altered maternal thyroid hormone levels during pregnancy, and lower infant birth weight (Chevrier et al., 2010; Harley et al., 2011; Harley et al., 2010).

A prospective cohort study from the Netherlands reported that brominated fire retardants (BFRs) were correlated with worse fine manipulative abilities and attention, but better coordination, visual perception, and behavior depending on the specific PBDE congener or other BFR (Roze et al., 2009). The conflicting data may be due to other unmeasured developmental toxicants such as methyl mercury.

Herbstman and colleagues prospectively followed a 9/11 cohort of mothers and their infants/children evaluating cord blood PBDE levels and neurodevelopmental testing. Depending on the specific PBDE congener, the researchers found that children who had the highest quintile of cord blood concentrations of BDEs 47, 99, or 100, had significantly lower developmental scores compared with children who were in the lower 80% of exposure. After adjustment for potential confounders, children with higher concentrations of BDEs 47, 99, or 100 scored lower on tests of mental and physical development at 12, 48, and 72 months. Associations were significant for 12-month Psychomotor Development Index (BDE-47), 24-month Mental Development Index (MDI) (BDE-47, 99, and 100), 36-month MDI (BDE-100), 48-month full-scale and verbal IQ (BDE-47, 99, and 100), performance IQ (BDE-100), and 72-month performance IQ (BDE-100) (Herbstman et al., 2010).

Flame-retarding compounds have often been compared to PCBs in their adverse perturbations of thyroid hormone. Transplacental transfer of maternal thyroid hormone is essential for normal fetal brain development, and even subtle variations in thyroid hormone may result in neurodevelopmental impairment (Janssen, 2005).

Solvents

Solvents are carbon-based substances that dissolve other substances. They are present in products such as paints, varnishes, lacquers, adhesives, glues, and cleaning agents (NIOSH, 2013). Solvents are also used in the production of dyes, polymers, plastics, textiles, printing inks, agricultural products, and pharmaceuticals (NIOSH, 2013). There are many different classes of organic solvents (including chlorinated hydrocarbons, aliphatic hydrocarbons, aromatic hydrocarbons, alcohols, glycols, ethers, esters, ethers, and ketones). According to NIOSH, 9.8 million workers in the United States were exposed to organic solvents in the first half of the 1970s (NIOSH, 1987). Because solvents are used in many applications, they have become predominant contaminants of industrial waste sites and nearby soil and groundwater (Stillerman et al., 2008).

The acute neurotoxic effects of organic solvent exposure in animal models include central nervous system depression, respiratory arrest, and at high concentrations, death (Desrosiers et al., 2012). Organic solvents recognized as carcinogens by NIOSH include benzene, carbon tetrachloride, trichloroethylene, and 1,1,2,2-tetrachloroethane (Desrosiers et al., 2012). A summary of epidemiological studies shows an association between solvents and the development of multiple sclerosis and systemic sclerosis (Miller et al., 2010).

Other health effects of solvents continue to be studied, most notably reproductive effects. Research studies have demonstrated a significant association between maternal occupational exposure to organic solvents and major congenital malformations such as cardiovascular anomalies (including ventricular septal defect), neural tube defects, and gastrointestinal abnormalities (such as diaphragmatic hernia), among others (Khattak et al., 1999; McMartin, Chu, Kopecky, Einarson, & Koren, 1998).

Phthalates

Phthalates are carbon-based compounds used in plastics to make them flexible and durable (US EPA, 2007). High-molecular-weight phthalates are primarily used in the manufacturing of polyvinyl chloride, which is present in medical equipment (such as IV tubing), flooring and wall coverings, and food storage products (Agency for Toxic Substances and Disease Registry, 2002). Low-molecular-weight phthalates are solvents used to develop cosmetics, lacquers, and varnishes (Agency for Toxic Substances and Disease Registry, 2001). Exposures to phthalates occur in a variety of ways. The main route of exposure is via ingestion, as phthalates commonly leach into foods heated in plastic containers. Phthalate exposure via inhalation can occur when nail polish or hair spray volatilizes. Phthalates can be absorbed into the bloodstream from IV tubing. Dermal exposures from lotions and other cosmetics also need to be considered. Finally, phthalates have been identified and quantified in both dust and indoor air in home environments (Rudel, Camann, Spengler, Korn, Brody, 2003).

An epidemiological review of health effects from developmental phthalate exposure found childhood phthalate exposure increased the risk of allergic disease and airway inflammation (Bornehag & Nanberg, 2010). Prenatal exposures to certain phthalates significantly increased the risk of childhood asthma in an inner city cohort (Whyatt et al., 2014).

Additionally, *in utero* exposure has been associated with altered genital development (specifically reduced male anogenital distance) and behavior development (such as ADHD or internalizing behaviors, such as social withdrawal or somaticizing) (Braun, Sathyanarayana, & Hauser, 2013). The increased incidence of cryptorchidism, hypospadias, and low sperm count is hypothesized (based on animal modeling), to be due in part to gestational exposure to certain phthalates (Sharpe & Skakkebaek, 2008).

Water Contaminants

An epidemiological study looked at contaminated drinking water events between 1997 and 2007 and examined birth records for New Jersey during that time period. Associations between maternal exposure to contaminated water were identified, including a 14% increase in low birth weight as well as a 10% increase in prematurity (Currie, Graff, Meckel, Neidell, & Schlenker, 2013). Perchlorate, a by-product of jet fuel, is found in approximately 4% of US public water systems, and in one study, higher levels of maternal perchlorate were associated with lower IQ levels at age 3 (Taylor et al., 2014).

With increasing human population, water utilities have struggled to meet the rising demand for treated water. Before treatment, water usually contains dissolved organic and inorganic material, mostly from industrial waste. To disinfect, water is commonly treated with chlorination. As a result, chlorinated by-products are present in treated water, including trihalomethanes (THM) and haloacetic acids (HAA). These chlorinated by-products exhibit greater toxicity than their precursors by virtue of their increased lipophilicity; thus they have a better ability to permeate biological membranes (Tillner et al., 2013). As a result, they can cause adverse health effects in humans, damaging the central nervous system, liver, and kidneys and increasing cancer risk (US EPA, 2013b).

There have been a number of incidents over the past few decades of chemicals accidentally leaching into the water supply. A recent example occurred in West Virginia in early 2014, when a tank storing crude 4-methylcyclohexanemethanol (MCHM) leaked into the Elk River. The tank,

---

Box 35.5 Camp Lejeune—Example of Accidental Water Contamination

Contamination of the drinking water at the Camp Lejeune Marine Corps Base in North Carolina from 1953 to 1987 was primarily due to the solvents PCE (perchloroethylene or tetrachloroethylene) and TCE (trichloroethylene). Other contaminants in the drinking water included benzene and the TCE degradation products trans-1, 2-DCE (t-1, 2-dichloroethylene), and vinyl chloride. Water contamination was traced to a variety of sources, including an off-base dry cleaners and military activities (Agency for Toxic Substances and Disease Registry, 2014).

The ATSDR recently released the results of a case-control study of children born from 1968 to 1985 to mothers who had consumed Camp Lejeune's contaminated drinking water. Based on water-modeling exposures and documented birth defects or childhood cancers, the researchers concluded that first trimester exposure to benzene or TCE increased the risk of neural tube defects (odds ratio [OR] respectively = 4.1 and 2.4). Exposure to TCE (OR = 1.6) or vinyl chloride (OR = 1.6) during early gestation increased the risk of childhood hematopoietic cancers (Ruckart, Bove, & Maslia, 2013).

Mortality outcomes of active duty and other military personnel who were stationed at Camp Lejeune from 1975 to 1985 were evaluated and compared with a similar unexposed cohort from Camp Pendleton, California. There were elevated hazard ratios for cancers of the kidney, liver, esophagus, and cervix; multiple myeloma; Hodgkin's lymphoma; and amyotrophic lateral sclerosis (ALS) (Bove, Ruckart, Maslia, & Larson, 2014).

---

owned by Freedom Industries, was located about 1.5 miles upstream from the intake pipe for Charleston, West Virginia water supply system (Tullo, Kemsley, Hogue, & Morrissey, 2014).

Air Pollution

Air pollution exposure (both outdoor and indoor), has been responsible for increasing morbidity and mortality worldwide. Air pollution consists of the following: particulate matter and gases (including carbon monoxide [CO], ozone [O_3], nitrogen dioxide [NO_2], and sulfur dioxide [SO_2]). Air pollution has been implicated in many studies over the past 20 years as a cause of cardiovascular and pulmonary disease in adults (Adar, Filigrana, Clements, & Peel, 2014; Uzoigwe, Prum, Bresnahan, & Garelnabi, 2013).

Several studies support the links between maternal exposure to air pollution and adverse birth outcomes. A meta-analysis using information from 14 centers and approximately three million births found that exposure to

particulate matter (PM 10 micron and 2.5 micron) from air pollution is associated with low birth weight at term (Dadvand et al., 2013). Two case-controlled
studies support the association between gestational and/or early life exposures
with autism (Becerra et al., 2013; Volk et al., 2013). Additionally, epidemiological studies indicate associations between gestational particulate matter (PM
10 and PM 2.5) exposure and congenital heart defects (Agay-Shay et al., 2013;
Padula et al., 2013).

Household air pollution (HAP) is derived from burning various biomass
fuels to cook or heat the home, such as wood and coal in North America or
dung, crop residue, or kerosene in developing countries. Combustion of these
products results in release of small particulate matter, carbon monoxide, and

---

Box 35.6 Health Effects of Fracking

Hydraulic fracturing or "fracking" is a complex process that extracts natural gas from
deep within the earth by drilling into rock formations and pumping water and chemicals that "fracture" the rocks and release natural gas. According to the US EPA, there
are five stages during fracking that may have an adverse effect on water supply and
quality. Concerns exist about the chemical additives and other particulate substances
that are added to water to facilitate the fracking process. Natural substances (such as
heavy metals and radioactive materials in the rock) may be unintentionally mobilized
and contaminate the water. Furthermore, disinfection by-products are formed after
the water has gone through the wastewater treatment cycle.

Recent research has found that even though fracking wastewater is diluted up to
10,000 times more than municipal wastewater, the higher concentrations of halides
present in the fracking wastewater can form toxic disinfection by-products, exceeding levels allowed for drinking water treatment plants (Parker, Zeng, Harkness,
Vengosh, & Mitch, 2014). At present, the US EPA does not regulate the injection of
fracking chemicals under the Safe Drinking Water Act (US EPA, 2014b).

Air quality and pollution is also of concern. Fracking releases methane from the
rock, which contributes to global warming. Hazardous and criteria air pollutants are
released either as part of the fracking process or from the machinery and trucks used
in this industry. Overall, 40% of US methane and the majority of industrially produced volatile organic compounds (VOCs) are produced or released from the oil and
natural gas industries (Weinhold, 2012).

There are few epidemiological studies evaluating prenatal exposure to natural gas
development and adverse birth outcomes. A recent study showed positive associations of density and proximity to fracking sites (within a 10-mile radius of maternal
residence) to congenital heart defects (CHD). Either benzene or components of air
pollution are the possible toxicants, given numerous studies implicating them as contributors to CHD (McKenzie et al., 2014).

endotoxins. The adverse health effects mirror those from tobacco use and include pneumonia, COPD, asthma, cancer, TB, and cardiovascular disease. Household air pollution is a significant problem in developing countries, and technological strategies have been developed (including more renewable fuels and fuel-efficient biomass cook stoves). In the United States, those who live in impoverished and/or rural areas are most likely to be exposed to HAP. For the average American, precautions should be provided regarding the use of an indoor wood stove that is not properly ventilated and recommendations to avoid burning paper (which releases dioxins) (Mortimer et al., 2012).

Bisphenol A

Bisphenol A is a carbon-based synthetic compound that is the building block for many plastic-based products, including polycarbonate and polyester. It is most commonly used in food packaging, paper receipts, and as a dental sealant. Research over the past 25 years has found that when plastic containers are exposed to high temperatures (such as in a microwave), BPA molecules can shed and leach out. As a result, BPA can be ingested and absorbed into the human body. The CDC has found that traces of BPA (between 33–80 ng/kg of weight) are present in the vast majority of Americans; this level is 1,000 times lower than the threshold found to cause deleterious health effects (as recommended by the US EPA and the European Union's Food Safety Authority (Biello, 2008; CDC, 2013a). However, endocrine disruptors can act in the PPB level, which may pose concern for current BPA exposures.

Bisphenol A has a chemical structure similar to both estrogen and DES and is a known endocrine disruptor (Figure 35.1).

According to one review article, there is robust evidence that BPA is an "ovarian toxicant" (Peretz et al., 2014). Research has found that either in animal models or humans, BPA perturbs ovarian meiosis, germ cell nest breakdown, follicle transition, steroidogenesis, and oocyte quality. In animal models, BPA is a "uterine toxicant" in that it perturbs endometrial cellular proliferation, uterine receptivity, and uterine gene expression and increases implantation failure.

In addition to interacting with estrogenic pathways, BPA has been found to interact with over 1,200 specific genes/proteins including those influencing progesterone, androgen, and thyroid hormone receptors, as well as growth hormone, prolactin, tumor necrosis factor, interleukin, cytochrome P450, and insulin-like growth factor (Singh & Li, 2012).

Evolving toxicological and epidemiological research is supporting the role of early life BPA exposures in perturbation of neurodevelopment, sexual

A. Estradiol

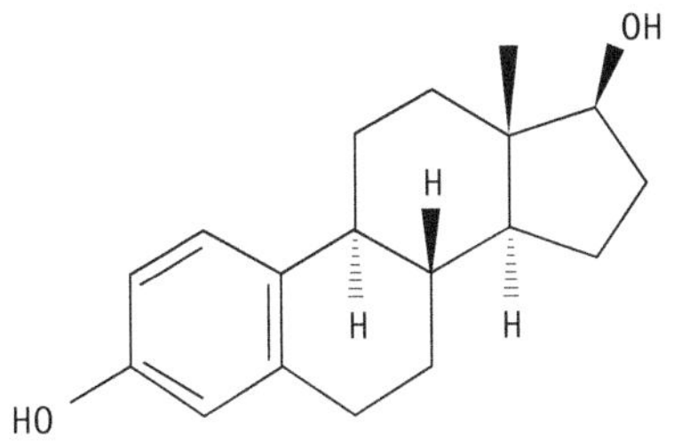

B. Diethylstilbestrol (DES)

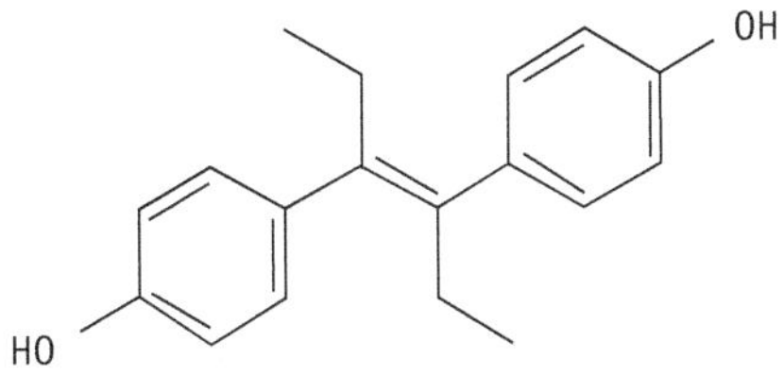

C. Bisphenol A

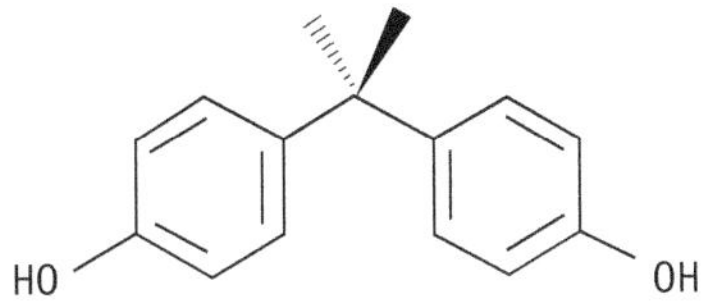

FIGURE 35.1. Chemical structures of estradiol (a), diethylstilbestrol (DES) (b), and bisphenol A (c).

A. Estradiol. *Source:* Description—English: Structure of estradiol; Date— June 29, 2007; *Source*—own work; Author—NEUROtiker This image was obtained in the public domain. The person who associated a work with this image has dedicated the work to the public domain by waiving all of his or her rights to the work worldwide under copyright law, including all related and neighboring rights, to the extent allowed by law.

All the information in each box was sourced and compiled by Drs. Berenji and Perron.

B. Diethylstilbestrol (DES)
Source: Description—English: Structure of Diethylstilbestrol; Date—January 25, 2015, *Source*—own work; Author—Kopiersperre(talk)

differentiation/behavior, and immune function (Kundakovic & Champagne, 2011). In addition to epigenetic mechanisms, animal research has demonstrated that BPA may influence neurodevelopment through inactivation of the X-chromosome (Kumamoto & Oshio, 2013).

Arsenic

Arsenic is a heavy metal that has been used as a medicinal agent, a pigment, and a pesticide. It is usually combined with other metals (such as copper or lead) to yield a highly durable alloy. Both organic and inorganic arsenic are identified contaminants in food (e.g. shellfish, rice) and water (Gilbert-Diamonda, Cottingham, Gruber, & Punshon, 2011). Most arsenic in groundwater is the result of natural erosion. While organic arsenic is relatively innocuous, inorganic arsenic is toxic at high concentrations. It can lead to serious health effects, including neurological, dermatologic, gastrointestinal, renal, pulmonary, and hematopoietic complications in adults (US EPA, 2012a).

A recent study demonstrated that long-term, low-level exposure to arsenic in groundwater can lead to neurological damage in adults, including lower scores in global cognition, processing speed, short-term memory formation, language, visuospatial skills, and executive functioning (O'Bryant, Edwards, Menon, Gong, & Barber, 2011). Prenatal exposures to high levels of arsenic via contaminated drinking water is well known to be associated with an elevated risk of respiratory disease, impaired lung function,

FIGURE 35.1. Continued

This image was obtained in the public domain. The person who associated a work with this image has dedicated the work to the public domain by waiving all of his or her rights to the work worldwide under copyright law, including all related and neighboring rights, to the extent allowed by law.

All the information in each box was sourced and compiled by Drs. Berenji and Perron.

C. Bisphenol A (BPA)
Source: Description—English: Skeletal Structure of Bisphenol A; Date—March 20, 2013; *Source*—own work; Author—darkness3560. This image was obtained in the public domain. The person who associated a work with this image has dedicated the work to the public domain by waiving all of his or her rights to the work worldwide under copyright law, including all related and neighboring rights, to the extent allowed by law.

All the information in each box was sourced and compiled by Drs. Berenji and Perron.

various cancers, and cardiovascular disease later in life (Farzan, Karagas, & Chen, 2013).

The research confirming the robust associations found in animal studies between developmental arsenic exposure and adverse birth outcomes in humans is beginning to emerge. In a Taiwanese population, biomarkers of maternal arsenic exposure were associated with adverse birth outcomes, including a significant risk of lower 1-minute Apgar scores (Chou et al., 2014). Another study found a significant association between expression of a placental gene and low infant birth weight (Fei, Koestler, Li, & Giambelli, 2013).

Special Topic: Breast Cancer and the Environment

That breast cancer risk is associated with age, reproductive history, breast-feeding, dietary choices, obesity, alcohol use, family history, breast density, certain benign breast lesions, ionizing radiation exposure, and use of hormonal medications is well-accepted (American Cancer Society, 2014a). Less appreciated is the research showing that environmental chemicals and toxicant exposures during vulnerable windows of susceptibility (*in utero*, early childhood, puberty, and lactation) likely play a significantly larger role in the development of breast cancer than once thought (Fenton, 2006; Gray, 2010; Hiatt, 2011).

Epidemiological evidence for the causal pathway from toxicant exposure to breast cancer is sparse because of the long latency from exposure to disease, the methodological weakness of retrospective studies, the complexity of chemical mixtures that humans are exposed to, and the ethical issues precluding deliberate exposure of human subjects to known toxicants (Gray, 2010; Hiatt, 2011). Consequently, much of the support linking environmental chemical exposure to breast cancer comes from animal bioassays.

Breast cancer outcomes in humans can be anticipated by identifying those chemicals that are carcinogenic in animals. As of 2007, among chemicals tested in animal cancer bioassays, 216 have been found to be associated with mammary gland tumors in at least one animal study; 29 are produced in the United States in volumes exceeding one million pounds per year; 35 are air pollutants; 25 have been associated with occupational exposures affecting more than 5,000 women per year; and 73 have been present in consumer products or as contaminants of food (Rudel, Attfield, Schifano, & Brody, 2007). Very few of the chemicals identified as animal mammary gland carcinogens or endocrine disruptors have ever been included in a human breast cancer study; the limited existing studies are often plagued by a lack of accurate measures of exposure (Brody et al., 2007).

Bisphenol A is an example of a high-volume, endocrine-disrupting chemical. It acts as an agonist for the nuclear estrogen receptors ER-alpha and ER-beta and is similar in structure to DES and estradiol (Prins & Calderon, 2010). Examination of mammary gland tissue from rodents exposed to BPA during susceptible windows of development revealed a substantial increase in the number of hyperplastic ducts in adulthood that progressed to carcinoma in situ (Murray, Maffini, & Ucci, 2007). The rodents also have increased susceptibility to known carcinogens and increased sensitivity to estrogen exposure in puberty (Durando, Kass, & Piva, 2007; Soto, Vandenberg, & Maffini, 2008).

Atrazine, a widely used herbicide in the United States, is another endocrine disruptor of concern due to its significant contamination of ground and surface water (Natural Resources Defense Council, 2009). Numerous rodent studies have shown that atrazine alters the developing mammary gland, makes it more susceptible to tumorigenesis or hyperplasia, and changes lactational ability. The likely mechanism of action in rodents is perturbation of hypothalamic control of luteinizing hormone and prolactin (Raynor & Fenton, 2011).

Additional evidence that exposure to environmental chemicals is associated with breast cancer comes from therapeutic, incidental, or occupational exposures. Recently, three cohort studies of DES-exposed and -unexposed women were combined, allowing evaluation of several reproductive outcomes, including breast cancer (Hoover et al., 2011). Prenatally exposed women, especially those with clinical evidence of vaginal epithelial changes at a young age (which is a marker of high DES dose and exposure early in gestation) had significantly higher risks than those without vaginal epithelial changes. The authors found a 1.7% excess risk for breast cancer in women over the age of 40 attributable to prenatal DES exposure.

Additional support for early life exposure to toxicants and later breast cancer comes from an analysis of DDT and its metabolite levels in a cohort of pregnant women between 1959 and 1967, a time of peak DDT use in the United States (Cohn, Wolff, Cirillo, & Sholtz, 2007). High levels of serum DDT compounds predicted a statistically- significant five-fold increased risk of breast cancer before the age of 50 among women who were born after 1931 and in particular were under the age of 14 at time of exposure. Women not exposed to DDT before 14 years of age showed no association between DDT and breast cancer ($p = .02$ for difference by age).

Early puberty, a known risk factor for breast cancer, is associated with exposure to certain endocrine disruptors, especially those found in personal care products (such as phthalates) (Hiatt, 2011; Wolff et al., 2010).

A 2007 comprehensive and systematic review of the current human evidence was carried out by Brody and coauthors; they found the evidence supports an association between exposure to polycyclic aromatic hydrocarbons (combustion products) and breast cancer in women with suboptimal DNA repair genetic variations. There were also strong associations between exposure to PCBs and breast cancer in women who were carriers of certain genetic variants (Brody et al., 2007). The evidence linking dioxins and organic solvents to breast cancer was considered sparse and methodologically limited, but was suggestive of an association (Warner, Mocarelli, & Samuels, 2011).

A recent follow-up of a cohort exposed to dioxins during a 1976 industrial accident in Italy found the hazard ratio (HR) for breast cancer, was increased, but not significantly (adjusted HR = 1.44, 95% confidence interval [CI]: 0.89, 2.33) (Warner et al., 2011).

The majority of studies evaluating the associations between occupation and resultant breast cancer have been inconclusive. A large population-based, case-control study was conducted in France looking at occupational exposures and risk of breast cancer (Villeneuve et al., 2011). An elevated incidence of breast cancer was found in women working in the manufacture and use of chemicals, such as nurses (OR 2.1 [1.3–3.4]), women who worked 10 or more years in the manufacture of motor vehicles (OR 2.6 [1.0–6.3]) or in the manufacture of other nonmetallic mineral products such as ceramics, cement, or stone products (OR 2.8 [1.1–7.4]). There was some indication of a dose-response trend with duration of employment in the latter industry. Conversely, women working in agriculture were at decreased risk (OR 0.7 [0.6–0.9]) (Villeneuve et al., 2011). A Canadian case-control study found an increased risk of breast cancer for women employed in agriculture, bars and gambling, automotive plastics manufacturing, food canning, and metalworking industries (Brophy et al., 2012). Premenopausal breast cancer was particularly high for women employed in the automotive plastics (OR 4.76 [1.58–14.4]) and food canning (OR 5.70 [1.03–31.5]) sectors.

Special Topic: Maternal and Paternal Occupational Exposures and Birth Defects

The National Birth Defects Prevention Study (NBDPS) is one of the premier observational studies looking at birth defect outcomes among US-born offspring, analyzing data from infants born between 1997 and 2011 (CDC, 2014b). Background information from the respective mothers and fathers has also been collected to better understand what potential risk factors may lead to birth defects. Studies have been conducted using the NBDPS data to identify whether there are associations between maternal/paternal occupational exposures and birth defects (see Boxes 35.7 and 35.8).

Another study reviewing the same data in NBDPS found maternal exposure to organic solvents 1 month prior to conception through the first trimester of pregnancy was a significant risk factor for congenital heart defects in the offspring (Gilboa et al., 2012). This same study group also examined the relationship between maternal solvent exposure and risk of neural tube defects and found periconception exposure to chlorinated solvents was associated with an increased risk of neural tube defects, especially spina bifida (Desrosiers et al., 2012).

Box 35.7 National Birth Defects Prevention Study—Significant Associations Between Maternal Occupation and Birth Defects During the Critical Period (by Specific Condition)

Occupation	Birth Defect
Administrative support	Craniosynostosis
Chemical/semiconductor workers	Neural tube defects
Dry cleaners	Esophageal atresia
Electrical equipment operators	Encephalocele, Neural tube defects, Left ventricular outflow tract obstruction
Food servers/processors	Anomalous pulmonary venous return, Gastroschisis
Healthcare workers	Hydrocephalus, Transverse limb deficiency
Janitors, Cleaners	Anopthalmia/Microopthalmia, Anorectal atresia, Anotia/Microtia, Glaucoma, Oral clefts
Landscapers	Intestinal atresia
Managers	Anotia/Microtia
Manufacturing/Transportation Workers	Anotia/Microtia
Office, other	Cataract, Diaphragmatic hernia
Personal Service/Athletes	Cleft palate, Duodenal atresia/stenosis, Gastroschisis
Scientists	Anorectal atresia, Atrioventricular septal defect, Bladder exstrophy, Conotruncal defects

Source: Based on analysis of information in Table 5 of Herdt-Losavio et al. (2010).

Box 35.8 National Birth Defects Prevention Study—Significant Associations Between Paternal Occupation and Birth Defects During the Critical Period (by Specific Condition)

Occupation	Birth Defect
Teachers, Librarians, Artists	Anopthalmos/Micropthalmus, Anotia/Microtia, Cleft palate, Cleft lip, Bilateral renal agenesis or hypoplasia, Transverse limb deficiency, Hypoplastic left heart syndrome
Food service worker	Anotia/Microtia, Biliary Atresia, Transverse Limb Deficiency, Gastroschisis
Landscapers	Anencephaly, Biliary atresia, TAPVR, ASD
Janitors, Cleaners	Amniotic band syndrome, Craniofacial disruptions, Cleft lip
Laundry Workers	Anopthalmos/Micropthalmus
Hairdressers	Ventricular septal defect
Office Workers	Glaucoma, Hypospadias, Bladder exstrophy, Omphalocele
Shippers	Cleft lip
Farmers/Farmworkers	Anotia/Microtia
Sawmill Workers	Hypospadias
Construction Workers	Biliary atresia
Electronic Workers	Cleft lip and Cleft palate
Vehicle Mechanics	Hypospadias
Mechanics, Other	Biliary atresia, Ventricular septal defect, Atrial septal defect
Petroleum/Gas Workers	Intercalary limb deficiency, Atrial septal defect
Iron, Other Metal Workers	Single ventricle
Welders	Laterality defects with congenital heart disease
Chemical Workers	Cleft lip, Pulmonary valve stenosis
Food Processing Workers	Encephalocele, Hydrocephalus
Printers	Colonic atresia/stenosis, Tricuspid atresia
Material Moving Equipment Operators	Cleft lip, Craniosynostosis
Motor Vehicle Operators	Anencephaly, Anopthalmos/Micropthalmus, Glaucoma/Anterior chamber defects, Cleft lip and Cleft palate, Hypospadias, Transverse limb deficiency
Aircraft Operators, Crew	Anencephaly
Transportation Workers	Colonic atresia/stenosis

Source: Based on analysis of information in Table 3 of Desrosiers et al. (2012).

Precautionary Principle

We live in an ever-changing global environment. With the exponential growth in the number of chemicals and biologically modified compounds over the past 50 years, scientists are gradually developing a better understanding of how people are exposed and how these exposures, especially at low concentrations over long periods of time, can affect health. But in the meantime, how do we as a society best protect ourselves from these exposures, most of which are not even characterized? The concept of the precautionary principle (PP) has been devised to address these unknowns.

The PP proposes that "when an activity raises threats of harm to the environment or human health, precautionary measures should be taken even if some cause and effect relationships are not fully established scientifically" (Science and Environmental Health Newsletter, 1998). Initially developed as an environmental policy in Germany, it has evolved into a risk assessment strategy to address environmental and health impacts associated with new commercial products (UNESCO—World Commission on the Ethics of Scientific Knowledge and Technology, 2005). The PP is founded on biological plausibility, using available evidence from animal models and cross-sectional studies, to make reasonable conclusions about the health effects of a particular chemical or biological agent.

With the advent of new technology, the chemical properties of various hazards can now be assessed in vitro using high-throughput screening techniques. This evolving science, otherwise known as computational toxicology, applies mathematical and advanced computer models to screen thousands of chemicals for toxicity (EPA National Center for Computational Toxicology, 2014). In the coming years, environmental health professionals can use these technologies to identify potentially hazardous chemicals and develop risk assessment profiles. Hopefully the chemicals industry will use these models, as well, to reduce the likelihood of developing chemicals with endocrine-disrupting, carcinogenic, or allergenic properties.

Taking an Exposure History

Often, exposures that may be the precipitating factor leading to a patient's constellation of symptoms are inadequately explored in the clinical encounter. Symptoms may be nonspecific, and it is often difficult to directly connect them to a definitive exposure. The Agency for Toxic Substances and Disease

Registry (ATSDR), a subsidiary of the CDC, has long recognized the importance of taking a comprehensive exposure history to formulate a risk assessment. The ATSDR has developed a tutorial for healthcare providers in how to conduct an exposure history for evaluating those patients (Agency for Toxic Substances and Disease Registry, n.d.).

The basic tenets of such history-taking involve inquiring about what a person does during the course of her day. This includes asking about what a person does for a living currently and activities done outside of work (including hobbies). Past occupational history should also be obtained, including seasonal jobs, as well as military service. If a person does confirm presence of symptom(s), pertinent questions include Do your symptoms seem to be aggravated by certain activities around the home? A hobby or task? Do your symptoms change at all at work? (Agency for Toxic Substances and Disease Registry, n.d.).

CASE STUDY 1—CHEMIST EXPOSED TO VAPORS

A 32-year-old female chemist has been working at a chemical plant for the last 8 years in research and development. As part of her work, she spends more than 4 hours a day in the fume hood synthesizing new chemicals. She uses solvents, primarily toluene and xylene. Over the past few weeks, she has noticed persistent tingling sensations in both upper extremities.

Individuals who work with organic solvents at high concentrations can be at risk for neurologic sequelae. The concentration and duration of the exposure need to be taken into account. If the chemist spent even an hour working with those organic solvents in a fume hood that was not functioning properly, she likely inhaled a significant amount of the vapors. In this situation, it would be recommended that the chemist ask facilities management to evaluate the ventilation of the fume hood to ensure that it is working properly. Safety specialists (such as industrial hygienists) can assist in doing air monitoring. The chemist would need to be medically evaluated for her neurological symptoms. A work illness report should be filed, which will then be logged into the employer's Occupational and Safety Health Administration's "Log 300" (a compilation of reportable illnesses/injuries).

CASE STUDY 2—ONCOLOGY NURSE WORKING WITH ANTINEOPLASTIC DRUGS

A 52-year-old female oncology nurse works in the adult inpatient oncology unit. As part of her job, she administers antineoplastic agents to patients. She works primarily with lymphoma patients and administers medications including rituximab, cyclophosphamide, doxirubicin, and vincristine. She receives the drugs from the pharmacy and prepares the formulations wearing gloves in a biosafety cabinet. She then goes to the patient's room to administer the agents intravenously. As she is about to hook-up the vincristine IV bag, the IV tube disconnects, and the vincristine spills onto the patient's bed and floor and some of the vincristine spills onto the nurses hands, wrists, and forearms. The nurse is able to reconnect the tubing. She washes her hands afterward. About an hour later, she notices a rash on both her wrists and forearms. She is otherwise not in acute distress.

In this case, the employee should go see a healthcare provider (ideally occupational/employee health) for an assessment and treatment. Given the history, this is likely a work-related incident and a work injury/illness report should be filed. A full history and physical should be obtained. The healthcare provider should treat symptomatically and refer to an occupational dermatologist. Only a limited number of studies have examined acute and chronic health effects related to occupational exposure to antineoplastic agents, including reproductive effects and risk of cancer development (CDC, 2013b).

Home Exposures

The home environment is a potential source of chemical exposures. If built before 1978, there may be lead paint on the walls and doors. Currently in the United States, 24 million housing units have deteriorated lead paint and elevated levels of lead-contaminated house dust. Lead in the home setting is of particular concern to families with young children, because any lead exposure, no matter how small, can lead to neurological and cognitive deficits in addition to other systemic effects (CDC, 2014a).

Question your patients about the environment surrounding their workplace and/or home. For example, a patient who works as an administrative assistant at an accounting firm, which is in close vicinity to a chemical plant that produces pesticides, presented with persistent headaches, nausea, and vomiting. In assessing the patient, environmental exposures are considered potential causative agents for her symptoms. The careful history of a provider schooled in environmental health prevented missing pertinent occupational information in this clinical encounter. In this case, the employee was referred to an occupational/employee health physician for assessment and treatment.

Exposure Reduction Recommendations

Despite the limited epidemiological evidence implicating exposure to environmental chemicals with adverse human health effects meeting the Bradford Hill criteria for causation (including strength of association, temporality, biological plausibility), there is precautionary information that healthcare providers can use to advise patients to reduce the risk of exposure for themselves and their families. Exposures can be greatly reduced by eating organic produce and eliminating food packaging (canned food and plastic wrap), a source of BPA and phthalate exposures (Lu et al., 2006; Rudel et al., 2011).

Additional recommendations supported by evidence include the following (Children's Health Protection Advisory Committee Letters, 2013; Gray, 2010; Program on Reproductive Health and the Environment, 2014; Sathyanarayana, Focareta, Dailey, & Buchanan, 2012):

- Wash hands frequently with plain soap and water.
- Eat hormone free meat and dairy.
- Avoid mercury by only eating fish low in mercury.
- Reduce consumption of animal fat.
- Use stainless steel or glass containers.
- Remove shoes before coming in the home.
- Wet mop floors regularly and vacuum with HEPA filter.
- Avoid carpeting/furniture with flame retardants.
- Subscribe to integrated pest management techniques and avoid pesticide use/application in and around the home or on pets.
- Use no-/low-VOC paint products.
- Don't burn trash.
- Test homes for radon, use carbon monoxide monitors.
- Do not microwave in plastic containers.

- Eliminate phthalate-containing household items (PVC plastic), toys, personal care products.
- Eliminate products containing "fragrance."
- Use nontoxic cleaning products.
- Avoid chemical-based dry cleaning.
- Test well water for harmful substances and use a water filtration system that removes chemicals (http://water.epa.gov/drink/info/well/faq.cfm).
- Avoid car exhaust and gasoline fumes.
- Avoid skin-lightening creams from foreign countries, which may contain mercury.
- Avoid sources of lead: pica, certain hobbies/occupations.

Summary

Environmental health is an under-taught and underconsidered area of considerable importance in women's health. The research base is ever-expanding, and understanding the science behind exposures can help clinicians better diagnose and customize treatment regimens for their patients in cases of acute exposures. In such instances, emergent medical attention is warranted and, at times, input from the local Poison Control Center can be elicited. In addition, having a strong environmental science knowledge base can help interested clinicians expand their focus from the individual patient to the community at large. Serving in such an advocacy role further advances environmental health programs nationwide. From a public health standpoint, rigorous and enforceable environmental standards can have a far-reaching and long-lasting impact on the health of our population as well as future generations both locally and globally.

Free Educational Resources

Agency for Toxic Substances and Disease Registry course: http://www.atsdr.cdc.gov/csem/exphistory/docs/exposure_history.pdf

Arizona Center for Integrative Medicine online course with 6 hours of CME/CE http://integrativemedicine.arizona.edu/education/online_courses/enviro-med.html

Pediatric Environmental Health Specialty Units, Resources for Health Professionals http://www.pehsu.net/training.html

Program on Reproductive Health and the Environment, University of California, San Francisco: http://prhe.ucsf.edu/prhe/clinical_practice.html

REFERENCES

Adar, S. D., Filigrana, P. A., Clements, N., & Peel, J. L. (2014). Ambient coarse particulate matter and human health: A systematic review and meta-analysis. *Curr Envir Health Rpt, 1,* 258–274.

Agay-Shay, K., Friger, M., Linn, S., Peled, A., et al. (2013). Air pollution and congenital heart defects. *Environ Res, 124,* 28–34.

Agency for Toxic Substances and Disease Registry. (2001). *Toxicological profile for di-n-butyl phthalate.* September 2001. Retrieved August 14, 2014, from http://www.atsdr.cdc.gov/toxprofiles/tp.asp?id=859&tid=167

Agency for Toxic Substances and Disease Registry. (2002). *Toxicological profile for di(2-ethylhexyl)phthalate (DEHP).* September 2002. Retrieved August 14, 2014, from http://www.atsdr.cdc.gov/toxprofiles/tp.asp?id=684&tid=65

Agency for Toxic Substances and Disease Registry. (2014). *Background—Camp Lejeune.* January 2014. Retrieved September 29, 2014, from http://www.atsdr.cdc.gov/sites/lejeune/background.html

Agency for Toxic Substances and Disease Registry. (n.d.). *How to take an exposure history.* Retrieved August 14, 2014, from http://www.atsdr.cdc.gov/csem/exphistory/docs/exposure_history.pdf.

Alavanja, M. C., Ross, M. K., & Bonner, M. R. (2013). Increased cancer burden among pesticide applicators and others due to pesticide exposure. *CA, Can J Clin, 63*(2), 120–142.

American Cancer Society. (2014a). *Breast cancer, Causes, risk factors, and prevention topics.* January 2014. Retrieved September 28, 2014, from http://www.cancer.org/cancer/breastcancer/detailedguide/breast-cancer-risk-factors

American Cancer Society. (2014b). *DES exposure: Questions and answers.* February 2014. Retrieved September 28, 2014, from http://www.cancer.org/cancer/cancercaUSes/othercarcinogens/medicaltreatments/des-exposure

American College of Obstetricians and Gynecologists. (2013). Committee Opinion No. 575: Exposure to Toxic Environmental Agents. *Obstet Gynecol, 122,* 931–935.

American College of Occupational and Environmental Medicine. (2011). *Reproductive and developmental hazard management guidance.* April 2011. Retrieved September 28, 2014, from http://www.acoem.org/Reproductive_Developmental_Hazard_Management.aspx

Barr, D. B. (2007). Concentrations of xenobiotic chemicals in the maternal-fetal unit. *Reprod Toxicol, 23,* 260–266.

Barry, V., Winquist, A., & Steenland, K. (2013). Perfluorooctanoic acid (PFOA) exposures and incident cancers among adults living near a chemical plant. *Environ Health Perspect, 121*(11–12), 1313–1318.

Basu, N., & Head, J. (2010). Mammalian wildlife as complementary models in environmental neurotoxicology. *Neurotoxicol Teratol, 32*, 114–119.

Becerra, T., Wilhelm, M., Olsen, J., Cockburn, M., et al. (2013). Ambient air pollution and autism in Los Angeles County, California. *Environ Health Perspect, 121*(3), 380–386.

Biello, D. (2008). *Plastic (not) fantastic: Food containers leach a potentially harmful chemical.* February 2008. Scientific American. Retrieved September 29, 2014, from http://www.scientificamerican.com/article/plastic-not-fantastic-with-bisphenol-a/

Birnbaum, L., & Bergman, A. (2010). Brominated and chlorinated flame retardants: The San Antonio Statement. *Environ Health Perspect, 118*(12), A514–A515.

Blum, A. (2014). *Viewpoints: Flame retardants are the asbestos of our time.* April 2014. Retrieved September 29, 2014, from http://generationgreen.org/2011/04/flame-retardants-the-asbestos-of-our-time/

Bornehag, C. G., & Nanberg, E. (2010). Phthalate exposure and asthma in children. *Int J Androl, 33*, 333–345.

Bove, F., Ruckart, P., Maslia, M., & Larson, T. (2014). Evaluation of mortality among marines and navy personnel exposed to contaminated drinking water at USMC base Camp Lejeune: A retrospective cohort study. *Environ Health, 13*(1), 1–14.

Braun, J., Sathyanarayana, S., & Hauser, R. (2013). Phthalate exposure and children's health. *Curr Opin Pediatr, 25*(2), 247–254.

Brody, J., Moysich, K., Humblet, O., et al. (2007). Environmental pollutants and breast cancer. *Cancer, 109*(12 Suppl), 2667–2711.

Brophy, J., Keith, M., Watterson, A., Park, R., et al. (2012). Breast cancer risk in relation to occupations with exposure to carcinogens and endocrine disruptors: A Canadian case–control study. *Environ Health Perspect, 11*, 87.

C8 Science Panel. (2013). *Probable link reports.* November 2013. Retrieved September 29, 2014, from http://www.c8sciencUS_EPAnel.org/prob_link.html

C8 Science Panel. (2013). *The science panel.* November 2013. Retrieved September 29, 2014, from http://www.c8sciencUS EPAnel.org/panel.html

Centers for Disease Control and Prevention (CDC). (2009). *National report on human exposure to environmental chemicals.* 2009. Retrieved August 1, 2014, from http://www.cdc.gov/exposurereport/pdf/FourthReport_ExecutiveSummary.pdf

Centers for Disease Control and Prevention (CDC). (2010). *Guidelines for the identification and management of lead exposure in pregnant and lactating women.* November 2010. Retrieved July 20, 2014, from http://www.cdc.gov/nceh/lead/publications/leadandpregnancy2010.pdf

Centers for Disease Control and Prevention (CDC). (2012). Lead poisoning in pregnant women who used Ayurvedic medications from India—New York City, 2011–2012. *MMWR, 61*, 641–646.

Centers for Disease Control and Prevention (CDC). (2013a). *Factsheet—Bisphenol A.* July 2013. Retrieved September 29, 2014, from http://www.cdc.gov/biomonitoring/BisphenolA_FactSheet.html

Centers for Disease Control and Prevention (CDC). (2013b). *Occupational exposure to antineoplastic agents.* October 2013. Retrieved August 14, 2014, from http://www.cdc.gov/niosh/topics/antineoplastic

Centers for Disease Control and Prevention (CDC). (2014a). *Lead—Prevention tips.* June 2014. Retrieved August 14, 2014, from http://www.cdc.gov/nceh/lead/tips.htm

Centers for Disease Control and Prevention (CDC). (2014b). *National Birth Defect Prevention Study (NBDPS).* October 2014. Retrieved November 1, 2014, from http://www.cdc.gov/ncbddd/birthdefects/nbdps.html

Chang, E. T., Hans-Olov, A., & Boffetta, P. (2014). A critical review of perfluorooctanoate and perfluorooctanesulfonate. *Crit Rev Toxicol, 44*(Suppl 1), 1–81.

Chen, Z., Myers, R., Wei, T., Bind, E., et al. (2014). Placental transfer and concentrations of cadmium, mercury, lead, and selenium in mothers, newborns, and young children. *J Expo Sci Environ Epidemiol, 24*(5), 537–544.

Chevrier, J., Harley, K. G., Bradman, A., Gharbi, M., Sjödin, A., & Eskenazi, B. (2010). Polybrominated diphenylether (PBDE) flame retardants and thyroid hormone during pregnancy. *Environ Health Perspect, 118,* 1444–1449.

Children's Health Protection Advisory Committee Letters. (2013). Retrieved September 29, 2014, from http://www2.US_EPA.gov/sites/production/files/2014-05/documents/chpac-appendix-a-prenatal-exposure-messages-2013-12-30.pdf

Chou, W. C., Chung, Y. T., Chen, H. Y., Wang, C. J., et al. (2014). Maternal arsenic exposure and DNA damage biomarkers, and the associations with birth outcomes in a general population from Taiwan. *PLoS ONE, 9*(2), e86398.

Cohn, B., Wolff, M., Cirillo, P., & Sholtz, R. (2007). DDT and breast cancer in young women: New data on the significance of age at exposure. *Environ Health Perspect, 115*(10), 1406–1414.

Costa, L. G., & Giordano, G. (2007). Developmental neurotoxicity of polybrominated diphenyl ether (PBDE) flame retardants. *Neurotoxicology, 28,* 1047–1067.

Currie, J., Graff, Z. J., Meckel, K., Neidell, M., & Schlenker, W. (2013). Something in the water: Contaminated drinking water and infant health. *Can J Econ Can d'économique, 46*(3), 791–810.

Dadvand, P., Parker, J., Bell, M., Bonzini, M., et al. (2013). Maternal exposure to particulate air pollution and term birth weight: A multi-country evaluation of effect and heterogeneity. *Environ Health Perspect, 121*(3), 267–373.

Darnerud, P. O. (2008). Brominated flame retardants as possible endocrine disrupters. *Int J Androl, 31,* 152–160.

Department of Health and Human Services, NIOSH. (2011). *NIOSH pesticide poisoning monitoring program protects farmworkers.* December 2011. Publication Number 2012–108. Retrieved August 14, 2014, from http://www.cdc.gov/niosh/docs/2012-108/

Desrosiers, T. A., Herring, A. H, Shapira, S. K., Hooiveld, M., Luben, T. J., Herdt-Losavio, M. L., ... Olshan, A. F. (2012). Paternal occupation and birth defects: Findings from the National Birth Defects Prevention Study. *Occup Environ Med, 69,* 534–542.

Desrosiers, T., Lawson, C., Meyer, R., Richardson, D., et al. (2012). Maternal occupational exposure to organic solvents during early pregnancy and risks of neural tube defects and orofacial clefts. *Occup Environ Med, 69*(7), 493–499.

Diamanti-Kandarakis, E., Bourguignon, J., Giudice, L., et al. (2009). Endocrine-disrupting chemicals: An Endocrine Society Scientific Statement. *Endocrine Rev, 30*(4), 293–342.

Dickenson, C., Woodruff, T., Stotland, N., Dobraca, D., & Das, R. (2012). Elevated mercury levels in pregnant woman linked to skin cream from Mexico. *AmJ Obstet Gynecol, 209*(2), e4–e5.

Dingemans, M. M. L., van den Berg, M., & Westerink, R. H. S. (2011). Neurotoxicity of brominated flame retardants: (In)direct effects of parent and hydroxylated poly-brominated diphenyl ethers on the (developing) nervous system. *Environ Health Perspect, 119*, 900–907.

Durando, M., Kass, L., & Piva, J. (2007). Prenatal bisphenol A exposure induces pre-neoplastic lesions in the mammary gland in Wistar rats. *Environ Health Perspect, 115*(1), 80–86.

Emory, Rollins School of Public Health, Department of Epidemiology. (2014). *The Michigan PBB registry, research findings*. 2014. Retrieved September 29, 2014, from http://www.pbbregistry.emory.edu/Research/Research%20Findings.html

EPA National Center for Computational Toxicology. (2014). Retrieved August 14, 2014, from http://www2.epa.gov/aboutepa/about-national-center-computational-toxicology-ncct

Farzan, S., Karagas, M., & Chen, Y. (2013). In utero and early life arsenic exposure in relation to long-term health and disease. *Toxicol Appl Pharmacol, 272*(2), 384–390.

Fei, D., Koestler, D., Li, Z., & Giambelli, C. (2013). Association between in utero arsenic exposure, placental gene expression, and infant birth weight: A US birth cohort study. *Environ Health, 12*, 58.

Fenton, S. (2006). Endocrine disrupting chemicals and mammary gland develop-ment: Early exposure and later life consequences. *Endocrinology, 147*(6 Suppl), s18–s24.

Fonnum, F., & Mariussen, E. (2009). Mechanisms involved in the neurotoxic effects of environmental toxicants such as polychlorinated biphenyls and brominated flame retardants. *J Neurochem, 111*, 1327–1347.

Gilbert-Diamonda, D., Cottingham, K., Gruber, J., & Punshon, T. (2011). Rice consump-tion contributes to arsenic exposure in US women. *PNAS, 108*(51), 20656–20660.

Gilboa, S., Desrosiers, T., Lawson, C., Lupo, P., et al. (2012). Association between maternal occupational exposure to organic solvents and congenital heart defects, National Birth Defects Prevention Study, 1997–2002. *Occup Environ Med, 69*(9), 628–635.

Grandjean, P., & Landrigan, P. J. (2006). Developmental neurotoxicity of industrial chemicals. *Lancet, 368*(9553), 2167–2178.

Grandjean, P., & Landrigan, P. (2014). Neurobehavioural effects of developmental tox-icity. *Lancet, 13*(3), 330–338.

Gray, J. (2010). *State of the evidence: The connection between breast cancer and the envi-ronment*. San Francisco: Breast Cancer Fund.

Gulson, B., Jameson, C., Mahaffey, K., Mizon, K., & Korsch, M. (1997). Pregnancy increases mobilization of lead from maternal skeleton. *J Lab Clin Med, 130*(1), 51–62.

Harley, K. G., Huen, K., Schall, R. A., Holland, N. T., Bradman, A., & Barr, D. B. (2011). Association of organophosphate pesticide exposure and paraoxonase with birth outcome in Mexican-American women. *PLoS One, 6*, e23923.

Harley, K. G., Marks, A. R., Chevirer, J., Bradman, A., Sjodin, A., & Eskenazi, B. (2010). PBDE concentrations in women's serum and fecundability. *Environ Health Perspect, 118*, 699–704.

Herbstman, J., Sjödin, A., Kurzon, M., et al. (2010). Prenatal exposure to PBDEs and neurodevelopment. *Environ Health Perspect, 118*(5), 712–719.

Herdt-Losavio, M. L., Lin, S., Chapman, B. R., Hooiveld, M., Olshan, A., Liu, X., ... Druschel, C. M. (2010). Maternal occupation and the risk of birth defects: An overview from the National Birth Defects Prevention Study. *Occup Environ Med, 67*, 158–166.

Hiatt, R. (2011). Epidemiologic basis of the role of endocrine disruptors. In J. Russo (Ed.), *Environment and breast cancer*. New York: Springer.

Hoover, R. N., Hyer, M., Pfeiffer, R. M., et al. (2011). Adverse health outcomes in women exposed in utero to diethylstilbestrol. *N Engl J Med, 365*(14), 1304–1314.

Janssen, S. (2005). *Brominated flame retardants: Rising levels of concern*. June 2005 Retrieved September 29, 2014, from http://www.noharm.org/lib/downloads/bfrs/BFRs_Rising_Concern.pdf

Khattak, S., K-Moghtader, G., McMartin, K., et al. (1999). Pregnancy outcome following gestational exposure to organic solvents: A prospective controlled study. *JAMA, 281*, 1106–1109.

Kumamoto, T., & Oshio, S. (2013). Effect of fetal exposure to bisphenol A on brain mediated by X-chromosome inactivation. *J Toxicol Sci, 38*(3), 485–494.

Kundakovic, M., & Champagne, F. (2011). Epigenetic perspective on the developmental effects of bisphenol A. *Brain Behav Immun, 25*(6), 1084–1093.

Legler, J. (2008). New insights into the endocrine disrupting effects of brominated flame retardants. *Chemosphere, 73*, 216–222.

Lu, C., Toepel, K., Irish, R., et al. (2006). Organic diets significantly lower children's dietary exposure to organophosphorus pesticides. *Environ Health Perspect, 114*(2), 260–263.

McDiarmid, M. A., & Gehle, K. (2006). Preconception brief: Occupational/environmental exposures. *Matern Child Health J, 10*, S123–S128.

McKenzie, L., Guo, R., Witter R., Savitz, D., et al. (2014). Birth outcomes and maternal residential proximity to natural gas development in rural Colorado. *Environ Health Perspect, 122*(4), 412–417.

McMartin, K. I., Chu, M., Kopecky, E., Einarson, T. R., & Koren, G. (1998). Pregnancy outcome following maternal organic solvent exposure: A meta-analysis of epidemiologic studies. *Am J Ind Med, 34*, 288–292.

Mead, M. N. (2008). Contaminants in human milk: Weighing the risks against the benefits of breastfeeding. *Environ Health Perspect, 116*(10), A426–A434.

Mendola, P., & Louis, G. (2010). Environmental contaminants, female reproductive health and fertility. In T. J. Woodruff et al. (Eds.), *Environmental impacts on reproductive health and fertility* (pp. 161–172). Cambridge, England: Cambridge University Press.

Miller, F., Alfreddsson, L., Costenbader, K., et al. (2010). Epidemiology of environmental exposures and human autoimmune diseases: Findings from a National Institute of Environmental Health Sciences Expert Panel Workshop. *J Autoimmun, 39*(4), 259–271.

Mortimer, K., Gordon, S., Jindal, S., Accinelli, R., et al. (2012). Household air pollution is a major avoidable risk factor for cardiorespiratory disease. *Chest, 142*(5), 1308–1315.

Murray, T., Maffini, M., & Ucci, A. (2007). Induction of mammary gland ductal hyperplasias and carcinomas in situ following fetal bisphenol A exposure. *Reprod Toxicol, 23*(3), 383–390.

National Institute for Environmental Health Sciences (NIEHS). (n.d.). *Endocrine disruptors.* Retrieved July 18, 2014, from http://www.niehs.nih.gov/health/topics/agents/endocrine/

National Institute for Occupational Safety and Health (NIOSH). (2013). *Organic solvents.* December 2013. Retrieved August 14, 2014, from http://www.cdc.gov/niosh/topics/organsolv/

National Institute for Occupational Safety Health (NIOSH). (1987). *Organic solvent neurotoxicity.* March 1987. Retrieved August 14, 2014, from http://www.cdc.gov/niosh/docs/87-104/

National Research Council. (2000). *Scientific frontiers in developmental toxicology and risk assessment.* Washington, DC: National Academies Press.

National Toxicology Program. (n.d.). *About the NTP.* Retrieved June 27, 2014, from http://ntp.niehs.nih.gov/about/index.html

Natural Resources Defense Council. (2009). *Atrazine, poisoning the well.* August 2009. Retrieved September 29 2014, from http://www.nrdc.org/health/atrazine/

Newbold, R., & Heindal, J. (2010). Developmental exposures and implications for early and latent disease. In T. J. Woodruff et al. (Eds.), *Environmental impacts on reproductive health and fertility* (pp. 92–102). Cambridge: Cambridge University Press.

O'Bryant, S. E., Edwards, M., Menon, C. V., Gong, G., & Barber, R. (2011). Long-term low-level arsenic exposure is associated with poorer neuropsychological functioning: A project FRONTIER study. *Int J Environ Res Public Health, 8*, 861–874.

Padula, A., Trager, I., Carmichael, S., Hammond, K., et al. (2013). Ambient air pollution and traffic exposures and congenital heart defects in the San Joaquin Valley of California. *Paediatr Perinat Epidemiol, 27*(4): 329–339.

Painter, R. C., Roseboom, T. J., & Bleker, O. P. (2005). Prenatal exposure to the Dutch famine and disease in later life: An overview. *Reprod Toxicol, 20*(3) 20(3), 345–352.

Parker, K. M., Zeng, T., Harkness, J., Vengosh, A., & Mitch, W. A. (2014). Enhanced formation of disinfection byproducts in shale gas wastewater-impacted drinking water supplies. *Environ Sci Technol.* doi: 10.1021/es5028184. Published online September 9, 2014.

Peretz, J., Vrooman, L., Ricke, W., Hunt, P., et al. (2014). Bisphenol A and reproductive health: Update of experimental and human evidence, 2007–2013. *Environ Health Perspect, 122*(8), 775–786.

President's Cancer Panel. (2010). *Reducing environmental cancer risk: What we can do now.* Department of Health and Human Services, National Institutes of Health, National Cancer Institute.

Prins, G., & Calderon, E. (2010). Environmental contaminants and cancers of the reproductive tract. In T. J. Woodruff et al. (Eds.), *Environmental impacts on reproductive health and fertility* (pp. 194–213). Cambridge: Cambridge University Press.

Program on Reproductive Health and the Environment. (2014). *All that matters.* March 2014. Retrieved September 19, 2014, fromhttp://prhe.ucsf.edu/prhe/allthatmatters. html

Raynor, J., & Fenton, S. (2011). *Atrazine: An environmental endocrine disruptor that alters mammary gland development and tumor susceptibility.* New York: Springer.

Rodier, P. M. (2004). Environmental causes of central nervous system maldevelopment. *Pediatrics, 113*(4 Suppl), 1076–1083.

Rose, M., Bennett, D., Bergman, A., Fangstrom, P. I., & Hertz-Picciotto, I. (2010). PBDEs in 2–5-year-old children from California and associations with diet and indoor environment. *Environ Sci Technol, 44*(7), 2648–2653.

Roze, E., Meijer, L., Bakker, A., Van Braeckel, K., Sauer, P., & Bos, A. (2009). Prenatal exposure to organohalogens, including brominated flame retardants, influences motor, cognitive, and behavioral performance at school age. *Environ Health Perspect, 117*(12), 1953–1958.

Ruckart, P., Bove, F., & Maslia, M. (2013). Evaluation of exposure to contaminated drinking water and specific birth defects and childhood cancers at Marine Corps Base Camp Lejeune, North Carolina: A case–control study. *Environ Health, 12,* 1–10.

Rudel, R. A., Camann, D. E., Spengler, J. D., Korn, L. N., Brody, J. G. (2003). Phthalates, alkylphenols, pesticides, polybrominated diphenyl ethers, and other endocrine-disrupting compounds in indoor air and dust. *Environ Sci Technol, 37,* 4543–4553.

Rudel, R., Attfield, K., Schifano, J., & Brody, J. (2007). Chemicals causing mammary gland tumors in animals signal new directions for epidemiology, chemicals testing, and risk assessment for breast cancer prevention. *Cancer, 109*(12 Suppl), 2635–2666.

Rudel, R., Gray, J., Engel, C., et al. (2011). Food packaging and bisphenol A and bis(2-ethyhexyl) phthalate exposure: Findings from a dietary intervention. *Environ Health Perspect, 119*(7), 914–920.

Rusyniak, D., Furbee, R. B., & Pascuzzi, R. (2005). Historical neurotoxins: What we have learned from toxins of the past about diseases of the present. *Neurologic Clinics, 23,* 337–352.

Sathyanarayana, S., Focareta, J., Dailey, T., & Buchanan, S. (2012). Environmental exposures: How to counsel preconception and prenatal patients in the clinical setting. *Am J Obstet Gynecol, 207*(6), 463–470.

Schecter, A., Harris, T., Brummit, S., et al. (2008). PBDE and HBCD brominated flame retardants in the USA, Update 2008: Levels in human milk and blood, food, and environmental samples. *Epidemiology, 19,* S76.

Schettler, T. (2001). Toxic threats to neurologic development of children. *Environ Health Perspect, 109*(Suppl 6), 813–816.

Science and Environmental Health Newsletter. (1998). *The precautionary principle. The Networker*, *3*(1). March 1998. Retrieved November 1, 2014, from http://www.sehn.org/Volume_3-1.html

Sharpe, R., & Skakkebaek, N. (2008). Testicular dysgenesis syndrome: Mechanistic insights and potential new downstream effects. *Ferti Steril, 89*(2 Suppl) e33-e38.

Shaw, S., Blum, A., & Weber, R. (2010). Halogenated flame retardants: Do the fire safety benefits justify the risks? *Rev Environ Health, 25*(4), 261–305.

Singh, S., & Li, S. (2012). Bisphenol A and phthalates exhibit similar toxicogenomics and health effects. *Gene, 494*(1), 85–91.

Skinner, M., Manikkam, M., & Guerrero-Bosagna, C. (2010). Epigenetic transgenerational actions of environmental factors in disease etiology. *Trends Endocrinol Metab, 21*(4), 214–222.

Soto, A., Vandenberg, L., & Maffini, M. (2008). Does breast cancer start in the womb? *Basic Clin Pharmacol Toxicol, 18*(2), 125–133.

Stillerman, K. P., Mattison, D. R., Giudice, L. C., & Woodruff, T. J. (2008). Environmental exposures and adverse pregnancy outcomes: A review of the science. *Reprod Sci, 15*, 631–650.

Sutton, P., Perron, J., Giudice, L., & Woodruff, T. (2011). *Pesticides matter, a primer for reproductive health physicians*. December 2011. Retrieved September 29, 2014, from http://prhe.ucsf.edu/prhe/pdfs/pesticidesmatter_whitUS EPAper.pdf

Taylor, P. N., Okosieme, O. E., Murphy, R., et al. (2014). Maternal perchlorate levels in women with borderline thyroid function during pregnancy and the cognitive development of their offspring: Data from the Controlled Antenatal Thyroid Study. *J Clin Endocrinol Metab, 99*(11), 4291–4298.

Till, C., Koren, G., & Rovet, J. F. (2008). Workplace standards for exposure to toxicants during pregnancy. *CAJ Publ Health, 99*, 472–474.

Tillner, J., Hollard, C., Bach, C., Rosin, C., Munoz, J. F., & Dauchy, X. (2013). Simultaneous determination of polycyclic aromatic hydrocarbons and their chlorination by-products in drinking water and the coatings of water pipes by automated solid-phase microextraction followed by gas chromatography–mass spectrometry. *J Chromat A, 1315*, 36–46.

Trudeau, V., Kah, O., & Bourguignon, J. (2011). Neuroendocrine disruption: The emerging concept. *J Toxicol Environ Health B Crit Rev, 14*(5–7), 267–269.

Tullo, A. H., Kemsley, J., Hogue, C., & Morrissey, S. R. (2014). Obscure chemical taints water supply; Chemical contamination of West Virginia drinking water system raises scientific, policy shortcomings. *Chemical and Engineering News*. February 2014. Retrieved September 27, 2014, from http://water.epa.gov/drink/contaminants/basicinformation/disinfectionbyproducts.cfm

UNESCO—World Commission on the Ethics of Scientific Knowledge and Technology. (2005). *Precautionary principle*. March 2005. Retrieved September 29, 2014, from http://unesdoc.unesco.org/images/0013/001395/139578e.pdf

US Environmental Protection Agency (US EPA). (2007). *TEACH chemical summary—Phthalates*. March 2007. Retrieved August 14, 2014, from http://www.US EPA.gov/teach/chem_summ/phthalates_summary.pdf

US Environmental Protection Agency (US EPA). (2011). *EPA releases report containing latest estimates of pesticide use in the United States.* February 17, 2011. Retrieved August 14, 2014, from http://epa.gov/oppfead1/cb/csb_page/updates/2011/sales-usage06-07.html

US Environmental Protection Agency (US EPA). (2012a). *Arsenic compounds—Hazard summary.* December 2012. Retrieved September 29, 2014, from http://www.epa.gov/ttn/atw/hlthef/arsenic.html.

US Environmental Protection Agency (US EPA). (2012b). *Proposed Agricultural Worker Protection Standard: EPA—Illegal pesticide products.* May 2012. Retrieved August 14, 2014, from http://www.epa.gov/pesticides/health/illegalproducts/index.htm

US Environmental Protection Agency (US EPA). (2013a). *2006–2007 pesticide market estimates, table of contents (sections).* July 2013. Retrieved September 29, 2014, from http://www.US EPA.gov/opp00001/pestsales/07pestsales/table_of_contents2007.htm

US Environmental Protection Agency (US EPA). (2013b). *Basic information about disinfection byproducts in drinking water: Total trihalomethanes, haloacetic acids, bromate, and chlorite.* December 2013. Retrieved September 27, 2014, from http://water.epa.gov/drink/contaminants/basicinformation/disinfectionbyproducts.cfm

US Environmental Protection Agency (US EPA). (2014a). *Persistent organic pollutants, a global issue, a global response.* June 2014. Retrieved September 28, 2014, from http://www2.US EPA.gov/international-cooperation/persistent-organic-pollutants-global-issue-global-response#pops

US Environmental Protection Agency (US EPA). (2014b). *US EPA's study of hydraulic fracturing and its potential impact on drinking water resources.* March 2014. Retrieved September 29, 2014, from http://www2.US EPA.gov/hfstudy/hydraulic-fracturing-water-cycle

Uzoigwe, J., Prum, T., Bresnahan, E., & Garelnabi, M. (2013). The emerging role of outdoor and indoor air pollution in cardiovascular disease. *N Am J Med Sci, 5,* 445–453.

Villeneuve, S., Févotte, J., Anger, A., et al. (2011). Breast cancer risk by occupation and industry: Analysis of the CECILE study, a population-based case–control study in France. *Am J Ind Med, 54*(7), 499–509.

Volk, H., Lurmann, F., Penfold, B., Hertz-Picciotto, I., et al. (2013). Traffic-related air pollution, particulate matter, and autism. *JAMA Psychiatry, 70*(1), 71–77.

Warner, M., Mocarelli, P., & Samuels, S. (2011). Dioxin exposure and cancer risk in the Seveso Women's Health Study. *Environ Health Perspect,* 1701–1705.

Weinhold, B. (2012). The future of fracking: New rules target air emissions for cleaner natural gas production. *Environ Health Perspect, 120*(7), a272–a279.

Whyatt, R. M., Perzanowski, M. S., Just, A. C., et al. (2014). Asthma in inner-city children at 5–11 years of age and prenatal exposure to phthalates: The Columbia Center for Children's Environmental Health Cohort. *Environ Health Perspect, 122*(10):, 1141–1146.

Wolff, M., Teitelbaum, S., Pinney, S., et al. (2010). Investigation of relationships between urinary biomarkers of phytoestrogens, phthalates, and phenols and pubertal stages in girls. *Environ Health Perspect, 118*(7), 1039–1046.

Woodruff, T. J., Zota, A. R., & Schwartz, J. M. (2011). Environmental chemicals in pregnant women in the United States: NHANES 2003–2004. *Environ Health Perspect, 119,* 878–885.

World Health Organization. (2007). *Preventing disease through healthy environments: Exposure to mercury: A major public health concern.* Retrieved July 7, 2014, from http://www.who.int/phe/news/Mercury-flyer.pdf

Zoeller, T. (2010). Environmental chemicals targeting thyroid. *Hormones, 9*(1), 28–40.

36

Women, Soul Wounds, and Integrative Medicine

BEVERLY LANZETTA

It should be the obligation of all physicians to respond to, as well as attempt to relieve, all suffering if possible. Therefore, physicians should be able to communicate with their patients about their patients' spirituality as integral to the way their patients cope with suffering. To ask a patient about his or her spiritual beliefs is essential to knowing who the patient is, how the patient copes with illness, and how the patient can heal.

—Puchalski (1999).

In our various forms of contemporary analysis, we have yet to take a serious look at the effect spiritual suffering and soul wounds exert on women's health. An important fact that impedes the medical profession's recognition of the spiritual implications of women's health has to do with a Western cultural tendency to see suffering as a purely physical response to pain and to separate the spirit from the body. The effect of this split between the material and spiritual aspects of health continues to have enormous ramifications in physician care and in a woman's capacity for well-being and healing. Despite advances in understanding the cultural, economic, and racial factors that impact health, and the important strides made in recognizing gender in medicine, there continues to be a paucity of research on the more subtle violation to women's spirits and its impact on women's healthcare. This denial or refusal to discuss soul afflictions blocks women's ability to claim and name themselves as subjects of their own healing and limits the full range of medical options available to health professionals and their patients.

If spirituality is seen as just one more adjunct modality within the various complementary and alternative medical (CAM) options, it truncates the full ability of integrative medicine to actualize its potential as a healing art in two important ways. First, spirituality is selectively incorporated into the integrative model for reasons of understanding, information, or increased empathy between physicians and patients rather than being embraced as a comprehensive perspective on healing and an integral system of interpretation, diagnosis, and treatment.

Second, spirituality, when it is incorporated into Western medical models, tends to be researched and applied through a particular evidence-based lens. Research on spirituality in medicine has focused on the effect of external indicators of religious adherence or faith, such as prayer and meditation, or the efficacy of forgiveness, hope, and other virtues on health outcomes. While these studies have helped to expand the range of integrative medicine, they are not designed to take into account the more subtle but powerful care of the soul and wounding of the spirit that in traditional societies, such as the Hopi and Navajo, are always implicated in physical illness.

If integrative medicine recognizes that meaning in one's life is a positive factor in response to illness, then it must take into account how inner wounding effects the totality of women's health and healing. This chapter begins with a brief overview of current views on spirituality and integrative medicine. It then discusses a specific feminine path to healing—*via feminina*—and the destructive force of socially sanctioned violence—overt and subtle—against women's souls and its consequent physical and mental health effects. The chapter ends with positive resources for women's healing, including a description of a distinctive spiritual process of integration, the "dark night of the feminine," and some suggestions for healthcare practitioners.

Spirituality and Integrative Medicine

Integrative medicine, as practiced and defined today, is a vision of healthcare that focuses on health and healing rather than disease and values the relationship between patient and physician. It is premised on patients being treated as whole persons—minds and spirits, as well as physical bodies—who participate actively in their own health. Integrative medicine also honors the innate ability of the body to heal and integrates the best of CAM with the best of conventional medicine to facilitate long-term health outcomes (Maizes, Koffler, & Fleishman, 2002; Maizes, Schneider, et al., 2002).

One of the most significant and challenging dimensions of integrative medicine is the inclusion of spirituality in both physicians' and patients' understanding of health and healing. Numerous studies have demonstrated the positive effects prayer and meditation, and religious practice or faith in a higher power, exert on health outcomes, ability to cope with illness, and patients' reported increase of well-being (Bearon & Koenig, 1997; Benson & Stark, 1997; Dessio et al, 2004; Dossey, 1993, 1997; Levine et al., 2009; Musgrave et al., 2002). Increasingly, the spirituality of medicine—including energy medicine, mind–body medicine, therapeutic touch, homeopathy, and traditional forms of Asian healing modalities—is incorporated into the integrative model. All of these styles draw on the historical usage of "spirit" as that realm of reality associated with the breath of life. Without the spirit—the animating principle—there is no life. While many religions do not have a word corresponding to the term "spirituality," they nonetheless affirm the holiness of life and the realm of the spirit. Spirituality, then, can be defined as the core or inner life of the person, sometimes called the soul or spirit. In this definition, all beings—human and nonhuman—have an inner life and thus are imbued with spirit (Edmondson et al., 2005; Gabriel, 2000; Larson, 2003; Massey, 1996; Puchalski, 2002).

Today, spirituality is used in secular and religious contexts, and is applied across and within disciplines, including medicine and other healing arts. In a sense, "spirituality" has become a kind of universal code word to indicate the human search for meaning and purpose in life as a quest for transcendent truth. In contrast to religion, which is an institutional and culturally determined approach to faith, spirituality is found in all human societies through an individual experience of the divine, a connection to nature and, or through, religious practice.

A spiritual interpretation helps physicians recognize the spiritual needs and implications of their patients' ills, and thus to refer them to the appropriate professional. It also serves as a point of discussion with patients and a guiding analysis of their physical problems. A spiritual sensibility helps in healing by calling attention to the fact that healing involves physical and spiritual elements. The body may be repaired, but the soul may be pained or in need of sustenance. This ability to see the whole person and the type of healing that is required to bring full health is at the heart of the practice of the integrative physician.

The burgeoning field of integrative medicine is increasingly incorporating into medical school curriculums the centrality of the spirit in healing and health. At the same time, integrative medical practice is challenged to understand that spirituality is not another adjunct to medicine proper, another modality to include in the menu of complementary or alternative options. Rather, spirituality is a more fundamental, whole-life interpretation, as it is already inscribed in the structure of life itself—the human body, consciousness, and all living organisms. It involves an awareness of the whole person—both physician and patient—as having an inner life or soul, a life that responds to and is sustained by nonmaterial factors. A spiritual perspective in medicine also recognizes that the inner life can sustain wounds and illness as well as being a source of vitality and change.

Just as other medical and life situations follow stages of transformation, so too does the spirit or soul. In describing the spirit, we must keep in mind that it is not a monolithic, static, or finalized reality. Rather, the spirit is dynamic, continually changing and learning in response to stimuli from the physical, mental, emotional, and psychic realms.

In entering into the privacy and mystery of a person's healing, health professionals observe a depth of experience that is seldom discussed in our culture. There are times in every person's life where changes in spiritual outlook, wounding of the heart, or denial of illness, pain, and death impact on the spiritual journey. Many practitioners are struck by how profoundly people suffer spiritually and how difficult it is to heal this suffering when there is not a language and a socially sanctioned way of discussing the interior life. Further, physicians express concern that these topics are more suited to clergy, pastors, rabbis, and other religious professionals. Medical researchers also question how spirituality is defined and what role it should play in the overall curriculum of medical students, in medical practice, and in patient care. Foremost among these concerns is whether physicians are crossing an ethical divide by asking patients about their spiritual beliefs, taking spiritual surveys, or including religious practices in health care (Berry, 2005; Hall & Curlin, 2004; Hall et al., 2004; Post et al., 2000; Sloan, 2000, 2006).

Physicians, as well as their patients, move through changes in their spiritual lives, they are illumined, have moments of insight, feel compunction and sorrow, struggle through uncertainty and doubt, suffer loss of prestige or self-identity, and emerge with deeper integration and self-reliance. Because our culture tends to neglect the spiritual suffering or soul wound that underlies the process of healing, it is not part of conventional thought to speak about matters of the heart. Trained to be objective and emotionally neutral, physicians may lack the skills to discuss with patients the embarrassment, shame, or vulnerability that often accompanies illness and healing. The deeper truths of sustaining health may be shrouded in silence and mystery and in the need for forgiveness and reconciliation. It is the willingness of physicians and patients to open themselves to these sufferings and fears, and then to share them with others, that is vital to the whole healing process. Thus, it is important for physicians and patients to have permission to address questions of meaning and other significant life issues that traditionally have not been included in medical intake but are at the core of integrative medicine as a healing art.

Spiritual Suffering and Women's Health

Much of the pain patients experience is not just physical pain, but also spiritual. In fact, from my clinical experience with patients, I have found that spiritual suffering underlies most of the pain that patients and their families experience. Pain is multifactorial: physical, emotional, social, and spiritual.... The threat to one's physical body can also ... lead to spiritual or existential suffering, which can affect physical pain and manifest as physical symptoms.

—Puchalski (2006, p. 21)

Numerous studies of medieval and contemporary women illustrate a female or feminine spiritual consciousness. Whether this consciousness can be ascribed to cultural, historical, or ontological factors is still in question. Nonetheless, without making an essentialist argument, there are tendencies common enough across cultures and historical periods to demarcate the outlines of a feminine spirituality (see Bynum, 1984, 1991; Donnelly, 1982; Harvey & Baring, 1996; Jantzen, 1999, 2000; King, 1993; Newman, 1987, 2003; Petroff, 1994; Raphael, 1996; Wiethaus, 1993). Elsewhere, I have called this spiritual consciousness *via feminina*, or the way of the feminine, and contended that it speaks to a distinctive female path toward integration and healing (Lanzetta, 2005). One historical constant in women's spiritual expression is an emphasis on an embodied, rather than abstract, spirituality. Across cultures and diverse time periods, women consistently name and practice a spirituality of the body, evident through biological life cycles and experiences of birth, menstruation, menopause, and dying. This lived, organic relationship between body, spirit, and nature is present in ancient goddess religions, medieval women mystics, and indigenous traditions, as well as in contemporary women today. Attentiveness to the closeness of the spirit in everyday life places further emphasis on the interdependent relationship between body, mind, and spirit in sustaining women's health.

Research on other attributes associated with female spirituality indicate that women describe a more porous sense of self and are more closely attuned to and able to negotiate the permeable boundaries of body and spirit, mind and heart. Current research in neurobiology indicates that the female capacity to be relational, integrative, and holistic also has a biological basis in the brain. Studies indicate that the female brain excels in integrating and assimilating information from the two sides of the brain, recognizing emotional overtones, verbal and social skills, and empathy (Alkire, Head, & Yeo, 2005; Brizendine, 2007; LeVay, 1994; Rabinowicz, Dean, Petetot, & de

Courten-Myers, 1999; Sabbatini, 2000; Schlaepfer et al., 1995). As a state of consciousness, women's spirituality tends to be relational and "undivided, that is to say, integral and holistic" (King, 1993, p. 88). It emphasizes qualities of mutuality, intimacy, and receptivity; its expression of the spirit tends to be nurturing, generative, sacrificial, and merciful. Women's spirituality is also bounded by a fierce determination, resiliency, and commitment to children, family, society, and work. Virtues of intimacy, mutuality, communion, and receptivity, often dismissed by material culture as signs of weakness, are distinctive soul strengths that guide women into states of consciousness capable of healing and transforming.

The richness of women's embodied spirituality is evident in their variety and creative expression. Deep founts of healing and soul renewal are found in the impressive panoply of spiritual resources traditionally used by women. From ancient times, women's healing rituals, ceremonies of life, devotional arts, and religious chanting and dance have been sources of strength. Often segregated from male religious privilege, women developed practices of domestic healing, including blessing with oils and water, lighting of candles, tending of sacred fires, intuitive medicine, and herbal cures. Among these many forms, women's communities encouraged reverence for nature and a model of emotional and spiritual nourishment that today remain vital to women's health and ability to overcome illness and other difficult life struggles.

Creating distinctive patterns of female spirituality, women throughout the world find enormous reserves of meaning in religious symbols, archetypes, and rituals. These diverse practices include devotion of Hispanic Catholic women to *Nuestra Señora de Guadalupe*; sacred yarn painting of Huichol Indian women of Mexico; the work of women potters of South India; the work of Eastern Orthodox women iconographers; Jewish women's rituals such as candle lighting and *mikva* (ritual cleansing); traditional rug weaving by Navajo women; Hopi spider women story-telling; vision quest of Lakota women; herbal medicine and spirit healing used by African and Haitian women; and Muslim women's veneration of Bibi Fatima.

In addition to the positive impact women's spirituality can exert on health outcomes, it is vital for health professionals to recognize that women also suffer from certain types of spiritual oppression simply because they are female. By virtue of living in societies that have been historically male-dominated, women in the global community sustain specific types of spiritual sufferings and soul wounds that are not found to the same degree in men. Understanding their causes and alleviation is critical to healing. Studies show that the various forms of personal and social violence—or "intimate violence"—women encounter on a daily basis exert their most profound effects on a woman's inner life or spirit (see Fisher, 1988a; Fortune, 1989; Mananzan et al., 1996;

West, 1999). Domestic abuse, sexual politics, economic inequalities, and legitimate fear of rape, assault, and other types of intimate violence circumscribe the lives of women and girls on a daily basis. Even women who have never experienced overt physical or sexual violence remain alert to subtle forms of emotional diminishment, social control, or unequal share of child rearing, household and family responsibilities, and caregiving.

Recent statistics provide a shocking view of worldwide abuses committed against women in all countries around the globe.

To cite an example, the worldwide economic and social marginalization of women, and their historical status as a permanent underclass are violent acts that rob a woman of self-worth, creating hidden scars in her being. Further, the global dimensions of women's suffering—rape, trafficking in women, wife-beating, bride burning, infanticide of girl babies, as well as the more subtle forms of social, religious, and economic violence that rob women of dignity—impact on women's capacity to heal and restore themselves to wholeness (Lanzetta, 2005, p. 63).

Lest we think that American women are free of an assault on their integrity, every year in the United States alone, a woman is beaten every 18 minutes, 3 to 4 million are battered each year, and 4,000 are beaten to death by their partners (Lanzetta, 2005, p. 186; Tjaden & Thoennes, 2000; UN Department of Public Information, 1991). Intimate violence is designed to depersonalize women's bodies, rape their souls, and destroy their resistance. This acceptance of the violation of women in the domestic sphere is reflected in shocking acts of violence that dehumanize and objectify women's bodies.

Medical professionals are starting to recognize that abuse and other forms of soul violations are implicated in women's mental, physical, and spiritual health and must become part of their integrative diagnosis and treatment plan (Marcus, 2008; Nicolaidis et al., 2004). They are learning that soul injuries and violation of the feminine inevitably impact on women's inner life and physical health. Understanding the causes that generate these soul wounds is essential in designing healing outcomes. Aware of the unequal burden placed on women in societies and religious communities around the world, integrative medicine can advance women's healthcare by taking into account and analyzing the deeper spiritual causes and consequences of a subtle but equally powerful form of physical and soul illness—the oppression of women's spirit. "I refer to this as *spiritual oppression* and contend its recognition and healing is fundamental to women's health and healing. The core of this stance is that *women's spiritual oppression is the foundation of all her other oppressions*. What harms a woman's soul reverberates in her physical, emotional, and mental spheres, generating suffering in every area of her life." Similarly, violations of a woman's body and diminishment of her social power have a direct impact on the health and integrity of her spirit (Lanzetta, 2005, p. 68).

What is spiritual oppression? The word "oppression" signifies an unjust exercise of authority or power by one person, group, or institution over another. Because the oppression I am referring to here is spiritual in nature, these varied interactions of personal, societal, and institutional control over women exert their influence beyond external events to invade a woman's psyche, soul, and body. Further, these abuses cannot be fully understood without recognizing how profoundly connected they are to cultural and religious devaluations of women as inferior to men. This fundamental belief in women's spiritual inferiority inevitably permeates the cultural imagination and contributes to and fosters violent acts against women, as it most often remains unacknowledged and unnamed.

When I say that all forms of women's oppression are fundamentally spiritual oppression, I mean that acts of violence against women—overt or subtle—are directed first and foremost at the core of her nature—her inner life or spirit. Often fueled by unconscious motivations, spiritual oppression is the wrongful violation of the sanctity of a woman's self. Violence against women—personal and structural—can be seen as nothing less than a desire to harm or destroy women's unique and particular embodiment of the spirit.

Corporate forms of oppression are present when the medical community applies a model of Cartesian reductionism to the spiritual implications of women's health; dismisses or denies gender differences in research, diagnosis, and treatment plans; or trivializes women's ailments as symptomatic, psychosomatic, or hysterical. The social structures that allow the unequal distribution of healthcare and that exploit or dictate women's innate healing abilities effectively possess woman's inner life, for they control in what way and in what measure women are valued and their health concerns taken seriously.

The presence of spiritual suffering in a woman's life is the most significant indicator of her inability to handle illness and quiet the restlessness that divides her soul (see Fisher, 1988a). Elusive and difficult to grasp, spiritual violence invades the integrity of a woman's psyche and soul at such a primary level that most women cannot recognize or name what has harmed them. Unable to identify the source of their pain, women often blame themselves and develop strategies to protect their oppressors. This quality of soul suffering, which survives at the cost of women's spiritual diminishment, inflicts on women an unequal burden of sin and blame (Fiorenza, 1996; Russell, 1996; Smith, 1998; Traitler-Espiritu, 1996; West, 1999). Thus, without understanding the subtle ways in which her soul is violated and the fierceness that marks the site of her affliction, an integrative approach is unable to address the full range of women's healthcare options. Often unspoken, denied, and ridiculed, or dismissed as unimportant and emotional, women's soul wounds must be brought to consciousness to avoid the trivialization of their experience and for healing to occur.

Dark Night of the Feminine and Women's Healing

Within the inner life, a woman finds deep resources of healing. Foremost among these are statistical evidence of women's greater participation in prayer, religion, and other sources of meaning as well as women's capacity for determination, resiliency, and hope. In addition, women often undergo a unique spiritual healing process, what I call the "dark night of the feminine" that moves them from oppression and illness to liberation and healing (Lanzetta, 2003a, 2003b, 2005). I have constructed this term from the ancient notion that transformation and healing requires a period of deconstruction or letting-go of old beliefs, wounds, and traumas, followed by an intense period of reintegration and soul healing. My particular usage of the term "dark night" is borrowed from the writings of the sixteenth-century Spanish mystic, John of the Cross (1991).

John depicts the dark night (Spanish, *noche oscura*) as a transformative stage of soul suffering prior to self-integration and divine intimacy. Torn by a wrenching inability to assuage the desolation of this dark passage, a person feels worthless and abandoned in the eyes of society, self, or her religion. Yet a light so bright is illuminating the soul that it appears dark to the disordered and suffering spirit. The soul cannot see what it is or name what it knows. John says that this dark night is the secret teaching of love in which the soul of a person is released from suffering and is lifted up to a special realization of its original, undivided nature. Using different names and cosmological systems—great death, annihilation, dismemberment—the interior process of spiritual suffering and recognition of soul wounds, followed by the healing light of wisdom and integration, is found in all cultures and religions around the world. While there tends to be a sense in contemporary depictions that the "soul" or "spirituality" transcends illness, suffering, and disease, this is not the dominant view in traditional religions or civilizations.

The specific attribution of the word "feminine" to dark night experiences indicates that there is another or additional dimension that women face beyond traditional accounts of transformation found in the world's religions. This process of healing specifically locates a woman's struggle to achieve fullness of being within her soul's internalization of the misogyny particular to her culture, and of the violation of her womanhood. The night of the feminine is emphasized as a continuum of consciousness that brings women to experience and heal another level of alienation and fragmentation specifically associated with being *female*. This intensification of suffering precludes a breakthrough into a new life of integration in which a woman discovers herself as worthy of healing and as fundamentally good and whole.

Specific elements of this process include an experience of intense impasse, where a woman is caught between two worlds: she cannot go back to how family, society, or religion defined her, but she cannot go forward to a future as yet unimagined (FitzGerald, 1996). The dark night process also can involve feelings of anguish, grief, and anger; self- and other-betrayal of deep needs and awareness of personal indignities disguised as socially sanctioned forms of women's oppression. Other wounds women have to overcome in the process of healing include the experience of being "nothing"; loss of self-identity or self-worth, often accompanied by self-loathing, guilt, anger, and shame; and internalization of the abuse committed by partners, society, clergy, religions, and family (Fisher, 1988a; Friedman, 2004; Kobeisy, 2004; Mecham, 2004).

The addition of the night of the feminine to the vocabulary of healing emphasizes its distinctiveness in a woman's spirituality and refines our understanding of the relationship between the interior life and health. When I say it is a feminine night, I mean women suffer afflictions to their most receptive and intimate nature, both in terms of the negative wounding sustained from violations of women's dignity, and the positive touching of the light of wisdom, which opens the soul to deeper reserves of communion and oneness. It is a dark night of the feminine not only because it occurs in females, but because the experience itself is the healing of the injury women sustain to their integrity of soul. This interior process, whereby a woman consciously or unconsciously experiences the effects of the violation of her body and spirit as female, becomes an essential precursor to her healing and a positive resource in combating illness, pain, suffering, and dying. The term "dark night of the feminine" helps health professionals to realize that even though the causes and conditions of illness may be inscrutable or unknown, the light of wisdom is a powerful resource in women's freedom of being and soul healing.

While the "dark night of the feminine" is not explicitly named or perhaps even understood as a spiritual process, physicians recount how women's resistance to healing often is the result of profound feelings of self-loathing, worthlessness, guilt, fear, and grief, fueled by a belief that they have sinned, are being punished by God, or do not deserve to be helped.

To illustrate her conviction that physicians' knowledge of their patients' personal belief systems and spiritual practices can aid in treatment, Christina

M. Puchalski, associate professor of medicine at George Washington University School of Medicine, tells this story:

> I once had a patient diagnosed with HIV who felt she had brought the disease on herself, that she had sinned and God was punishing her. As a result, she did not want to go ahead with any treatment plan. I didn't realize why she was so adamant about not taking her medicines until I asked about her spiritual history. Because I asked her I was able to get her help from a trained chaplain. Had I not addressed those issues, I would never have been able to figure out a way to help her (cited in Gabriel, 2000).

Suggestions for Integrative Healthcare

Awareness of spiritual suffering and soul healing in women is a complex topic that requires new ways of interpreting, diagnosing, and understanding healing of the whole person. Not all medical professionals can or should be prepared for this interior work. Yet, for those who find the more subtle dimensions of healthcare to be important, it is hoped that the path of *via feminina* and the transformative process of the dark night of the feminine will be of benefit and lead to further research on the profound interrelationship between physical health and spiritual states of consciousness.

Central to the integrative physician is to be of service, and to practice medicine with a loving and compassionate heart. In this way, a rapport is established between the physician and the patient that creates an atmosphere of trust and openness. This is especially important with patients who may be suffering from soul illness or who are confronting a terminal disease. In keeping with the philosophy of doing no harm, the following guidelines may be helpful to physicians and other health providers.

- Be open to a sight and inner wisdom beyond the physical, thus seeing patients as whole people with bodies and souls.
- Consider spirituality as a potentially important component of every patient's physical well-being and mental health.
- Listen to the signs and symptoms of the inner life.
- Become aware of your own spirituality, suffering, and ability to deal compassionately with your own and another's pain.
- Raise questions that allow for patient's reflection on their faith or religious beliefs, spiritual suffering, and emotional hopes and fears.

- Respect patient's privacy regarding spirituality and religion; do not impose your beliefs or faith on others.
- Be particularly attentive to subtle forms of spiritual oppression, coercion, and physical and emotional abuse in women.
- Recognize how women's more permeable self and capacity for synthesis and integration may be implicated in certain types of illness but also is a source of strength and resiliency.
- Provide female patients with resources for healing and for understanding their journey of *via feminina* and the "dark night of the feminine."
- Refer patients to other experts, such as chaplains, spiritual directors, social workers, and psychologists when appropriate.
- Allow for and honor mystery.

REFERENCES

Alkire, M. T., Head, K., & Yeo, A. (2005). *Intelligence in men and women is a grey and white matter.* University of California, Irvine. *ScienceDaily*, January 22. Retrieved from http://www.sciencedaily.com/releases/2005/01/050121100142.htm

Bearon, L. B., & Koenig, R. (1990). Religious cognitions and use of prayer in health and illness. *Gerontologist, 30*, 249–253.

Benson, H., & Stark, M. (1997). *Timeless healing: The power and biology of belief.* New York, NY: Scribner.

Berry, D. (2005). Methodological pitfalls in the study of religiosity and spirituality. *West J Nurs Res, 27*, 628–647.

Brizendine, L. (2007). *The female brain.* New York, NY: Broadway Books.

Bynum, C. W. (1984). *Jesus as mother: Studies in the spirituality of the high middle ages.* Berkeley: University of California Press.

Bynum, C. W. (1991). *Fragmentation and redemption: Essays on gender and the human body in medieval religion.* New York, NY: Zone Books.

Dessio, W., Wade, C., et al. (2004). Religion, spirituality, and healthcare choices of African-American women: results of a national survey. *Ethn Dis Spring, 14*, 189–197.

Donnelly, D. H. (1982). The sexual mystic: Embodied spirituality. In M. E. Giles (Ed.), *The Feminist mystic and other essays on women and spirituality* (pp. 120–141). New York: Crossroad.

Dossey, L. (1993). *Healing words: The power of prayer and the practice of medicine.* San Francisco, CA: Harper San Francisco.

Dossey, L. (1997). *Prayer is good medicine: How to reap the healing benefits of prayer* San Francisco, CA: Harper San Francisco.

Edmondson, K. A., et al. (2005). Spirituality predicts health and cardiovascular responses to stress in young adult women. *J Relig Health, 44, 2.*

Fiorenza, E. S. (1996). Ties that bind: Domestic violence against women. In M. J. Mananzan et al. (Eds.), *Women resisting violence, Spirituality for life* (pp. 39–55). Maryknoll, NY: Orbis Books.

Fisher, K. (1988a). The problem of anger. In *Women at the well: Feminist perspectives on spiritual direction* (pp. 154–174). New York, NY: Paulist Press.

Fisher, K. (1988b). Violence against women: The spiritual dimension. In *Women at the well: Feminist perspectives on spiritual direction* (pp. 175–192). New York, NY: Paulist Press.

FitzGerald, C. (1996). Impasse and dark night. In J. W. Conn (Ed.), *Women's spirituality: Resources for Christian development* (pp. 410–435). New York, NY: Paulist Press.

Fortune, M. M. (1989). The transformation of suffering: A biblical and theological perspective. In J. C. Brown & C. R. Bohn (Eds.), *Christianity, patriarchy, and abuse: A feminist critique.* New York, NY: Pilgrim.

Friedman, M. E. (2004). Shame and illness: A Jewish perspective. *Yale Journal for Humanities in Medicine*, September 17. http://yjhm.yale.edu/archives/spirit2004/shame/mfriedman.htm

Gabriel, B. (2000). Is spirituality good medicine? Bridging the divide between science and faith. *AAMC Report, 9*, 13. http://www.aamc.org/newsroom/reporter/oct2000/spirit.htm

Hall, D., & Curlin, F. (2004). Can physicians' care be neutral regarding religion? *Acad Med, 79*, 677–679.

Hall, D., Koenig, H., et al. (2004). Conceptualizing "religion": How language shapes and constrains knowledge in the study of religion and health. *Pers Biol Med, 47*, 386–401.

Harvey, A., & Baring, A. (1996). *The divine feminine: Exploring the feminine face of god around the world.* Berkeley, CA: Conari Press.

Jantzen, G. M. (1999). *Becoming divine: Towards a feminist philosophy of religion.* Bloomington: Indiana University Press.

Jantzen, G. M. (2000). *Julian of Norwich: Mystic and theologian.* New York, NY: Paulist Press.

John of the Cross. (1991). The dark night. In *The collected works of St John of the Cross* (K. Kavanaugh & O. Rodriquez, Trans., pp. 353–457). Washington, DC: Institute of Carmelite Studies.

King, U. (1993). *Women and spirituality: Voices of protest and promise* (2nd ed.). University Park: Pennsylvania State University Press.

Kobeisy, A. N. (2004). Shame in the context of illness: An Islamic perspective. *Yale Journal for Humanities in Medicine*, September 14. http://yjhm.yale.edu/archives/spirit2004/shame/akobeisy.htm

Lanzetta, B. J. (2003a). *Julian and Teresa as cartographers of the soul: A contemplative feminist hermeneutic.* Paper delivered American Academy of Religion Annual Meeting, Atlanta, Georgia, November.

Lanzetta, B. J. (2003b). *The soul of woman and the dark night of the feminine in St Teresa of Avila*. Paper delivered American Academy of Religion Western Region (WESCOR), University of California Davis, March.

Lanzetta, B. J. (2005). *Radical wisdom: A feminist mystical theology*. Minneapolis, MN: Fortress Press.

Larson, D. B. (2003). Spirituality's potential relevance to physical and emotional health: A brief review of quantitative research. *J Psychol Theol, 31*, 37–51.

LeVay, S. (1994). *The sexual brain: The female brain*. Cambridge, MA: MIT Press.

Levine, G., Aviv, C., et al. (2009). The benefits of prayer on mood and well-being of breast cancer survivors. *Supportive Care Mar, 17*, 295–308.

Maizes, V., Koffler, K., & Fleishman, S. (2002). Revisiting the health history: An integrative medicine approach. *Int J Integr Med, 3*, 7–13.

Maizes, V., Schneider, C., et al. (2002). Integrative medical education: Development and implementation of a comprehensive curriculum at the University of Arizona. *Acad Med, 77*, 851–860.

Mananzan, M. J., et al. (Eds.). (1996). *Women resisting violence: Spirituality for life*. Maryknoll, NY: Orbis Books.

Marcus, E. N. (2008). Screening for abuse may be key to ending it. *New York Times*, May 20. http://www.nytimes.com/2008/05/20/health/20abus.html

Massey, E. A. (1996). Affirming spirituality and healing in medicine. *J Past Care, 50*, 235–237.

Mecham, M. P. (2004). Guilt in the context of illness: A protestant perspective. *Yale Journal of Humanities in Medicine*.

Musgrave, C, Allen, C., et al. (2002). Spirituality and health for women of color. *Am J Public Health, 92*, 557–560.

Newman, B. (1987). *Sister of wisdom: St Hildegard's theology of the feminine*. Berkeley: University of California Press.

Newman, B. (2003). *Gods and the goddesses: Vision, poetry, and belief in the middle ages*. Philadelphia: University of Pennsylvania Press.

Nicolaidis, C., et al. (2004). Violence, mental health and physical symptoms in an academic internal medicine practice. *J Gen Internal Med, 19*.

Petroff, E. A. (1994). *Body and soul: Essays on medieval women and mysticism*. New York: Oxford University Press.

Post, S. G., et al. (2000). Physicians and patient spirituality: Professional boundaries, competency, and ethics. *Ann Internal Med, 132*, 578–583.

Puchalski, C. M. (1999). Touching the spirit: The essence of healing. *Spiritual Life, 43*, 154–159. http://www.spiritual-life.org/id30.htm

Puchalski, C. M. (2002). Forgiveness: Spiritual and medical implications. *Yale J Human Med*.

Puchalski, C. M. (2006). *A time for listening and caring: Spirituality and the care of the chronically ill and dying*. New York, NY: Oxford University Press.

Rabinowicz, T., Dean, D. E., Petetot, J. M., & de Courten-Myers, G. M. (1999). Gender differences in the human cerebral cortex: More neurons in males; more processes in females. *J Child Neurol, 14*, 98–107.

Raphael, M. (1996). *Thealogy and embodiment: The post-patriarchal reconstruction of female sacrality.* Sheffield, England: Sheffield Academic Press.

Russell, Letty, M. (1996). Spirituality, struggle, and cultural violence. In M. J. Mananzan et al. (Eds.), *Women resisting violence, Spirituality for life* (pp. 20–26). Maryknoll, NY: Orbis Books.

Sabbatini, R. M. E. (2000, October–December). Are there differences between the brains of males and females? *Mind and Brain: Electronic Magazine on Neuroscience.*

Schlaepfer, T. E., Harris, G. J., Tien, A. Y., Peng, L., Lee, S., & Pearlson, G. D. (1995). Structural differences in the cerebral cortex of healthy female and male subjects: A magnetic resonance imaging study. Psychiatry Res, *61,* 129–135.

Sloan, R. P. (n.d.). *Field analysis of the literature on religion, spirituality, and health.* Metanexus. http://www.metanexus.net/tarp/pdf/TARP-Sloan.pdf

Sloan, R. P. (2000). Should physicians prescribe religious activities? *N Engl J Med, 342,* 1913–1916.

Sloan, R. P. (2006). *Blind faith: The unholy alliance of religion and medicine.* New York, NY: St. Martin's Press.

Smith, A. (1998). Christian conquest and the sexual colonization of native women. In C. J. Adams & M. M. Fortune (Eds.), *Violence against women and children: A Christian theological sourcebook* (pp. 377–403). New York, NY: Continuum.

Tjaden, P., & Thoennes, N. (2000). *Extent, nature and consequences of intimate partner violence: Findings from the National Violence Against Women Survey.* National Institute of Justice and the Centers of Disease Control and Prevention.

Traitler-Espiritu, R. (1996). Violence against women's bodies. In M. J. Mananzan et al. (Eds.), *Women resisting violence: Spirituality for life* (pp. 66–79). Maryknoll, NY: Orbis Books.

UN Department of Public Information. (1991). *Women: Challenges to the year 2000.* New York.

US Department of Justice, Bureau of Justice Statistics. (2006). *Intimate partner violence in the United States.* December.

West, T. C. (1999). *Wounds of the spirit: Black women, violence, and resistance ethics.* New York: New York University Press.

Wiethaus, U. (Ed.). (1993). *Maps of flesh and light: The religious experience of medieval women mystics* Syracuse, NY: Syracuse University Press.

37

Women's Health: Epilogue

TIERAONA LOW DOG AND VICTORIA MAIZES

The course of women's lives continues to change, challenging the health-care system to broaden its understanding of what constitutes "women's health." Women's health has typically been presented in a biologically defined manner, divided into functional, reproductive segments that revolve around menstruation. Unfortunately, this model falls short of recognizing the totality of women's experiences across the life span and has resulted in gaps in research, public policy, and delivery of comprehensive healthcare services. Women often see one provider during pregnancy, another for gynecological problems, a third for well-woman care, and an array of specialists who manage chronic diseases, with little coordination between services and caregivers. While this fragmentation of services is not unique to women, it is more pronounced among them. The emphasis that has been placed on reproduction has also, unfortunately, led to both societal and medical attributions of many female behaviors to hormonal fluctuations rather than the economic, environmental, and social causes that so deeply affect women's lives. These are the areas addressed in this final chapter.

Economics and Health

It is well known that the economic status of women is intimately intertwined with their health and well-being. While women have made tremendous gains toward economic equality over the last several decades, they remain disproportionately affected by poverty. In 2012, women's median annual paychecks reflected only 77 cents for every dollar earned by men; African American women earned only 66 cents and Latinas 54 cents (Entmacher, Robins, Vogtman, & Frohlich, 2013).

The poverty rate for female single head of household families is 40%, more than double the rate for male single head of household families (Entmacher et al., 2013). Married women with dependent children are also disadvantaged, as they are more likely to work fewer hours for lower pay as they take time off for family responsibilities. Studies show women remain the primary family caregivers, caring for sick children, parents, or partners, which often means working and earning less. These wage inequities follow women into their retirement years, reducing their Social Security benefits, pensions, savings, and other financial resources. Women often work in part-time positions that are less likely to offer health insurance and paid sick days. Taking time off to care for a sick child means loss of wages or even the loss of a job. It also means less time for personal healthcare.

While the exact numbers are not known, it is estimated that 1%–4% of women in the United States identify as lesbian or bisexual. Lesbian and bisexual women interface less with the healthcare system for numerous reasons including fear of discrimination, uncertainty around the need for routine health services, and lack of insurance coverage. Surveys have found that lesbians are 1.6 and bisexual women are 3.1 times more likely to be sexually assaulted than heterosexual women. Upon reflection, we realized that there are unique challenges that these women face and thus included the chapter "Lesbian, Bisexual, and Transgender Health" in this second edition.

If the misery of the poor be caused not by the laws of nature, but by our institutions, great is our sin.

—Charles Darwin

The Affordable Care Act signed into law in March 2010 not only ensured access to all people living in the United States, it helped to ensure that women would receive a comprehensive set of preventive healthcare services without having to pay any co-payments or a deductible. These services include annual well-woman visits that are age appropriate, including contraceptive methods counseling, screening for sexually transmitted diseases, interpersonal violence, and domestic abuse; preconception care; and many services necessary for prenatal care as well as breastfeeding support, supplies, and counseling (HRSA, 2012). The Act also prohibits insurance companies from discriminating against people based on sexual orientation and gender identity, allowing for coverage of same-sex spouses and their children. We feel that, while not perfect, this healthcare reform legislation will improve the lives of many women and their families.

Environmental Medicine

If we are going to live so intimately with these [agricultural] chemicals—eating and drinking them—taking them into the very marrow of our bones—we had better know something about their nature and their power.

—*Rachel Carson, Silent Spring*

The current focus on risk management through health behaviors addresses many elements of disease prevention, but falls short in acknowledging the role that environmental factors play in our health. In the 1962 book *Silent Spring*, Rachel Carson, a marine biologist and environmentalist, increased public awareness to the harm that might occur due to the indiscriminate use of pesticides. She called attention to our growing reliance on chemicals for which safety is incompletely understood. Women know that their womb provides the first environment for their child and that the responsibility for the nourishment, safety, and well-being of their children falls primary to them. Women are increasingly concerned about the accumulating evidence that from the air we breathe to the fish we eat and the water we drink, a broad range of compounds in the environment may be adversely affecting the health of our families and the health of our planet.

While there are zealots and skeptics on both sides of the issue, many scientists suspect that there is a link between environmental toxins and some of our most prevalent medical conditions, such as asthma, autism, cancer, neurodegenerative diseases, and infertility. Of particular concern are those compounds with the potential to disrupt normal endocrine, reproductive, central nervous, and immune function. Endocrine-disrupting compounds (EDCs), many of which act like estrogens in the body, may be associated with decreasing sperm counts and increasing birth defects in males and in females with estrogen-driven cancers and gynecological disorders such as endometriosis, recurrent miscarriage, infertility, and polycystic ovary syndrome. Recognizing that sensitivity to endocrine disruptors varies extensively across the life span, with specific windows of increased susceptibility, we strongly support expanding our biomonitoring capabilities to assess the level of harmful chemicals in the body. We feel it is critical to track long-term low-level exposure to environmental toxicants from infancy through old age to better determine at what point these crucial windows occur. Tighter regulatory standards for evaluating the safety of new industrial compounds should be rapidly implemented to safeguard public health as well as the health of other earth inhabitants. Because the environment and women's health are so intricately intertwined, we included a new chapter, "Environmental Exposures and Women's Health" in this edition of our book.

> *When an activity raises threats of harm to human health or the environment, precautionary measures should be taken even if some cause and effect relationships are not fully established scientifically In this context the proponent of an activity, rather than the public, should bear the burden of proof The process of applying the precautionary principle must be open, informed and democratic and must include potentially affected parties It must also involve an examination of the full range of alternatives, including no action.*
>
> —Wingspread Statement on the Precautionary Principle, January 1998

Women and Research

Historically, scientists have paid little attention to the study of sex differences at the basic *cellular* and *molecular* levels, as well as in clinical trials. The research community assumed that beyond the reproductive system, such differences either did not exist or were not relevant. Clinicians have assumed that information obtained from clinical studies conducted on male subjects could simply be extrapolated to women. Yet, as researchers unravel the complex interplay between DNA, hormones, and environment, this assumption, even on a mechanistic level, seems almost childishly simplistic. For instance, the dominant model of human response to stress has been the "fight or flight" response. No one considered that there could be any significant difference in the way men and women physiologically respond to stress. However, research shows that stressors in women can also cause the release of oxytocin, a hormone that buffers the fight or flight response and encourages women to tend children and affiliate with others (Taylor, 2000). This "tend and befriend" response to a threat reduces biological stress responses, including elevated heart rate, blood pressures, and hypothalamic-pituitary-adrenal axis stress responses, such as elevations in cortisol. This may explain why women are more likely than men to seek out and use social support in all types of stressful situations, including health-related concerns, relationship problems, and work-related conflicts.

Understanding why the prevalence of disease can vary so dramatically between men and women is another area ripe for investigation. Women are two times more likely than men to suffer from depression, a statistic that holds true throughout the world (Weissman & Olfson, 1995). Differences in brain structure and function, and hormonal fluctuations across the reproductive cycle, may differentially predispose women to depression. Research shows that estrogen modulates serotonin function and that women respond far better to serotonin reuptake inhibitors (SSRIs) than men (Young et al., 2009) and premenopausal women respond far better than postmenopausal women (Kornstein et al., 2000). However, gender differences in socialization, rates of violence against women, and women's disadvantaged social status, are also very likely to contribute to the greater prevalence in women. Depression, like most conditions, is likely a combination of both biology and environment.

> *While it is anatomically obvious why only males develop prostate cancer and only females get ovarian cancer, it is not at all obvious why, for example, females are more likely than males to recover language ability after suffering a left-hemisphere stroke or why females have a far greater risk than males of developing life-threatening ventricular arrhythmias in response to a variety of potassium channel-blocking drugs.*
>
> —Wizeman and Pardue (2001)

Sex and gender research is growing but is still in its infancy. Prior to 1990, the National Institutes of Health (NIH) devoted only 13% of its research funds toward studies of drug effects, diseases, and treatments that affect women as well as men, although women make up 52% of the world's population. Due to the glaring discrepancies in scientific research and the tireless work of women's health advocacy groups, the Office of Research on Women's Health (ORWH) was established in 1990 to ensure the inclusion of women and minorities in NIH-funded research. Its mission is to promote, stimulate, and support efforts to improve the health of women through biomedical and behavioral research on the roles of sex (biological characteristics of being female or male) and gender (social influences based on sex) in health and disease. A legislative mandate that women and minorities be included in all clinical research studies was incorporated into the NIH Revitalization Act of 1993.

There are tremendous opportunities and challenges that confront researchers who study the role of sex and gender in health and disease. New methodologies and models will need to be developed to enable scientists to investigate both male and female cell lines to determine whether stressors or medicines affect them differently. It is also critical that the editors of medical and scientific journals encourage authors to describe the sex ratios in their clinical trials and to what extent differences in outcomes were noted between the sexes. If no differences were identified, this should also be clearly stated. This type of research and reporting is crucial before generalized recommendations can be made for the public (IOM, 2001).

A thoughtful examination of, and recommendations for, a more inclusive and expansive scientific agenda on women's health research is found in the ORWH Agenda for Research on Women's Health for the 21st Century. http://orwh.od.nih.gov/research/resagenda.html

Women's Voices

It seems fitting to close this chapter with an acknowledgment of all the women, named and unnamed, throughout history from ancient times to the present, across cultures and ethnicities, who have tended the sick and broken, helped bring countless children into the world, and given comfort to those who were dying. In honor of this long tradition of healing, we chose women clinicians to write the chapters for this book. They came from many disciplines and traditions: traditional Chinese medicine, Ayurveda, naturopathy, psychology, public health, dietetics/nutrition, nursing, family practice, internal medicine (oncology, rheumatology, cardiology), obstetrics/gynecology, osteopathy, pediatrics, and psychiatry.

If health is more than the absence of disease—if it is, rather, a harmonious interplay between the physical, emotional, social, and spiritual aspects of one's life—then a biopsychosocial, or integrative, approach to women's health is the only one that makes sense. Moving beyond a medical system that is primarily focused on curing to one that also recognizes, embraces, and encourages healing is essential. Healing stretches beyond the boundaries of disease and cure into the realms of transcendence: purpose, hope, and meaning that form the very fabric of human experience and desire (Swinton, 2001). A union that marries the social, political, cultural, geographical, and economic factors of women's lives with conventional biomedical care—placing each individual woman within the larger story of her own life and experience—allows us to more fully appreciate the dynamic and unique nature of health. It was from within this philosophical stance that this second edition of *Integrative Medicine and Women's Health* was written with the hopes that it can serve as a model for helping improve the health and well-being of women across the life span and throughout the globe.

Women have always been healers. They were the unlicensed doctors and anatomists of western history. They were abortionists, nurses and counselors. They were pharmacists, cultivating healing herbs and exchanging the secrets of their uses. They were midwives, travelling from home to home and village to village. For centuries

women were doctors without degrees, barred from books and lectures, learning from each other, and passing on experience from neighbor to neighbor and mother to daughter. They were called "wise women" by the people, witches or charlatans by the authorities. Medicine is part of our heritage as women, our history, our birthright.
—Barbara Ehrenreich and Deirdre English, Witches, Midwives, and Nurses: A History of Women Healers

REFERENCES

American Chiropractic Association. (n.d.). Facts and statistics about chiropractic: General information about chiropractic care. Retrieved May 1, 2009, from http://www.acatoday.org/level1_css.cfm?T1ID=21

American Massage Therapists Association. (2009). *Massage therapy industry fact sheet* Retrieved May 1, 2009, from http://www.amtamassage.org/news/MTIndustryFactSheet.html

American Medical Association. (1997). *Women in medicine data source* Chicago, IL: American Medical Association.

Carson, R. (1962). *Silent Spring.* Boston, MA: Houghton Mifflin Harcourt Publishers.

Ehrenreich, B. & English, D. (2010). *Witches, Midwives, and Nurses: A History of Women Healers*, 2nd edition. The Feminist Press at CUNY.

Entmacher, J., Robins, K. G., Vogtman, J., & Frohlich, L. (2013). *Insecure and unequal: Poverty and income among women and families 2000–2012.* National Women's Law Center, September.

Health and Human Services. (2006). *2004 national sample survey of registered nurses.* Retrieved May 1, 2009, from http://bhpr.hrsa.gov/healthworkforce/rnsurvey04/

Health and Human Servies. (2010). Affordable Care Act: Essential Services. Retrieved June 17, 2015 from www.hhs.gov/opa/affordable-care-act/health-services-and-benefits/essential-health-benefits/ .

Institute of Medicine. (2001). Exploring the Biological Contributions to Human Health: Does Sex Matter? Retrieved June 15, 2015, from https://www.iom.edu/Reports/2001/Exploring-the-Biological-Contributions-to-Human-Health-Does-Sex-Matter.aspx

Institute for Women's Policy Research. (2003). *Single mothers and their children suffered most in the last year with persistently high poverty: Gender wage gap stagnant.* Press release, September 26. Washington, DC: Institute for Women's Policy Research.

Kornstein, S. G., Schatzberg, A. F., Thase, M. E., et al. (2000). Gender differences in treatment response to sertraline versus imipramine in chronic depression. *Am J Psychiatry, 157*, 1445–1452.

Swinton, J. (2001). *Spirituality and mental health care: Rediscovering a "forgotten" dimension.* Philadelphia, PA: Kingsley.

Taylor, S. E., Klein, L. C., Lewis, B. P., Gruenewald, T. L., Gurung, R. A., & Updegraff, J. (2000). Biobehavioral responses to stress in females: Tend-and-befriend, not fight-or-flight. *Psychol Rev, 107*(3), 411–429.

Weissman, M. M., & Olfson, M. (1995). Depression in women: Implications for health care research. *Science, 269,* 799–801.

The Wingspread Statement on the Precautionary Principle (1998). Retrieved June 17, 2015, from http://www.sehn.org/state.html

Society for Women's Health Research. *Women and men: 10 differences that make a difference.* Retrieved April 20, 2009, from http://www.womenshealthresearch.org/site/PageServer?pagename=hs_sbb_10diff

Young, E. A., Kornstein, S. G., Marcus, S. M., et al. (2009). Sex differences in response to citalopram: A STAR*D report. *J Psychiatr Res, 43,* 503–511.

INDEX

Note: Page numbers followed by b or f indicate a box or table on the designated page.

Mediterranean diet (*Cont.*)
  for obesity, 20
  during pregnancy, 254
  in vitro fertilization and, 239
Melatonin
  for acid reflux, 5
  breast cancer and, 400
  for FM/CFS, 567
  for irritable bowel syndrome, 517–518
Membrane sweeping, for labor induction, 270
Menopause, 340–366. *See also*
    Postmenopausal women
  acupuncture and, 134, 364
  adjunctive therapies for, 163
  antidepressant medications, 44
  anxiety with, 453t
  Ayurveda for, 150
  bioidentical/natural hormones, 359, 360t
  case study, 340–341
  depression and, 347
  dietary supplements for, 43–44, 347–348
  energy medicine for, 162, 164
  evaluation of, 341
  herbal medicines for, 44, 210, 348–358,
    350, 359
  homeopathy for, 172–174
  hormone testing, 342–343
  hormone therapy for, 43–44, 110–111, 309,
    358, 360–361
  hot flashes in, 341, 345–358, 363–365
  hypnosis and, 365, 394t
  ideal prescribing route, 361
  IF for hot flashes, 24
  mind-body therapies for, 90–91, 364–365
  nutritional approach, 345–346
  physical activity and, 64, 68, 346
  progesterone for, 360t, 361–362
  soy protein and, 13
  stress management and, 346–347
  TCM and, 129, 131, 132, 135, 364
  testosterone for, 362–363
  traditional Chinese medicine for, 44, 132,
    350, 359
  type-2 diabetes and, 366
Menstrual camps
  Chinese medicine and, 132
  herbal teas for, 263
  homeopathy and, 170
Menstruation
  Ayurveda and, 141
  bloating and, 509
  chasteberry for, 208, 298, 350

Chinese medicine and, 131
dong quai and, 351
IBS symptoms during, 509
progesterone and, 211
spirituality and, 797
traditional Chinese medicine and, 131
Mentha suaveolens essential oil
  for vaginitis, 227t
Mercury toxicity, 16, 258, 758, 759b
Metabolic syndrome. *See also* Insulin
  resistance
  cardiovascular disease and, 639t
  caution against using, 293
  diagnosis, 640t
  Mediterranean diet for, 20
  metformin for, 292
  mind-body practices for, 116
  for PCOS, 292–293, 294, 299
  physical activity for, 57
  sugar and, 11
Metformin
  for metabolic syndrome, 292
  PCOS and, 292
  possible risk factors, 38
Micronutrients, 16, 18t
Migraine headaches
  acupuncture for, 541
  anti-inflammatory
    diet for, 534, 544
  autogenics for, 540
  background, 525, 527
  biofeedback for, 540, 543
  caffeine and, 528, 534
  comorbidities, 529–530
  conventional treatments
    for, 530–533
  craniosacral therapy for, 541
  dietary supplements for, 534–539
  elimination diet for, 534
  estrogen-associated, 528–529
  herbal medicine for, 534–535, 538–539
  homeopathy for, 541–542
  hypnotherapy for, 540
  mind-body therapies for, 541
  nutritional approach, 533, 534
  physical activity for, 540–541
  PMR for, 540
  preventive therapies, 533
  sleep regulation for, 542
  SMT for, 184, 189
  symptoms, 526t
  triggers, 527